Disease and Mortality in Sub-Saharan Africa

Second Edition

Disease and Mortality in Sub-Saharan Africa

Second Edition

Editors

Dean T. Jamison

Richard G. Feachem

Malegapuru W. Makgoba

Eduard R. Bos

Florence K. Baingana

Karen J. Hofman

Khama O. Rogo

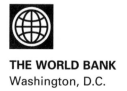

THE WORLD BANK
Washington, D.C.

ISBN-10: 0-8213-6397-2
ISBN-13: 978-0-8213-6397-3
eISBN: 0-8213-6398-0
DOI: 10.1596/978-0-8213-6397-3

Library of Congress Cataloging-in-Publication data has been applied for.

Contents

Tables

Foreword

More attention is now focused on improving the health of the population of Sub-Saharan Africa than at any previous time. In the years since the publication of the first edition of *Disease and Mortality in Sub-Saharan Africa* in 1991, numerous reports have been issued by national governments, development agencies, and researchers addressing the health status of African populations and proposing strategies to more effectively combat poor health with improved delivery of health services to prevent and cure diseases. Prime among these was the World Bank's 2005 report *Improving Health, Nutrition and Population Outcomes in Sub-Saharan Africa—The Role of the World Bank*, which gave rise to the publication of this book. Increased funding for health from governments, multilateral and bilateral donors, as well as new public-private partnerships and foundations has become available for assisting African countries to deliver more effective health interventions. The Millennium Development Goals have focused the attention of the world on achieving a clear set of goals—several of which are directly concerned with improving health outcomes—to be achieved by 2015.

Yet the sobering reality is that life expectancy has decreased by almost five years for the continent as a whole since the 1991 publication, and by much more in some countries. As the chapters in this volume document, children under five are dying at unacceptably high rates from causes for which effective interventions exist, and adult mortality from infectious diseases has risen to extraordinary levels. HIV/AIDS has spread from eastern Africa to the rest of the continent, affecting southern African countries the most. Malaria mortality of children increased during the 1990s, and TB has reemerged as a leading cause of death for adults, largely due to the spread of AIDS. Not surprisingly, at this time Sub-Saharan Africa is not on track to reach any of the health Millennium Development Goals.

It is important to recognize that not all trends have been negative. The prevalence of HIV/AIDS has significantly decreased in several African countries, including Uganda, one of the worst-affected countries at the time of the publication of the first edition. Measles mortality has been virtually eliminated in the countries of southern Africa in the past decade. Enormous strides continued to be made in the control of onchocerciasis during the 1990s. Although many factors contributed to these successes, a common theme in these and other successful programs has been the emphasis on the monitoring of disease indicators and the effectiveness of programs to address them. Without knowledge of disease incidence, prevalence, and severity, setting policies for prioritizing interventions risks misallocating resources to combat causes of ill health that contribute little to the overall health status of a population. Good epidemiological information does not ensure good policy decisions or effective implementation, but without reliable epidemiological data, efforts to design cost-effective strategies and to implement technologies are no more than theoretical exercises.

Since the publication of the first edition of *Disease and Mortality in Sub-Saharan Africa*, many new sources of health and demographic information have become available, including data on trends in HIV infection from antenatal clinic surveillance sites, the first set of African life tables from a growing number of demographic surveillance sites, injury statistics from a small number of injury mortality surveillance registers, and cancer data from cancer registers. Improved methods for estimating the incidence of several other diseases, including tuberculosis, maternal mortality, and chronic diseases, have also improved the reliability of health statistics. Verbal autopsy studies have linked with demographic surveillance sites, adding to our knowledge on changes in the cause-of-death composition in several countries.

Notwithstanding these advances in health statistics, a theme that emerges from all the chapters in this volume is that too little is known about trends in the diseases and conditions included here in order to monitor and evaluate the effectiveness of programs intended to produce better health outcomes. As we get closer to the 2015 end point of the Millennium Development Goals, reaching the goals will become increasingly challenging. The continued improvement of disease surveillance and other regularly published health information remains as important a priority for African health systems as it was for the first edition.

Callisto Madavo
Former Vice-President
Africa Region
The World Bank

Acknowledgments

This publication consists of the contributions of 70 authors, coordinated by a group of editors at the World Bank (Florence Baingana, Eduard Bos, and Khama Rogo), the U.S. National Institutes of Health (Karen Hofman and Dean Jamison), the Global Fund to Fight AIDS, Tuberculosis, and Malaria (Richard Feachem), and the South African Medical Research Council (Malegapuru Makgoba). Management of the publication was carried out jointly at the World Bank and, for a subset of chapters, at the South African Medical Research Council.

The editors are grateful to the chapter authors, named at the beginning of each of their respective chapters, who worked tirelessly to produce the various drafts and revisions.

The editors thank the following reviewers of draft chapters: Larry Barat (World Bank, USA), George Bicego (South Africa CDC, South Africa), Gretchen Birbeck (Michigan State University, USA, and The Gambia), Martien Borgdoff (The Netherlands), Julie Cliff (Mozambique), Jerry Coovadiah (University of Natal, South Africa), Andrew Grulich (University of New South Wales, Australia), David Gwatkin (World Bank, USA), Kenneth Hill (Johns Hopkins University, USA), Adnan Hyder (Johns Hopkins University, USA), Jean-Claude Mbanya (Yaounde University, Cameroon), Samuel Lantei Mills (World Bank, USA), Pindile Mntla (Medical University of Southern Africa, South Africa), David Ndetei (Nairobi University, Kenya), Steven Obaro (Imperial College School of Medicine, UK), Robert Redfield (University of Maryland, USA), Brian Robertson (Cape Town University, South Africa), Daniel M. Sala-Diakanda (IFORD, Cameroon), Eugene Sobngwi (Yaounde University, Cameroon), David Thomas (Fred Hutchinson Cancer Research Center, USA), and Mark Wainberg (McGill University, Canada).

The publication of this volume was made possible by the generous support of the government of the Netherlands through the Bank-Netherlands Partnership Program (BNPP) at the World Bank. The editors are grateful to Julie McLaughlin and Ok Pannenborg of the Africa Region of the World Bank for initiating and subsequently overseeing the whole process leading to the publication of this book. Administrative and logistical support was provided by Carole Roberts of the South African Medical Research Council and Richard Babumba of the World Bank. Rifat Hasan of the World Bank guided the manuscript through the final stages and produced an "Executive Summary" for distribution at the High-Level Forum on the Health Millennium Development Goals meeting in Paris, 2005. Anne-Sophie Ville and Willyanne DeCormier Plosky also provided support.

The editors are also grateful to the World Bank and the Fogarty International Center of the U.S. National Institutes of Health, which allowed the editors and authors from these institutions to dedicate staff time to contribute to this publication.

Contributors

Volume Editors

Dean T. Jamison, Professor, Institute for Global Health, University of California, San Francisco

Richard G. Feachem, Executive Director, Global Fund to Fight AIDS, Tuberculosis, and Malaria; and Director, Institute for Global Health, University of California, San Francisco and Berkeley

Malegapuru W. Makgoba, Vice-Chancellor and Principal, University of KwaZulu-Natal, South Africa

Eduard R. Bos, Lead Population Specialist, Human Development Network, The World Bank, Washington, DC

Florence K. Baingana, Senior Health Specialist, Human Development Network, The World Bank, Washington, DC

Karen J. Hofman, Director, Division of Advanced Studies and Policy Analysis, Fogarty International Center, National Institutes of Health, Washington, DC

Khama O. Rogo, Lead Specialist, Africa Region, The World Bank, Washington, DC

Chapter Authors

Jacob Adetunji, Technical Adviser, U.S. Agency for International Development, Washington, DC

Atalay Alem, Psychiatrist, Amanuel Psychiatric Hospital, Faculty of Medicine, Addis Ababa University, Ethiopia

Uche Amazigo, Director, African Programme for Onchocerciasis Control, Ouagadougou, Burkina Faso

Agbessi Amouzou, PhD Candidate, Department of Population Dynamics, John Hopkins University, Baltimore, Maryland

Florence K. Baingana, Senior Health Specialist, The World Bank, Washington, DC

Todd Benson, Research Fellow, Food Consumption and Nutrition Division, International Food Policy Research Institute, Washington, DC

Bruce Benton, Public Health Adviser, Human Development Department, Africa Region, The World Bank, Washington, DC

Fred Binka, Executive Director, INDEPTH Network, Accra, Ghana

Eduard R. Bos, Lead Population Specialist, Human Development Network, The World Bank, Washington, DC

Cynthia Boschi-Pinto, Medical Officer, Department of Child and Adolescent Health and Development, World Health Organization, Geneva

Brett Bowman, Senior Researcher, Institute for Social and Health Sciences, University of South Africa

Debbie Bradshaw, Director, Burden of Disease Research Unit, Medical Research Council, South Africa

Rodolfo A. Bulatao, Independent Consultant, Washington, DC

Jesse Bump, Consultant, Onchocerciasis Coordination Unit, Human Development Department, Africa Region, The World Bank, Washington, DC

Zvavahera Chirenje, Lecturer/Consultant, Department of Obstetrics and Gynaecology, College of Health Sciences, University of Zimbabwe, Harare

Samuel J. Clark, Assistant Professor, Department of Sociology, University of Washington, Seattle; Research Associate, Institute of Behavioral Science, University of Colorado at Boulder; and Research Officer, MRC/Wits Rural Public Health and Health Transitions Research Unit (Agincourt), School of Public Health, University of the Witwatersrand, South Africa

Albertino Damasceno, Professor of Cardiology, Faculty of Medicine, Eduardo Mondlane University, Mozambique

Don de Savigny, Head of Unit, Clinical and Intervention Epidemiology, Swiss Tropical Institute, Basel, Switzerland

Norman Duncan, Chair, Department of Psychology, University of the Witwatersrand, South Africa

Christopher Dye, Coordinator, Tuberculosis Monitoring and Evaluation, Stop TB Department, World Health Organization, Geneva

Max Essex, Chair, Department of Immunology and Infectious Diseases, Harvard AIDS Institute, and the Botswana-Harvard AIDS Institute Partnership, Harvard School of Public Health, Boston, Massachusetts

Demissie Habte, International Director, James P. Grant School of Public Health, BRAC University, Bangladesh

Anthony D. Harries, Technical Adviser, HIV Care and Support, Ministry of Health, Lilongwe, Malawi

Yusuf Hemed, Coordinator, MEASURE Evaluation, Dar es Salaam, Tanzania

Kenneth Hill, Professor, Department of Population and Family Health Sciences, Johns Hopkins University, Baltimore, Maryland

Karen J. Hofman, Director, Division of Advanced Studies and Policy Analysis, Fogarty International Center, National Institutes of Health, Bethesda, Maryland

S. Mehran Hosseini, Epidemiologist, Stop TB Department, World Health Organization, Geneva

Rachel Jenkins, Director, World Health Organization–United Kingdom Collaborating Centre, Institute of Psychiatry, Kings College London

Elly Katabira, Neurologist, Department of Neurology, Makerere Medical School, Kampala, Uganda.

Keith P. Klugman, Codirector, Medical Research Council Respiratory and Meningeal Pathogens Research Unit, National Institute of Communicable Diseases, University of the Witwatersrand, Johannesburg, South Africa; and Professor, Department of Global Health, Rollins School of Public Health and Division of Infectious Diseases, School of Medicine, Emory University, Atlanta, Georgia

Olive Kobusingye, Adviser, Violence and Injury Prevention, and Disabilities, World Health Organization Regional Office for Africa, Brazzaville, Congo

Claudio F. Lanata, Senior Researcher, Instituto de Investigación Nutricional, Lima, Peru

Bernhard Liese, Public Health Adviser, Human Development Department, Africa Region, The World Bank, Washington, DC

Alan D. Lopez, Professor and Head of School, School of Population Health, University of Queensland, Herston, Australia

Shabir A. Madhi, Codirector, Medical Research Council Respiratory and Meningeal Pathogens Research Unit, National Institute of Communicable Diseases, University of the Witwatersrand, Johannesburg, South Africa

Dermot Maher, Medical Officer, Stop TB Department, World Health Organization, Geneva

Jean-Claude Mbanya, Endocrine and Diabetes Unit, Department of Internal Medicine and Specialities, Faculty of Medicine and Biomedical Sciences, University of Yaoundé I, Yaoundé, Cameroon

Anthony Mbewu, President, Medical Research Council, South Africa; and Visiting Professor in Medicine and Cardiology, University of Cape Town, South Africa

Souleymane Mboup, Professor of Microbiology, Laboratory of Bacteriology and Virology, CHU Le Dantec, Université Cheikh Anta Diop, Dakar, Senegal

Walter Mendoza, Researcher, Instituto de Investigación Nutricional, Lima, Peru

Fred Mhalu, Professor of Microbiology and Immunology, Muhimbili University College of Health Sciences, Dar es Salaam, Tanzania

Mark A. Miller, Director, Division of International Epidemiology and Population Studies, Fogarty International Center, National Institutes of Health, Bethesda, Maryland

Nokuzola Mqoqi, National Cancer Registry and Cancer Epidemiology Research Group, National Health Laboratory Service, Johannesburg, South Africa

Rosemary Musonda, Director, National AIDS Council, Lusaka, Zambia

Philip Mwalali, International Health Consultant and Medical Adviser, African Economic Foundation, Los Angeles, California

Pierre Ngom, Senior Research Adviser, Family Health International, Nairobi, Kenya

Wilfred Nkhoma, Regional Adviser (Tuberculosis), World Health Organization, Harare, Zimbabwe

Mounkaila Noma, Chief, Epidemiology and Vector Elimination Unit, African Programme for Onchocerciasis Control, Ouagadougou, Burkina Faso

Judy A. Omumbo, Research Fellow, Public Health Group, Kenya Medical Research Institute-Wellcome Trust Collaborative Program, Nairobi, Kenya

John Oucho, Professor of Demography and Chairman, African Population and Environment Institute, Nairobi, Kenya

Max Parkin, Chief, Unit of Descriptive Epidemiology, International Agency for Research on Cancer, Lyons, France

Kaushik Ramiaya, Consultant Physician and Assistant Medical Administrator, Shree Hindu Mandai Hospital, Dar es Salaam, Tanzania

Chalapati Rao, Lecturer, School of Population Health, University of Queensland, Herston, Australia

Khama O. Rogo, Lead Specialist, Africa Region, The World Bank, Washington, DC

Felix M. Salaniponi, Programme Director, National Tuberculosis Control Programme, Ministry of Health, Lilongwe, Malawi

Osman A. Sankoh, Manager, Communications and External Relations, INDEPTH Network Secretariat, Accra, Ghana

Mohamed Seedat, Director, Institute for Social and Health Sciences, University of South Africa, and South African Medical Research Council-University of South Africa Crime, Violence and Injury Lead Programme

Azodoga Seketeli, Medical Entomologist, Former Director, African Programme for Onchocerciasis Control, Ouagadougou, Burkina Faso

John T. Sentz, Research Assistant, Division of International Epidemiology and Population Studies, Fogarty International Center, National Institutes of Health, Bethesda, Maryland

Meera Shekar, Senior Nutrition Specialist, Human Development Network, The World Bank, Washington, DC

Donald Silberberg, Professor of Neurology, University of Pennsylvania, Philadelphia

Freddy Sitas, Director, Cancer Research and Registers Division, The Cancer Council of New South Wales, Australia

Robert W. Snow, Professor, Tropical Public Health, Centre for Tropical Medicine, University of Oxford, United Kingdom; and Head, Public Health Group, Kenya Medical Research Institute-Wellcome Trust Collaborative Program, Nairobi, Kenya

Geoff Solarsh, Professor and Head of School, Monash University School of Rural Health, Bendigo, Australia

Lara Stein, Acting Director, National Cancer Registry and Cancer Epidemiology Research Group, National Health Laboratory Service, Johannesburg, South Africa

Krisela Steyn, Director, Chronic Diseases of Lifestyle Unit, Medical Research Council, South Africa

Ian M. Timaeus, Head, Centre for Population Studies and Professor of Demography, London School of Hygiene and Tropical Medicine

Henry Wabinga, Professor, Kampala Cancer Registry, Department of Pathology, Makerere University, Kampala, Uganda

Laurent Yaméogo, Coordinator, Office of Programme Director, African Programme for Onchocerciasis Control, Ouagadougou, Burkina Faso

Honorat Zouré, Biostatistic and Mapping, African Programme for Onchocerciasis Control, Ouagadougou, Burkina Faso

Abbreviations and Acronyms

ADR	adverse drug reactions
AFB	acid-fast bacilli
AIDS	acquired immune deficiency syndrome
AMMP	Adult Morbidity and Mortality Project
anti-GAD	glutamic acid decarboxylase antibodies
APOC	African Programme for Onchocerciasis Control
AR	androgen receptor
ARI	acute respiratory infections
ARV	antiretroviral
AUDIT	Alcohol Use Disorders Identification Test
BCG	bacillus Calmette-Guérin
BMI	body mass index
BOMA	Burden of Malaria in Africa
BOSTID	Board of Science and Technology for International Development
CBR	community-based rehabilitation
CDTI	community-directed treatment with ivermectin
CHD	coronary heart disease
CHMR	child mortality rate
CI	confidence interval
CIESIN	Center for International Earth Science Information Network
CIN	cervical intraepithelial neoplasia
CM	cerebral malaria
CMD	common mental disorders
CMO	chronic otitis media
CNS	central nervous system
CRF	circulating recombinant forms
CRS	congenital rubella syndrome
CSO	Central Statistical Office
CTL	cytolytic T cell
CVD	cardiovascular disease
CWIQ	Core Welfare Indicators Questionnaire
DALY	disability-adjusted life year
DCCT	Diabetes Control and Complication Trial
DCM	dilated cardiomyopathy
DHS	Demographic and Health Survey

DMSSA-1	*Disease and Mortality in Sub-Saharan Africa,* first edition
DMSSA-2	*Disease and Mortality in Sub-Saharan Africa,* second edition
DOTS	directly observed treatment, short course
DSS	demographic surveillance system
DTP	diphtheria, tetanus, pertussis
EAEC	entero-adherent pathogenic *Escherichia coli*
EIR	entomological inoculation rates,
EMF	endomyocardial fibrosis
EmOC	emergency obstetric care
EPI	Expanded Program on Immunization
EPTB	extrapulmonary tuberculosis
ETEC	enterotoxigenic *Escherichia coli*
FAO	Food and Agriculture Organization of the United Nations
FCS	fuzzy climate suitability
FWCW	Fourth World Conference on Women
GAVI	Global Alliance for Vaccines and Immunization
GHQ	general health questionnaire
GIS	Geographical Information System
GBD	global burden of disease
GDM	gestational diabetes mellitus
GDP	gross domestic product
GHQ	General Health Questionnaire
HAART	highly active antiretroviral therapy
HAV	hepatitis A virus
HBIG	hepatitis B immunoglobin
HBV	hepatitis B
HES	hypereosinophilic syndrome
HHV8	human herpesvirus-8
Hib	*Haemophilus influenzae* type B
HIC	high-income country
HIPC	heavily indebted poor country
HIV	human immunodeficieny virus
HMIS	health management information systems
HPV	human papillomavirus
HSCL	Hopkins Symptom Checklist
ICA	islet cell antibodies

ICD-10	*International Statistical Classification of Diseases and Related Health Problems*, 10th revision	PA-ICPD	Programme of Action of the International Conference on Population and Development
IDD	iodine deficiency disorder	PCP	*Pneumocystis carinii* pneumonia
IFG	impaired fasting glycemia	PEM	protein-energy malnutrition
IGT	impaired glucose tolerance	PMDF	proportion of deaths of women of reproductive ages due to maternal causes
IHD	ischemic heart disease		
IMR	infant mortality rate	PPP	international dollars
INCLEN	International Clinical Epidemiology Network	PRSP	poverty reduction strategy paper
IPD	invasive pneumococcal disease	PSE	Present State Examination
IPT	isoniazid preventive treatment	PTB	pulmonary tuberculosis
IPTT	Initiative for Technology Transfer	PTSD	posttraumatic stress disorder
IPV	inactivated poliovirus vaccine	PYO	person-years of observation
IQI	interquartile intervals	RAMOS	Reproductive Age Mortality Studies
IQR	interquartile ranges	REMO	Rapid Epidemiological Mapping of Onchocerciasis
IUATLD	International Union against TB and Lung Disease		
IUGR	intrauterine growth retardation	RHD	rheumatic heart disease
IVIG	intravenous immunoglobulin	RR	relative risk
LBW	low birthweight	RTI	road traffic injury
LMIC	low- to middle-income country	SADC	Southern African Development Community
LRTI	lower respiratory tract infections	SAVVY	Sample Vital Registration and Verbal Autopsy
MDG	Millennium Development Goal	SIR	Susceptible-Infected-Removed
MDR	multidrug resistance	SIV	simian immunodeficiency virus
MICS	Multiple Indicator Cluster Surveys	SMA	severe malarial anemia
MMR	maternal mortality ratio	SRQ-25	Self Report Questionnaire—25 item version
MOTT	mycobacteria other than *tuberculosis*	SSRI	selective serotonin reuptake inhibitor
MR	mental retardation	STD	sexually transmitted disease
NCD	noncommunicable disease	TB	tuberculosis
NDS	National Demographic Survey	TCA	tricyclic antidepressant
NEPAD	New Partnership for Africa's Development	TFR	total fertility rate
NGDO	nongovernmental development organization	TMP-SMX	trimethoprim-sulfamethoxazole
NGO	nongovernmental organization	TT	tetanus toxoid
NIMSS	National Injury Mortality Surveillance System	U5MR	under-five mortality rate
NNRTI	nonnucleoside reverse transcriptase inhibitor	UKPDS	United Kingdom Prospective Diabetes Study
NNT	neonatal tetanus	UNAIDS	Joint United Nations Programme on HIV/AIDS
NRTI	nucleoside analogue reverse transcriptase inhibitor	UNDP	United Nations Development Programme
		UNICEF	United Nations Children's Fund
NVP	nevirapine	URTI	upper respiratory tract infection
OCP	Onchocerciasis Control Programme	VA	verbal autopsy
OEPA	Onchocerciasis Elimination Program for the Americas	VAD	vitamin A deficiency
		VAPP	vaccine-associated paralytic poliomyelitis
OPV	oral poliovirus vaccine	VR	vital statistics registration system
OR	odds ratio	WFS	World Fertility Survey
ORT	oral rehydration therapy	WHO	World Health Organization
OSD	onchocercal skin disease	YLD	years lived with disability

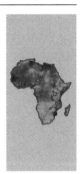

Chapter 1

Changing Patterns of Disease and Mortality in Sub-Saharan Africa: An Overview

Florence K. Baingana and Eduard R. Bos

Fifteen years have passed since the first edition of *Disease and Mortality in Sub-Saharan Africa* (*DMSSA-1*) was published. Its main purpose was to assist the World Bank's work in the health sector by describing conditions and diseases that contributed most to the overall burden of disease and by identifying ways to prevent and manage these causes of ill health. The volume was timely because of the adverse effect the economic downturn of the early 1980s had on health in Africa and because of the need to evaluate the impact of primary health care strategies that had been promoted in the preceding decade. Epidemiologic information coming from demographic surveillance sites that had not previously been fully compared and disseminated provided a new source for assessing trends in mortality. All this occurred against a backdrop of increasing concern about how the human immunodeficiency virus/acquired immune deficiency syndrome (HIV/AIDS), then still a relatively new and geographically more limited disease, could potentially affect health and development in Africa.

In the years since the publication of *DMSSA-1* in 1991, epidemiological and demographic changes have occurred that require an update if the volume is to remain useful for policy makers in addressing the "Key Concerns" shown in box 1.1. The most significant impact on disease and mortality in Africa has been the growth of the HIV/AIDS epidemic, which has infected more than 30 percent of adults in some countries while spreading across the continent. Its impact has changed trends in many of the diseases covered in this volume and dramatically worsened the overall level of mortality in many African countries. The potential impact of HIV/AIDS was anticipated in *DMSSA-1;* the current volume documents the burden the disease is currently inflicting on Africa.

APPROACH

Although the second edition (hereafter called *DMSSA-2*) has the same overall objective of informing policy makers (at the World Bank as well as in countries and among other development partners), the approach taken to compile the information was quite different from that for the first edition. *DMSSA-1* was organized in three broad sections, covering patterns of mortality, diseases and conditions, and longitudinal studies of mortality in demographic surveillance sites. In *DMSSA-2,* the number of chapters covering diseases and conditions has been expanded from 8 to 17 (out of a total of 24 chapters), with greater emphasis on emerging noncommunicable conditions and injuries. The section discussing the demographic surveillance sites has been dropped, and the information from the sites is now covered in a synthesis chapter that enables a better comparative perspective. The number of authors and editors has increased along with the number of chapters: there are now 24 chapters with one to eight authors each (for a total of 70); most chapters have at least one author from Sub-Saharan Africa.

CONDITIONS NOT COVERED IN *DMSSA-1*

DMSSA-1 emphasized communicable diseases, which are responsible for the largest disease burden and cause the highest number of deaths. The burden of communicable diseases has increased since the publication of the first edition, largely owing to the rapid rise in HIV/AIDS. Noncommunicable diseases, however, are also becoming a significant burden in several countries, leading to dual burdens of disease. *DMSSA-1* combined cardiovascular disease and cancers in one chapter; *DMSSA-2* expands the coverage of noncommunicable diseases (NCDs) substantially. Chapters on the following diseases and conditions have been added:

Developmental Disorders. This chapter discusses the higher rates of severe mental retardation, visual impairment, and hearing impairment found in Sub-Saharan Africa than in more developed regions. An estimated 47 percent of visual and 50 to 66 percent of hearing impairments in Sub-Saharan Africa are found to be preventable. Risk factors include congenital disorders, perinatal and neonatal conditions, infections, environmental toxins, accidents, injuries, and malnutrition.

Lifestyle and Related Risk Factors for NCDs. Increased use of tobacco and increased consumption of fats, sugar, alcohol, and animal products are critical risk factors for many NCDs. At the same time, the amount of physical exercise has been decreasing, leading to a sedentary lifestyle that is associated with obesity, diabetes, and hypertension. This chapter provides an overview of the risk factors for the NCDs discussed in subsequent chapters.

Diabetes Mellitus. Three million people in Sub-Saharan Africa were afflicted with type 2 diabetes as of 1994, but that number is projected to increase by two- or threefold by 2010. The highest prevalence is found among populations of Indian descent, urban populations, and those with a family history of diabetes, obesity, or physical inactivity. The chapter includes a discussion of studies of diabetes onset and mortality in Tanzania and Zimbabwe. Challenges to the provision of health care for diabetes in Sub-Saharan Africa include short consultation times, inadequately trained staff, nonexistent referral systems, inadequate levels of staff, and poor record keeping.

Cancers. Cancers have been a low priority in Sub-Saharan Africa, yet the probability of a 65-year-old woman developing cancer in Sub-Saharan Africa is only 20 percent lower than in Western Europe. Factors affecting cancer incidence and mortality include increases in the prevalence of tobacco consumption; HIV-induced immunosuppression; increased use of alcohol; the high prevalence of cancer-associated agents like papilloma viruses, hepatitis B virus, and human herpes virus 8; and exposure to aflatoxins. The top three cancers for men are Kaposi's sarcoma, liver cancer, and prostate cancers; for women, cervical cancer, breast cancer, and Kaposi's sarcoma.

Cardiovascular Diseases. Cardiovascular disorders are the second most common cause of adult deaths in Sub-Saharan Africa, as well as a major cause of chronic illness and disability. Half of cardiovascular disease (CVD) deaths occur among people 30 to 69 years of age, which is 10 or more years younger than in more developed regions. Incidence of stroke in Sub-Saharan Africa is estimated to be about 1 per 1,000. Survival outcomes are poor, due to delayed hospitalization, absence of thrombolysis and angioplasty, and low socioeconomic status and illiteracy. Rheumatic heart disease, still prevalent among children and teenagers, is a disease of poverty that is related to overcrowding, poor housing, and undernutrition.

Mental Health, Alcohol and Substance Abuse. Depression in Sub-Saharan Africa is estimated to have an incidence rate of 15 to 18 percent and a lifetime prevalence rate of 18 to 30 percent. Common mental disorders (depression and anxiety) have a point prevalence rate that ranges from 1 to 5 percent. The point prevalence rate for schizophrenia is the same as in other parts of the world, ranging from 2 to 5 per 1,000 population, with a lifetime prevalence of 7 to 9 per 1,000. The Sub-Saharan Africa region, the most conflict-affected region of the world, has seen rates of post-traumatic stress disorder (PTSD), anxiety, and depression range from 20 to 60 percent, and alcohol abuse has seen a sharp increase. In South Africa, suicide is found to be much more frequent among those who are HIV positive.

Neurological Disorders. The prevalence of epilepsy in Sub-Saharan Africa ranges from 2.2 to 58.0 per 1,000 people. Stroke has been found to be as common in Sub-Saharan Africa as in the West. The leading causes of neurological disorders are infections during pregnancy, neonatal infections, and sequelae to the disorders that cause high under-five mortality. Challenges to the management of neurological disorders include the lack of adequately trained personnel able to recognize and manage the disorders, lack of equipment necessary to confirm a neurological diagnosis, and unavailability of the common drugs that would control epilepsy.

Violence and Injuries. Intentional injuries (violence) resulted in the deaths of more than 300,000 people in Africa in 2000. Intentional injuries also are estimated to result in at least 6.2 million disabled or incapacitated people, 20 times the number of deaths. Road traffic injuries, burns, drowning, war, and homicide are the major causes of injury mortality in Sub-Saharan Africa.

KEY DEVELOPMENTS SINCE *DMSSA-1*

This section deals with the changes in the overall socioeconomic environment that have had a major impact on prevalence of diseases in Sub-Saharan Africa, such as economic and demographic developments, as well as the changes in how health in Africa is addressed by development organizations.

The Impact of HIV/AIDS

A striking feature of *DMSSA-2* is the documentation of the direct impact of HIV/AIDS on the epidemiology of almost all infectious diseases included in this volume, as well as on overall adult and child mortality. According to the United Nations' (UN) 2004 projections, life expectancy at birth has dropped by three years since 1990 for the region as a whole; for countries most affected by HIV/AIDS, the drop in life expectancy has been 20 years or more.

As shown in the chapters in this volume, HIV is linked to worsening trends in many diseases, for both adults and children. For example, Madhi and Klugman (chapter 11) state that as much as 45 percent of hospitalizations and 80 percent of deaths due to lower respiratory tract infections occur among HIV-infected children, and strides made in reducing childhood mortality from lower respiratory tract infections during the 1980s and the early 1990s have been reversed. In chapter 13, on tuberculosis, Dye and his colleagues discuss how people latently infected with *Mycobacterium tuberculosis* are at greater risk of developing active tuberculosis if their immune systems are also weakened with HIV infection. Consequently, the tuberculosis caseload has increased by a factor of five or more in the countries of eastern and southern Africa most affected by HIV.

Malaria has a two-way relationship with HIV/AIDS. Anemia resulting from malaria increases the risk for HIV infection through increased use of blood transfusions. In the review of malaria (chapter 14), Snow and Omumbo report an odds ratio for HIV infection of 3.5 for malaria patients transfused once, 21.5 for those transfused twice, and 43.0 for those transfused three times during a single admission. HIV infection, in turn, increases the risk of malaria, which is associated with higher density of parasitemia and more severe symptoms of malaria in adults.

HIV/AIDS not only affects the incidence of communicable diseases but is also a risk factor for several noncommunicable diseases. As discussed in chapter 10, children with HIV infection are at special risk for developmental disabilities. Low birthweight, prematurity, poverty, malnutrition, and micronutrient deficiencies, more frequently seen in HIV-infected children, are likely to compromise early child development. Maternal-child interaction is also affected;

even HIV-uninfected children of HIV-infected mothers are at higher risk for cognitive and language delays.

Kaposi's sarcoma, now ranked first for male cancers and third for female cancers in the region, is also associated with HIV/AIDS. Prior to the epidemic, this was a rare cancer, but it has increased twentyfold, and in countries with a high prevalence of HIV, Kaposi's sarcoma is the leading cancer in children.

As discussed by Mbewu and Mbanya (chapter 21), 30 percent of those living with HIV show evidence of cardiac involvement. Mental health also shows the impact of HIV/AIDS: psychiatric sequelae of HIV/AIDS include depression, anxiety disorders, manic symptoms, and atypical psychosis.

Maternal HIV infection compromises the provision of care and undermines global cognitive development even in the uninfected children. HIV-infected infants demonstrate lower mental and motor development (Baingana, Thomas, and Comblain 2005). Other effects of HIV on the nervous system are discussed in chapter 23.

The direct impact of HIV on the incidence of and mortality from both communicable and noncommunicable diseases is documented in the chapters that follow. HIV/AIDS further affects health and mortality because of the social and economic consequences of the disease, including a large increase in the number of orphans, the burden on health services, the impact on human resources for health, and the impoverishing consequences of the disease. The extraordinary impact of HIV/AIDS has created a "development crisis" that extends far beyond its epidemiological effects.

The Socioeconomic Context

Growth in GDP per capita in low-income countries in Sub-Saharan Africa has continued to lag behind most other regions (figure 1.1), and real per capita GDP growth was negative for the period 1991 to 2000. Growth accelerated during the first few years of the twenty-first century but still lagged behind that of all other regions except Latin America and the Caribbean in 2004; the World Bank predicts that it will remain slow until 2015. In the 1980s, per capita income expressed in purchasing power parity (PPPs, international dollars) was higher in Africa than in other low-income countries, but it has gradually deteriorated (figure 1.2) and, as of 2004, was well below that of other low-income countries (World Bank 2005c).

Although some countries experienced rapid growth, more countries showed declines in real per capita income (expressed in US$) during both the 1980s and 1990s

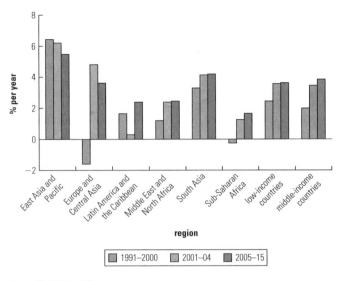

Figure 1.1 Real GDP per Capita Growth, by Region, 1991–2015

Source: World Bank 2005a.

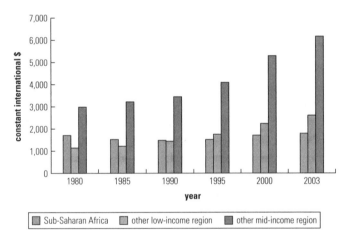

Figure 1.2 Real GDP per Capita, by Developing Region, 1980–2003

Source: World Bank 2005c.

(table 1.1). Growth rates have also been more volatile: of the 45 Sub-Saharan African countries, only 5 consistently recorded real per capita growth rates above 2 percent per year (Botswana, Cape Verde, Mauritius, the Seychelles, and Swaziland), whereas nearly three-quarters of the countries experienced at least one year of per capita growth lower than minus 10 percent (World Bank 2005a).

Closely linked to the low level of economic growth is the lack of progress in reducing poverty. Although most of the world is on track to achieve the Millennium Development Goal (MDG) of a 50 percent reduction in the number of people living below $1 per day, poverty has been on the increase in Sub-Saharan Africa: in 1990, 44.6 percent of the

Table 1.1 Gross National Income, per Capita, 1980, 1990, 2003 *(current US$)*

Country	1980	1990	2003	Percentage change 1980–90	Percentage change 1990–2003
Angola	—	820	740	—	−10
Benin	410	370	440	−10	19
Botswana	1,120	2,750	3,530	146	28
Burkina Faso	290	330	300	14	−9
Burundi	220	220	90	0	−59
Cameroon	620	950	630	53	−34
Cape Verde	—	980	1,440	—	47
Central African Republic	340	470	260	38	−45
Chad	240	270	240	13	−11
Comoros	—	550	450	—	−18
Congo, Dem. Rep. of	600	220	100	−63	−55
Congo, Rep. of	820	880	650	7	−26
Côte d'Ivoire	1,140	780	660	−32	−15
Equatorial Guinea	—	350	—	—	—
Eritrea	—	—	190	—	—
Ethiopia	—	170	90	—	−47
Gabon	4,800	4,800	3,340	0	−30
Gambia, The	380	310	270	−18	−13
Ghana	420	380	320	−10	−16
Guinea	—	460	430	—	−7
Guinea-Bissau	150	220	140	47	−36
Kenya	440	380	400	−14	5
Lesotho	500	650	610	30	−6
Liberia	530	—	110	—	—
Madagascar	450	240	290	−47	21
Malawi	190	200	160	5	−20
Mali	270	270	290	0	7
Mauritania	450	540	400	20	−26
Mauritius	—	2,300	4,100	—	78
Mozambique	—	170	210	—	24
Namibia	—	1,720	1,930	—	12
Niger	440	310	200	−30	−35
Nigeria	780	270	350	−65	30
Rwanda	250	370	220	48	−41
São Tomé and Principe	—	430	300	—	−30
Senegal	530	720	540	36	−25
Seychelles	2,080	5,020	7,490	141	49
Sierra Leone	380	200	150	−47	−25
Somalia	100	130	—	30	—
South Africa	2,550	2,890	2,750	13	−5
Sudan	470	570	460	21	−19
Swaziland	960	1,190	1,350	24	13
Tanzania	—	190	300	—	58
Togo	450	440	310	−2	−30
Uganda	—	320	250	—	−22
Zambia	630	450	380	−29	−16
Zimbabwe	950	880	—	−7	—
All Sub-Saharan Africa (unweighted)	734	825	860	12	4

Source: World Bank 2005c.
Note: — = not available.

population lived below the $1 per day line; this had increased to 46.4 percent by 2003.

There is little doubt that slow economic growth and increasing poverty are related to slow progress in health outcomes. Wagstaff and Claeson (2004) summarized findings on income, coverage of interventions related to health, and health outcomes, documenting that higher incomes lead to improved access to and use of preventive and curative interventions, such as antenatal care, immunizations, use of treated bednets, and receipt of therapy for diarrhea and medicines for reducing fever. Income is also an important determinant of access to nutritious food, which, in turn, leads to lower levels of malnutrition, a key risk factor for many childhood diseases.

While some countries at lower-middle levels of income have achieved good health outcomes, such examples are rare for the countries with the lowest incomes. A basic package of health interventions would in the case of the poorest low-income Sub-Saharan African countries overwhelm public health budgets, and prospects for scaling up public health services from domestic resources are unfavorable.

The Demographic Context

Sub-Saharan Africa is the "youngest" of the World Bank regions, as measured by the proportion of the population below age 15 and by the median age of the population. About 44 percent of the population is younger than 15 (compared with 28 percent globally), and the median age of the population is just 17.5 years (compared with 27 years globally; figures 1.3, 1.4). In countries such as Uganda and Niger, the proportion below age 15 is close to 50 percent of the population. Fertility in Sub-Saharan Africa continues to be the highest in the world despite some decline in recent years. From 1990 to 2003 the total fertility rate (TFR) declined somewhat, but it is still higher now than in any other region in 1990 (figure 1.5).

The youthfulness of the population reflects fertility and mortality rates, which in turn have an impact on the epidemiological characteristics of the population. High fertility and high adult mortality lead to a high proportion of young people, who are much less likely to be vulnerable to chronic diseases that typically affect the adult and elderly populations. Epidemiology and demography thus interact to generate the overall disease and mortality patterns in which infectious diseases are dominant over noncommunicable diseases and conditions.

Population growth averaged 2.5 percent during 1990 and 2003 for the region as a whole, exceeding 3 percent in

Figure 1.3 Population below Age 15, 2003

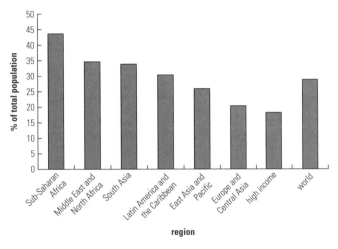

Source: United Nations 2005.

Figure 1.4 Median Age of Population, 1990 and 2003

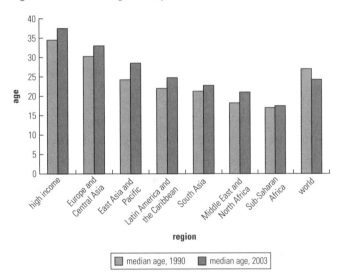

Source: United Nations 2005.

Figure 1.5 Total Fertility Rate, 1990 and 2003

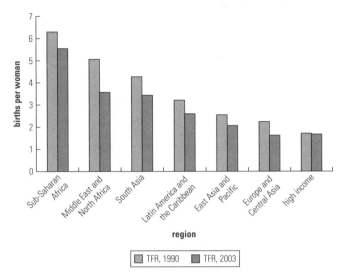

Source: United Nations 2005.

Figure 1.6 Age Pyramid for Botswana, 2005, with and without AIDS

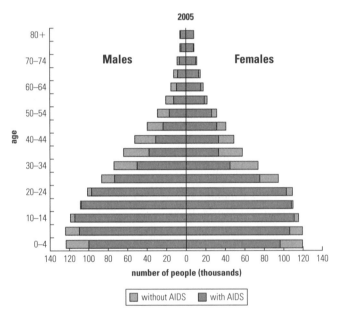

Source: U.S. Census Bureau 2004.

countries such as Chad, the Republic of Congo, The Gambia, and Niger. At a rate of 2.5 percent, the population would double in less than 28 years. However, population growth rates are projected to fall precipitously in countries in which HIV/AIDS has infected a large number of people. World Bank projections for the region as a whole show the population growth rate declining to 2.0 percent during 2000–10, and 1.9 percent during 2010–15. In the most affected countries in southern Africa, World Bank projections show a decline to between 0.2 and 0.5 percent growth per year. Other agencies that have published demographic projections show an even greater impact of AIDS mortality, leading to population decline by 2010 in some countries. Due to the high mortality of AIDS during the young adult

years, age structures of the affected countries will become characterized by an unusually small number of adults, as shown in the age pyramid for Botswana (figure 1.6).

Increasing International Attention to Health in Sub-Saharan Africa

In the years since the publication of *DMSSA-1*, the attention being paid to health conditions in Sub-Saharan Africa has rapidly increased, as evidenced by the number of studies

Box 1.2 The Health-Related Millennium Development Goals and Indicators

- Goal 1: Eradicate extreme poverty and hunger
  - Target is to cut in half the proportion of people who suffer from hunger between 1990 and 2015. Progress is measured by the prevalence of underweight children under five years of age.
- Goal 4: Reduce child mortality
  - Target is to reduce the under-five mortality rate by two-thirds between 1990 and 2015.
- Goal 5: Improve maternal health
  - Target is to reduce the maternal mortality ratio by three-quarters between 1990 and 2015.

- Goal 6: Combat HIV/AIDS, malaria, and other diseases
  - Target is to have halted and begun to reverse the spread of these diseases by 2015.
- Goal 7: Ensure environmental sustainability
  - Target is to cut in half the proportion of people without sustainable access to safe drinking water by 2015.
- Goal 8: Develop a global partnership for development
  - Target is to provide access to affordable essential drugs in developing countries.

and reports, new initiatives that draw attention to particular diseases, and increased financing from donor countries, foundations, and multilateral agencies.

Many reports have either explicitly focused on Africa or have focused on health conditions in poor countries, leading to a strong emphasis on Africa. Among the more prominent recent studies are the 2001 report *Macroeconomics and Health: Investing in Health for Economic Development* (Commission on Macroeconomics and Health 2001); the 2005 report *Our Common Interest* (Commission for Africa 2005); and World Bank studies and publications, such as the 1998 publication *Better Health in Africa: Experiences and Lessons Learned,* the 2005 report *Improving Health, Nutrition, and Population Outcomes in Sub-Saharan Africa: The Role of the World Bank,* and the *Global Monitoring Report 2005: Millennium Development Goals—From Consensus to Momentum* (World Bank 1998, 2005b, 2005a, respectively).

New initiatives and partnerships formed or strengthened during recent years have similarly provided advocacy for increased attention to diseases of the poor, generally with a focus on Africa. Among these are partnerships that focus on neglected diseases that mostly affect Sub-Saharan Africa, such as guinea worm, trypanosomiasis, onchocerciasis, and schistosomiasis. Other global partnerships have increased the availability of pharmaceuticals at lower costs, through pooled procurement, for diseases such as malaria and tuberculosis and for vaccine-preventable diseases. Foundations and funds, such as the Bill & Melinda Gates Foundation or the Global Fund to Fight AIDS, Malaria, and Tuberculosis, have made large amounts of new financing available to address diseases that disproportionately affect Sub-Saharan

Africa. Traditional donors, such as bilateral development agencies, the World Bank, and regional development banks, have also increased financing for health, and the joint WHO–World Bank High-Level Forum on the Health MDGs is considering new mechanisms to expand the availability of resources to combat communicable diseases.

An important influence on priorities for the global health agenda are the MDGs, endorsed by 147 heads of state at the UN Millennium Summit of September 2000. The goals include numerical targets that are to be achieved between 1990 and 2015. Of the eight goals, three are directly concerned with mortality and morbidity, and six have been identified as "health related" (box 1.2). The focus of the MDGs on achieving health outcomes has increased the awareness of the lack of progress in Sub-Saharan Africa. Other low- and middle-income regions show progress toward some of the MDGs (although current trends indicate that not a single World Bank region is making sufficient progress to reach all of them). Sub-Saharan Africa is not on track to achieve a single one of the targets. Halfway through the period from 1990 to 2015, not a single Sub-Saharan Africa country is on track for the under-five mortality rate target, and only one in four would achieve the malnutrition target on current trends. The increased focus on monitoring of trends has also provided evidence that many countries in the region have worse indicators than they did 15 years ago.

Expanding Data Collection Efforts

Efforts to collect more data on health outcomes have intensified over the past decade, and as a result *DMSSA-2* is more empirically based than the previous edition. Household surveys, including the Demographic and Health Surveys, the UNICEF Multiple Indicator Cluster Surveys, the World Bank's Living Standards Measurement Surveys, and other surveys conducted by the World Health Organization as well as by country statistical offices, have vastly increased the availability and quality of the data.

Demographic surveillance sites have joined in an alliance, called the INDEPTH Network, which has published standardized reports on demographic indicators, including a set of life tables. The network, which has grown to include 20 African sites, supports cross-site collaboration, capacity building, and dissemination of the collected data. Another area in which surveillance has greatly improved is HIV surveillance in antenatal clinics. Through annual reports of the data, such surveillance has been used to document the sharp increases in HIV prevalence among pregnant women in southern African countries, as well as the decline in HIV prevalence in Uganda. Other areas of improvement over the past decade include the surveillance and reporting of cancers, from an increased number of cancer registries, and injuries, from injury surveillance systems. Advances have also been achieved in malaria mapping and in the estimation of diabetes and lung disease incidence.

Nevertheless, the availability of morbidity and mortality data is far from sufficient for monitoring disease outbreaks, the impact of health interventions, or even annual monitoring of incidence and prevalence of most diseases. Routine vital registration is still absent in almost all countries (except Mauritius and the Seychelles), although progress has been made in mortality registration in South Africa. One consequence of this lack is the general unavailability or reliability of the denominators needed to estimate overall mortality or cause-specific rates. Efforts to expand the coverage of vital registration beyond urban areas would have substantial payoffs for improving the quality of epidemiological information.

Human Resources for Health: A Worsening Crisis?

Human resources have been described as "the heart of the health system in any country," and "the most important aspect of health care systems" (Hongoro and McPake 2004). The recent study *Human Resources for Health: Overcoming the Crisis*, by the Joint Learning Initiative (2004), suggests that both the number and the skill levels of health workers in Sub-Saharan Africa are far below what is needed to reduce mortality (table 1.2). The region has 25 percent of

Table 1.2 Overview of Health Worker Vacancy Rates for Four Countries

Health worker	Vacancy rates (percent)			
	Ghana	Lesotho	Namibia	Malawi
Doctors	42.6	7.6	26.0	36.3
Nurses	25.5	48.1	2.9	2.9
Auxiliary nurses	—	5.4	0.6	18.4
Doctor specialists	72.9	0.0	25.7	—
Other staff	—	29.9	25.3	62.8

Source: Hongoro and McPake 2004.
Note: — = not available.

the world disease burden, but only 1.3 percent of the share of the world's health workforce (Commission for Africa 2005). Central to the problem are issues of supply, demand, and mobility (transnational, regional, and local). These include large differences in remuneration and nonrewarding work in the low-income countries juxtaposed with a growing demand for skilled workers, in particular, nurses, in the high-income countries (Joint Learning Initiative 2004). The problem of low staff numbers is compounded by low morale and skills and the maldistribution of staff geographically. Further challenges are the wars and other internal conflicts that adversely affect health infrastructure, services, and personnel retention. The HIV epidemic increases the workload, and AIDS mortality has reduced the number of health workers. In countries such as Malawi and Zambia, it is estimated that the illness of health workers has increased five- to sixfold (Padarath et al. 2003).

Conflicts, Refugees, and Internally Displaced People

In the years since *DMSSA-1* was published, the continent has undergone numerous armed conflicts, including civil wars and genocide. Since 1980, more than 30 wars have plagued Africa. It is estimated that as of the end of 2003, 16 million people in Sub-Saharan Africa had been displaced through conflict (WHO 2002). Low-income countries are disproportionately affected by conflicts. Fifteen countries in the region had a major conflict between 1990 and 2003 (UNICEF 2005). Table 1.3 illustrates the relative global burden of conflict-related deaths by region.

Injuries due to collective violence are concentrated in Sub-Saharan Africa. In the last decade, the bulk of lives lost to war injuries in Africa have resulted from conflicts in the Democratic Republic of Congo, Liberia, and Rwanda. The

Table 1.3 Conflict-Related Deaths by Region
(per 100,000 people)

Region	No. of deaths
High-income countries	0.0
Low-income countries	6.2
WHO Africa region	32.0
WHO Eastern Mediterranean region	8.1
WHO European region	4.2

Source: WHO 2002.

legacy of war in the form of landmines continues to contribute to mortality in the continent. As of October 2004, 1.2 million Sudanese had been uprooted from their homes, many killed by militias, and those who found their way into Chad faced disease, poor nutrition, and inadequate shelter. In a typical five-year war, the under-five mortality increases by 13 percent and adult mortality even more. During the first five years of peace, the average under-five mortality was found to be 11 percent higher than the corresponding level before the war. Sexual violence during conflicts increases the spread of HIV (UNICEF 2005).

In Sub-Saharan Africa, for children who survive the first four years of life, injury becomes the most likely cause of disability and death. Most intentional injuries are caused by war; it is estimated that 120,000 to 200,000 child soldiers age 5 to 16 years are participating in conflicts, putting them at risk for bullet and shrapnel wounds, burns, and land mine injuries (UNICEF 2005). Psychosocial and mental disorders resulting from conflicts had affected 15.5 percent of the population in Rwanda five years after the genocide; depression, anxiety, and PTSD can range from 20 to 60 percent in conflict-affected populations (Baingana, Thomas, and Comblain 2005).

The most dramatic outbreak of a diarrhea epidemic occurred in July 1994 among Rwandan refugees in Goma, Democratic Republic of Congo, when almost 50,000 refugees died (see chapter 9). Conflicts have also had an impact on immunization rates. From 1990 to 2000 the vaccination rates for diptheria, pertussis, and tetanus (DPT) in the Central African Republic fell from 82 percent to 29 percent, and in the Democratic Republic of Congo, from 79 percent to 33 percent (see chapter 12). The probability of surviving from age 15 to age 60 in 2000 was less than 50 percent in almost half of the Sub-Saharan Africa countries, due in part to the conflicts.

REFERENCES

Baingana, F., R. Thomas, and C. Comblain. 2005. *HIV/AIDS and Mental Health.* Health Nutrition and Population electronic discussion paper. http://www.worldbank.org.

Commission for Africa. 2005. *Our Common Interest: Report of the Commission for Africa.* London: Commission for Africa. http://www.commissionforafrica.org.

Commission on Macroeconomics and Health. 2001. *Macroeconomics and Health: Investing in Health for Economic Development.* Geneva: WHO.

Feachem, R. G., and D. T. Jamison. 1991. *Disease and Mortality in Sub-Saharan Africa.* Washington, DC: World Bank.

Hongoro, C., and B. McPake. 2004. "How to Bridge the Gap in Human Resources for Health." *Lancet* 364: 29–34.

Joint Learning Initiative. 2004. *Human Resources for Health: Overcoming the Crisis.* Cambridge, MA: Harvard University Press.

Padarath A., C. Chamberlain, D. McCoy, A. Ntuli, M. Rowson, and R. Loewenson. 2003. "Health Personnel in Southern Africa: Confronting Maldistribution and Brain Drain." Discussion paper 3, Equinet Africa, *Training and Research Support Centre (TARSC)*, Harare, Zimbabwe. http://www.equinetafrica.org/bibl/resources.php.

UNICEF (United Nations Children's Fund). 2005. *The State of the World's Children: Childhood under Threat.* New York: UNICEF.

United Nations. 2005. *World Population Prospects: The 2004 Revision.* New York: United Nations.

U.S. Census Bureau. 2004. International Programs Center, AIDS surveillance database. http://www.census.gov/ipc/www/hivaidsn.html.

Wagstaff, A., and M. Claeson. 2004. *The Millennium Development Goals for Health: Rising to the Challenges.* Washington, DC: World Bank.

World Bank. 1998. *Better Health in Africa: Experiences and Lessons Learned.* Washington, DC: World Bank.

———. 2005a. *Global Monitoring Report 2005: Millennium Development Goals—From Consensus to Momentum.* Washington, DC: World Bank.

———. 2005b. *Improving Health, Nutrition and Population Outcomes in Sub-Saharan Africa.* Washington, DC: World Bank.

———. 2005c. *World Development Indicators 2005.* Washington, DC: World Bank. http://devdata.worldbank/dataonline/.

WHO (World Health Organization). 2002. *World Report on Violence and Health.* Geneva: WHO.

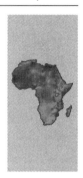

Chapter 2

Levels and Trends in Mortality in Sub-Saharan Africa: An Overview

Jacob Adetunji and Eduard R. Bos

One of the major achievements of the twentieth century in Sub-Saharan Africa is the unprecedented decline in mortality and the corresponding increase in the expectation of life at birth. At the dawn of the twentieth century, Sub-Saharan Africa was characterized by extremely high under-five mortality levels and by low life expectancy at birth. By the end of the century, however, mortality among children under five had decreased from about 500 per 1,000 live births to about 150 (World Bank 2005). Similarly, the average length of life, which was less than 30 years about 100 years ago, had increased to more than 50 years by the early 1990s. Much of the mortality decline happened in the second half of the twentieth century, the fastest rate of decline occurring in the first decades after World War II (Hill 1991). In the 1990s, mortality decline stalled for the region overall, with many countries experiencing reversals in the upward trend in life expectancy largely because of AIDS mortality.

This overview focuses on the period between 1960 and 2005. This period roughly corresponds to the postcolonial era in many countries in the region, in which large economic and social changes occurred. Some of these changes were beneficial to the health of the population (such as economic growth and increasing access to health interventions),

whereas others are associated with increasing exposure to risk factors that lead to increased morbidity and mortality (such as increasing exposure to risks for noncommunicable diseases or the spread of new and reemerging communicable diseases). Therefore, monitoring mortality levels and trends in the Sub-Saharan region provides not only a direct reflection of the health status of populations but also an indirect gauge of the effects of economic, political, and epidemiological turbulence that faced the region.

INDICATORS OF MORTALITY LEVELS AND TRENDS

In this overview chapter, two indicators of mortality are used to assess levels and trends for Sub-Saharan Africa, its subregions, and countries. The infant mortality rate, calculated as the proportion of newborns in a given period that do not survive to their first birthday, is a standard measure not affected by age structure and therefore suitable to use for comparisons over time and across regions. Life expectancy at birth, calculated as the average number of years a newborn would live if subject to the mortality rates for a given year, is used to compare the force of mortality across the entire age spectrum. The dearth of reliable data is one of the main problems confronting the study of mortality levels and trends in Sub-Saharan Africa. Although vital registration systems exist in most countries in the region, they usually do not produce reliable data. In the absence of reliable vital registration systems and good quality census data that are needed for direct calculation of infant and child mortality rates, demographers have developed indirect methods for obtaining these vital statistics from incomplete and often defective data. However, over the past 30 years, information available for the study of mortality patterns, particularly among children under age five, has improved dramatically. The improvement in information is largely due to the implementation of large-scale household survey programs, such as the World Fertility Surveys (WFS) program of 1972–84, the Demographic and Health Surveys (DHS), and UNICEF's Multiple Indicator Cluster Surveys (MICS). Of all these survey programs, the DHS has had the largest impact on data availability, analysis, and report dissemination. About 70 DHS surveys have been conducted in 33 of the 46 major countries in Sub-Saharan Africa.

Apart from the DHS-type surveys, Sub-Saharan Africa has an extensive network of longitudinal study sites. At least 19 such study sites exist in the region and their data have been invaluable in deriving mortality estimates by age as well as model life tables that show how the age pattern of African mortality differs from the model life tables constructed by Coale and Demeny (1983) and United Nations model life tables (INDEPTH Network 2001). The main problem with this source is that most of these longitudinal study sites are based in rural settings and are scattered throughout the whole region and therefore provide estimates of unknown generalizability. The locations of the sites are neither systematically planned to represent the Sub-Saharan Africa region nor do they adequately represent the countries in which they are located.

In this chapter the estimates for countries and subregions are those issued most recently by the United Nations Population Division; the estimates are based on a variety of sources, including surveys, censuses, and demographic modeling. The delineation of geographic subregions used are those defined by the United Nations.

MORTALITY LEVELS AND TRENDS

The following section will provide a comparison of indicators of mortality trends discussed above, first comparing trends in life expectancy and infant mortality in Sub-Saharan

Table 2.1 Life Expectancy at Birth for World and UN Regions, 1960–2005

Region	1960–69	1970–79	1980–89	1990–99	2000–04
World	52.5	58.1	61.4	63.7	65.4
Sub-Saharan Africa	42.4	46.3	49.0	47.6	45.9
Asia	48.5	56.4	60.4	64.0	67.3
Europe	69.6	71.0	72.0	72.6	73.7
Latin America and Caribbean	56.8	60.9	64.9	68.3	71.5
Northern America	70.1	71.6	74.3	75.5	77.6
Oceania	63.7	65.8	69.3	71.5	74.0

Source: United Nations 2005.

Africa and other regions, followed by a comparison of these mortality indicators for subregions within Sub-Saharan Africa.

Sub-Saharan Africa Relative to Other, Less Developed Regions

Sub-Saharan Africa is, by far, the region of the world with the highest level of mortality. Overall life expectancy at birth is 46 years, whereas in Asia, the region with the second lowest life expectancy, it is 67.

As shown in table 2.1, the disparity between Sub-Saharan Africa and other regions of the world has widened since the 1960s. In that decade the difference in life expectancy with the Asian region was only 6 years, but this has grown to almost 21 years now. And, whereas all other regions have experienced uninterrupted increases in life expectancy, in Sub-Saharan Africa life expectancy peaked in the early 1990s at 50 years, and has since fallen back by almost 4 years.

Declines in infant mortality rates in Sub-Saharan Africa started to slow down considerably in the 1990s. These slow declines have meant that Sub-Saharan Africa has lagged more and more behind other regions and hence the mortality gap has widened (table 2.2).

Subregional Differences in Mortality

In Sub-Saharan Africa as a whole, infant mortality rates declined from 149 per 1,000 live births in the 1960s to about 101 in 2005—a 32 percent decline over a period of 35 years. Toward the end of the last decade of the twentieth century, the decline in infant mortality rates leveled off, decreasing only slightly for the region as a whole.

Table 2.2 Infant Mortality Rates for World and UN Regions, 1960–2005

(per 1,000 live births)

Region	1960–69	1970–79	1980–89	1990–99	2000–04
World	119	93	78	66	57
Sub-Saharan Africa	149	130	115	107	101
Asia	123	96	77	63	54
Europe	33	23	17	11	9
Latin America and Caribbean	96	75	52	35	26
Northern America	24	16	9	7	7
Oceania	49	43	36	32	29

Source: United Nations 2005.

Table 2.3 Infant Mortality Rates for Sub-Saharan Africa and UN Subregions, 1960–2005

(per 1,000 live births)

Region, subregion	1960–69	1970–79	1980–89	1990–99	2000–04
Sub-Saharan Africa	149	130	115	107	101
Eastern Africa	144	124	112	101	93
Middle Africa	156	131	121	122	116
Southern Africa	90	78	58	47	45
Western Africa	165	145	128	119	114

Source: United Nations 2005.

In regard to subregional disparities, infant mortality rates are highest in West Africa and in Middle Africa and have consistently been so from 1960 (table 2.3). The infant mortality rate declined somewhat faster in West Africa, and as a result, Middle Africa is currently the subregion with the highest rate. Of all subregions of Sub-Saharan Africa, countries in Southern Africa have had the lowest infant mortality rates. For example, in 1960 the rate was 42 percent lower than in other subregions, and even with increasing overall mortality in the 1990s, the infant mortality rate in Southern Africa was still less than half the average for Sub-Saharan Africa in 2000.

Life expectancy at birth has increased 3.5 years for the continent as a whole since 1960, but it is now lower in Southern Africa than in the 1960s (table 2.4). All the subregions reached peak levels of life expectancy about 1990, but they have since shown a decline, largely due to AIDS mortality. Nowhere has the decrease in life expectancy been steeper and greater than in Southern Africa, where 40 years of increases in life expectancy were reversed in a period of 10 years.

Table 2.4 Life Expectancy at Birth for Sub-Saharan Africa and UN Subregions, 1960–2005

Region, subregion	1960–69	1970–79	1980–89	1990–99	2000–04
Sub-Saharan Africa	42.4	46.3	49.0	47.6	45.9
Eastern Africa	43.4	47.3	49.4	46.7	45.7
Middle Africa	41.0	45.3	47.0	44.3	43.4
Southern Africa	50.7	54.4	59.6	59.6	47.7
Western Africa	40.3	43.9	47.1	47.2	46.3

Source: United Nations 2005.

Country Differences in Mortality

Figure 2.1 illustrates the differences in the levels and trends in the infant mortality rate in selected Sub-Saharan Africa countries. The rates vary from 15 in Mauritius, to 165 in Sierra Leone, and the rates of change from 1960 to the present differ from about 20 percent in the Democratic Republic of Congo, Liberia, Rwanda, and Sierra Leone to over 50 percent in countries in Southern Africa. It is noteworthy, however, that infant mortality has declined in all countries since 1960.

Figure 2.2 shows country patterns in life expectancy at birth. The range in current levels is about 35 years, from a high of 72 in Mauritius to a low of 37 in Zimbabwe and Zambia. Recent trends are clearly negative in many countries, where increases in adult mortality resulting from AIDS have led to a decline in overall life expectancy. Most of these countries experienced the highest life expectancies during 1985 to 1990 and have since declined to below the levels in 1960.

Figure 2.1 Infant Mortality Rate in Selected Countries, 1960–2005

(per thousand)

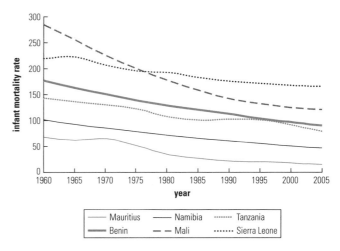

Source: Adapted from United Nations 2005.

Figure 2.2 Life Expectancy in Selected Countries

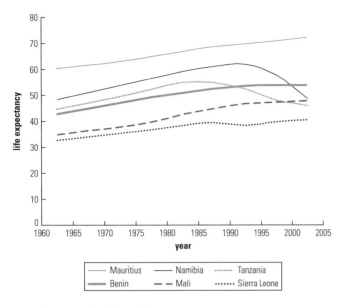

Source: Adapted from United Nations 2005.

REFERENCES

Coale, A., and P. Demeny. 1983. *Regional Model Life Tables and Stable Populations.* New York: Academic Press.

Hill, A. 1991. "Infant and Child Mortality: Levels, Trends and Data Deficiencies." In *Disease and Mortality in Sub-Saharan Africa,* ed. R. G. Feachem and D. T. Jamison, 37–74. New York: Oxford University Press.

INDEPTH Network. 2001. *Population and Health in Developing Countries.* Vol. 1. Ottawa: International Development Research Centre.

United Nations. 2005. *World Population Prospects. The 2004 Revision.* New York: United Nations.

World Bank. 2005. *World Development Indicators.* Washington, DC: World Bank.

Chapter **3**

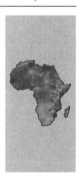

Trends in Child Mortality, 1960 to 2000

Kenneth Hill and Agbessi Amouzou

Under-five mortality, the probability of dying between birth and age five expressed per 1,000 live births, and infant mortality, the probability of dying before age one expressed per 1,000 live births, are widely used as measures of children's, and more broadly a population's, well-being. Reduction of the under-five mortality rate (U5MR) by two-thirds between 1990 and 2015, equivalent to an annual average rate of reduction of 4.3 percent, is one of the six health-related Millennium Development Goals (MDGs). Data indicate that some 11 million children under the age of five die annually in the world as a whole, and more than 10 million of these deaths occur in the developing world. Sub-Saharan Africa is the region most affected and accounts for more than one-third of deaths of children under the age of five (Hill et al. 1999). Some two-thirds of the child deaths in the developing world are caused by diseases (predominantly acute respiratory infections, diarrhea, and malaria) for which practical, low-cost interventions, including immunization, oral rehydration therapy (ORT), and antibiotics, exist (Jones et al. 2003).

The quality and quantity of data on child mortality have increased dramatically over the last 30 years, particularly in Sub-Saharan Africa. However, the quantity, timeliness, and quality of available information vary widely by country. Figure 3.1 contrasts the data availability for the Republic of Congo and Kenya. The only information available for the Republic of Congo is a set of indirect estimates derived from data collected by the 1974 census, effectively covering only the period 1960 to 1970. Kenya, in contrast, has estimates from several censuses, a World Fertility Survey (WFS), a National Demographic Survey (NDS), and three Demographic and Health Surveys (DHSs). For the Republic of Congo, there exists no possibility of consistency checks, and there has been no empirical basis for estimating child mortality since about 1970. For Kenya, however, the different data sources provide a large number of estimates, not all of which are mutually consistent, for overlapping time periods and a considerable density of observations covering the early 1960s to the late 1990s.

The multiplicity and in some cases inconsistency of U5MR estimates from different sources has made the determination of national trends problematic. Hill and Yazbeck (1994), and subsequently Hill and colleagues (1999), developed and applied an explicit, objective, and replicable

Figure 3.1 Contrasting Data Availability: The Republic of Congo and Kenya
(per 1,000 births)

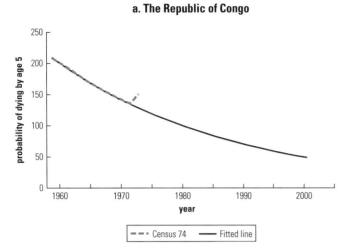

a. The Republic of Congo

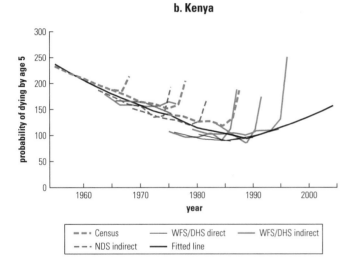

b. Kenya

Source: Updated version of database compiled by Hill and colleagues (1999).

methodology to derive a single consistent time series of estimates for infant and under-five mortality from the assembled data.

In this chapter, the estimates by Hill and colleagues (1999) for countries of Sub-Saharan African are updated. Country data that have become available since that study are added in order to provide more complete information about levels and trends of under-five mortality since 1990.

DATA SOURCES AND METHODS

In countries with accurate registers of births and deaths, infant mortality year by year is measured by the infant mortality rate (IMR), the ratio of deaths of infants under one

year to births in the same year obtained from civil registration data. The mortality of children after infancy is typically obtained from civil registration information on deaths of young children by age and from population census information on the size of the population of those ages exposed to the risk of dying.[1] Thus, civil registration data provide all the information needed to measure infant mortality, which can therefore be readily calculated annually, but measurement of mortality after infancy requires additional information on population sizes.

In countries where the registration of vital events is not complete, the registration of infant deaths is often less complete than the registration of births, with the result that the registered IMR underestimates the true value. In these countries, estimates of infant and under-five mortality are typically obtained instead from one or more of three types of survey data. Most similar to registration data is that obtained from the longitudinal or prospective sample survey. A sample of the national population is followed over a period of time, with all vital events being recorded. Such data provide the basis for calculating the conventional IMR as the ratio of infant deaths to births, and also provide the basis for calculating mortality rates after infancy, since population numbers are also available. Such surveys have not been widely used, partly because they are expensive to mount, and partly because they require careful supervision over an extended period to provide good data on trends.

The second data source is a retrospective sample survey that collects full birth histories. Each mother is asked for information on the date of birth and, if relevant, the age at death of every live-born child she has had. In the 1970s and early 1980s the WFS program, and more recently the DHS project, collected such data in many developing countries. Both IMRs and U5MRs for periods up to 15 years before the survey can be calculated from the data, dividing deaths for given ages and time periods by exposure to risk (expressed as person-years of life lived) of the reported children (Somoza 1980). However, the collection of such information by surveys is complex and requires high levels of interviewer quality and training. The surveys are therefore quite expensive and can cover only relatively small samples.

The third data source is a retrospective survey that collects summary birth histories. Each woman surveyed is asked for very simple information: her age, the total number of children she has borne, and the number of those children that have died; in short, a summary birth history with no information about individual children. For a particular age group of women, the proportion of children dead depends primarily on two things: the level of under-five mortality, and the distribution of the children by how long they had been exposed to risk. William Brass (1964) first developed a method for deriving estimates of child mortality from such data. The Brass method and developments of it (Sullivan 1972; Trussell 1975; United Nations 1983) adjust the proportions of children dead by age group of mother for an estimated exposure distribution in order to arrive at pure measures of under-five mortality and of reference dates for these measures. The adjustment process assumes certain patterns of fertility and under-five mortality by age, and results can be quite sensitive to the choices made. The methodology is better suited to estimating under-five mortality than infant mortality (Hill 1991).

Hill and colleagues (1999) reviewed more completely methods for measuring under-five mortality in countries lacking accurate vital registration data, and Hill (1991) reviewed their various advantages and disadvantages.

Data Used

The basic data used in this chapter are observations of U5MR derived from full or summary birth histories. A summary birth history provides seven observations of U5MR, one for each five-year age group of mothers between ages 15 and 49. A full birth history typically provides three observations of U5MR, for the periods 0 to 4, 5 to 9, and 10 to 14 years before the survey, although observations are sometimes also calculated for the periods 15 to 19 and 20 to 24 years before the survey. The observations used are the same as those used by Hill and colleagues (1999), updated with observations that have become available more recently.

Observations for time periods since the early 1990s come primarily from DHS surveys conducted since 1995 and from Multiple Indicator Cluster Surveys (MICS) conducted in 2000. A DHS is a nationally representative survey; such surveys have been conducted in many developing countries, and an increasing number of countries have conducted more than one survey. A typical DHS survey records full birth histories of women of reproductive age (15 to 49) along with the survival status of each child ever born to them. Thus, DHS data provide a basis for both direct and indirect estimation of child and infant mortality. The survey reports tabulate direct estimates for at least the three five-year periods preceding the survey. In this chapter we have also used the birth history data as a basis for indirect estimation using the Manual X version of the Brass technique

of estimation of child mortality from information on children ever born and children surviving (see United Nations 1983). The MICS surveys are also nationally representative surveys, conducted by UNICEF in many countries in Sub-Saharan Africa. Most MICS surveys record only summary birth histories for each woman of reproductive age, thus allowing only indirect estimation of infant and child mortality. Only one country in the region—South Africa—is thought to have vital registration data that are complete enough to provide valid estimates of the IMR (Rob Dorrington, personal communication 2004). These estimates are not used here, since there is no satisfactory way of knowing at what point in the recent past the infant mortality information became complete.

Nine of the Sub-Saharan African countries that Hill and colleagues (1999) included in their study have no information on child mortality more recent than that already analyzed. Seven countries—Angola, Comoros, Gabon, Guinea-Bissau, Somalia, São Tomé and Principe, and South Africa—that they did not include are in the present analysis. The database they used has been updated with direct or indirect estimates of infant and child mortality based on recent data for 27 countries. Some small countries—Cape Verde, Djibouti, Equatorial Guinea, Mauritius, Réunion, and the Seychelles—are not included because they did not have appropriate data or were not regarded as being representative of Sub-Saharan Africa. In sum, a total of 153 data sets covering 42 countries of Sub-Saharan Africa are included in this analysis.

Methodology for Estimation of Trends

The methodology adopted in this chapter is that used by Hill and colleagues (1999; see appendix 3A for a detailed description). The chapter focuses primarily on under-five mortality; all the observations used come from full or summary birth history data collected by censuses or surveys, and it is argued that such methods of data collection provide better estimates of U5MR than of IMR. For each country, many observations with a range of time reference dates are available. These observations are not typically mutually consistent, so some approach is needed to obtain a set of estimates from the various observations. In our approach, a regression model is fitted to the observations of U5MR by reference date. The model assumes that at the country level the rate of change of U5MR is constant over defined time periods, the time periods themselves being determined by the number of observations available. Thus, a country with a large number of observations can have a more flexible time trend of U5MR than a country with few observations. Estimates of U5MR are then derived from the model for specified time points from 1960 to 2000. It is these estimates that are described below. The appendix shows country examples of observations and the time trends fitted to them.

RESULTS

The U5MR is widely recognized as an important indicator of development. In high-mortality settings, it is preferable to the IMR as a single index because the U5MR captures the substantial mortality risk after 12 months of age (Hill 1995). Consequently, this section focuses on changes in U5MR derived from the country-specific analyses undertaken in this chapter, rather than on changes in the IMR. However, for completeness we do present country estimates of the levels of infant mortality in 2000, but it must be emphasized that these estimates are derived from the U5MR estimates using the Coale-Demeny model life table system (Coale and Demeny 1983). Tables 3B.1 and 3B.2 in appendix 3B show country-specific estimates of U5MR and IMR, respectively, for five-year time points from 1960 to 2000. Table 3B.1 also shows the number of censuses or surveys for each country on which the estimates are based, and gives a subjective assessment of the quality of the estimates, based on their consistency. Figure 3B.1 provides graphs of available estimates plotted against time for one example country in each category.

Levels and rates of change in U5MR over the 40 years from 1960 to 2000, estimated using the methodology described above, are summarized here in the form of box plots[2] for major regions of Sub-Saharan Africa, and for Sub-Saharan Africa as a whole. The United Nations (UN) definitions of regions—Middle, Eastern, Southern, and Western—are used (see tables 3B.1 and 3B.2 for countries included in each region).

The model in equation 3.1 is used to estimate U5MR levels for the mid-point of years ending in 0 or 5.

$$\ln({}_5q_0)_i = b_0 + b_1(date)_i + b_2(postk1)_i \\ + b_3(postk2)_i + b_4(postk3)_i + \cdots + \varepsilon_i \quad (3.1)$$

Change is then measured between estimated values over five-year periods, 1960–65, 1965–70, and so on. Rates of change are calculated as

$$_5r_{n-5} = \frac{1}{5} \times \ln\left(\frac{_5q_0[n]}{_5q_0[n-5]}\right) \quad (3.2)$$

where $_5r_{n-5}$ is the rate of change between year $n-5$ and year n, and $[n]$ represents a year ending in 0 or 5.

Note that in this section, the unit of analysis is the country, not the child. A country will appear in the analysis for a particular time point only if the U5MR is supported by an observation within two years of that time point. Thus country–time point estimates are selected for data availability, so that, for example, the countries contributing to estimates for 1990 will not be the same as the countries contributing to estimates for 1995. Any association between levels and rates of change of U5MR on the one hand and data availability on the other may cause a bias.

Estimated Level of U5MR and IMR in 2000

Estimated levels of U5MR and IMR in 2000 are shown in figure 3.2. The U5MR ranges from 47 per 1,000 births (South Africa) to 314 per 1,000 (Sierra Leone); the median is 153 per 1,000. For the median country, among 100 children born,

Figure 3.2 Estimated Levels of Under-Five and Infant Mortality, by Region of Africa, 2000
(per 1,000 births)

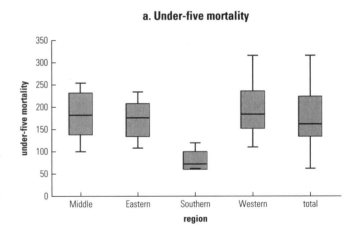

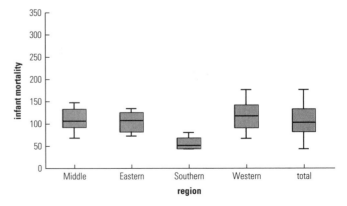

Source: Tables 3B.1 and 3B.2.

more than 15 die before their fifth birthday. The comparable figure for the developing world as a whole is less than 100 per 1,000, and for the more developed world, less than 10 per 1,000. The interquartile range is from 124 to 217, indicating continuing high child mortality in the majority of countries covered. Infant deaths account for almost two-thirds of under-five deaths. The median IMR is 101 per 1,000 with an interquartile range from 80 to 133 per 1,000.

There is considerable variability in the level of U5MR and IMR by region. The Middle and Western Africa regions have the highest median level of U5MR at 174 per 1,000 live births, followed by the Eastern region with a median of 168 per 1,000. The Southern region exhibits a comparatively low rate of U5MR of 58 per 1,000. The Western region has the highest level of IMR (a median of 117 per 1,000), followed by the Middle and the Eastern, which have similar rates (medians of 105 per 1,000). The Southern region has the lowest level of IMR (a median of 46 per 1,000). The Western region has the highest variability between countries in infant and under-five mortality, and the Southern region has the lowest.

Trends in U5MR

Figure 3.3 presents levels of U5MR at time points separated by five years, from 1960 to 2000. For Sub-Saharan Africa as a whole, U5MR declined from 1960 to 2000. However, most of the decline took place between 1965 and 1990, during which period the median U5MR dropped from 232 to 165 per 1,000. Since 1990 the downward trend has stalled. This overall trend also characterizes each region, although at different levels and speeds. The countries of the Western region had the highest U5MR in 1960, with a median value of about 291 per 1,000 live births. This level fell below 183 per 1,000 by 1990. The Middle region had a median rate of 268 per 1,000 in 1960 and experienced a decline to 164 per 1,000 in 1990. The median in the Eastern region oscillated around 200 per 1,000 prior to 1975 before declining to 170 per 1,000 in 1990. The Southern region had the lowest median U5MR in 1960 (about 200 per 1,000) and experienced the sharpest decline, to about 70 per 1,000 by 1990. The Western and Southern regions thus experienced the fastest declines from 1960 to 1990, with the countries of the Middle and Eastern regions showing the slowest improvement. Declines appear to have stalled in all regions in the 1990s.

Figure 3.4 summarizes the annual rates of change in U5MR over five-year periods. For Sub-Saharan Africa as a whole, rates of decline averaged about 1 percent in the 1960s, increasing to close to 2 percent between 1970 and 1985, dropping back to about 1 percent between 1985 and 1990, and averaging less than 1 percent during the 1990s. These rates of decline are much below the average annual

Figure 3.3 Trends in Under-Five Mortality, by Five-Year Period and Region, 1960–2000 *(per 1,000 births)*

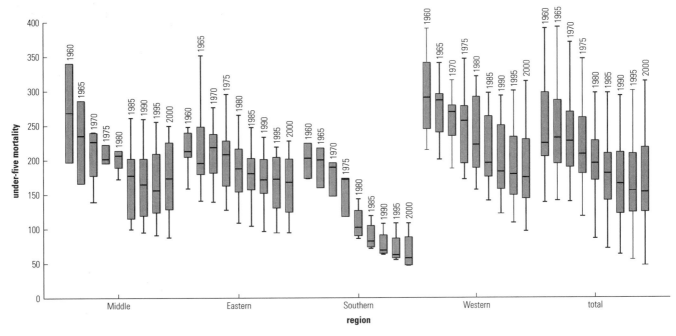

Source: Table 3B.1.

Note: See endnote 2 for a description of a box plot.

Figure 3.4 Annual Rate of Change in Under-Five Mortality, by Five-Year Period, 1965–2000

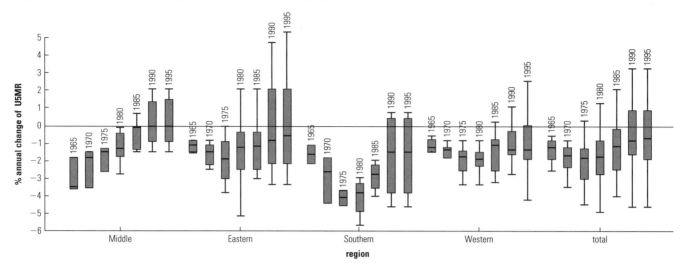

Source: Table 3B.1.
Note: See endnote 2 for a description of a box plot.

decline of 4.3 percent required between 1990 and 2015 to reach MDG targets. Indeed, between 1960 and 2000, the median rate of decline in U5MR approached the required rate of decline in only one region (Southern) for only one five-year period. Also, these rates of decline average only about half those of the developing world as a whole. The relatively poor performance of Sub-Saharan Africa in the 1990s is underlined by the observation that a large number of countries, especially in the Middle, Eastern, and Southern regions, have a positive rate of change in the 1990s, indicating increasing U5MRs. In the Middle Africa region, the estimates indicate increases in U5MR for Cameroon and Chad and a stall in the Democratic Republic of Congo (see the country-specific estimates in table 3B.1). In the Eastern Africa region, the rise or stall is observed in Burundi, Kenya, Rwanda, Zambia, and Zimbabwe. In the Southern region, Botswana and Swaziland are adversely affected, whereas in the Western region, Burkina Faso, Côte d'Ivoire, Mauritania, and Sierra Leone show increases. All these countries have one or more things in common: they are seriously affected by the human immunodeficiency virus and acquired immune deficiency syndrome (HIV/AIDS) epidemic or have suffered an economic crisis or political instability that created a civil war. It is likely that these factors have played a major role in the poor health performance observed in these countries and in Sub-Saharan Africa as a whole.

Age Patterns of Under-Five Mortality

Birth histories, such as those collected by the DHSs, provide information not only about childhood mortality levels

but also about the age pattern of that mortality. The birth history data can be used to calculate the probability of dying in the first year of life (the IMR) and the probability of dying between exact ages one and five (the child mortality rate, or CHMR). Long data series for the developed world indicate that as under-five mortality declines, CHMR tends to decline faster than IMR, leading to an increased concentration of mortality risk in the first year of life (Hill 1991). The historical experience of the developed world also shows substantial variation in the relationship between IMR and CHMR between populations (Coale and Demeny 1983).

Figure 3.5 plots recorded CHMR against recorded IMR for each DHS survey included in this analysis for three

Figure 3.5 Relationships between CHMR and IMR, by Country *(per 1,000 live births)*

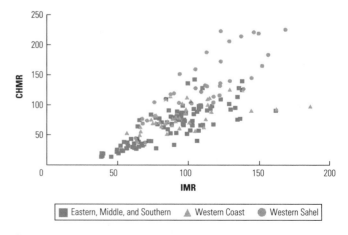

Source: Updated version of database compiled by Hill and colleagues (1999).

five-year periods prior to the survey, that is, for periods 0 to 4, 5 to 9, and 10 to 14 years before data collection. Inspection of an early version of this figure using different symbols for observations from countries for five different regions of Sub-Saharan Africa (Eastern, Southern, Middle, Western Coast, and the western Sahel, using UN definitions of regions except for the additional breakdown of Western Africa into coastal and Sahelian countries) suggested no clear differences of pattern for the countries of Eastern, Southern, and Middle Africa, but possibly different patterns for the Western Coast and the western Sahel. Different symbols are therefore used to identify points in figure 3.5 for the Western Coast, the western Sahel, and the other areas. Although there is a considerable amount of scatter, countries of the western Sahel appear in general to have higher CHMR relative to IMR than other countries, but the differences appear to decline as IMR drops. Western Coast countries appear to have broadly similar patterns to the countries of the Eastern, Middle, and Southern regions at lower levels of IMR, but lower CHMR at higher levels of IMR.

To explore differences in age patterns more fully, the natural log of CHMR was regressed on the IMR for each of three groups of countries: Eastern, Middle, and Southern as one group, Western Coast as another, and western Sahel as the third. Predicted values of CHMR for each group for given values of IMR were obtained.[3] Figure 3.6 shows the summarized age patterns of under-five mortality for the three groups.

As can be seen, the broad pattern of the relationship between CHMR and IMR is similar for populations of Eastern, Middle, and Southern Africa on the one hand and the populations of Sahelian West Africa on the other, except that for a given level of IMR the CHMR in the former group of countries is about 30 per 1,000 lower than in the latter group. The Western Coast, however, appears to have a very different pattern, with lower CHMR at higher levels of IMR and higher CHMR at lower levels of IMR than the other areas.

A final model was estimated relating the log of CHMR to IMR using dummy variables to identify populations of coastal Western Africa and of the western Sahel, plus a dummy variable to identify estimates with a reference period of 1990 or earlier and a dummy variable to identify estimates for the period 0 to 4 years before a survey (as opposed to 5 to 9 or 10 to 14 years before a survey). The fitted model is as follows:

$$\ln(\text{CHMR}) = 2.66 + 0.0147(\text{IMR}) + 0.2252(\text{West Coast})$$
$$+ 0.3880(\text{Sahel}) + 0.1250(1990 \text{ or earlier})$$
$$+ 0.1167(0\text{--}4 \text{ years before survey}) \qquad (3.4)$$

As expected from the previous analysis, the Western Coast and western Sahel dummy variables are positive and highly significant. The dummy variables for estimates with a reference date of 1990 or earlier and for the period 0 to 4 years before the survey are also both positive and significant, although only at a 5 percent level. That the reference date variable is positive implies that, controlling for region and level of IMR, mortality risks between ages one and five fell faster in Sub-Saharan Africa in the 1990s than previously, perhaps because of successful measles vaccination programs. It is puzzling that the coefficient for the dummy variable identifying estimates for the five years immediately before the survey is positive. Two errors thought to affect birth histories are a tendency to round age at death up from under one year to "one year," thus tending to inflate CHMR at the expense of IMR, and a tendency to differentially omit deaths of very young children, thus tending to reduce IMR but without any effect on CHMR. Our prior expectation was that both these errors would be more prevalent the further before the survey of the event being reported, thus tending to increase CHMR relative to IMR for time periods 5 to 9 or 10 to 14 years before the survey more than in the time period 0 to 4 years before the survey. The data suggest the opposite, but we have no ready explanation for why that might be so.

Figure 3.6 Estimated Relationships between CHMR and IMR, by Region
(per 1,000 live births)

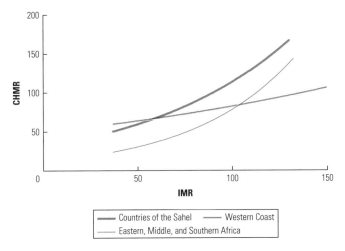

Source: Updated version of database compiled by Hill and colleagues (1999).

DISCUSSION

Improvements in data sources relevant to the measurement of infant and child mortality in Sub-Saharan Africa have made it possible to use a standard methodology to estimate levels and trends in U5MR for most countries over at least some portion of the last 40 years. This exercise reveals that Sub-Saharan Africa has performed rather poorly in terms of child mortality reduction over the period. The average annual decline in U5MR of less than 2 percent per year is only about half the average for the developing world overall and less than half the rate needed to meet MDGs. The median U5MR for Sub-Saharan Africa in the year 2000 also exceeded the developing world median by a substantial margin. The countries of Sub-Saharan Africa have performed unevenly over the period in reducing infant and child mortality, both by region and by time period. About 1960, countries of Western Africa had high U5MR, on average close to 300 per 1,000 children; countries of Eastern and Southern Africa had somewhat lower risk, on average close to 200 per 1,000; and the countries of Middle Africa had an intermediate risk, on average about 250 per 1,000. Since 1960, the countries of Western and Southern Africa appear to have achieved the most rapid declines in U5MR, and across all regions the period between 1975 and 1985 appears to have seen the fastest improvements. Rates of decline were lower prior to 1975 and have slowed practically to zero since 1990, and a quarter of all countries actually experienced increases.

The populations of Sub-Saharan Africa have experienced changes in many areas other than child survival since 1960. There have been improvements in literacy and formal education, fluctuating but generally rising standards of living, rapid population growth and urbanization, widespread political instability and civil strife, and since the mid-1980s the devastating HIV/AIDS epidemic. Further analysis is required to understand better how all these other changes have affected child mortality, why Sub-Saharan Africa has performed worse than other developing regions in reducing infant and child mortality, why the period 1975 to 1985 was the period of most rapid improvement, and why the U5MR decline has stalled since 1990. The period of most rapid improvement, between 1975 and 1985, occurred in a period during which a number of low-cost interventions (oral rehydration therapy, vaccines) were developed and distributed widely with the support of international agencies and aid programs. The poor performance in the 1990s has coincided with rapid expansion of the HIV epidemic, which has almost certainly been a factor in the child mortality increases, along with a "loss of focus" (Jones et al. 2003) on the part of international agencies.

A handful of inexpensive interventions of demonstrated effectiveness could have, with universal coverage, prevented well over half the 4.4 million deaths of children under age five estimated to have occurred in Sub-Saharan Africa in 2000 (Jones et al. 2003). Efforts to reduce the U5MR through the widespread use of these inexpensive interventions may have been responsible for the rapid declines seen between 1975 and 1985 in Sub-Saharan Africa and the developing world more broadly. Renewed emphasis on these same interventions, with a small number of recent additions, such as micronutrient supplementation, can still have a major impact today.

APPENDIX 3A: METHODOLOGY AND DETAIL RESULTS

There are many ways in which a set of estimates can be obtained from a series of observations and in which extrapolations forward or backward to any desired time point can be made. The simplest procedure is hand smoothing: drawing a freehand curve through a set of observations and extending its general trend onward to some specified time point for which an estimate or projection is required. Such a procedure is unlikely to be objective—different analysts would almost inevitably draw different lines, particularly for extrapolations beyond the earliest or latest observations. An alternative would be to use hand smoothing for the period covered by observations and then apply a model to extrapolate; this is essentially what was done in both the United Nations (1988, 1992) reports on under-five mortality in the developing world. With this method, the hand smoothing is still subjective, and it is hard to specify the extrapolation model satisfactorily.

Regression analysis offers a set of possible approaches: robust regression, locally weighted least squares, weighted least squares, or ordinary least squares. Such regression techniques offer a greater degree of objectivity than hand smoothing but still require the choice of model specification. Each approach has advantages and disadvantages. Ordinary least squares makes few assumptions about the nature of errors, but the results are heavily influenced by outliers. Robust regression essentially underweights outlying observations that have an inordinate influence on the fitted line, but no prior information about the likely accuracy of particular types of observation is used. Locally weighted least squares fits a nonparametric trend to a set of observations, but provides no basis for extrapolation. Weighted least squares requires the use of predetermined weights, introducing a subjective element into the analysis but at the same time allowing the incorporation of prior knowledge about the likely accuracy of different methods of measurement.

Weighted Least Squares with Linear Splines

The approach adopted here is that used by Hill and colleagues (1999). A regression line is fitted to the relationship between IMRs or U5MRs and their reference dates using weighted least squares. The basic model assumes that the *rate* at which infant or under-five mortality changes is linear in time, that is, that mortality risk changes at a constant annual percentage rate over some defined time period. The dependent variable is the logarithm of either the IMR or the U5MR. The independent variables used are date variables. The simplest model relates the logarithm of each estimate of the risk of dying to the date of the estimates; this model implies a constant rate of change in mortality over the entire period studied. Figure 3A.1a shows a hypothetical example of such a simple model for under-five mortality. More complex models can allow the rate of change of mortality to vary over the period; figure 3A.1b is an example of where the relationship between the U5MR and time is allowed to change two times, reflecting two "knot" points (defined every time a sum of weights reaches five, as explained below). Clear changes in trend are indicated in this instance.

Linear Splines and "Knots"

The model used in this chapter allows the rate of change of infant or under-five mortality to vary according to the number of independent observations available. At the country level, U5MR is modeled using linear splines, whereby the rate of change in U5MR over time is assumed to be constant for some period, but then is allowed to change at some time point or "knot." This model, shown as equation 3A.1, relates the log of U5MR (by using logs the rate of change is held constant) to a date variable and additional variables measuring time since a series of knot dates. The number and location of these knot dates are determined by the number and location in time of observations available for a particular country. Knots are defined working backward in time from the most recent observation. Observations of particular

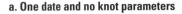

Figure 3A.1 Fitted Trends Using Different Numbers of Knot Parameters
(per 1,000 births)

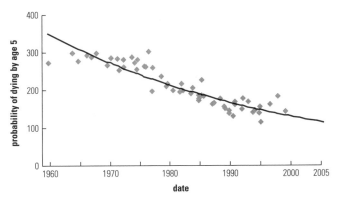

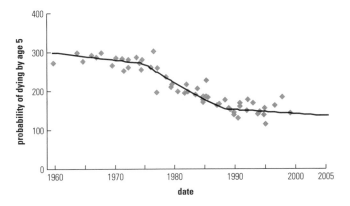

Source: Illustrative country data.

types (for example, an observation derived from a full birth history for the period zero to four years before the survey) are assigned weights reflecting a priori judgments of their likely validity. The weights for successive observations are summed, and a knot is defined every time the sum of weights reaches a multiple of five. This definition of a knot is based on the idea that five years of vital registration, or one set of indirect or direct estimates such as one DHS, are sufficient to define one trend or slope. The weights assigned to five years of vital registration, or to one set of direct or indirect estimates, sum to five. Thus, the process of allowing a knot to be defined when weights sum to five means, in effect, that each DHS, WFS, or other such survey, and each five-year period of vital registration defines a particular slope.

The only exception to this procedure is for the last knot defined (the earliest knot in time). For this last knot, the remaining weights must sum to at least five to ensure that the first date variable is based on observations whose weights sum to at least five. The more acceptable observations there are for a particular country, the more knots there will be and the more flexible the trend in infant or under-five mortality over time will be.

The underlying model used is

$$\ln(_nq_0)_i = b_0 + b_1(date)_i + b_2(postk1)_i + b_3(postk2)_i \\ + b_4(postk3)_i + \cdots + e_i \qquad (3A.1)$$

The variable *date* is simply the calendar year; *postk*1 is *date* minus the date of the earliest defined knot if positive, or zero otherwise, and picks up any change in trend after the first knot (recall that the knots are defined from the present backward into the past, but the earliest knot is defined to ensure at least five observations between it and the start of the series); *postk*2 is *date* minus the date of the second defined knot if positive, or zero otherwise, and picks up any change in trend after the second knot; and so on. Thus, the number of slope-changing time variables varies with the number and weight of the observations over time. The coefficients on *postk*1, *postk*2, and so on, can be interpreted as changes in the rate of change of infant or under-five mortality with time in that particular period. Thus, the rate of change in period 1 is b_1; in period 2, $(b_1 + b_2)$; in period 3, $(b_1 + b_2 + b_3)$; and so on. Referring back to figure 3.1, only a single date variable with no slope-changing variables would be used to fit a trend in U5MR for the Republic of Congo, since the data weights only sum to five. For Kenya, the date variable and seven slope-changing variables would be used, since the data weights sum to 42.5 (figure 3.1b).

It should be noted that the error term e_i is assumed to be normally distributed around the logarithm of the mortality indicator. As a result, estimates of mortality obtained by exponentiating an estimated value of the logarithm of the mortality indicator will be biased upward by an amount that will depend on the goodness of fit of the model. This is a relatively benign bias in the sense that the infant or under-five mortality estimates obtained will tend to be on the high side, and the poorer the fit of the model the more on the high side the estimates will be.

Weights

Weighted least squares regression is used to fit equation 3A.1 to each country's data. Weighted least squares is used because a substantial body of evidence suggests different validity weights for different types of observations. For example, it is generally thought that the quality of retrospectively reported information deteriorates with the length of time elapsed since the events (Som 1973).

Each estimate from vital registration or a prospective survey is given a "standard" validity weight of 1.0. For vital registration, the weight is justified by the typically large number of events involved and by the lack of any substantial lag between event and report; for prospective surveys, the weight is justified by the lack of lag and by the accuracy enforced by the data collection methodology. Estimates derived from birth histories are assigned standard weights that vary with the length of time before the survey to which the estimate refers, on the grounds that recent information is more likely to be more accurate than information for periods further in the past. Specifically, estimates for the 5 years before the survey are given a weight of 2.0; for periods 5 to 9 years before the survey, 1.8; and for periods 10 to 14 years before the survey, 1.2.

Weights for indirect estimates based on the proportions dead of children ever born vary by the age group of the mother; estimates based on reports of young women are given low weight—zero for women age 15 to 19 and 0.2 for women age 20 to 24—because of the well-known selection problems that affect such estimates (early childbearing is often highest among the poor, who also suffer the highest U5MRs). Estimates based on reports of women in the age groups 25 to 29, 30 to 34, and 35 to 39 are given the highest weights, 1.2 each. Then, as age increases the weights decline slowly, on the grounds that information about events longer ago is more prone to error, such that estimates for the age group 40 to 44 get a weight of 0.8, and those for the age group 45 to 49 get a weight of 0.4.

Note that it is these weights that are summed to determine the location of knots described earlier. The under-five mortality estimates from a particular survey collecting birth histories have a combined weight of five, as do the estimates from a particular survey providing indirect measures. In cases in which a particular survey contributes two types of estimates (for example, a DHS survey that provides both direct estimates from the birth history and indirect estimates from children ever born and children surviving), the two sets of weights are reduced to half their standard level, so that the data source is not overly weighted. The observation-specific weights described earlier are essentially based on the authors' judgment and experience. However, robust regression techniques can be used to estimate robust weights for particular types of observations; these estimated robust weights can then be compared with the observation-specific weights.[4]

Applying the Methodology

The intention of the methodology is to provide a transparent and largely objective way of fitting a smoothed trend to a set of observations and of extrapolating the trend to cover the period from 1960 to the present. However, subjective judgments are involved at every step.

In step 1 of the smoothing and extrapolation process, the regression model in equation 3A.1 is fitted to observations of U5MR using appropriate date variables and standard validity weights as defined above. Results from step 1 depend on the standard validity weights applied to different types of data. The standard validity weights are objective in the sense that they are invariant across data sets or across countries, but they are subjective in the sense that different analysts would choose different values.

In step 2, results from step 1 are critically examined and data sets that are clearly aberrant are identified, such as indirect estimates that are clearly inconsistent with the majority of other sources. The weights for the entire aberrant data set are reduced by a constant factor that is generally zero (giving no weight to estimates from that data set). Step 1 is then repeated using these revised weights.

This second step involves subjective choices as well. Most important is the decision as to whether to underweight entire data sets and, if so, by how much. The decision to underweight some data sets relative to others can have a large effect on the sequence of under-five mortality estimates

obtained. In the process followed in this chapter, this decision is made on the basis of graphical inspection. If the estimates from one source are clearly higher or lower than the bulk of available estimates or if their time trend is clearly different, a constant factor of zero (giving zero weight to the entire data set) might be used. If the estimates fluctuate a lot or display some other undesirable characteristic a constant factor between zero and one might be used, thus reducing the standard weight for the entire data set. It is this decision that is most likely to introduce substantial differences in results between analysts. In the analysis reported here, it is assumed that errors are more likely to result in underestimates of under-five mortality than in overestimates. Thus, when two data sets indicate very different levels, other things being equal, the set indicating higher mortality is assumed more likely to be right.

APPENDIX 3B: ESTIMATES OF U5MRs AND IMRs AND DATA SOURCES

Tables 3B.1 and 3B.2 present the estimates of U5MRs and IMRs, respectively. Countries are categorized into four groups depending on the number of surveys available and the consistency of the under-five mortality estimates obtained from those surveys. Data sources for each country are given in table 3B.3. Figure 3B.1 shows an example of a country in each category.

Table 3B.1 Estimates of Under-Five Mortality, by Country and Year
(per 1,000 births)

Region and country	No. of censuses and surveys	Category	Under-five mortality rate								
			1960	1965	1970	1975	1980	1985	1990	1995	2000
Middle											
Angola	2	C	—	—	—	—	262	261	260	255	249
Cameroon	3	C	258	235	214	196	172	150	141	156	173
Central African Republic	3	C	340	286	240	202	189	177	164	152	141
Chad	3	C	—	—	—	233	214	196	195	209	226
Congo, Democratic Republic of	1	C	276	257	239	222	207	202	202	202	202
Congo, Republic of	2	C	197	166	139	—	—	—	—	—	—
Gabon	1	C	—	—	—	—	104	99	95	91	87
São Tomé and Principe	1	D	—	—	—	—	112	115	120	124	128
Eastern											
Burundi	5	A	248	237	227	214	190	186	183	192	201
Comoros	2	D	—	—	—	174	154	136	121	107	94
Eritrea	1	C					206	177	152	131	112
Ethiopia	4	B	259	248	238	228	218	209	201	193	185
Kenya	9	A	204	179	158	139	115	104	97	114	134
Madagascar	3	C	138	141	149	159	170	181	174	147	125
Malawi	7	A	361	351	330	296	265	247	233	210	189
Mozambique	3	D	309	292	276	261	247	233	221	208	197
Rwanda	5	A	206	190	209	226	216	188	168	192	220
Somalia	1	C	—	—	—	—	195	203	211	219	227
Tanzania	7	B	240	228	218	203	175	157	157	151	142
Uganda	5	A	223	194	187	186	185	180	160	153	150
Zambia	5	A	213	195	181	162	150	166	184	204	227
Zimbabwe	8	D	158	149	139	127	109	84	74	94	123
Southern											
Botswana	6	B	173	159	147	118	95	71	63	65	68
Lesotho	4	B	203	200	190	173	158	144	131	120	109
Namibia	3	C	244	200	164	134	110	90	74	59	47
South Africa	1	C	—	—	—	—	86	74	64	55	48
Swaziland	4	A	224	217	196	172	143	119	108	108	108
Western											
Benin	3	C	298	274	252	232	214	199	184	170	156
Burkina Faso	4	A	315	296	278	261	242	223	211	223	236
Côte d'Ivoire	5	A	349	286	235	192	172	156	158	179	203
Gambia, The	4	A	367	340	315	269	227	192	164	143	125
Ghana	5	B	214	201	188	171	157	141	122	109	97
Guinea	2	C	—	—	—	335	297	263	232	188	153
Guinea-Bissau	1	D	—	—	—	—	286	267	250	233	218
Liberia	4	B	284	276	269	252	235	219	204	191	178
Mali	4	A	518	451	392	341	297	265	252	240	229
Mauritania	3	D	223	213	205	196	188	181	182	187	193
Niger	3	D	—	—	—	287	291	296	293	273	249
Nigeria	3	D	279	255	234	214	196	179	165	153	143
Senegal	5	A	297	288	279	265	216	175	150	148	148
Sierra Leone	4	A	390	393	370	346	321	297	286	300	314
Togo	3	C	267	240	215	194	175	158	152	148	143

Source: Authors' calculations.

Notes: — = no observed data available for that year or for years around it. The "Category" column indicates a subjective judgment of the quality of the estimates available for a given country. The categories are as follows: A = four or more surveys with broadly consistent results; B = four or more surveys with broadly inconsistent results; C = three or fewer surveys with broadly consistent results; D = three or fewer surveys with broadly inconsistent results.

Table 3B.2 Estimates of Infant Mortality, by Country and Year
(per 1,000 births)

Region and country	Infant mortality rate								
	1960	1965	1970	1975	1980	1985	1990	1995	2000
Middle									
Angola	—	—	—	—	156	155	154	152	150
Cameroon	153	139	127	117	104	93	88	96	105
Central African Republic	194	166	145	127	121	115	109	103	98
Chad	—	—	—	138	127	117	117	124	133
Congo, Democratic Republic of	162	153	145	137	130	128	128	127	127
Congo, Republic of	133	114	97	—	—	—	—	—	—
Gabon	—	—	—	—	75	72	69	67	64
São Tomé and Principe	—	—	—	—	80	82	85	87	90
Eastern									
Burundi	147	140	134	127	114	112	110	115	120
Comoros	—	—	—	118	106	95	85	77	69
Eritrea					138	120	105	92	80
Ethiopia	173	166	159	152	146	140	135	130	126
Kenya	122	108	97	87	73	67	63	72	83
Madagascar	86	87	92	97	103	109	105	91	78
Malawi	205	200	189	171	157	149	142	131	121
Mozambique	178	169	162	155	149	142	136	131	125
Rwanda	122	114	124	134	128	113	102	115	130
Somalia	—	—	—	—	117	121	125	130	135
Tanzania	142	135	129	121	106	96	96	93	88
Uganda	132	116	112	112	111	109	98	94	92
Zambia	126	117	109	99	92	101	111	121	134
Zimbabwe	97	92	86	80	70	56	50	61	78
Southern									
Botswana	118	110	102	84	69	54	48	50	52
Lesotho	136	135	128	118	109	100	92	85	78
Namibia	147	126	109	94	82	70	59	49	40
South Africa	—	—	—	—	63	56	49	43	38
Swaziland	150	145	132	117	100	84	77	77	77
Western									
Benin	177	162	149	138	127	118	111	103	96
Burkina Faso	181	171	163	155	146	137	132	137	143
Côte d'Ivoire	236	192	157	130	118	107	109	122	136
Gambia, The	208	194	181	159	139	123	109	99	90
Ghana	127	119	113	104	96	87	77	69	63
Guinea	—	—	—	191	172	156	142	121	104
Guinea-Bissau	—	—	—	—	191	179	167	156	146
Liberia	190	185	180	168	157	147	137	129	121
Mali	293	254	222	194	172	157	151	146	140
Mauritania	149	143	137	132	127	123	123	127	130
Niger	—	—	—	170	173	176	174	162	147
Nigeria	166	151	138	127	117	108	100	94	88
Senegal	172	167	163	157	134	114	102	101	101
Sierra Leone	220	222	210	197	184	172	167	173	180
Togo	158	142	128	116	106	97	94	91	89

Source: Authors' calculations.

Notes: — = no observed data available for that year or for years around it.

Table 3B.3 Countries and Data Sources

Region and country	Data sources
Middle	
Angola	MICS, 2000
Cameroon	WFS, 1978; DHS, 1991, 1998
Central African Republic	Census, 1975, 1988; DHS, 1995
Chad	Census, 1993; DHS, 1997; MICS, 2000
Congo, Democratic Republic of	Census, 1984; MICS, 1996
Congo, Republic of	Census, 1974
Gabon	DHS, 2001
São Tomé and Principe	MICS, 2000
Eastern	
Burundi	DS, 1970; PCS, 1979; DHS, 1987; Census, 1990; MICS, 2000
Comoros	DHS, 1996; MICS, 2000
Eritrea	DHS, 1995
Ethiopia	DS, 1981; Census, 1984; FFS, 1990; DHS, 2000
Kenya	Census, 1960; DS, 1977; WFS, 1977; Census, 1979; DS, 1983, 1988, 1993; Census,1989; DHS, 1998
Madagascar	Vital Reg., 1960–61, 1963–72; DS, 1966; DHS, 1992, 1997
Malawi	PCS, 1970; Census, 1977; MDS, 1982; FFS, 1984; Census, 1987; DHS, 2000, 1992
Mozambique	Census, 1970, 1980; DHS, 1997
Rwanda	DS, 1970, 1978; NFS, 1983; DHS, 1992, 2000
Somalia	MICS, 2000
Tanzania	Census, 1967; DS, 1973; Census, 1978, 1988; DHS, 1991, 1994, 1996, 1999
Uganda	Census, 1969; DHS, 1988; IHS, 1992; DHS, 1995, 2000
Zambia	Census, 1969; SCP, 1974; Census, 1980; DHS, 1992, 1996
Zimbabwe	Census, 1969, 1982; RHS, 1984; ICD, 1987; DHS, 1988; Census, 1992; DHS, 1994, 1999
Southern	
Botswana	Vital Reg., 1982–87; Census, 1971, 1981; DHS, 1984, 1988; Census, 1991; MICS, 2000
Lesotho	CES, 1968; DS, 1971; Census, 1976; WFS, 1977
Namibia	DHS, 1992, 2000
South Africa	DHS, 1998
Swaziland	Census, 1966, 1976, 1986; MICS, 2000
Western	
Benin	WFS, 1982; DHS, 1996, 2001
Burkina Faso	PES, 1976; Census, 1985; DHS, 1992, 1999
Côte d'Ivoire	MRS, 1978; WFS, 1980; DHS, 1994, 1998
Gambia, The	Census, 1973, 1983, 1993; MICS, 2000
Ghana	Census, 1971; FS, 1979; DHS, 1988, 1993, 1998
Guinea	DHS, 1992, 1999
Guinea-Bissau	MICS, 2000
Liberia	PGS, 1969, 1970; Census, 1974; DHS, 1986
Mali	Census, 1976; DHS, 1987, 1995, 2001
Mauritania	WFS, 1981; MICS, 1996; DHS, 2000
Niger	DHS, 1992, 1998; MICS, 2000
Nigeria	WFS, 1981; DHS, 1990, 1999
Senegal	WFS, 1978; DHS, 1986, 1992, 1997, 1999
Sierra Leone	Pilot Census, 1973; Census, 1974, 1985; MICS, 2000
Togo	DS, 1971; DHS, 1988, 1998

Source: Authors' compilation.

Note: CES = Consumption and Expenditure Survey; DS = Demographic Survey; FS = Fertility Survey; FFS = Family Formation Survey; ICD = Inter-Censal Demographic Survey; IHS = Integrated Household Survey; MRS = Multiple Round Survey; NFS = National Fertility Survey; PCS = Population Change Survey; PES = Population Enumeration Survey; PGS = Population Growth Survey; RHS = Retrospective Health Survey; SCP = Sample Census of Population; Vital Reg. = vital registration.

Figure 3B.1 Examples of "Quality" Categories for Selected Countries
(per 1,000 births)

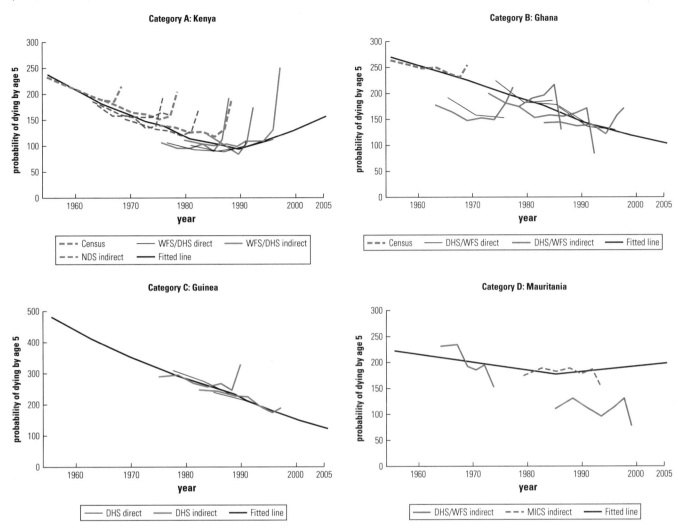

Source: Updated version of database compiled by Hill and colleagues (1999).

NOTES

1. Theoretically, in a population with perfect registration of vital events and no migration, the mortality of children after infancy could also be measured purely from civil registration data. However, in practice, registration is not perfect, and migration is not negligible, so mortality in childhood is calculated from deaths from civil registration data and from exposure to risk according to a census or population estimate.

2. A box plot summarizes the distribution of a variable. The box is a rectangle, the top and bottom of which mark the 75th and 25th percentiles, respectively, with the median observation (in this case, the median country) as a cross-bar within the box. The "whiskers" for each box are the lines protruding above and below, and indicate the range of the data above and below the upper and lower quartiles.

3. The robust regression coefficients for the regions were as follows (all coefficients were significant at the 0.001 level or better). Eastern, Middle, and Southern Africa: $\ln(CHMR) = 2.50 + 0.0179(IMR)$; coastal West Africa: $\ln(CHMR) = 3.90 + 0.0049(IMR)$; West Sahelian Africa: $\ln(CHMR) = 3.46 + 0.0122(IMR)$.

4. See Hill et al. (1999) for an example of use of robust regression to estimate the weights.

REFERENCES

Brass, W. 1964. "Uses of Census or Survey Data for the Estimation of Vital Rates." E/CN.14/CAS.4/V57. Paper presented at the African Seminar on Vital Statistics, Addis Ababa, December 14–19.

Coale, A. J., and P. Demeny. 1983. *Regional Model Life Tables and Stable Populations.* 2nd ed. New York: Academic Press.

Hill, K. 1991. "Approaches in the Measurement of Childhood Mortality: A Comparative Review." *Population Index* 57 (3).

———. 1995. "Age Patterns of Under-Five Mortality in the Developing World." *Population Bulletin of the United Nations* 39.

Hill, K., R. Pande, M. Mahy, and G. Jones. 1999. *Trends in Child Mortality in the Developing World: 1960–1996.* New York: UNICEF.

Hill, K., and A. Yazbeck. 1994. *Trends in Under-Five Mortality, 1960–90: Estimates for 84 Developing Countries.* Washington, DC: World Bank.

Jones, G., R. Steketee, R. Black, Z. Bhutta, S. Morris, and the Bellagio Child Survival Study Group. 2003. "How Many Child Deaths Can We Prevent This Year?" *Lancet* 362: 65–71.

Som, R. K. 1973. *Recall Lapse in Demographic Surveys.* Bombay: Asia Publishing House.

Somoza, J. L. 1980. *Illustrative Analysis: Infant and Child Mortality in Colombia.* World Fertility Survey Scientific Reports 10. London: World Fertility Survey.

Sullivan, J. M. 1972. "Models for the Estimation of the Probability of Dying between Birth and Exact Ages of Early Childhood." *Population Studies* 26 (1): 79–97.

Trussell, T. J. 1975. "A Re-estimation of the Multiplying Factors for the Brass Technique for Determining Childhood Survivorship Rates." *Population Studies* 29 (1): 97–108.

United Nations. 1983. *Manual X: Indirect Techniques for Demographic Estimation.* Population Studies 81. New York: United Nations.

———. 1988. *Mortality of Children under Age 5. World Estimates and Projections, 1950–2025.* Population Studies, No. 105. Department of International Economic and Social Affairs. New York: United Nations.

———. 1992. *Under-Five Mortality since the 1960s: A Database for Developing Countries.* New York: United Nations.

Chapter 4

Levels and Trends of Adult Mortality

Debbie Bradshaw and Ian M. Timaeus

Adult mortality remains a neglected public health issue in Sub-Saharan Africa. A lack of empirical data about the levels of mortality experienced by adults in this region has fueled this neglect, combined with the focus on maternal and child health, which has the highest incidence of disease and subsequent mortality. This picture is changing. The high mortality of adults in the African region is now being recognized more widely, and a response has begun to emerge, particularly with regard to the impact of the AIDS epidemic and high mortality due to malaria.

The Global Burden of Disease studies of 1990 and 2000 estimate that Sub-Saharan Africa has the highest burden of disease in the world (Murray and Lopez 1996; WHO 2000). These and related studies have revealed high levels of adult mortality resulting from the multiple burdens of disease experienced by the populations in the region (Murray, Yang, and Qiao 1992). The studies show that fast-growing epidemics of human immunodeficiency virus and acquired immune deficiency syndrome (HIV/AIDS) and certain noncommunicable diseases coexist with the conditions related to underdevelopment, such as malaria, malnutrition, and tuberculosis. In addition, they highlight the increasing road traffic injury burden and the less predictable toll of mortality due to war and violence.

Health sector reforms have swept the continent during the last 20 years and given primary health care priority in attempts to provide accessible health care to rural communities and contain costs. However, the strategies of primary health care have focused largely on maternal and child health and the provision of acute care. These strategies have yet to overcome the challenges posed by the health needs of adults, such as the management of chronic conditions and, more recently, the provision of treatment for AIDS. The imperative of these challenges has been obscured by the lack of good data on the levels of adult mortality and its trends and causes. Although childhood and maternal mortality once faced the same problem, survey-based techniques, including indirect methods of estimation and the widespread collection of birth histories, have improved the situation in this regard.

SOURCES OF DATA

Vital registration systems are the ideal source of data with which to monitor mortality levels and trends. However, the statistics systems of most Sub-Saharan Africa countries continue to be underdeveloped; few countries are able to provide adequate vital statistics. In 2001 the World Health Organization (WHO) contacted all member states in Sub-Saharan Africa to try to obtain death statistics for a global assessment of the burden of disease (Kowal, Rao, and Mathers 2003). Just 9 out of 46 member states provided such data. Furthermore, coverage of registration was less than 60 percent in most of these 9 countries, with only Mauritius and the Seychelles providing vital registration data that were more than 90 percent complete. These two island states make up a tiny fraction of the population of Sub-Saharan Africa. Adequate vital statistics are far more widespread in other regions, particularly Europe and the Americas, and 60 percent of the countries for which the WHO could not obtain registration data are in Sub-Saharan Africa. Data series of any time length are particularly rare. Due to a lack of appropriate direct data, the Adult Mortality in Developing Countries project, which studied trends in adult mortality in 27 developing countries (Hill 2003), included only 2 countries from mainland Sub-Saharan Africa (Benin and Zimbabwe). Among the mainland countries, South Africa is an exemplary country because of the government's determined efforts in the last decade to improve its statistics. The lack of reliable mortality data had been dubbed the "black hole of vital statistics" (Botha and Bradshaw 1985), but national efforts during the 1990s resulted in over 90 percent of the adult deaths being registered (Dorrington et al. 2001). Yet, even in South Africa, the production of timely cause-of-death statistics remains a challenge.

The pervasive lack of vital registration data makes it necessary to derive estimates of mortality using indirect demographic techniques based on survey and census data. The most readily accessible data that can be used to estimate adult mortality come from the Demographic and Health Surveys (DHS). At least one such survey has been conducted in most African countries, and many of the African surveys include sibling histories that were developed to obtain estimates of maternal mortality (Rutenberg and Sullivan 1991). Unfortunately, almost all DHS samples are too small to enable the study of age-specific mortality in adulthood or mortality trends in any detail. Moreover, concerns exist about both the reliability and validity of reports on the survival of respondents' siblings. Although Bicego (1997) found good correspondence with other data, Stanton, Abderrahim,

and Hill (1997) suggest that sibling survival may progressively underestimate adult mortality as the time since the event lengthens. These authors conclude that sibling histories can at best provide an estimate of adult mortality in the few years before the data were collected. Comparison of successive sets of sibling history data in the three African countries that have collected them in two DHS surveys also supports this conclusion (Timaeus and Jasseh 2004). Apart from the DHS surveys, several other international programs of surveys have been conducted in Sub-Saharan Africa during the past decade. However, although the Multiple Indicator Cluster Surveys (MICS) conducted by UNICEF are an important source of child mortality estimates, they have not included questions on adult mortality. Moreover, data from the World Health Survey have yet to become available.

Data on adult mortality can be collected in national censuses either by including questions about recent deaths in households or by asking about the survival of the parents of household members. Only some African countries have a tradition of asking one or both sets of questions in their censuses, and few additional countries responded to the growing concern about adult mortality from AIDS and other causes by adding them to their schedule for the 2000 census. Even fewer countries have yet published these data. Although reporting of recent deaths can often be incomplete and subject to reference period and age reporting errors, a range of methods exists for the evaluation of such information and, in favorable circumstances, the correction of inadequate data (Bennett and Horiuchi 1984; Brass 1975; Hill 1987). Data on the survival of parents can be used to estimate conventional life table indexes by means of the orphanhood method (Brass and Hill 1973; Timaeus 1992). The method can be used to estimate the historical trend in mortality and has been refined in various ways in order to produce more up-to-date estimates (for example, Timaeus 1991). Moreover, adjustments can be made to orphanhood data to correct for the biases introduced by the excess mortality of orphans who have been vertically infected with HIV (Timaeus and Nunn 1997).

Two consecutive censuses can also be used to estimate adult mortality from intercensal cohort survival or age-specific growth (Preston and Bennett 1983). The ratio resulting from matching age groups in the second population to the first population provides a summary measure of adult mortality. This requires that the population be closed to migration and that the census coverage be the same in both censuses. Few, if any, Sub-Saharan Africa countries come close to meeting either of these conditions. Thus, the method has not been used much or with great success.

Demographic surveillance of local populations has been used for many years in a handful of African populations to study mortality and provide a framework for epidemiological research and the trial of health interventions (for example, Pison and Langaney 1985). In response to the spread of HIV in Africa, many more such longitudinal surveillance systems have been established recently in which vital events are monitored at regular intervals (Gregson et al. 1997; Hosegood, Vanneste, and Timaeus 2004; Nunn et al. 1997; Sewankambo et al. 2000; Todd et al. 1997; Tollman et al. 1999; Urassa et al. 2001). Almost all these sites, however, cover only small and select populations. Therefore, they are of little use for the estimation of adult mortality in national populations. The partial exception is the surveillance system organized by the Adult Morbidity and Mortality Project (AMMP) in Tanzania, which covers three districts that include both rural and urban areas, although it is not statistically representative of the population of the country as a whole (Kitange et al. 1996).

Because of the shortage of reliable empirical estimates, *World Population Prospects* (United Nations 2003) uses estimates of child mortality and assumptions about the age pattern of mortality taken from a family of model life tables to determine life expectancy in all of mainland Sub-Saharan Africa. The system of model life tables adopted by the United Nations (UN) Population Division implicitly defines the level of adult mortality. In most of these countries the Population Division simply has assumed that non-AIDS mortality at all ages conforms to a Princeton North model life table. These models are derived from historical data largely on northern Europe (Coale, Demeny, and Vaughan 1983) and are fitted to an estimate of under-five mortality (United Nations 2002). In a few countries, Princeton West models (Coale, Demeny, and Vaughan 1983) or UN Far Eastern models (United Nations 1982) have been used in the same way. Moreover, Sub-Saharan Africa is the only area in which data are completely lacking for a few countries and mortality in them has to be guessed from estimates for neighboring countries. The UN Population Division bases its estimates of AIDS deaths in high-prevalence African countries on those produced by the Joint United Nations Programme on HIV/AIDS (UNAIDS) using epidemiological models fitted to HIV seroprevalence data collected in antenatal clinics (UNAIDS Reference Group 2002). Although these models are based on careful review of the data coming out of a range of research studies, at present no attempt is made by any of the UN agencies to use empirical data on mortality in national populations to estimate AIDS deaths in particular countries.

The WHO reviewed the various estimates and observed substantial variations, depending on the different procedures and judgments made (Lopez et al. 2002). It produced its own set of life table estimates for 191 countries in 2000 based on its own mortality database and a new family of model life tables, which in turn were based on an extension of the Brass logit system (Murray et al. 2003). Although the basis of these life tables was measures of mortality from direct registration wherever possible, the only mainland Sub-Saharan Africa countries for which such data were adopted were Zimbabwe and South Africa and in addition, for Tanzania, where the AMMP surveillance data for part of the country were used.

For the rest of Africa, the WHO, like the UN Population Division, was forced to estimate adult mortality and life expectancy by extrapolation from estimates of child mortality. It did this by modeling the relationship between adult and child mortality in its database of more than 1,800 life tables, using its modified logit life table system. Given the lack of such data, however, this database includes few life tables from Sub-Saharan Africa and few with levels of child mortality as high as those that are typical of the African region. Thus, although the WHO's estimates are based on models developed using contemporary developing country data, there is no guarantee that they will be more accurate for Africa than those made by the UN Population Division using model life tables based on historical data on high-mortality Western populations. Moreover, like the Population Division, the WHO was unable to locate any up-to-date mortality data on some eight African countries. To produce the final life tables, mortality levels were estimated without HIV/AIDS, and then estimates of the additional adult AIDS deaths were added, based on the impact observed in the direct estimates from the demographic surveillance sites in Tanzania and the national vital registration systems of Zimbabwe and South Africa (Salomon and Murray 2001).

MORTALITY LEVELS

Table 4.1 shows estimates of adult mortality based on the WHO life tables for Africa in 2000 (Lopez et al. 2002). The index presented is the probability of dying between exact ages 15 and 60 ($_{45}q_{15}$). It refers to a particular year but can be interpreted as the probability that someone who had survived childhood would die before old age if he or she went through life subject to the age-specific death rates of the year in question. This measure has been adopted by

Table 4.1 Probabilities of Dying between Ages 15 and 60 ($_{45}q_{15}$) in Sub-Saharan Africa

WHO region and country	Male	Female	WHO region and country	Male	Female
Southern Africa			*Western Africa*		
Angola	0.492	0.386	Algeria	0.155	0.119
Botswana	0.703	0.669	Benin	0.384	0.328
Lesotho	0.667	0.630	Burkina Faso	0.559	0.507
Malawi	0.701	0.653	Cape Verde	0.210	0.121
Mozambique	0.674	0.612	Côte d'Ivoire	0.553	0.494
Namibia	0.695	0.661	Gambia, The	0.373	0.320
South Africa	0.567	0.502	Ghana	0.379	0.326
Swaziland	0.627	0.587	Guinea	0.432	0.366
Zambia	0.725	0.687	Guinea-Bissau	0.495	0.427
Zimbabwe	0.650	0.612	Liberia	0.448	0.385
Eastern Africa			Mali	0.518	0.446
Burundi	0.648	0.603	Mauritania	0.357	0.302
Eritrea	0.493	0.441	Niger	0.473	0.408
Ethiopia	0.594	0.535	Nigeria	0.443	0.393
Kenya	0.578	0.529	Senegal	0.355	0.303
Rwanda	0.667	0.599	Sierra Leone	0.587	0.531
Tanzania	0.569	0.520	Togo	0.460	0.406
Uganda	0.617	0.567	*Indian Ocean*		
Central Africa			Comoros	0.381	0.325
Cameroon	0.488	0.559	Madagascar	0.385	0.322
Central African Republic	0.620	0.573	Mauritius	0.228	0.109
Chad	0.449	0.361	Seychelles	0.268	0.122
Congo, Dem. Rep. of	0.571	0.493			
Congo, Rep. of	0.475	0.406			
Equatorial Guinea	0.339	0.280			
Gabon	0.380	0.330			
São Tomé and Principe	0.269	0.226			

Source: Authors' calculations; data from Lopez et al. 2002.

many international agencies, including the WHO, as a good indicator of the overall level of adult mortality. Unlike life expectancy at age 15, it is not influenced by death rates at age 60 and over, which are very difficult to measure in countries with defective vital statistics systems. One limitation of the measure is that it is heavily influenced by death rates in the upper part of the 45-year age range. This reduces its sensitivity to trends in death rates in early adulthood. In addition, without supplementary data or assumptions, neither sibling history data, which refer mainly to young adults, nor orphanhood data, which refer largely to middle-aged parents, can provide robust measures of adult mortality across the whole of this wide age range.

In its estimates of mortality, the WHO found that of the 40 countries with the highest mortality, 37 were from the Sub-Saharan region. The level of adult mortality is highly variable across African countries. Southern and Eastern Africa have particularly high adult mortality, whereas mortality in Western Africa is lower and the Indian Ocean Islands, which accommodate relatively small populations, have the lowest rates. According to these WHO estimates, the probability of surviving from exact age 15 to exact age 60 in 2000 was less than 50 percent in nearly half of the countries in Sub-Saharan Africa. Most of these are countries affected severely by the HIV/AIDS epidemic, but the list also includes war-torn countries, such as Sierra Leone. The

Figure 4.1 Probabilities of Dying between Exact Ages 15 and 60 in Sub-Saharan Africa, by Sex

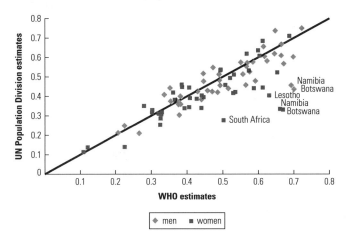

Source: Authors' calculations from United Nations 2003 and Lopez et al. 2002.
Note: WHO estimates are for 2000; UN Population Division estimates are for 1995–2000.

estimates suggest that adult men have consistently higher mortality than adult women in Sub-Saharan Africa, with the female advantage in survivorship being smallest in the very high mortality countries and largest in the low-mortality island states.

The estimates of adult mortality produced by the WHO for 2000 and those made by the United Nations Population Division for the period 1995–2000 are compared in figure 4.1. It is clear that the WHO estimates tend to be significantly higher than those issued by the Population Division for both men and women. The discrepancies are especially large in several countries in the Southern African region, but are also significant for men and of borderline significance for women ($p = 0.059$) in the other countries of the region. As much of Africa is experiencing rising adult mortality from HIV/AIDS, one would expect the WHO's 2000 estimates to be slightly higher than those made by the Population Division for a period on average 2.5 years earlier. However, HIV/AIDS can explain only a small part of the discrepancies between the two sets of estimates. Instead, they are rooted in part in differences in what is assumed about the level of child mortality by the two organizations, in part in the use of different model life tables to extrapolate from child to adult mortality, and in part in different assumptions about the scale of AIDS mortality in particular countries. One cannot readily quantify the relative importance of these contributions to the scatter revealed by figure 4.1. It seems likely, however, that the large discrepancies between the estimates for some southern African countries result at least in part from different assumptions about the severity of AIDS mortality in them.

TRENDS IN ADULT MORTALITY

There is growing evidence of rising trends in adult mortality in the countries in Sub-Saharan Africa. The eastern and southern African regions have been particularly hard hit by the AIDS epidemic, and the available data show large increases in adult mortality rates. For example, data from Malawi show that adult mortality was declining until the mid-1980s but that this trend was reversed in the 1990s (table 4.2). These results are based on the intercensal survival method but are broadly consistent with estimates based on recent household deaths and DHS sibling history data (Blacker 2004). They suggest that mortality for men and women were at similar levels, rather than women having lower mortality, but long-standing evidence exists to suggest that Malawi may be exceptional in this regard (Timaeus 1993, 1998).

Analyses of data from censuses in Kenya also suggest that a reversal in the trend in adult mortality occurred in that country during the 1990s (table 4.3). The orphanhood estimates of person-years lived indicate that slight improvements were made between the 1970s and 1980s but that an even larger decline occurred in the next decade. In this country, the mortality of women is lower than that of men.

Table 4.2 Probabilities of Dying between Ages 15 and 60 ($_{45}q_{15}$), by Sex, according to Intercensal Survival, Malawi

Period	Males	Females
1966–77	0.391	0.344
1977–87	0.243	0.290
1987–98	0.487	0.429

Source: Blacker 2004.

Table 4.3 Orphanhood Estimates of Person-Years Lived and Lost at Ages 35–75 (Men) and 25–75 (Women), Kenya

	Hypothetical Intercensal Cohorts		
	1969–79	1979–89	1989–99
Males 35–75			
Years lived	31.0	32.5	29.6
Years lost	9.0	7.5	10.4
Females 25–75			
Years lived	43.4	44.8	42.8
Years lost	6.6	5.2	7.2

Source: Blacker, Kizito, and Obonyo 2003.

Analysis of a range of data sources from Zimbabwe, including vital registration data, has also shown a marked rise in the adult mortality rates during the 1990s (Feeney 2001). This is in keeping with the rising prevalence of HIV observed in antenatal clinics during the late 1980s and early 1990s. Trends in the probability of dying between ages 30 and 65, $_{35}q_{30}$, are shown in figure 4.2. The estimates from vital registration, household deaths, and survival of parents are reasonably consistent, although the last of these series may underestimate somewhat for the earlier period and place the subsequent rise in mortality slightly too early. Mortality probably fell during the 1970s and early 1980s, but age-specific death rates and probabilities of death subsequently rose by 200 to 300 percent between the late 1980s and late 1990s for both adult men and adult women.

Analysis of a range of data sources from South Africa that also include vital registration data shows that adult mortality rates were fairly constant during the 1980s, followed by an increase in the late 1990s (Timaeus et al. 2001). Trends in $_{45}q_{15}$, the probability of surviving from 15 to 60, are shown in figure 4.3 and reveal the initial signs of the impact of the major HIV epidemic that emerged during the 1990s. More recent data collated from the national population register show that there has been a continued rise in the number of adult deaths registered in South Africa (figure 4.4) and the increase has followed the distinct age pattern associated with AIDS. However, improved registration of deaths and improved registration on the population register could

Figure 4.3 Conditional Probabilities of Dying between Ages 15 and 60 in South Africa, by Sex, from Different Data Sources, 1980–2000

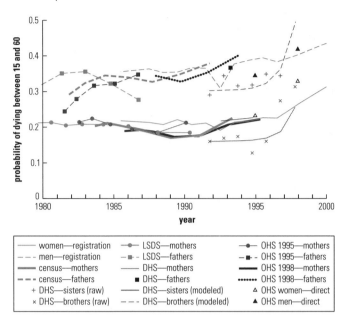

Source: Timaeus et al. 2001.

Note: DHS = Demographic and Health Survey, 1998; LSDS = Living Standards and Development Study, 1993; and OHS = October Household Study.

account for some of this increase. Taking into account these improvements as well as population growth, the increase in deaths of persons at ages 15 years or more has been approximately 40 percent. Age-specific rates can be calculated for South Africa from these data by adjusting for underregistration of deaths (Dorrington, Moultrie, and Timaeus 2004). This can only be done for the years up to 2001, the date of the most recent census, which provides an estimate of the population against which to assess the underregistration. It confirms that a large rise in the mortality of young adults has occurred. The relative increase in mortality rates has been greater for women than for men, although starting from a lower base. Also, the increase for women occurs at a younger age than that for men.

Comparison of the empirically based estimates presented in figure 4.3 with those in table 4.1 suggest that the modeling procedure used by the WHO to estimate adult mortality in South Africa in 2000 has produced severe overestimates, particularly for women. This highlights the uncertainty attached to estimates of adult mortality made from data on children and to projections using epidemiological models fitted to HIV data. It may be the case that the WHO also overestimated women's mortality in the other southern African countries for which it published much higher estimates than the UN (figure 4.1). However, the estimates

Figure 4.2 Conditional Probabilities of Dying between Ages 30 and 65 in Zimbabwe, by Sex, from Different Data Sources, 1969–90

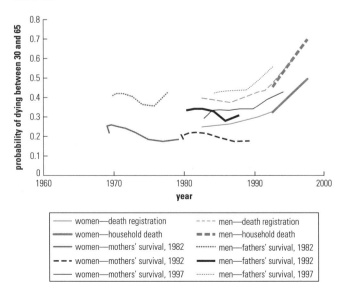

Source: Feeney 2001.

Figure 4.4 Age Distribution of Reported Adult Deaths on the National Population Register of South Africa, by Sex, 1998–2003

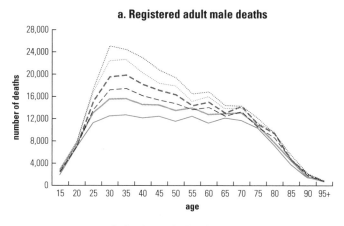

a. Registered adult male deaths

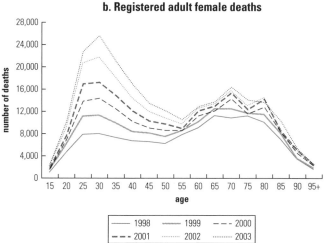

b. Registered adult female deaths

—— 1998	—— 1999	– – – 2000
– – 2001	······· 2002	········ 2003

Source: Bradshaw et al. 2004.

in table 4.1 are not consistently exaggerated. For example, the estimates for Zimbabwe produced by the WHO are broadly consistent with the most up-to-date empirical estimates shown in figure 4.2.

Although the rise in adult mortality in South Africa by 2000 remained moderate at the national level, adult mortality had already risen far more in some parts of the country. Data from a demographic surveillance site in a rural area of one of the provinces that has been most severely affected by HIV/AIDS show that a massive rise in adult mortality occurred between the mid-1990s and 2000. By the latter year the probability of dying between exact ages 15 and 60 reached 58 percent for women and 70 percent for men (Hosegood, Vanneste, and Timaeus 2004). Moreover, this site collects information on causes of death using verbal autopsies. As they are based on a review of symptoms, these data are less liable than the official statistics to attribute AIDS deaths to other causes. They show that the huge rise in adult mortality,

which is concentrated among young adults, as in the national statistics, can be accounted for entirely by AIDS deaths.

Church records from northern Namibia have been used to estimate the mortality experience of the parishioners (Notkola, Timaeus, and Siiskonen 2004). Adult mortality did not change much during the 1980s but increased rapidly from about 1994. In 2000 the death rates of women at ages 20–64 were 3.5 times higher than in 1993; for men they were 2.5 times higher.

An analysis of the sibling histories collected prior to 1997 in 11 DHS surveys in Sub-Saharan Africa showed that, although adult mortality was falling or stagnant in Western Africa and in Namibia in the 1980s, it had begun to rise sharply in Eastern Africa (Timaeus 1998, 1999). Moreover, four of the six Eastern African countries considered were characterized by unusually high mortality of young adults relative to older adults. Unfortunately, DHS surveys collect sibling histories only from women of reproductive age (although respondents report on siblings older than themselves) and the surveys cover rather small samples for the study of adult mortality, especially at ages 45–59. Thus, these surveys lack the statistical power to enable one to produce meaningful estimates of how the age pattern of mortality in adulthood is evolving in each country as the overall death rate rises. Timaeus and Jasseh (2004) incorporate the results of more recent DHS surveys into an analysis based on 26 studies in 23 countries. They attempt to sidestep the relatively small size of DHS samples by estimating a common age pattern of mortality increase across all the countries in which HIV has become present while determining the size of that mortality increase separately for each country. Their smoothed summary estimates of the level and trend in the probability of dying between ages 15 and 60 are shown in table 4.4 and by the WHO region in figure 4.5, which also plots the WHO's own estimates of the same index for the year 2000 (Lopez et al. 2002).

The results of the analysis by Timaeus and Jasseh (2004) show that the fastest rises in adult mortality have occurred in South Africa, Zimbabwe, Zambia, Uganda, Guinea, and Cameroon. Adult mortality has risen relatively slowly or continued to fall in the Sahel. A significant change in the trend about four years after the development of a generalized HIV/AIDS epidemic is observed in 16 of the 19 countries in which the sibling histories cover the relevant period. Of the three countries in which HIV has become prevalent but mortality has not risen markedly, the data for Nigeria are known to be of poor quality, but it is unclear why Ethiopia and Rwanda do not conform to the usual pattern. The increase in mortality is concentrated among women age

Figure 4.5 Trend in the Estimates of the Probabilities of Dying between Ages 15 and 60 ($_{45}q_{15}$), by Sex and WHO Region, from DHS Sibling Histories

(per 1,000 people)

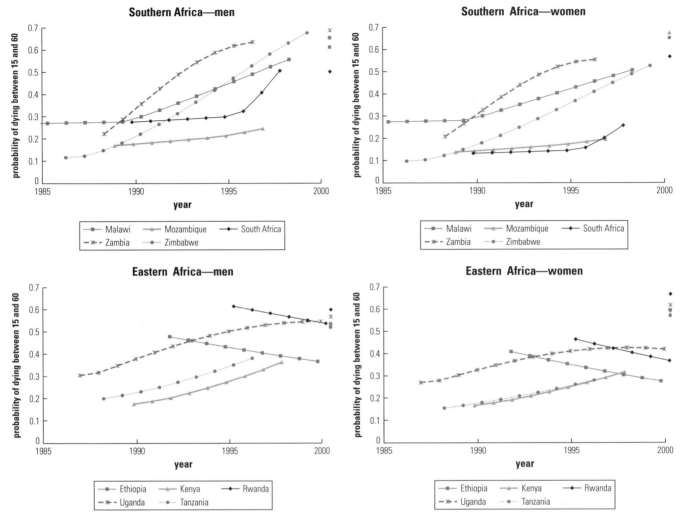

Source: Timaeus and Jasseh 2004.

25 to 39 and men age 30 to 44. On average, men's death rates have risen by about a third more than those of women. However, as women are dying at younger ages and African populations have grown rapidly during the last few decades, the sex differential in the number of AIDS deaths is small.

Extrapolation of the trend in the sibling history estimates forward to 2000 and comparison of them with those made by the WHO (also shown in figure 4.5) reveal that they are in quite good agreement for some countries, including high mortality countries, such as Malawi, Zambia, and Zimbabwe. For men, the WHO estimates are much higher than predicted by the sibling history estimates in Mozambique and in countries where the prevalence of HIV infection is fairly low, that is to say Chad and western African countries such as Benin, Burkina Faso, and Mali. For

women, the discrepancies between the two series are larger and more widespread. They extend to South Africa, the eastern African countries and, to a lesser extent, Côte d'Ivoire, Guinea, and Togo in western Africa. These discrepancies might result from severe underreporting of dead siblings in the DHS. However, it is unclear why this should be more serious in lower mortality countries and, in some cases, for sisters alone. Alternatively, the UN agencies may tend to overestimate adult mortality in Africa. An analysis comparing the numbers of orphans implied in the estimates by the Population Division with empirical data gathered by the DHS on the proportions of children orphaned provides evidence in support of the latter interpretation (Grassly et al. 2004). The DHS data find far fewer orphans than are predicted by models based on the Population Division and

Figure 4.5 (*Continued*)

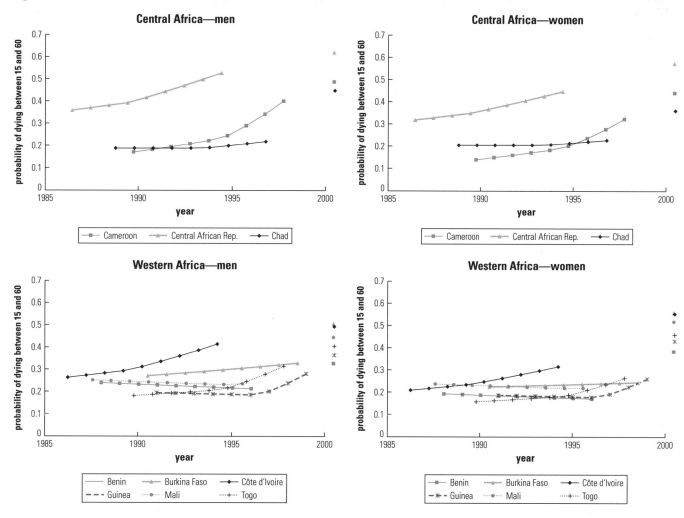

UNAIDS estimates of mortality. Just as in the comparison of the sibling history estimates with the WHO estimates presented here, these discrepancies tend to be larger for maternal orphans than paternal orphans and larger in low-mortality countries than in high-mortality countries. This pattern of discrepancies suggests that, rather than the problem being underreporting of orphanhood in DHS or exaggeration of the scale of AIDS mortality, the model life table systems used by the UN agencies may systematically overestimate background adult mortality in Sub-Saharan Africa, especially for women.

CONCLUSION

The lack of good quality vital registration data in Sub-Saharan Africa has resulted in uncertainty in the levels of adult mortality. Estimates of adult mortality vary, depending on the data source, the methodology used, and the assumptions made. Despite the uncertainties in the data, the evidence shows that adult mortality rates are generally high, reflecting poor levels of health in the region. By the mid-1990s the levels of adult mortality do appear to have become far more varied among the regions and countries and between the genders than they had been a decade earlier. Many countries have shown an increase, with death rates reaching unprecedented heights. This is in stark contrast to the findings by Hill (2003) that adult mortality has been declining in most developing countries—at a rate of 1 percent per year for men and 2 percent per year for women. Estimates of adult mortality for some countries in Sub-Saharan Africa are by far the highest in the world.

Because of the inadequacy of vital statistics in Sub-Saharan Africa, both the UN Population Division and the WHO estimate adult mortality and life expectancy in the countries of the region by extrapolating from estimates of child mortality using model life tables and adding in an estimate of AIDS deaths based on antenatal clinic data. Enough is known about adult mortality in Africa to make it clear

Table 4.4 Estimates of the Probability of Dying between Ages 15 and 60($_{45}q_{15}$), from DHS Sibling Histories
(per person)

Country	Women				Men			
	1985	1990	1995	2000	1985	1990	1995	2000
Benin	0.201	0.187	0.173	—	0.250	0.232	0.216	—
Burkina Faso	—	0.225	0.237	0.251	—	0.271	0.305	0.346
Cameroon	—	0.147	0.226	—	—	0.179	0.276	—
Central African Republic	0.308	0.367	0.469	—	0.348	0.418	0.558	—
Chad	—	0.206	0.219	—	—	0.189	0.207	—
Côte d'Ivoire	0.204	0.252	0.340	—	0.257	0.319	0.452	—
Ethiopia	—	0.433	0.342	0.266	—	0.503	0.423	0.359
Guinea	—	0.189	0.180	0.325	—	0.197	0.188	0.357
Kenya	—	0.175	0.262	—	—	0.185	0.292	—
Malawi	0.275	0.306	0.435	—	0.272	0.306	0.464	—
Mali	0.244	0.230	0.219	—	0.259	0.244	0.236	—
Mozambique	—	0.147	0.181	—	—	0.181	0.224	—
Namibia	0.172	0.183	—	—	0.318	0.336	—	—
Niger	0.251	0.198	—	—	0.252	0.199	—	—
Nigeria	—	0.076	0.114	0.179	—	0.093	0.140	0.233
Rwanda	—	—	0.458	0.363	—	—	0.610	0.533
Senegal	0.165	0.163	—	—	0.186	0.184	—	—
South Africa	—	0.135	0.147	—	—	0.280	0.302	—
Tanzania	0.127	0.184	0.266	—	0.166	0.236	0.360	—
Togo	—	0.162	0.204	—	—	0.187	0.238	—
Uganda	0.274	0.339	0.416	0.415	0.310	0.395	0.511	0.545
Zambia	0.149	0.339	0.547	—	0.159	0.372	0.623	—
Zimbabwe	0.094	0.187	0.378	0.566	0.113	0.232	0.486	0.726

Source: Timaeus and Jasseh 2004.

Notes: — = not available. Estimates extrapolated to 2000 are presented for countries conducting a survey in 1998 or later.

that age patterns of mortality vary markedly between different populations in the region. The assumption that a fixed relationship between adult and child mortality holds across the continent is bound to produce estimates that are badly in error in particular countries, even if they are unbiased overall. In addition, evidence from DHS orphanhood data (Grassly et al. 2004), DHS sibling histories (Timaeus and Jasseh 2004), and earlier surveys and censuses (Timaeus 1993) all suggest that in recent years the Population Division's extrapolations using Princeton North model life tables have overestimated non-AIDS adult mortality in large parts of the region. The WHO's estimates infer the relationship between child and adult mortality from a database of populations that tend to have lower mortality than is typical of Africa and appear to suffer from very similar limitations to those produced by the Population Division.

Given the limitations of the demographic and epidemiological data, there are inevitably large errors in some of the estimates of AIDS mortality made by UNAIDS and the WHO. Nevertheless, the evidence that adult mortality is now rising in most of Sub-Saharan Africa is clear cut. Moreover, the empirical evidence as to the size and speed of the rise in adult mortality in different countries in the region and the evolving age pattern of the mortality impact is consistent with predictions from epidemiological surveillance data and models of the impact of HIV/AIDS on adult mortality in most countries. The annual toll of AIDS deaths in Sub-Saharan Africa continues to grow rapidly, and the urgency of responding to the poor health conditions in the region has been exacerbated by the emergence of the HIV/AIDS epidemic.

In some African countries significant numbers of people have been dying from AIDS since the 1980s. In such countries it is difficult to imagine what would have happened to rates of mortality by today in the absence of AIDS. Thus, it is no longer viable to estimate and forecast mortality by adding an estimate of AIDS deaths to a separate estimate of non-AIDS mortality. Instead, new approaches for making mortality estimates and projections are required that can be calibrated to data on both the prevalence of HIV infection and all-cause adult mortality.

While existing data do signal the broad scale of the impact of AIDS on the mortality of adult populations in Sub-Saharan Africa, they are clearly not sufficiently detailed, reliable, or timely to provide the description of changes in level and age pattern that is urgently needed to monitor the impacts of programs that are being funded by African governments, the Global Fund, the World Bank, and bilateral donors. The fundamental cause of the uncertainty about levels of adult mortality and the impact on them of AIDS in Africa remains the limitations of epidemiological monitoring and demographic data systems in the region. The rollout of antiretroviral care and treatment activities throughout the continent should have a major impact (short, middle, and long term) on mortality dynamics and the demographic landscape of the region. More than ever before, better epidemiological and demographic data are required to evaluate the impact of health programs and to assess whether these efforts are effective in reducing the mortality of young adults.

National statistical offices, technical advisers, donors, and researchers are urged to assign more priority to the collection of adult mortality data in this region. In addition to responding to the poor levels of adult health, reinvigorating vital registration and statistics is essential in the long term and must also be placed high on the health and development agenda. An effective registration system is the only way of producing detailed annual series of mortality statistics, including those on causes of death. Moreover, as countries in Sub-Saharan Africa experience the phenomenon of aging, improved vital registration systems will be critical to provide information about mortality trends at older ages, which are largely unknown at present and difficult to investigate using methods based on survey data. Thus, countries are encouraged to establish expert teams to critically review their national civil registration systems in regard to their legal framework, organizational issues, system design, training needs, and quality control issues and to implement strategies for their improvement.

Given the stresses on governments in the region (in part due to the impacts we are trying to measure), it is also vital to propose ways in which survey data, census data, and demographic surveillance data might be expanded and better used to track and understand changes in mortality while vital registration still remains defective. Demographic and epidemiological surveillance in localized sites has proved invaluable and can yield relatively reliable statistics on causes of death. However, it needs to be balanced by other sources that can provide nationally representative data. Although sibling history data have serious limitations, in particular their limited statistical precision in all but the largest surveys, they have proved useful. We believe that countries should continue to collect these data. Moreover, they should collect them repeatedly, as this greatly increases the scope for assessment of the quality of the statistics that result. However, the crucial source of demographic data for planning, particularly at the subnational or district level, is the population census. All African governments are faced with either the reality or the threat of massive rises in adult mortality and they should all include questions about household deaths by age and sex and about orphanhood in their 2010-round censuses. A major drive is needed on the part of the United Nations agencies and donor organizations to support African governments in this, so as to ensure that question and form design, enumerator training, data capture, and the analysis of these data are all conducted successfully.

REFERENCES

Bennett, N., and S. Horiuchi. 1984. "Mortality Estimation from Registered Deaths in Less Developed Countries." *Demography* 21: 217–33.

Bicego, G. 1997. "Estimating Adult Mortality Rates in the Context of the AIDS Epidemic in Sub-Saharan Africa: Analysis of DHS Sibling Histories." *Health Transition Review* 7 (Suppl. 2): 7–22.

Blacker, J. 2004. "The Impact of AIDS on Adult Mortality: Evidence from National and Regional Statistics." *AIDS* (Suppl. 2): S10–26.

Blacker, J., P. Kizito, and B. Obonyo. 2003. "Projecting Kenya's Mortality: Using Spectrum to Project the AIDS and Non-AIDS Components." Paper presented at the Conference on Empirical Evidence for the Demographic and Socioeconomic Impact of AIDS, Durban.

Botha, J. L., and D. Bradshaw. 1985. "African Vital Statistics—A Black Hole?" *South African Medical Journal* 67: 977–81.

Bradshaw, D., R. Laubscher, R. Dorrington, D. Bourne, and I. M. Timaeus. 2004. "Unabated Rise in Number of Adult Deaths in South Africa." *South African Medical Journal* 94 (4): 278–79.

Brass, W. 1975. *Methods for Estimating Fertility and Mortality from Limited and Defective Data.* Chapel Hill, NC: International Program of Laboratories for Population Statistics.

Brass, W., and K. H. Hill. 1973. "Estimating Adult Mortality from Orphanhood." In *International Population Conference, Liège, 1973.* Vol. 3. Liège: International Union for the Scientific Study of Population.

Coale, A. J., P. Demeny, and B. Vaughan. 1983. *Regional Model Life Tables and Stable Populations.* London: Academic Press.

Dorrington, R. E., D. Bourne, D. Bradshaw, R. Laubscher, and I. M. Timaeus. 2001. *The Impact of HIV/AIDS on Adult Mortality in South Africa.* Cape Town: Medical Research Council. http://www.mrc/bod/bod.htm.

Dorrington, R., T. A. Moultrie, and I. M. Timaeus. 2004. *Estimation of Mortality Using the South African Census 2001 Data.* Monograph 11.

Cape Town, South Africa: Centre for Actuarial Research, University of Cape Town. http://www.commerce.uct.ac.za/care/Monographs/Monographs/Mono11.pdf.

Feeney, G. 2001. "The Impact of HIV/AIDS on Adult Mortality in Zimbabwe." *Population and Development Review* 27: 771–80.

Grassly, N. C., J. J. C. Lewis, M. Mahy, N. Walker, and I. M. Timaeus. 2004. "Comparison of Survey Estimates with UNAIDS/WHO Projections of Mortality and Orphan Numbers in Sub-Saharan Africa." *Population Studies* 58: 207–17.

Gregson, S., R. M. Anderson, J. Ndlovu, T. Zhuway, and S. K. Chandiwana. 1997. "Recent Upturn in Mortality in Rural Zimbabwe: Evidence for an Early Demographic Impact of HIV-1 Infection?" *AIDS* 11: 1269–80.

Hill, K. 1987. "Estimating Census and Death Registration Completeness." *Asian and Pacific Population Forum* 1 (3): 8–13, 23–24.

———. 2003. "Adult Mortality in the Developing World; What We Know and How We Know It." Paper presented at the Training Workshop on HIV/AIDS and Adult Mortality in Developing Countries, New York, September. Organized by the United Nations Population Division, Department of Economic and Social Affairs, UN/POP/MORT/2003/1. http://www.un.org/esa/population/publications/adultmort/HILL_Paper1.pdf.

Hosegood, V., A. M. Vanneste, and I. M. Timaeus. 2004. "Levels and Causes of Adult Mortality in Rural South Africa: The Impact of AIDS." *AIDS* 18: 663–71.

Kitange, H. M., H. Machibya, J. Black, D. M. Mtasiwa, G. Masuki, D. Whiting, N. Unwin, et al. 1996. "Outlook for Survivors of Childhood in Sub-Saharan Africa: Adult Mortality in Tanzania." *British Medical Journal* 312: 216–20.

Kowal, P., C. Rao, and C. Mathers. 2003. *Report on a WHO Workshop: Minimum Dataset on Ageing and Adult Mortality in sub Saharan Africa.* Geneva: WHO.

Lopez, A. D., O. B. Ahmad, M. Guillot, B. D. Ferguson, J. A. Salomon, C. J. L. Murray, and K. H. Hill. 2002. *World Mortality in 2000: Life Tables for 191 Countries.* Geneva: WHO.

Murray, C. J. L., B. D. Ferguson, A. D. Lopez, M. Guillot, J. A. Salomon, and O. Ahmad. 2003. "Modified Logit Life Table System: Principles, Empirical Validation, and Application." *Population Studies* 57: 165–82.

Murray, C. J. L., and A. D. Lopez. 1996. *The Global Burden of Disease: A Comprehensive Assessment of Mortality and Disability from Diseases, Injuries and Risk Factors in 1990 and Projected to 2020.* Vol. 1 of the Global Burden of Disease and Injury series. Cambridge, MA: Harvard University Press.

Murray, C. J. L., G. Yang, and X. Qiao. 1992. "Adult Mortality: Levels, Patterns, and Causes." In *The Health of Adults in the Developing World*, ed. R. G. A. Feachem, T. Kjellstrom, C. J. L. Murray, O. Mead, and M. A. Phillips. New York: Oxford University Press.

Notkola, V., I. M. Timaeus, and H. Siiskonen. 2004. "Impact on Mortality of the AIDS Epidemic in Northern Namibia Assessed Using Parish Registers." *AIDS* 18: 1061–65.

Nunn, A. J., D. W. Mulder, A. Kamali, A. Ruberantwari, J.-F. Kengeya-Kayondo, and J. Whitworth. 1997. "Mortality Associated with HIV-1 Infection over Five Years in a Rural Ugandan Population: Cohort Study." *British Medical Journal* 315: 767–71.

Pison, G., and A. Langaney. 1985. "The Level and Age Pattern of Mortality in Bandafassi (Eastern Senegal): Results from a Small-Scale and Intensive Multi-Round Survey." *Population Studies* 39: 387–405.

Preston, S. H., and N. G. Bennett. 1983. "A Census-Based Method for Estimating Adult Mortality." *Population Studies* 37: 91–104.

Rutenberg, N., and J. Sullivan. 1991. "Direct and Indirect Estimates of Maternal Mortality from the Sisterhood Method." In *Proceedings of the Demographic and Health Surveys World Conference, Washington, D.C.* Vol. 3. Columbia, MD: IRD/Macro International.

Salomon, J. A., and C. D. L. Murray. 2001. "Modeling HIV/AIDS Epidemics in Sub-Saharan Africa Using Seroprevalence Data from Antenatal Clinics." *Bulletin of the World Health Organization* 79: 586–692.

Sewankambo, N. K., R. H. Gray, S. Ahmad, D. Serwadda, F. Wabwire-Mangen, F. Nalugoda, N. Kiwanuka, et al. 2000. "Mortality Associated with HIV Infection in Rural Rakai District, Uganda." *AIDS* 14: 2391–400.

Stanton, C., N. Abderrahim, and K. Hill. 1997. *DHS Maternal Mortality Indicators: An Assessment of Data Quality and Implications for Data Use.* Demographic and Health Surveys Analytical Report 4. Calverton, MD: Macro International.

Timaeus, I. M. 1991. "Estimation of Mortality from Orphanhood in Adulthood." *Demography* 28: 213–27.

———. 1992. "Estimation of Adult Mortality from Paternal Orphanhood: A Reassessment and a New Approach." *Population Bulletin of the United Nations* 33: 47–63.

———. 1993. "Adult Mortality." In *Demographic Change in Sub-Saharan Africa*, ed. K. A. Foote, K. H. Hill, and L. G. Martin. Washington, DC: National Academy Press.

———. 1998. "Impact of the HIV Epidemic on Mortality in Sub-Saharan Africa: Evidence from National Surveys and Censuses." *AIDS* 12 (Suppl. 1): S15–27.

———. 1999. "Mortality in Sub-Saharan Africa." In *Health and Mortality: Issues of Global Concern*, ed. J. Chamie and R. L. Cliquet. New York and Brussels: United Nations Population Division and Population and Family Study Centre, Flemish Scientific Institute.

Timaeus, I. M., R. E. Dorrington, D. Bradshaw, N. Nannan, and D. Bourne. 2001. "Adult Mortality in South Africa, 1980–2000: From Apartheid to AIDS." Paper presented at the Population Association of America's annual meeting, Washington, DC, March 29–31.

Timaeus, I. M., and M. Jasseh. 2004. "Adult Mortality in Sub-Saharan Africa: Evidence from Demographic and Health Surveys." *Demography* 41: 757–72.

Timaeus, I. M., and A. J. Nunn. 1997. "Measurement of Adult Mortality in Populations Affected by AIDS: An Assessment of the Orphanhood Method." *Health Transition Review* 7 (Suppl. 2): 23–43.

Todd, J., R. Balira, H. Grosskurth, P. Mayaud, F. Mosha, G. ka-Gina, A. Klokke, et al. 1997. "HIV-Associated Adult Mortality in a Rural Tanzanian Population." *AIDS* 11: 801–7.

Tollman, S. M., K. Kahn, M. Garenne, and J. S. Gear. 1999. "Reversal in Mortality Trends: Evidence from the Agincourt Field Site, South Africa, 1992–1995." *AIDS* 13: 1091–97.

UNAIDS (Joint United Nations Programme on HIV/AIDS) Reference Group on Estimates, Modelling and Projections. 2002. "Improved Methods and Assumptions for Estimation of the HIV/AIDS Epidemic and Its Impact: Recommendations of the UNAIDS Reference Group on Estimates, Modelling and Projections." *AIDS* 16: W1–W16.

United Nations. 1982. *Model Life Tables for Developing Countries.* New York: United Nations.

———. 2002. *World Population Prospects: The 2000 Revision.* Vol. 3: *Analytical Report.* New York: United Nations.

———. 2003. *World Population Prospects: The 2002 Revision; Datasets in Excel and PDF Formats.* New York: United Nations.

Urassa, M., J. T. Boerma, R. Isingo, J. Ngalula, J. Ng'weshemi, G. Mwaluko, and B. Zaba. 2001. "The Impact of HIV/AIDS on Mortality and Household Mobility in Rural Tanzania." *AIDS* 15: 2017–23.

WHO (World Health Organization). 2000. *The World Health Report 2000—Health Systems: Improving Performance.* Geneva: WHO.

Chapter **5**

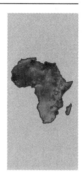

Causes of Death

Chalapati Rao, Alan D. Lopez, and Yusuf Hemed

Consistent estimates of cause-specific mortality are essential for understanding the overall epidemiological profile of disease in a population. The principal data source for these estimates is civil registration systems. Adequately functioning systems that produce statistics on causes of death on a regular basis exist in only about one-third of all countries of the world (Lopez et al. 2002). In Sub-Saharan Africa, very little information has been available on cause-specific mortality, let alone data from civil registration systems, as described in the previous edition of this book (Feachem and Jamison 1991). Estimates at that time were derived largely from independent disease-specific epidemiological studies and were not examined within the context of an overall demographic "envelope" of mortality, as is required to ensure that claims about causes of death are not exaggerated.

Over the past decade, much progress has been made in the collection of mortality statistics from a wide array of sources. These include data from previously existing sources that were uncovered during a systematic search, as well as data from new data collection ventures that were established to fill these data gaps. Although we are still a long way from having satisfactory empirical data that can be directly used to derive national and regional cause-specific mortality estimates, the expansion in available data suggests that estimates of causes of death can now be made with somewhat greater confidence. The absence of complete vital registration data in virtually all countries of the region nonetheless means that we need to rely on epidemiological research and demographic surveillance to generate model-based estimates of deaths by cause.

Such an estimation process is complex and involves two stages. First, a demographic estimate of overall mortality by age and sex is required. Second, a cause-specific mortality structure is fitted to this estimate. Many assumptions are required, and an attempt has been made here to delineate these clearly, so that they can be kept in mind when interpreting the results.

DATA SOURCES

The previous edition of this book provided information on cause-specific mortality in the form of a set of estimates for the entire region, disaggregated over seven broad disease categories, and in six age groups. These estimates were essentially derived from linear models relating mortality levels to broad causes of death (Preston 1976), with very little attempt to incorporate other epidemiological information. The authors stated that the large proportion of deaths lumped under other causes reflected the weakness of the estimates, and suggested great caution in interpreting or using them (Feachem, Jamison, and Bos 1991).

Building on previous experience, researchers have made much more comprehensive attempts over the past decade to collect and analyze information in order to estimate the cause-specific mortality structure for Sub-Saharan Africa as part of the Global Burden of Disease (GBD) Study (Mathers, Stein et al. 2002; Murray and Lopez 1996). Discussed here are the results of two major data collection efforts that were undertaken to estimate the burden of premature mortality in Africa. The first effort involved a search for, and analysis of, epidemiological literature on causes of death in the region. The second effort involved a similar exercise using data from national vital records.

Review of Epidemiological Literature

Much of the earlier attempts to estimate causes of death in the region drew on published and unpublished reports based on epidemiological studies. Adetunji, Murray, and Evans (1996) conducted a major review of epidemiological studies to identify usable cause-specific mortality data. They identified a total of 48 research studies from 16 countries that met specific criteria related to data definition and data quality issues for inclusion in the analysis. The main criteria for inclusion was that the study should have reported the relative magnitude of all causes of death and not focus on a single or a few causes without mention of other causes within the sample. Other criteria refer to methods used to derive the cause of death, age groups reported, site, and period of the study. Reports from South Africa were excluded from this analysis, since the data overlapped with that available from vital records. About 80 percent of the reports were based on information from hospital records, verbal autopsy interviews, or both. A majority of the studies (again 80 percent) focused on causes of maternal and child mortality, whereas causes of adult male deaths were relatively neglected. The authors presented results in the form of cause composition of mortality for three distinct cause groups: communicable diseases and maternal, perinatal, and nutritional conditions (group 1); noncommunicable diseases (group 2); and injuries (group 3). These cause groups were the same as those used in the GBD Study. The results of their review of deaths of children younger than five years are summarized in table 5.1.

Table 5.1 Proportion of Deaths Due to Diseases and Injuries in Children under Five Years, by Source of Data

Method	No. of studies	No. of deaths	Gp 1 (%)	Gp 2 (%)	Gp 3 (%)	Others[a] (%)	Total
Verbal autopsy (surveys)	13	4,964	68	4	0	28	100
Verbal autopsy and hospital records	3	1,139	54	16	0	30	100
Verbal autopsy (prospective studies)	4	1,906	62	1	0	37	100
Vital registration	3	11,878	52	19	0	29	100
Hospital records	1	2,419	75	0	0	25	100
Other multiple sources	3	1,288	86	9	1	4	100
Hospital autopsy	1	953	73	15	9	12	100

Source: Adetunji, Murray, and Evans 1996.
a. Includes ill-defined conditions and cause unknown.

The high proportion of deaths for which the cause was unknown raises serious questions about data quality. The largest number of deaths in this review was in the vital records for Abidjan, Côte d'Ivoire (1987–92). However, these too have high proportions of "other" causes (29 percent). A detailed analysis of specific causes based on the data from these studies suggested that respiratory infections, diarrhea, malnutrition, and anemia were the leading causes of death in this age group.

At ages 5 to 14 years (see table 5.2), the largest number of deaths was also in the vital records from the same source, although the total number of deaths registered is very small. In such situations, deriving a meaningful estimate of even the proportions across broad cause groups is difficult, because paucity in numbers is coupled with high proportions of ill-defined causes (44 percent). Nevertheless, the results suggested that malaria, diarrheal diseases, and malnutrition were the leading causes of death among school-age children.

Table 5.2 Proportion of Deaths Due to Diseases and Injuries in Children Age 5 to 14 Years, by Source of Data

Method	No. of studies	No. of deaths	Gp 1 (%)	Gp 2 (%)	Gp 3 (%)	Others[a] (%)	Total
Verbal autopsy (surveys)	1	25	88	0	0	12	100
Vital registration	2	2,817	38	12	6	44	100
Hospital records	1	713	67	0	21	12	100
Hospital autopsy	1	52	56	15	12	17	100

Source: Adetunji, Murray, and Evans 1996.
a. Includes ill-defined conditions and cause unknown.

For ages above 15 years, epidemiological studies on causes of death concentrate on causes of maternal mortality. Adetunji, Murray, and Evans (1996) reviewed information from 21 studies and identified 3,818 deaths due to maternal causes. About 80 percent of these studies were based on hospital records. This could have two possible implications. On the one hand, hospital-based studies could overestimate maternal mortality, as high risk and emergency cases are likely to be concentrated in hospitals. On the other hand, better emergency care in hospitals may avert more deaths than would have occurred in the community. Notwithstanding these possible biases, the causes as documented in hospital records are likely to be more reliable than those from community-based studies. The pooled results suggested hemorrhage (19 percent), puerperal sepsis (13 percent), hypertensive disorders of pregnancy (7.8 percent), and ruptured uterus (7 percent) as the leading causes of maternal mortality in Sub-Saharan Africa, at least among women referred to hospitals.

Adetunji, Murray, and Evans (1996) also documented three sources of data on causes of adult mortality; two from vital records in Lagos (1977) and Abidjan (1987–92), and one from the Adult Morbidity and Mortality Project (AMMP) in Tanzania (1992). The data from Lagos predate the HIV/AIDS period and record accidents and violence as the leading cause of adult deaths (26.3 percent). In Abidjan, the data suggest hypertensive disease (31 percent), diarrheal disease (11 percent) and HIV/AIDS (10.5 percent) as the leading causes. Data from the AMMP are available by sex and show HIV/AIDS to be the leading cause in both sexes (higher proportions in women) and injuries in males and pregnancy-related causes to be the other significant conditions. All these results suggest that hypertensive disease, HIV/AIDS, pregnancy-related causes, and injuries are the leading causes of death among adults in Sub-Saharan Africa.

We have described this review in some detail in part because it was the most comprehensive previous attempt to estimate causes of death in Africa, and in part to show that compiling information from various sources, despite the enormous effort involved, still results in substantial uncertainty about the cause structure of mortality owing to biases in the way the data were collected and the high proportions of unspecified causes in the reports. However, these epidemiological studies were designed to focus on one or a few specific causes of mortality, yielding useful information on incidence, duration, and case-fatality rates. These indexes were used by independent researchers to infer mortality specific to that cause at the population level,

and such epidemiological estimates for individual causes are useful to build the overall cause-specific mortality picture.

Information from Vital Records

Another data collection effort was centered on the acquisition of vital records data. The World Health Organization (WHO) conducted a comprehensive search for these data over the period 2001–02, as part of the data collection for the GBD 2000 project (Kowal, Rao, and Mathers 2003). Few countries in Africa have vital registration systems that are more than 50 percent complete. Coverage is about this level in Kenya and Zimbabwe (Lopez et al. 2002), and close to 90 percent in South Africa (Dorrington et al. 2001). In Mozambique a major exercise was undertaken to improve mortality registration and cause-of-death attribution in four cities (Cliff et al. 2003). The ministries of health in Botswana, Eritrea, and Zambia collect and collate information on causes of death from health facility data and from vital records, essentially in urban areas. The AMMP in Tanzania has built up a comprehensive district-level mortality surveillance system that operates currently in three districts (Hai, Morogoro, and Dar es Salaam) and has compiled information on causes of death over a 10-year period. Vital records data from the city of Antananarivo have been systematically compiled over a 12-year period to describe urban causes of death in Madagascar (Waltisperger, Cantrelle, and Ralijaona 1998). Data from all these countries have been collated and analyzed at the WHO.

Vital records data, although impressive in overall numbers of deaths for which information on cause is available, have their own limitations. First, coverage is incomplete, and it is not possible to map these data to an underlying population to make an assessment of death rates. Second, there is no indication of the bases used for cause-of-death attribution, whether physician attribution at the time of death, hospital records, verbal autopsy, or lay reported information. The proportionate distribution of causes of death are therefore examined in this chapter according to the GBD groups at different ages, as was done in the earlier analyses using data from epidemiological studies.

Included in these tabulations are the proportionate distributions for two epidemiological subregions in Sub-Saharan Africa (AFR D and AFR E),[1] as estimated by the GBD cause-of-death study. These subregions group countries with similar estimated levels of child and adult mortality, as described in detail later in the section on the GBD estimation process. For comparison purposes, and so

Table 5.3 National Vital Records Data: Proportionate Distribution of Cause of Death of Children under Five

Country	Year of data collection	No. of deaths	Gp 1 (%)	Gp 2 (%)	Gp 3 (%)	Ill-defined[a] (%)
Botswana	1998	1,443	80	10	1	9
Kenya	2001	53,478	88	4	1	7
Madagascar	1984–95	49,250	83	7	2	8
Mozambique	2001	6,712	78	6	3	13
South Africa	1996	29,043	75	8	8	9
Tanzania[b]	1998–2000	1,338	88	2	0	9
Zambia	1999–2000	32,586	94	2	2	2
Zimbabwe	1995	17,786	86	7	3	5
GBD AFR D	2000	2,134,635	96	2	2	—
GBD AFR E	2000	2,265,960	95	3	2	—

Source: Authors.
Note: — = not available.
a. As part of the GBD approach, deaths from ill-defined categories are reallocated to specific categories.
b. For Tanzania, information collected in the AMMP project was used.

Table 5.4 National Vital Records Data: Proportionate Distribution of Cause of Death at Age 5 to 14 Years

Country	Year of data collection	No. of deaths	Gp 1 (%)	Gp 2 (%)	Gp 3 (%)	Ill-defined[a] (%)
Botswana	1998	129	53	30	9	4
Kenya	2001	11,240	75	9	5	12
Madagascar	1984–95	5,362	57	19	12	12
Mozambique	2001	1,013	68	12	13	7
South Africa	1996	5,160	19	19	53	10
Tanzania	1998–2000	653	73	8	12	6
Zimbabwe	1995	1,842	47	22	25	6
GBD AFR D	2000	248,012	67	6	27	—
GBD AFR E	2000	314,283	74	6	20	—

Source: Authors.
Note: — = not available.
a. As part of the GBD approach, deaths from ill-defined categories are reallocated to specific categories.

their plausibility may be judged, these figures are included here with available local data.

Among children under five, the highest proportion of deaths, as expected, is from group 1 causes (perinatal conditions, communicable diseases, and malnutrition), ranging from 75 percent in the South African data set to 94 percent in the data from Zambia. A reassuring feature of these vital records data is the relatively low proportion of deaths not classified in any of the three cause groups. In the GBD estimates, unclassifiable deaths at ages below five years are reallocated to group 1 (Murray and Lopez 1996). Hence, we estimate that about 95 percent of deaths at these ages are due to group 1 causes, which approximates the upper end of the range of observed proportions from this cause category from the vital records data sets (table 5.3).

As age increases, the proportion of deaths due to noncommunicable diseases and injuries rises. In global comparisons, this shift in cause composition across ages is less evident in Sub-Saharan Africa than in other regions, due to the catastrophic HIV/AIDS epidemic. At ages 5 to 14 years, the South African data set suggests a low proportion of deaths due to group 1 causes, which may be because the population covered by registration is urban, with higher socioeconomic status (expressed as GDP per capita) than the national average (table 5.4). Another possible cause for low group 1 proportions is that the coverage of vital registration in South Africa is only 90 percent, and the missed deaths could be group 1 deaths. However, such corrections would result only in marginal changes in the specific

proportions of the groups. Again, from all the data sets, the proportion of deaths due to ill-defined causes is low. In the GBD estimation process, these deaths due to ill-defined causes at ages above five years are reallocated proportionately across group 2 causes. In comparison, group 1 proportions in the estimates again approximate the higher end of the range of observations in the local data.

Much more complex is to estimate cause-specific mortality for the young adult (15 to 44 years) age group. At these ages in Sub-Saharan Africa, a triple burden of cause-specific factors exists, namely, the HIV/AIDS epidemic; high incidence rates of injury and violence, especially among males; and the high burden of maternal mortality among females. These aspects of cause-specific mortality are evident from the results of the epidemiological literature review discussed earlier. Table 5.5 shows the group-specific proportions from vital records at these ages. The proportion of deaths in vital records due to injuries at these ages appears to be low in most countries, given the wars and violence in the region. The GBD estimates of war-related deaths are included in deaths due to violence and marginally increase the proportions of deaths due to injuries. Also, the relatively low proportion of deaths due to group 1 causes in the Madagascar data set could be because the population covered was urban, or that HIV prevalence, transmission, and mortality is low in Madagascar (Ravaoarimalala et al. 1998). Group 1 conditions appear to cause a major proportion of mortality at these ages.

Local data for deaths at older ages (45 years and older) from all sites have significantly higher proportions of unclassifiable

Table 5.5 National Vital Records Data: Proportionate Distribution of Cause of Death at Age 15 to 44 Years

Country	Year of data collection	No. of deaths	Gp 1 (%)	Gp 2 (%)	Gp 3 (%)	Ill-defined[a] (%)
Botswana	1998	2,658	76	19	3	2
Kenya	2001	69,910	75	11	6	8
Madagascar	1984–95	23,056	39	40	13	9
Mozambique	2001	8,008	71	12	9	8
South Africa	1996	83,482	25	22	43	10
Tanzania	1998–2000	3,943	72	11	9	9
Zimbabwe	1995	30,124	59	13	8	19
GBD AFR D	2000	913,976	69	13	18	—
GBD AFR E	2000	1,879,690	82	7	11	—

Source: Authors.
Note: — = not available.
a. As part of the GBD approach, deaths from ill-defined categories are reallocated to specific categories.

Table 5.6 National Vital Records Data: Proportionate Distribution of Cause of Death at 45 Years of Age and Older

Country	Year of data collection	No. of deaths	Gp 1 (%)	Gp 2 (%)	Gp 3 (%)	Ill-defined[a] (%)
Botswana	1998	2,082	44	48	2	4
Kenya	2001	64,729	57	27	3	13
Madagascar	1984–95	45,166	18	63	3	16
Mozambique	2001	5,843	45	30	5	20
South Africa	1996	167,828	13	64	7	15
Tanzania	1998–2000	4,811	48	32	4	16
Zimbabwe	1995	28,173	30	35	5	31
GBD AFR D	2000	1,337,672	28	67	5	—
GBD AFR E	2000	1,683,816	37	58	5	—

Source: Authors.
Note: — = not available.
a. As part of the GBD approach, deaths from ill-defined categories are reallocated to specific categories.

deaths, approaching 31 percent in Zimbabwe (table 5.6). At these ages, one would normally expect higher proportions of deaths from noncommunicable diseases, which is reflected in the data. There is a possibility of misclassification between group 2 and group 1, since in some instances individuals with long-standing noncommunicable diseases develop infectious complications during terminal stages, which tend to be more readily identified and classified as the underlying cause of death. The estimates are close to the upper end of the range of proportions of group 2 conditions from local data.

From the above analyses, vital registration data would seem to be useful in understanding general patterns of cause-specific mortality at broad-cause-group level. However, biases introduced by incomplete or selective coverage and difficulty in identifying specific causes beyond the broad-cause-group level preclude their usage directly in the estimation process. In situations of incomplete data, the process of estimating mortality from specific causes entails the synthesis of information from different data sources or, if necessary, by drawing on other regional or international cause-specific mortality patterns.

GBD Process for Estimating Cause-Specific Mortality

The GBD Study method of estimating cause-specific mortality in populations without detailed information on the levels or cause structure of mortality is essentially based on three sequential steps:

1. The first step is to derive an overall envelope of mortality, in terms of estimated numbers of deaths, for each age-sex group within the population. In practical terms, a model

life table–based age-specific risk of mortality is applied to a national age-sex population estimate. The purpose of this step is to provide an upper limit or "demographic envelope," to constrain cause-of-death estimates within the bounds of demographic plausibility.

2. The second step is to use cause-of-death models to predict a GBD group-specific (broad causes) proportionate composition of mortality for each age-sex group and to apply the proportions to the mortality envelope derived in step 1 to derive an age-sex GBD group-specific envelope of mortality.

3. The third step is to fit a condition-specific cause structure of mortality for each broad-cause group onto their respective envelopes as derived in step 2 to derive estimates of deaths from specific conditions by age and sex for the population.

In the current analysis, separate estimates were developed for each country in Sub-Saharan Africa, and they were summed up to generate two subregional population aggregations. The classification of WHO member states into the mortality strata was carried out using population estimates for 1999 (United Nations Population Division 1998) and estimates of child mortality (defined as $_5q_0$, the risk of dying between birth and age 5) and adult mortality (defined as $_{45}q_{15}$, the risk of dying between ages 15 and 60) based on WHO analyses of mortality rates for 1999 (Mathers, Stein et al. 2002). Five mortality strata were defined in terms of quintiles of the distribution of $_5q_0$ and $_{45}q_{15}$ (both sexes combined). Adult mortality $_{45}q_{15}$ was regressed on $_5q_0$ and the regression line used to divide countries with high child

Figure 5.1 Global Mortality Strata for GBD 2000 Regions

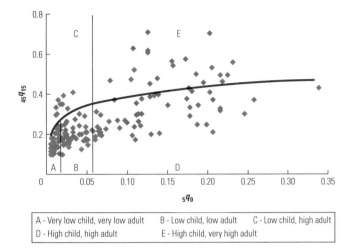

A - Very low child, very low adult	B - Low child, low adult	C - Low child, high adult
D - High child, high adult	E - High child, very high adult	

Source: Mathers, Stein et al. 2002.

mortality into high adult mortality (stratum D) and very high adult mortality (stratum E), as in figure 5.1. Stratum E includes the countries in Sub-Saharan Africa where HIV/AIDS has had a substantial impact.

A fundamental principle in the estimation process is to maintain internal consistency between the overall demographic envelope of mortality and the cause composition within the envelope. In other words, the mortality due to specific causes within an age group should exactly sum up to the life table–derived envelope of mortality. Such constraints call for significant assumptions and judgments; hence, the final estimates should be interpreted based on these choices. With the high estimated levels of HIV/AIDS mortality in the region, judgments regarding burden due to competing causes of death are based on evidence from vital records and epidemiological estimates for specific diseases. However, preceding these issues is the process of deriving the life tables for estimating the mortality envelope by age and sex and the use of cause-of-death models for allocating deaths to broad-cause groups.

Life Tables

Detailed age-specific mortality rates are required to construct life tables for populations. Such rates are not available for any country within Sub-Saharan Africa. Attempts at estimating death rates based on recall of deaths in censuses and surveys have generally led to implausibly low death rates (Brass 1968). The best available data on mortality risk are levels of child mortality derived from Demographic and Health Surveys (DHS) conducted in most countries within the region during the 1990s. These estimates are derived using data from birth histories collected from women respondents

age 15 to 49 years. In a few countries, information on sibling survival, subsequently analyzed to derive estimates of adult mortality, has also been collected and compiled.

A new modified logit model life table system (Murray et al. 2003) allows for predicting an abridged life table using as inputs true or estimated levels of child and adult mortality or, if necessary, using only levels of child mortality. Recent work by Murray and colleagues has resulted in development of a validated life table system that uses a single global standard that represents the full range of mortality patterns seen in contemporary human populations; the system generates better predictions of age-specific mortality rates than the Coale-Demeny or original Brass systems.[2]

A set of 1,802 life tables, based on empirical data from national mortality registration systems between 1901 and 1999, were used to develop and test this model. These life tables were based on observed mortality risks in HIV-free populations, and hence, predicted life tables from the model can be used to estimate HIV-free age-specific mortality. In this context, estimates of child mortality from DHS surveys for the 52 countries in Sub-Saharan Africa were used to develop HIV-free envelopes of mortality at the national level. Steps 2 and 3 as described earlier were carried out for each country to construct a cause-specific mortality estimate without accounting for HIV, and as a final step, epidemiological estimates of HIV mortality were added on to derive the overall national age-, sex-, and cause-specific mortality estimate (Lopez et al. 2002). Figure 5.2 shows, by way of example, the final age-specific death rates for Zambia, for the year 2000. Note the markedly high death rates at young adult ages, including the deaths due to AIDS.

Compositional cause-of-death models have been developed around the relationship between cause-specific mortality and total mortality by age, as observed from patterns of causes of death recorded in nations with good vital registration systems (Salomon and Murray 2002). For each age-sex group an income variable for each observed country-year of data has been added to the model to strengthen the predicted proportionate composition by the three GBD cause groups. The models have been built using an empirical data set of 1,576 country-years of observations from 58 countries for the years 1950 to 1998. A set of regression equations have been developed that predict the cause composition of mortality by age, for a given input of total mortality by age and an estimate of national per capita gross domestic product (GDP). For each country, the estimate of total mortality by age and sex derived from the life tables (from step 1) and the national GDP are used as inputs, and the model produces an implied cause composition of

Figure 5.2 Estimated Age-Specific Death Rates for Zambia, 2000

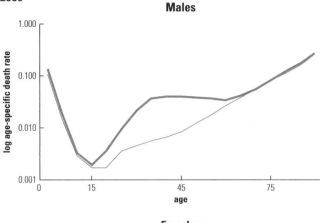

Males

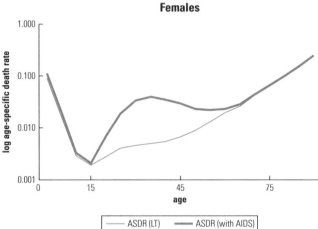

Females

| ——— ASDR (LT) | ▬▬▬ ASDR (with AIDS) |

Source: Authors.

Note: ASDR = age-specific death rate; LT = from model life tables for Zambia, 2000; graphs are in logarithmic scale.

Figure 5.3 Model-Based Predictions of GBD Cause–Group Composition of Mortality by Age and Sex, Zambia, 2000

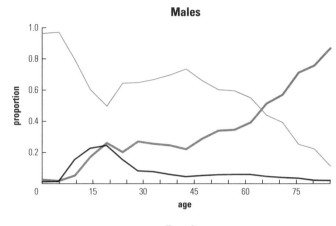

Males

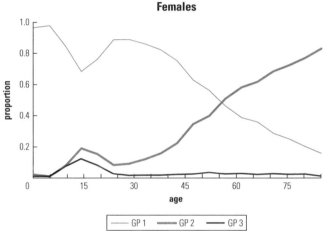

Females

| ——— GP 1 | ▬▬▬ GP 2 | ▬▬▬ GP 3 |

Source: Authors.

mortality by age and sex. Since the empirical data set for developing the regression equations does not include any information on mortality in countries experiencing AIDS epidemics, it is difficult to predict with confidence the proportions of deaths due to group 1 causes at different ages. Wherever possible, the outputs of the model were validated against compositional structures from available vital records data from the country or region and from small-scale longitudinal population surveillance systems. An example of the model outputs is shown in figure 5.3, depicting the predicted proportionate composition by age for males and females, respectively.

Communicable diseases (group 1) account for a large proportion of deaths at all ages up to about age 60. The proportions derived from the model are used to derive GBD group-specific numbers of deaths for each age group from the life table–derived total numbers of deaths in each age group. After this, information from vital records or specific disease epidemiological studies are used to construct the detailed cause-of-death estimates.

Epidemiological Estimates

Cause-of-death models in combination with life table–derived mortality risks and national population estimates provide an estimate of the numbers of deaths by age, sex, and broad-cause group. Estimating the numbers of deaths due to specific causes within each broad group—for example, the composition within group 1 due to different infectious diseases and perinatal disorders at infant ages or the composition within group 2 due to neoplasms, cardiovascular diseases, and other noncommunicable diseases at adult ages—is the next stage. The mass of epidemiological evidence on mortality due to different infectious diseases and maternal causes over the past two decades has been invaluable in this estimation process. Researchers have critically examined data from different studies and used them to derive independent epidemiological estimates of cause-specific mortality for the region. It is useful to examine in brief the results of these independent estimation exercises and to assess their plausibility with reference to an overall demographic envelope of mortality. We have included in this discussion results from such estimation exercises available for Africa in 2003. There is a need to conduct similar estimations for other important conditions, such as tuberculosis and road traffic accidents.

Malaria. Malaria is one disease that has been extensively researched in Africa. Snow and his colleagues initially estimated malaria mortality in the region for 1990 and later refined their approach to produce another set of estimates for 1995 (Snow et al. 1999). They integrated evidence from research on several aspects of the epidemiology of malaria. First, they used a detailed analysis of environmental factors that affect the distribution, seasonality, and transmission intensity to develop an epidemiological stratification of the continent into five regions based on climatic suitability for the existence and stability of malarial transmission. In the next step, they used geographical information systems to define at-risk populations within regions suitable for transmission based on different transmission scenarios as described. A specially constructed population database for more than 4,000 administrative units in Africa (Deichmann 1996) was used in this step. Finally, direct estimates of fatal risks for malarial mortality were selected from over 200 empirical data sources on the health impact of malaria, and these were combined with estimates of at-risk populations to derive age-specific estimates of deaths due to malaria in the region, as summarized in table 5.7. The median estimates were taken as the guideline for the GBD estimates for the entire region.

Diarrheal Diseases. Estimates of death rates due to diarrheal disease from epidemiological studies vary widely across populations, and within populations over time. Also,

complex interactions between intrinsic factors, such as nutritional status, and extrinsic factors, such as exposure to multiple infections, make the attribution of death to a single underlying cause extremely difficult. Kosek, Bern, and Guerrant (2003) reviewed 34 studies in 21 countries to derive an estimate of diarrheal mortality rates. Studies were included only if diarrheal deaths were ascertained through active surveillance, and in the selected studies only a primary cause listed as diarrhea was considered as a diarrheal death. As a result, they estimated a mortality rate of 4.9 per 1,000 children under five per year (95 percent confidence interval (CI), 1.0–9.1) in countries with high levels of overall child mortality. On a global scale, this appears as a decline from an estimated rate of 13.6 per 1,000 in 1982 (Snyder and Merson 1982).

In view of different cause-of-death attribution strategies in different settings, proportionate mortality due to diarrhea is considered as an alternate approach to estimating the number of deaths due to this cause. Morris, Black, and Tomaskovic (2003) developed a prediction model to estimate the distribution of deaths among children under five by cause. The model estimated that about 20 percent of all under-five deaths in Sub-Saharan Africa would be caused by diarrhea.

Table 5.8 shows the total population of children under age five in the region, and the estimate of diarrheal deaths on applying the median observed death rate of 4.9 per 1,000 (Kosek, Bern, and Guerrant 2003), and a proportionate mortality of 20 percent (Black, Morris, and Bryce 2003).

Vaccine-Preventable Diseases. Despite expansion in immunization services in the developing world, vaccine-

Table 5.7 Epidemiological Estimates of Malaria Mortality in Nonpregnant African Population, 1995

| Age group | Estimated deaths | | |
	Lower bound	Median	Upper bound
0 to 4	578,214	765,775	1,010,337
5 to 9	109,986	145,747	192,233
10 to 14	34,427	45,349	60,215
≥15	22,018	32,730	43,444
Total	744,645	986,601	1,306,229

Source: Adapted from Snow et al. 1999.

Table 5.8 Estimates of Diarrheal Deaths of Children under Five, 2000

Estimate based on death rates		
Under-five population in Sub-Saharan Africa		127,856,836
Estimated diarrheal death rate		4.9 per 1,000
Estimated diarrheal deaths	639,284	
Estimate based on proportionate mortality		
Under-five total deaths		4,475,675
Estimated diarrheal proportionate mortality		20%
Estimated diarrheal deaths	895,135	
GBD estimate	626,734	

Source: Estimate based on death rates adapted from Kosek, Bern, and Guerrant 2003; estimate based on proportional mortality from Black, Morris, and Bryce 2003; GBD estimate from WHO 2003.

preventable diseases remain significant causes of mortality in Africa. Stein and colleagues (2003) conducted an epidemiological exercise to estimate measles mortality. They used national-level information on vaccine coverage from health surveys and estimates of disease incidence, vaccine efficacy, and case fatality from specific epidemiological studies to develop a static model by which to estimate regional and global measles mortality. They estimated a total of 452,000 deaths due to measles in Sub-Saharan Africa in the year 2000, of which approximately three-fourths would occur among children under five.

Crowcroft and colleagues (2003) developed a model by which to estimate cases and deaths due to pertussis for the year 1999. Parameters used in the model included vaccine coverage and efficacy data and estimates of case-fatality ratios from epidemiological studies. Two coverage scenarios were used in the model, at levels below and above 70 percent, based on information from WHO reports adjusted by survey data where available. For each scenario, a different age structure was used to represent a range of possible patterns of infection in susceptible children. The model assumed a vaccine efficacy of 95 percent for preventing death. They estimated 170,000 deaths due to whooping cough in the African region in 1999.

Lower Respiratory Infections. Acute respiratory infections (ARI) are the third leading cause of death globally among children under five years of age. Much uncertainty surrounds the ascertainment of pneumonia as the underlying cause of death, principally from verbal autopsy–based studies in developing countries. In these settings, significant comorbidity exists in the form of measles, whooping cough, diarrheal diseases, or malaria. Williams and colleagues (2002) developed a model to predict the proportion of ARI mortality for a given level of under-five mortality. A review of 49 studies provided data on the level of child mortality and the proportion of deaths due to ARI. The researchers fitted a log linear curve to the data; from the resultant equation they estimated the number of deaths due to ARI for all countries, using WHO estimates of country-specific under-five mortality in the year 2000. Through this model they estimated a total of 794,000 deaths due to ARI in the region in the year 2000. The authors demonstrated that differences between predicted proportions from the model and observed proportions from verbal autopsy studies could be explained by the variability inherent with the use of verbal autopsy methods, induced by such comorbidity.

Maternal Mortality. Hill, AbouZahr, and Wardlaw (2001) in collaboration with researchers at the WHO collated available evidence on country-specific maternal mortality in the form of vital registration records, DHS-type sibling survival surveys, and special Reproductive Age Mortality Studies to develop a statistical model to predict the proportion of deaths of women of reproductive ages due to maternal causes (PMDF). The PMDF was found superior to the maternal mortality ratio (MMR) as the dependent variable for estimating the number of deaths from maternal causes, mainly because of its applicability to a demographic "envelope" of deaths at maternal ages. Also, information from national-level sisterhood surveys were found to yield more robust measures of PMDF than MMR to use as inputs in the construction of the model. Independent variables chosen to predict national PMDF were general fertility rate, female literacy, per capita income, percentage of deliveries attended by skilled attendants, country-specific estimates of HIV prevalence, and variables for region and level of vital registration in individual countries. The predicted PMDF for each country was then applied to age- and sex-specific mortality estimates from *World Population Prospects* (United Nations Population Division 1998), to derive the absolute numbers of deaths due to maternal causes. Based on the model, Hill, AbouZahr, and Wardlaw (2001) predicted a total of 272,500 maternal deaths in Sub-Saharan Africa for 1995, with a mean MMR of 1,006 per 100,000 live births.

HIV/AIDS. The Joint United Nations Programme on HIV/AIDS (UNAIDS) and the WHO established an Epidemiology Reference Group to work toward making estimates and projections of mortality on a biennial basis. Country-level information on prevalence of infection among attendants at antenatal clinics and sexually transmitted disease clinics and prevalence among other high-risk groups, such as intravenous drug users, homosexual males, and commercial sex workers, has been used to monitor epidemics at the country level. Using these data, an epidemiological model was developed that included the following parameters:

1. the initial rate (r) of spread of HIV as determined by the reproductive potential
2. the peak prevalence (f) as determined by the fraction of population at risk of infection
3. the final epidemic prevalence (ϕ) as determined by the behavioral response of the population
4. the start date of epidemics in individual countries.

A negative value of φ indicates that people become less likely to adopt risky behavior in response to observed AIDS mortality or prevention programs. Hence, apart from prevalence data from sentinel sites, behavioral surveys are essential to assess the potential of HIV epidemics and to estimate the size of at-risk populations.

An assessment of factors that affect survival of adults suggested that an overall median survival time of 9 years, with a range of uncertainty of 8 to 11 years, and a Weibull distribution of the survival function were used in the modeling process. For children, the survival curve was built to account for two periods of high mortality, which are infancy, when HIV frequently overwhelms the immature immune system, and after age nine years, when the response to HIV infection resembles that in adults. Overall, the survival curve for children predicts 40 percent survival from HIV-related mortality at five years of age.

The UNAIDS/WHO model was used to develop country-specific point estimates of HIV/AIDS mortality for 2001 (WHO and UNAIDS 2002). The estimated regional death toll from this disease for Sub-Saharan Africa stands at a total of 2.2 million deaths. Policy decisions aimed at addressing this epidemic should include activities aimed at improving such measurements.

Cancers. Ferlay and colleagues (2001) at the International Agency for Research in Cancer developed a data set of worldwide estimates of cancer incidence, mortality, and prevalence for the year 2000, which they called the Globocan 2000. Their mortality estimates were based on vital registration data where available; for other regions they used information from survival models derived from available cancer registry data (Sankaranarayan, Black, and Parkin 1998). These mortality estimates did not correct for underreporting in vital registration or for possible misclassification of causes of death.

As part of the GBD 2000 Study, Mathers, Shibuya et al. (2002) used relative interval survival data from the Surveillance Epidemiology and End Results (SEER) Program at the National Cancer Institute in the United States to develop an age-period-cohort survival model, which was further adjusted for levels of economic development. The model was then applied to age-, sex-, and site-specific incidence estimates from cancer registries that were compiled for the Globocan 2000 and from other specific incidence studies. The model was useful to smooth out random variations in observed incidence and survival rates that resulted from small numbers of cases or cases lost to follow up. The estimated cancer survival rates by site, age, and sex for different regions in the world were used as key inputs to estimate the distribution of cancer deaths by site. Estimates of cancer mortality by region were then developed (Shibuya et al. 2002), correcting for levels of overall mortality in regions with incomplete coverage of registration, and also correcting for the likely differences in cause-of-death patterns that would be expected in uncovered and often poorer subpopulations. As a result, the GBD 2000 Study estimated a total of 572,000 deaths due to cancer within the region.

War. Deaths due to war within Sub-Saharan Africa merit attention as an avoidable burden. Murray and colleagues (2002) used a comprehensive analysis of media reports, vital registration records, and adjustments based on observed relationships between direct and indirect mortality to estimate the global burden of mortality due to armed conflict. Keeping in mind the limitations of estimates based largely on qualitative analysis of media reports, conservative estimates were used for some of the major conflicts in the world. According to these estimates, armed conflicts had resulted in an overall death toll of about 77,000 for Sub-Saharan Africa for the year 2001.

Estimating Cause-Specific Mortality

Using all the various dimensions of cause-specific mortality estimation for Sub-Saharan Africa—available data from vital records, specific studies, and global disease epidemiological extrapolations for the region—we have prepared estimates of causes of death in Sub-Saharan Africa based on the GBD approach. Figure 5.4 summarizes the estimation process for countries within the region.

As mentioned earlier, predicted proportions for broad-cause groups by age and sex were validated against information from country-specific vital records where available and for neighboring or epidemiologically similar countries where possible. Also, wherever applicable, cause-specific proportions from vital records for specific causes were used in deriving population-level estimates for these causes. The resultant cause-specific structure was finally adjusted with disease-specific mortality estimates to produce the overall numbers of deaths by age, sex, and cause. National estimates were summed up to totals for two subregions and for Sub-Saharan Africa as a whole. During this process of synthesizing epidemiological estimates into the overall demographic and cause-of-death model based on the broad-cause group

Figure 5.4 Summary of GBD Process for Estimating Cause-Specific Mortality in African Countries

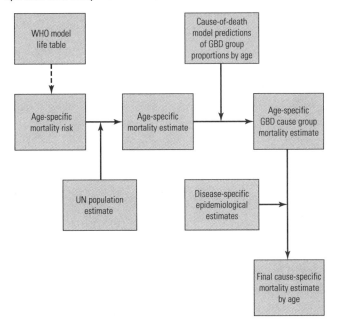

Source: Authors.

envelope of mortality, some of the disease-specific estimates described earlier were reduced to meet these envelope constraints.

RESULTS AND DISCUSSION

Distinct differences exist between countries belonging to the two epidemiological subregions, essentially divided by the level of HIV/AIDS-related mortality within them.

Overall, we estimate that about 10.8 million deaths (table 5.9) occurred in the year 2002 in the region, or just under 20 percent of global mortality. The age structure of mortality roughly divides into 46 percent of deaths occurring before the age of 15 years, another 36 percent between the ages of 15 and 59 years, and the remaining 18 percent at age 60 and above.

It is not surprising, therefore, that five of the six estimated leading causes of mortality in Sub-Saharan Africa are

Table 5.9 GBD Estimates of Leading Causes of Death, by Sex, 2000

Cause of death in all persons (10,778,044)	Total deaths (%)	Cause of death in males (5,557,783)	Total deaths (%)	Cause of death in females (5,220,261)	Total deaths (%)
1 HIV/AIDS	20.4	1 HIV/AIDS	19.4	1 HIV/AIDS	21.6
2 Malaria	10.1	2 Lower respiratory infections	10.3	2 Malaria	11.0
3 Lower respiratory infections	9.8	3 Malaria	9.3	3 Lower respiratory infections	9.3
4 Diarrheal diseases	6.5	4 Diarrheal diseases	6.6	4 Diarrheal diseases	6.3
5 Perinatal conditions	5.1	5 Perinatal conditions	5.8	5 Perinatal conditions	4.5
6 Measles	4.1	6 Measles	4.0	6 Measles	4.2
7 Cerebrovascular disease	3.3	7 Tuberculosis	3.8	7 Cerebrovascular disease	4.1
8 Ischemic heart disease	3.1	8 Ischemic heart disease	3.1	8 Ischemic heart disease	3.1
9 Tuberculosis	2.8	9 Cerebrovascular disease	2.6	9 Tuberculosis	1.8
10 Road traffic accidents	1.8	10 Road traffic accidents	2.4	10 Pertussis	1.6
11 Pertussis	1.6	11 Violence	1.9	11 Road traffic accidents	1.2
12 Violence	1.2	12 Pertussis	1.5	12 Maternal hemorrhage	1.1
13 COPD	1.1	13 War	1.5	13 Nephritis and nephrosis	1.1
14 Tetanus	1.0	14 COPD	1.3	14 Tetanus	1.0
15 Nephritis and nephrosis	0.9	15 Tetanus	1.0	15 Diabetes mellitus	1.0
16 Malnutrition	0.9	16 Malnutrition	1.0	16 Malnutrition	0.8
17 War	0.8	17 Drownings	0.9	17 Maternal sepsis	0.8
18 Syphilis	0.8	18 Syphilis	0.9	18 COPD	0.8
19 Diabetes mellitus	0.7	19 Nephritis and nephrosis	0.8	19 Syphilis	0.8
20 Drownings	0.6	20 Prostate cancer	0.7	20 Hypertensive heart disease	0.8
21 All other specific causes	23.2	21 All other specific causes	21.4	21 All other specific causes	23.2

Source: Authors.
Note: COPD = chronic obstructive pulmonary disease.

Table 5.10 GBD Estimates of Leading Causes of Death in AFR D and AFR E, 2000

Cause of death in AFR D persons (4,634,295)	Total deaths (%)	Cause of death in AFR E persons (6,143,749)[a]	Total deaths (%)
1 Malaria	11.6	1 HIV/AIDS	28.4
2 Lower respiratory infections	11.3	2 Malaria	8.9
3 HIV/AIDS	9.8	3 Lower respiratory infections	8.6
4 Diarrheal diseases	7.4	4 Diarrheal diseases	5.8
5 Perinatal conditions	6.1	5 Perinatal conditions	4.4
6 Measles	5.6	6 Cerebrovascular disease	3.1
7 Cerebrovascular disease	3.7	7 Tuberculosis	3.0
8 Ischemic heart disease	3.5	8 Measles	2.9
9 Tuberculosis	2.6	9 Ischemic heart disease	2.8
10 Pertussis	2.2	10 Road traffic accidents	1.6
11 Road traffic accidents	2.1	11 Violence	1.3
12 Tetanus	1.4	12 War	1.2
13 Violence	1.2	13 Pertussis	1.2
14 COPD	1.1	14 COPD	1.1
15 Malnutrition	1.0	15 Nephritis and nephrosis	0.8
16 Nephritis and nephrosis	1.0	16 Malnutrition	0.8
17 Syphilis	0.9	17 Syphilis	0.8
18 Drownings	0.8	18 Tetanus	0.7
19 Diabetes mellitus	0.8	19 Diabetes mellitus	0.7
20 Hypertensive heart disease	0.6	20 Congenital anomalies	0.6
21 All other specific causes	25.3	21 All other specific causes	21.3

Source: Authors.
Note: COPD = chronic obstructive pulmonary disease.
a. AFR E subregion includes countries with high HIV prevalence.

those that cause deaths at childhood ages, namely, infectious diseases and conditions originating in the perinatal period (also see table 5.10). About 20 percent of the estimated 2.2 million deaths due to HIV/AIDS are also predicted to occur in childhood. Although the rank order of tuberculosis is almost similar in males (7) and females (9), the estimated number of deaths in males (about 210,000) is more than double that predicted in females (95,000). Similarly, road traffic accidents, chronic obstructive pulmonary disease, and war were estimated to cause more than double the number of deaths in males than in females. In the entire region, maternal conditions are estimated to cause 4.4 percent of deaths in females.

A subregional disaggregation of the magnitude of cause-specific mortality sheds more light on the epidemiological variation possible in Sub-Saharan Africa. Two-thirds of the total mortality occurs in countries within the AFR E region, which contains just over half (54 percent) of the regional population. A comparison of the rank structure of leading causes of death between the two epidemiological subregions, AFR D and AFR E, is shown in table 5.10.

The threefold difference in rank and percentage of deaths caused by HIV/AIDS between the two regions translates into a nearly fourfold difference in absolute numbers of deaths. There is reasonable similarity in the rank order and magnitude of the other leading causes, when deaths due to all ages are combined. The importance of war as a cause of death at all ages in AFR E stands out, being ranked as the 12th leading cause.

At childhood ages, the rank structure and proportion of deaths from individual leading causes is almost similar in the two regions, and between males and females, except for the HIV/AIDS subregional difference mentioned earlier. Overall, the subregional proportions of child mortality are nearly equal; 48 percent of deaths occur in AFR D, and 52 percent occur in AFR E. Sex differentials too are slight, with 52 percent of deaths in males and 48 percent in females.

Table 5.11 shows the leading causes of child deaths for the two subregions together. As expected, estimated leading causes in Sub-Saharan Africa are infectious diseases, perinatal conditions, and malnutrition. Two important implications of these observations are that childhood mortality remains a

Table 5.11 GBD Estimates of Leading Causes of Death at Age 0 to 14 Years, 2000

Cause of death in males (2,594,761)	Total deaths (%)	Cause of death in females (2,368,129)	Total deaths (%)
1 Malaria	18.1	1 Malaria	22.0
2 Lower respiratory infections	17.2	2 Lower respiratory infections	14.2
3 Diarrheal diseases	12.7	3 Diarrheal diseases	12.6
4 Perinatal conditions	12.4	4 Perinatal conditions	9.8
5 HIV/AIDS	8.5	5 Measles	9.1
6 Measles	8.4	6 HIV/AIDS	9.0
7 Pertussis	3.3	7 Pertussis	3.6
8 Road traffic accidents	2.0	8 Tetanus	1.8
9 Tetanus	1.7	9 Protein-energy malnutrition	1.5
10 Protein-energy malnutrition	1.6	10 Road traffic accidents	1.3
11 All other causes	14.2	11 All other causes	15.0

Source: Authors.

Table 5.12 GBD Estimates of Leading Causes of Death at Age 15 to 59 Years, Subregional Comparison, 2000

Cause of death in AFR D persons (1,352,164)	Total deaths (%)	Cause of death in AFR E persons (2,536,058)	Total deaths (%)
1 HIV/AIDS	25.8	1 HIV/AIDS	54.1
2 Tuberculosis	6.7	2 Tuberculosis	5.3
3 Lower respiratory infections	5.6	3 Lower respiratory infections	3.2
4 Violence	3.5	4 War	2.7
5 Road traffic accidents	3.5	5 Violence	2.6
6 Cerebrovascular disease	3.1	6 Road traffic accidents	1.9
7 Ischemic heart disease	2.6	7 Cerebrovascular disease	1.8
8 Malaria	2.3	8 Ischemic heart disease	1.5
9 Syphilis	2.2	9 Maternal hemorrhage	1.3
10 Maternal hemorrhage	1.9	10 Malaria	1.2

Source: Authors.

major cause of burden in Sub-Saharan Africa and that there is no difference in the magnitude of the burden between different populations within the region.

When comparing mortality during adulthood, however, there are sizable differences, both between the two subregions and, within each subregion, between males and females. The mortality differences between the two subregions, as seen from the leading causes for both sexes combined, are shown in table 5.12.

The most striking feature is that the estimated number of deaths at these ages in AFR E is nearly double that estimated for AFR D. Readers will recall that the number of childhood deaths in the two regions is nearly equal. From table 5.12 it is clear that in AFR E, the HIV/AIDS epidemic and in specific countries, armed conflicts are the causes of the excess mortality. Clearly, the number of deaths from each of the leading causes is significantly higher in AFR E, despite a somewhat similar rank structure of causes apart from HIV/AIDS and war.

As observed at childhood ages, the difference between mortality in males and that in females is minimal (52 to 48). The leading causes of mortality in each sex in AFR E are shown in table 5.13.

Apart from the high burden of mortality due to infectious diseases, it is evident that injury-related causes of death among males, pregnancy-related causes among females, and cardiovascular diseases in both sexes are major issues to be dealt with. The high mortality due to HIV/AIDS in both sexes has a major bearing on the occurrence of orphanhood within these countries.

Table 5.13 GBD Estimates of Leading Causes of Death in AFR E at Age 15 to 59 Years: Comparison between Males and Females, 2000

Cause of death in males (1,308,048)	Total deaths (%)	Cause of death in females (1,228,010)	Total deaths (%)
1 HIV/AIDS	50.3	1 HIV/AIDS	58.1
2 Tuberculosis	7.4	2 Lower respiratory infections	3.8
3 War	4.8	3 Tuberculosis	3.2
4 Violence	4.2	4 Maternal hemorrhage	2.6
5 Road traffic accidents	2.8	5 Cerebrovascular disease	2.0
6 Lower respiratory infections	2.7	6 Maternal sepsis	1.9
7 Ischemic heart disease	1.8	7 Abortion	1.4
8 Cerebrovascular disease	1.7	8 Hypertensive disorders of pregnancy	1.4
9 Malaria	1.1	9 Malaria	1.4
10 Syphilis	1.0	10 Ischemic heart disease	1.2

Source: Authors.

Table 5.14 GBD Estimates of Leading Causes of Death at Age 60 Years and Older: Comparison between Males and Females, 2000

Cause of death in males (953,391)	Total deaths (%)	Cause of death in females (973,542)	Total deaths (%)
1 Ischemic heart disease	13.4	1 Cerebrovascular disease	17.0
2 Cerebrovascular disease	10.8	2 Ischemic heart disease	13.4
3 Lower respiratory infections	6.5	3 Lower respiratory infections	5.6
4 COPD	6.1	4 Nephritis and nephrosis	3.8
5 Prostate cancer	4.0	5 Diabetes mellitus	3.7
6 Tuberculosis	3.1	6 COPD	3.5
7 HIV/AIDS	2.9	7 Hypertensive heart disease	3.2
8 Nephritis and nephrosis	2.9	8 Diarrheal diseases	2.6
9 Diarrheal diseases	2.3	9 HIV/AIDS	2.3
10 Diabetes mellitus	1.9	10 Cervix uteri cancer	2.3

Source: Authors.
Note: COPD = chronic destructive pulmonary disease.

The subregional differences in mortality among the elderly is similar to that observed in children: 47 percent in AFR D and 53 percent in AFR E. The leading causes of death at these ages are similar for the two mortality strata. For convenience, the discussion here will focus on the difference in the cause-of-death structure between the two sexes, aggregated for both regions together or, in other words, for Sub-Saharan Africa.

As expected, in both sexes, cardiovascular diseases are estimated as the leading causes of mortality among the elderly (table 5.14). Among males, chronic obstructive pulmonary disease and prostate cancer are other leading causes, whereas in women, kidney disorders and diabetes mellitus are major causes of mortality. Cirrhosis of the liver is estimated as the 11th leading cause in males; the corresponding rank for women is taken by breast cancer. The presence

of lower respiratory infections, tuberculosis, diarrheal diseases, and HIV/AIDS among the leading causes of death in both sexes, even among the elderly, clearly defines the importance of communicable disease control in African countries.

CONCLUSION

Estimating cause-specific mortality in Sub-Saharan Africa poses a major epidemiological challenge. The availability of data and information on causes of death has increased within the region, and the results lead us to a few important observations. First, childhood mortality is a major cause of the high premature mortality rates in Africa, accounting for nearly half the total mortality in the region. As a corollary, the observed leading causes of childhood mortality—malaria, diarrheal diseases, measles, lower respiratory tract infections, and conditions originating in the perinatal period—require immediate attention.

Second, the young adult population in countries within the AFR E mortality subregion is at significant risk of possible premature death from HIV/AIDS, armed conflict and other forms of violence, road traffic accidents, tuberculosis, and, among women, causes related to pregnancy and childbearing.

Third, nearly a fifth of the mortality in the region occurs among individuals age 60 years and older. The proportion of deaths at these ages is much less than that observed in developed countries. For instance, in Australia, over 80 percent of deaths occur above the age of 60 years (ABS 2003). However, in Sub-Saharan Africa, the absolute number of deaths itself—1.92 million—merits attention to the health needs of the elderly. At these ages, cardiovascular disease, chronic obstructive pulmonary disease, cancers (prostate cancer in males, cervix and breast cancer in females), and, notably, infectious diseases are the major causes of mortality.

It is generally accepted that statistics from complete vital registration systems are the "gold standard" for national mortality statistics. Although cause-of-death information from vital records is subject to some biases on account of quality of cause-of-death attribution within the system, there is ample global evidence to justify a reliance on such data for national cause-specific mortality analysis and estimation.

It is heartening to note that countries within the region are making special efforts to improve vital registration systems. The process, however, involves huge resources, and can be expected to take decades before data of reasonable quality from national vital registration systems will be available for such estimation exercises. It has been observed in Kenya, South Africa, and Zimbabwe that although the coverage of registration of vital events by age and sex can be improved rapidly by instituting certain administrative reforms, obtaining information on the cause of death remains elusive, on account of deaths occurring at home in the absence of medical attention in remote areas.

An alternative system that has been tested and found effective has been sample registration, as has been employed in India and China. A representative sample of villages or population clusters is routinely monitored for vital events, and upon death, a formal verbal autopsy procedure is employed to ascertain its probable cause. Initiatives such as the Health Metrics Network (established by the WHO) are currently devising a framework for testing and establishing the Sample Vital Registration and Verbal Autopsy method of obtaining information on causes of death for national mortality estimation purposes. This is the most viable interim solution to meet requirements of data for both health policy as well as for monitoring the impact of health programs and interventions. The GBD method of estimation, with the extensive use of models and extrapolations from specific epidemiological studies, may not be useful for the monitoring function.

Another area of data collection that warrants attention at this stage is the function of physician certification of cause of death and the implementation of guidelines, based on the International Classification of Diseases, for coding and classification of causes of death. Capacity building in these areas will assist national health information systems in providing useful information on causes of death, at least in urban areas, where a significant number of deaths would occur in hospitals or where the deceased may have been attended by a physician in the time immediately preceding death.

Undoubtedly, there is vast uncertainty about causes of death in Africa, but enough is currently known to prepare preliminary estimates, adhering to a rigorous scientific framework for evaluation of data quality and ensuring substantial prudence in interpreting the findings. What data are available suggest that further, massive responses to the HIV epidemic are needed and that major communicable diseases and maternal health require scaled-up investments. Prevention of injuries, in part from war, would contribute much to the improvement of health and survival of young adult males. But what is most urgently needed is investment in cost-effective methods to monitor mortality if we are not to be similarly ignorant about health conditions in Africa 10 years hence.

NOTES

1. **AFR D** (high child and high adult mortality): Algeria, Angola, Benin, Burkina Faso, Cameroon, Cape Verde, Chad, Comoros, Equatorial Guinea, Gabon, The Gambia, Ghana, Guinea-Bissau, Liberia, Madagascar, Mali, Mauritania, Mauritius, Niger, Nigeria, São Tomé and Principe, Senegal, Seychelles, Sierra Leone, Togo. **AFR E** (high child and very high adult mortality): Botswana, Burundi, Central African Republic, Côte d'Ivoire, Democratic Republic of Congo, Eritrea, Ethiopia, Kenya, Lesotho, Malawi, Mozambique, Namibia, the Republic of Congo, Rwanda, South Africa, Swaziland, Uganda, Tanzania, Zambia, Zimbabwe.

2. The Coale-Demeny system is a system of model life tables that predicts age-specific mortality rates based on two parameters only, the level of (usually child) mortality in any age group and some idea of the relationship between infant and child mortality, which define the family (N, S, E, W). The Brass logit system is a relational model life table system that predicts the set of age-specific death rates from knowledge of any two rates (usually child and adult ages 15–59) and the choice of a survival curve as standard.

REFERENCES

ABS (Australian Bureau of Statistics). 2003. *Deaths Australia*. Vol. 3302. Annual report. Canberra: ABS.

Adetunji, J. A., C. J. Murray, and T. Evans. 1996. "Causes of Death in Africa: A Review." Paper presented at a meeting of the Population Association of America, New Orleans, May.

Black, R. E., S. S. Morris, and J. Bryce. 2003. "Where and Why Are 10 Million Children Dying Every Year?" *Lancet* 361: 2226–34.

Brass, W. 1968. *Demography of Tropical Africa*. Princeton, NJ: Princeton University Press.

Cliff, J., J. Sacarlal, O. Augusto, A. Nóvoa, M. Dgedge, G. Machatine, and H. Cossa. 2003. *Estudos das principais causas de morte registadas, nas citades des Maputo, Beira, Chimoio e Nampula, em 2001*. Maputo City, Mozambique: Ministerio de Saude.

Crowcroft, N. S., C. Stein, P. Duclos, and M. Birmingham. 2003. "How Best to Estimate the Global Burden of Pertussis?" *Lancet Infectious Diseases* 3: 413–18.

Deichmann, U. 1996. African Population Database. Digital Database and Documentation. National Center for Geographical Information and Analysis, University of California, Santa Barbara. http://www.glowa-volta.de/cd_v3.1/landuse/populat/africa.htm.

Dorrington, R., D. Bourne, D. Bradshaw, R. Laubscher, and I. Timaeus. 2001. *The Impact of HIV/AIDS on Adult Mortality in South Africa*. Cape Town: Medical Research Council.

Feachem, R. G., and D. T. Jamison, eds. 1991. *Disease and Mortality in Sub-Saharan Africa*. New York: Oxford University Press.

Feachem, R. G., D. T. Jamison, and E. R. Bos. 1993. "Changing Patterns of Disease and Mortality in Sub-Saharan Africa." In *Disease and Mortality in Sub-Saharan Africa*, ed. R. G. Feachem and D. T. Jamison. New York: New York University Press.

Ferlay, J., F. Bray, P. Pisani, and D. M. Parkin. 2001. *Globocan 2000: Cancer Incidence, Mortality and Prevalence Worldwide*. Version 1. IARC CancerBase 5. Lyons: IARC Press.

Hill, K., C. AbouZahr, and T. Wardlaw. 2001. "Estimates of Maternal Mortality for 1995." *Bulletin of the World Health Organization* 79 (3): 182–98.

Kosek, M., C. Bern, and R. Guerrant. 2003. "The Global Burden of Diarrhoeal Disease, as Estimated from Studies Published between 1992 and 2000." *Bulletin of the World Health Organization* 81 (3): 197–204.

Kowal, P., C. Rao, and C. D. Mathers. 2003. *Report on a WHO Workshop: Minimum Dataset on Ageing and Adult Mortality in Sub Saharan Africa*. Geneva: WHO.

Lopez, A. D., O. B. Ahmad, M. Guillot, B. D. Ferguson, J. A. Salomon, C. J. L. Murray, and K. H. Hill. 2002. *World Mortality in 2000: Life Tables for 191 Countries*. Geneva: WHO.

Mathers, C. D., K. Shibuya, C. Boschi-Pinto, A. D. Lopez, and C. J. Murray. 2002. "Global and Regional Estimates of Cancer Incidence and Mortality by Site. I. Application of Regional Cancer Survival Model to Estimate Cancer Mortality Distribution by Site." *BMC Cancer* 2 (1): 36.

Mathers, C. D., C. Stein, D. Mafat, C. Rao, M. Inoue, N. Tomijima, C. Bernard, A. D. Lopez, and C. J. L. Murray. 2002. "Global Burden of Disease 2000. Version 2: Methods and Results." GPE discussion paper 50, WHO, Geneva.

Morris, S. S., R. E. Black, and L. Tomaskovic. 2003. "Predicting the Distribution of Under-Five Deaths by Cause in Countries without Adequate Vital Registration Systems. *International Journal of Epidemiology* 32 (6): 1041–51.

Murray, C. J. L., B. D. Ferguson, A. D. Lopez, M. Guillot, J. A. Salomon, and O. Ahmad. 2003. "Modified Logit Life Table System: Principles, Empirical Validation, and Application." *Population Studies* 57 (2): 165–82.

Murray, C. J. L., G. King, A. D. Lopez, N. Tomijima, and E. G. Krug. 2002. "Armed Conflict As a Public Health Problem." *British Medical Journal* 324 (7333): 346–49.

Murray, C. J. L., and A. D. Lopez, eds. 1996. *The Global Burden of Disease*. Cambridge, MA.: Harvard University Press.

Preston, S. H. 1976. *Mortality Patterns in National Populations: With Special Reference to Recorded Causes of Death*. New York: Academic Press.

Ravaoarimalala, C., R. Andriamahenina, B. Ravelojaona, D. Rabeson, J. Andriamiadana, J. F. May, F. Behets, and A. Rasamindrakotroka. 1998. "AIDS in Madagascar. II. Intervention Policy for Maintaining Low HIV Infection Prevalence." *Bulletin de la Société de Pathologie Exotique*. 91 (1): 71–73.

Salomon, J. A., and C. J. L. Murray. 2002. "The Epidemiologic Transition Revisited: Compositional Models for Causes of Death by Age and Sex." *Population and Development Review* 28 (2): 205–28.

Sankaranarayan, R., R. J. Black, and D. M. Parkin. 1998. *Cancer Survival in Developing Countries*. IARC Scientific Publications 145. Lyons: IARC Press.

Shibuya, K., C. D. Mathers, C. Boschi-Pinto, A. D. Lopez, and C. J. Murray. 2002. "Global and Regional Estimates of Cancer Incidence and Mortality by Site. II. Results of the Global Burden of Disease 2000." *BMC Cancer* 2 (1): 37.

Snow, R. W., M. Craig, U. Deichmann, and K. Marsh. 1999. "Estimating Mortality, Morbidity, and Disability Due to Malaria among Africa's Non-Pregnant Population." *Bulletin of the World Health Organization* 77 (8): 624–40.

Snyder, J. D., and M. H. Merson. 1982. "The Magnitude of the Global Problem of Acute Diarrhoeal Disease: A Review of Active Surveillance Data." *Bulletin of the World Health Organization* 60: 604–13.

Stein, C. E., M. Birmingham, M. Kurian, P. Duclos, and P. Strebel. 2003. "The Global Burden of Measles in the Year 2000—A Model That Uses Country Specific Indicators." *Journal of Infectious Diseases* 187 (Suppl. 1): S8–14.

United Nations Population Division. 1998. *World Population Prospects: The 1998 Revision*. New York: United Nations.

Waltisperger, D. M., P. Cantrelle, and O. Ralijaona. 1998. *La mortalite a Antananarivo de 1984 a 1995*. Paris: Centre Population et Développement.

WHO (World Health Organization). 2003. *World Health Report 2003—Shaping the Future*. Geneva: WHO.

WHO (World Health Organization) and UNAIDS (Joint United Nations Programme on HIV/AIDS). 2002. "Improved Methods and Assumptions for Estimation of the HIV/AIDS Epidemic and Its Impact: Recommendations of the UNAIDS Reference Group on Estimations, Modeling and Projections." *AIDS* 16: W1–W14.

Williams, B. G., E. Gouws, C. Boschi-Pinto, J. Bryce, and C. Dye. 2002. "Estimates of World-Wide Distribution of Child Deaths from Acute Respiratory Infections." *Lancet* 2: 25–32.

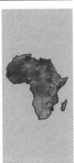

Chapter 6

Population and Mortality after AIDS

Rodolfo A. Bulatao

The acquired immune deficiency syndrome (AIDS) affects population size and composition in several ways. In particular age groups, deaths increase directly from AIDS and may also increase indirectly, as orphans, for instance, face higher mortality risks. Fertility can be affected, not only biologically but also from changes in sexual behavior. Communities may be weakened, and migration may alter the geographic distribution of the population.

This chapter draws on the work of agencies that produce global population projections to discuss the overall population effect of AIDS in Sub-Saharan African countries. It does not attempt to elucidate all the mechanisms involved—each of which deserves separate attention. Instead, the chapter focuses on the broad demographic impact. Decades after the start of the epidemics, estimates of this impact generally ignore all subtle and indirect effects and cover only the additional mortality directly from AIDS. Even this impact is highly uncertain. There is general agreement on substantial impact but no consensus on how substantial and long lasting it is.

APPROACH AND DATA

The projections of demographic impact to be considered come from three agencies: the Population Division of the United Nations (UN), the U.S. Census Bureau, and the World Bank. Each agency has produced population projections for most countries for some time. Up to 50 Sub-Saharan countries or territories are covered, although the smallest ones are left out in some data series. For at least a decade, these agencies have explicitly incorporated the effect of AIDS in selected countries. In general, mortality due to AIDS is added to a life table for a given country, and then overall mortality is projected into the future together with other vital parameters in order to project population. Possible effects of AIDS on fertility (for example, Zaba and Gregson 1998) and migration, except for indirect effects of mortality change, are not modeled.

The projections vary not only because of the mortality assumptions but also because of assumptions about initial population size and composition and fertility and migration trends. These differences are not detailed here. A recent description and results are in United Nations 2003a, 2003b, 2004; for the other two sets of projections, recent descriptions are difficult to find, but one might consult earlier descriptions in McDevitt 1999, Bos and colleagues 1994, and National Research Council 2000. Results are in Stanecki 2004 and World Bank 2004.

Although the approach to incorporating AIDS mortality in the projections is similar across agencies, important details are different. Agencies differ in how initial levels of mortality are estimated and projected and how AIDS mortality is projected.

United Nations Population Division

The Population Division of the UN seeks to apply country life tables where available but mostly uses UN model life tables. These are projected with reference to life expectancy, with gains expected to diminish as life expectancy rises. In the medium scenario (the only one considered here), the annual gain is 0.4 years for males and 0.5 years for females from a life expectancy level for both sexes combined of 60 years, but the gain shrinks to 0.1 years for males and 0.2 years for females when life expectancy reaches 75 years.

AIDS mortality is added to the life tables for 38 of the 50 countries or territories in Sub-Saharan Africa. The remainder, with reported low prevalence of the human immunodeficiency virus (HIV) or no data from UNAIDS, are island countries, except for Mauritania, Niger, Senegal, and Somalia. A criterion of HIV prevalence no higher than 1 percent appears to be used in excluding countries, but the size of the affected population is also taken into account. (This is noticeable mainly outside Sub-Saharan Africa, because AIDS mortality is also added for China.)

To add AIDS mortality, a separate projection of HIV/AIDS in the population is necessary. The procedure begins with reported levels of HIV prevalence among adults. With appropriate assumptions, the UN back-calculates the incidence of HIV and distributes cases by sex and age. From the size of the infected population and the remaining, susceptible population, the UN estimates the trend in subsequent infections. It derives mortality associated with AIDS given assumptions about the progression of the infection and adds additional mortality from perinatal infections. Life tables are adjusted for the additional mortality.

The Population Division has described the procedure for estimating AIDS mortality, which follows the recommendations of the Joint United Nations Programme on HIV/AIDS (UNAIDS) Reference Group on Estimates, Modelling and Projections (UNAIDS Reference Group 2002), in *World Population Prospects: The 2004 Revision* (United Nations 2004, 136–79). Calculations start with estimates of HIV prevalence over time, mainly estimates for pregnant women from antenatal clinics. The future trend of AIDS mortality is basically an extrapolation, with appropriate adjustments, from this trend. HIV prevalence estimates as of 2001 are taken from UNAIDS Reference Group 2002. For Djibouti, Gabon, Guinea, and Liberia, UNAIDS (2002) reports no estimate, and the UN Population Division makes its own. The source of estimates prior to 2001, used to establish a trend, is not specified, but is presumably the database maintained by the U.S. Census Bureau and similar sources. Although an attempt is made to match the UNAIDS (2002) estimate for 2001, fitting a trend sometimes leads to an HIV prevalence figure that varies from it, by a maximum of 2 percentage points (for Botswana) or 12 percent (for Uganda).

U.S. Census Bureau

The U.S. Census Bureau follows a similar but not identical procedure (Stanecki 2004). Usually, a life expectancy target is set in the future without considering AIDS, and logistic curves represent the trend to this target, with appropriate life tables generated to match it. AIDS mortality is added for 37 Sub-Saharan countries. In contrast to the countries covered by the UN Population Division, the Census Bureau does not introduce AIDS-specific deaths for Equatorial Guinea, The Gambia, and Sudan but does cover Niger and Senegal. The criterion for inclusion is national HIV prevalence above 1 percent (as estimated by UNAIDS for 1999), HIV prevalence of 5 percent or more in low-risk urban populations, or a prevalence trend that suggests the latter level will soon be reached.

Instead of modeling the AIDS epidemic in each country separately, the bureau takes a shortcut. It defines five epidemic scenarios, progressively more severe, ranging from a "low" to a "super high" epidemic, each starting at an indefinite date. These scenarios are developed using a program labeled iwgAIDS (Stanley et al. 1991), which models the spread of HIV infections, the development of AIDS, and subsequent deaths in a population. Each scenario incorporates the effect of increased condom use and shows HIV prevalence eventually plateauing and declining.

Each country is assigned to a scenario, or more precisely to an interpolated scenario between an assigned pair of these five. The assignment is made by matching the reported trend in HIV prevalence in urban areas to scenario trends. Total country prevalence is then used to determine dates for the epidemic. It is assumed that HIV prevalence will peak in 2010 and AIDS mortality will decline to zero by 2070. AIDS deaths are therefore added to the life table, from the projected epidemic, up to 2070, at which time the life table reverts to what it would be without the epidemic.

Uganda is treated as a special case, because of a reported decline in prevalence from the mid-1990s, which violates the assumption of a 2010 peak. Separate epidemics are modeled: a high one up to 1995 and a low one from 2005 on, with an interpolated epidemic in the intervening period.

The initial HIV national prevalence levels used are similar to those adopted by UNAIDS, relying heavily on reported infections among pregnant women. In this, the bureau projections resemble those of the UN Population Division. However, the future trend imposed on prevalence is unusual. The year 2010 represents a later peak to the epidemics than projected by the UN, in most cases. Peak incidence, in 55 percent of the Sub-Saharan cases in the UN projections, is before 1995, and in 95 percent of the cases before 2000. Although prevalence tends to peak later than incidence, this is unlikely to adequately account for the long delays between UN incidence peaks and Census Bureau prevalence peaks.

World Bank

World Bank mortality projections begin with life tables that already incorporate AIDS. However, these life tables, developed by the World Health Organization (WHO) for 2000, are constructed in a familiar way, with AIDS mortality being added to mortality from all other causes.

The WHO takes estimates of child mortality ($_5q_0$) and adult mortality ($_{45}q_{15}$) and expands them into life tables for each country, using the Brass logit approach (Murray et al. 2000; Lopez et al. 2001). The child mortality estimates were selected from survey and census estimates after systematic review of available statistics (Ahmad, Lopez, and Inoue 2000). The adult mortality estimates were more problematic. For Africa, plausible national estimates in the literature prior to 1990 (to exclude the effect of AIDS) were used, supplemented where necessary with UN estimates (United Nations 1998), and projected forward to 1999 and, later, 2000.

To add AIDS mortality, the WHO begins with reported HIV prevalence (based, as usual, on pregnant women) and works backward to HIV incidence and then forward to obtain an overall AIDS mortality level. (The researchers caution, based on preliminary work for Zimbabwe, that "these models may overestimate the level of the epidemic" [Salomon, Gakidou, and Murray 1999, 8], a point we return to below.) An age pattern of deaths, based on limited data from Tanzania, South Africa, and Zimbabwe (Lopez et al. 2001), is imposed, and AIDS mortality is then added to the life table.

In projecting mortality forward from the initial life tables taken from the WHO, the World Bank does not attempt to model the HIV/AIDS epidemics in any way, but simply assumes that their effect will gradually be reduced to zero by 2020 at the latest (depending on the country), at which time country mortality trends resume a standard pattern used in the Bank's projections.

Comparisons

Counterfactual projections that include no effect of AIDS are useful in assessing impact. Only the UN Population Division provides detailed results for such a scenario. The bureau has run such scenarios and provides brief descriptions but quite limited numerical information on the results (Stanecki 2004). The World Bank has no such scenario. Most comparisons to be made, therefore, will rely on the UN no-AIDS scenario.

It is not obvious from the approach taken in each projection set which should show the greatest current impact of AIDS on population and mortality. For future impact, however, a possible order emerges. Because the Census Bureau assumes a relatively late peak to the epidemics, one might expect greater demographic impact in its projections. Because the World Bank assumes a fairly direct decline in mortality impact, with the elimination of this impact by 2020 instead of the Census Bureau's projection of 2070, one might expect these projections to show the least future impact. This depends crucially on specific parameters, however, and the results of comparisons need not be uniform across countries.

EFFECTS ON POPULATION SIZE, DECOMPOSED

Population trends taking AIDS into account are illustrated for 2000–50 in figure 6.1, which compares results from the three agencies. An additional line represents the special UN scenario with no AIDS mortality. For Sub-Saharan Africa as a whole, the three projections of total population are well below the no-AIDS scenario practically from 2000 and fairly close to each other up to about 2015. By 2020, some divergence appears, with the Census Bureau projection 0.1 percent above the UN projection and the World Bank projection 2.5 percent below it. Divergence increases as the projections lengthen, so that by 2050 the Census Bureau

Figure 6.1 Projected Population, Sub-Saharan Africa and Three Selected Countries *(thousands)*

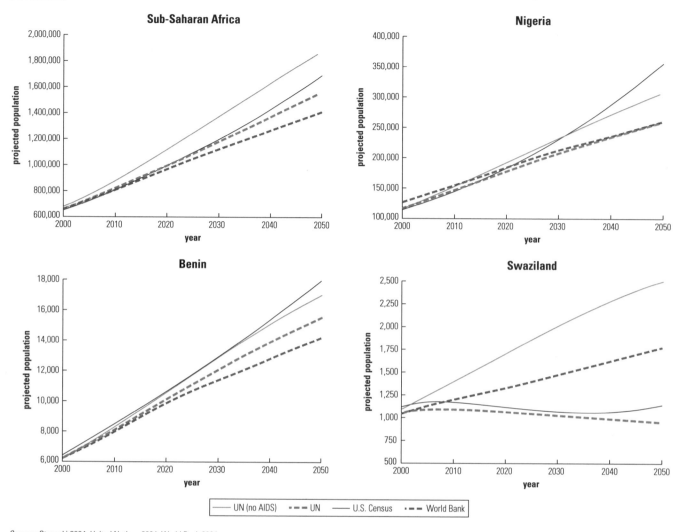

Sources: Stanecki 2004; United Nations 2004; World Bank 2004.

projection is 8.6 percent above the UN projection and the World Bank projection is 9.4 percent below. This is the reverse of the relative impact one would expect from comparing methodologies.

Three countries are shown in figure 6.1: Nigeria, with the largest regional population and an HIV prevalence rate intermediate for the region (5.4 percent infected of adults 15 to 49 years old, as reported by UNAIDS [2004] for 2003); Benin, with low HIV prevalence, for the region, of 1.9 percent in 2003; and Swaziland, with one of the highest HIV prevalence rates, for the region or the world, of 38.8 percent in 2003. For these individual countries, greater divergence in projections is evident than for the region as a whole, some of it clearly not due to AIDS mortality. The Census Bureau, for instance, projects a larger population than in the no-AIDS projection for Nigeria by 2035, as well as a larger population for Benin all the way back to 1990. Although AIDS does

affect population size, its effects are entangled with, and may be overwhelmed by, assumed change (or lack of change) in other parameters, particularly fertility.

Fertility assumptions are indeed quite variable across the projection sets. The UN projection and the no-AIDS scenario, but not the other two projections, have similar total fertility rates by design. World Bank estimates of total fertility in Sub-Saharan countries for 2000–05 range from 21 percent below to 23 percent above UN estimates, with a tendency to be lower rather than higher. Census Bureau estimates, in contrast, range from 37 percent lower to 53 percent higher than UN estimates, with a decided tilt toward being higher. The variation tends to increase, in percentage terms, for later years, at least up to around 2025. Higher bureau and lower Bank fertility projections appear to counteract the effect on projected population of longer-lasting epidemics for the Census Bureau than for the Bank.

Table 6.1 Effects of Demographic Factors in Producing Differences between Projections

Comparison and indicator	2020 population					2050 population				
	Total	Base population	Births	Deaths	Net migrants	Total	Base population	Births	Deaths	Net migrants
UN vs. no AIDS										
Sub-Saharan Africa	0.890	0.976	1.014	0.901	0.998	0.830	0.976	1.026	0.923	0.989
Country maximum	1.000	1.000	1.052	1.000	1.004	1.000	1.000	1.105	1.000	1.000
Country minimum	0.591	0.907	1.000	0.624	0.981	0.370	0.907	1.000	0.646	0.951
U.S. Census vs. no AIDS										
Sub-Saharan Africa	0.891	0.971	1.020	0.910	0.988	0.901	0.971	1.067	0.930	0.978
Country maximum	1.252	1.161	1.232	1.043	1.091	1.484	1.161	1.242	1.027	1.098
Country minimum	0.516	0.637	0.758	0.633	0.803	0.322	0.637	0.844	0.620	0.783
World Bank vs. no AIDS										
Sub-Saharan Africa	0.868	0.985	0.983	0.898	0.998	0.752	0.985	0.984	0.922	0.989
Country maximum	1.034	1.122	1.115	1.029	1.070	1.100	1.122	1.090	1.013	1.034
Country minimum	0.660	0.791	0.861	0.709	0.916	0.515	0.791	0.850	0.798	0.955

Source: Calculated from data in United Nations 2004; Stanecki 2004; and World Bank 2004. See note 1 at the end of the text.
Note: An effect of 0.89, for instance, means that the specified factor by itself reduces one projected population to 89 percent of the comparison population. Maximum and minimum effects are across 48 countries (the Seychelles and Saint Helena having incomplete data).

Ideally the effect of fertility assumptions would be discounted by running parallel scenarios with and without AIDS, as the UN has done. Such scenarios are not available, at least not in sufficient detail, for the other two sets of projections, but we do attempt to separate the effects of the fertility and mortality assumptions. We decompose the ratio of populations from two separate projections into multiplicative factors representing differences in the assumed base population and in fertility, mortality, and migration assumptions.[1] This decomposition does not specifically identify AIDS impact, but it at least helps us separate out the fertility and mortality effects.

Table 6.1 shows the results for 2020 and 2050. The comparison between the UN projection and the no-AIDS scenario (also from the UN) has some interesting points. The projected total population for 2020 is 89 percent of the projection without AIDS (as the first "Total" column shows). Therefore, the overall reduction in population due to AIDS is 11 percent by 2020, 17 percent by 2050. Most of this is due to mortality, but other effects also contribute. Part is due to differences in the base population, the population assumed for the start of the projection in 2000. The UN estimates that AIDS had already produced some demographic effect before 2000, reducing regional population by over 2 percent. The largest such effect across countries is 9 percent, for Zimbabwe.

Births also have an effect—a positive one in the UN projection, in contrast to the no-AIDS scenario. The effect is small for the region as a whole, at 1.4 percent in 2020, rising to 2.6 percent by 2050. It is, however, positive for each country where some effect of AIDS is modeled. Since the same total fertility is assumed country by country in the UN projection and its no-AIDS scenario, this result deserves some explanation.

Crude birth rates differ between the projections, as figure 6.2 illustrates. For the region as a whole, the difference is relatively slight, but for countries severely affected by AIDS, the difference can be much larger, as in the projection for Botswana. AIDS raises the crude birth rate because of its effect on the age structure. Figure 6.3 shows the distribution by age group of women of reproductive age in Botswana. Whereas, without AIDS, the age distribution is projected, over 50 years, to gradually become rectangular over the range of 15 to 49 years, with AIDS it remains skewed toward those under 35. This translates into a higher crude birth rate because fertility is higher among women under 35 years. The fertility advantage of younger women is assumed to decline over time, but the decline does not entirely offset the relative increase, when AIDS is taken into account, in proportions of younger women. The effect is entirely distributional and does not involve any assumptions about the biological impact of HIV, which, if it were taken into account, might moderate the result somewhat. AIDS does not increase the number of births, but these results indicate that it does increase the ratio of births to the population.

Figure 6.2 Projected Crude Birth Rate, Sub-Saharan Africa and Botswana

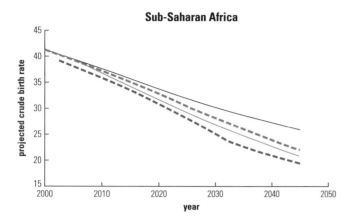

Sub-Saharan Africa

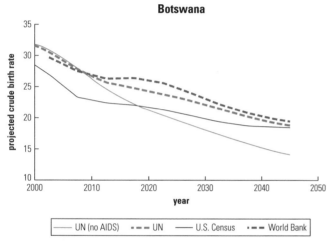

Botswana

— UN (no AIDS)   = = = UN   — U.S. Census   = ·= · World Bank

Sources: Stanecki 2004; United Nations 2004; World Bank 2004.

Figure 6.3 Distribution of Women of Reproductive Age in the UN Projection and the No-AIDS Scenario, Botswana

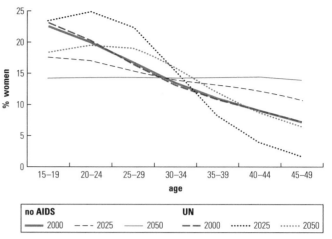

no AIDS			UN		
—— 2000	– – – 2025	—— 2050	= = = 2000	······ 2025	······· 2050

Source: United Nations 2004.

Figure 6.4 Mortality Effects on Population, Relative to the No-AIDS Scenario, in Different Projections

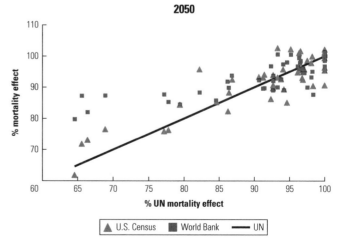

2020

2050

▲ U.S. Census   ■ World Bank   —— UN

Sources: Calculated from Stanecki 2004, United Nations 2004, and World Bank 2004.

The Census Bureau also shows a generally positive births effect. Part of this, as for the UN, may be due to the effect of AIDS on the age structure, but a larger part is simply higher assumed fertility than in the no-AIDS scenario. As expected, the births effect is negative for the World Bank.

The direct effect of mortality on population size in the projections is of course negative and much larger in the absolute than the effect of fertility, implying a reduction in population size for the region, if the UN projection is compared with the no-AIDS scenario, of 10 percent by 2020 and 8 percent by 2050. For the region as a whole, the mortality effect is roughly comparable, if the U.S. Census Bureau projections or the World Bank projections are compared with the same standard. We expected the Census Bureau to show a stronger mortality effect than the World Bank, given the assumption of longer-lasting epidemics, but the reverse is the case, except when the most affected countries are considered.

Figure 6.4 shows the mortality effects for individual countries—with the most affected countries toward the lower left—when assessed for 2020 and for 2050. Although the agencies generally agree about which countries are more affected by AIDS mortality, their estimates of the degree of this effect vary, particularly for the most affected countries. For countries where the UN estimates that AIDS mortality reduces population in 2020 by at least 20 percent, the Census Bureau estimates that the population reduction on average is 5 percentage points less, and the World Bank estimates that it is 8 percentage points less. For countries where the UN estimates a population reduction of at least 20 percent by 2050, the Census Bureau estimates an average reduction that is 3 percentage points less, and the World Bank a reduction of 13 percentage points less.

These comparisons involve not only AIDS mortality but mortality generally. It is likely, however, that the differences have to do mainly with variation in AIDS mortality than in mortality from all other causes, although this cannot be established. At any rate, the results fail to substantiate any general agreement about the demographic effect of AIDS mortality.

LIFE EXPECTANCY

Looking at other mortality indexes does not help further specify the AIDS effect but does provide additional perspectives on the severity of the impact. Figure 6.5 shows some projected life expectancy trends. For Sub-Saharan Africa as a whole, the UN Population Division indicates that by 2000–05 life expectancy had already fallen 8.8 years short of what it would be without AIDS and that the relative deficit will grow to a maximum of 10.4 years by 2010–15 before beginning to shrink slowly. The Census Bureau suggests that the current deficit is slightly smaller, and the World Bank suggests it will shrink slightly faster. For the region as a whole, there is not great disagreement about life expectancy trends.

For individual countries, however, the differences among projections can be substantial. The UN projections start (in 2000) with a much higher estimate of life expectancy for Nigeria than the other two projections, a gap that is generally maintained over time. For Benin, the Census Bureau

Figure 6.5 Projected Life Expectancy, Sub-Saharan Africa and Three Selected Countries

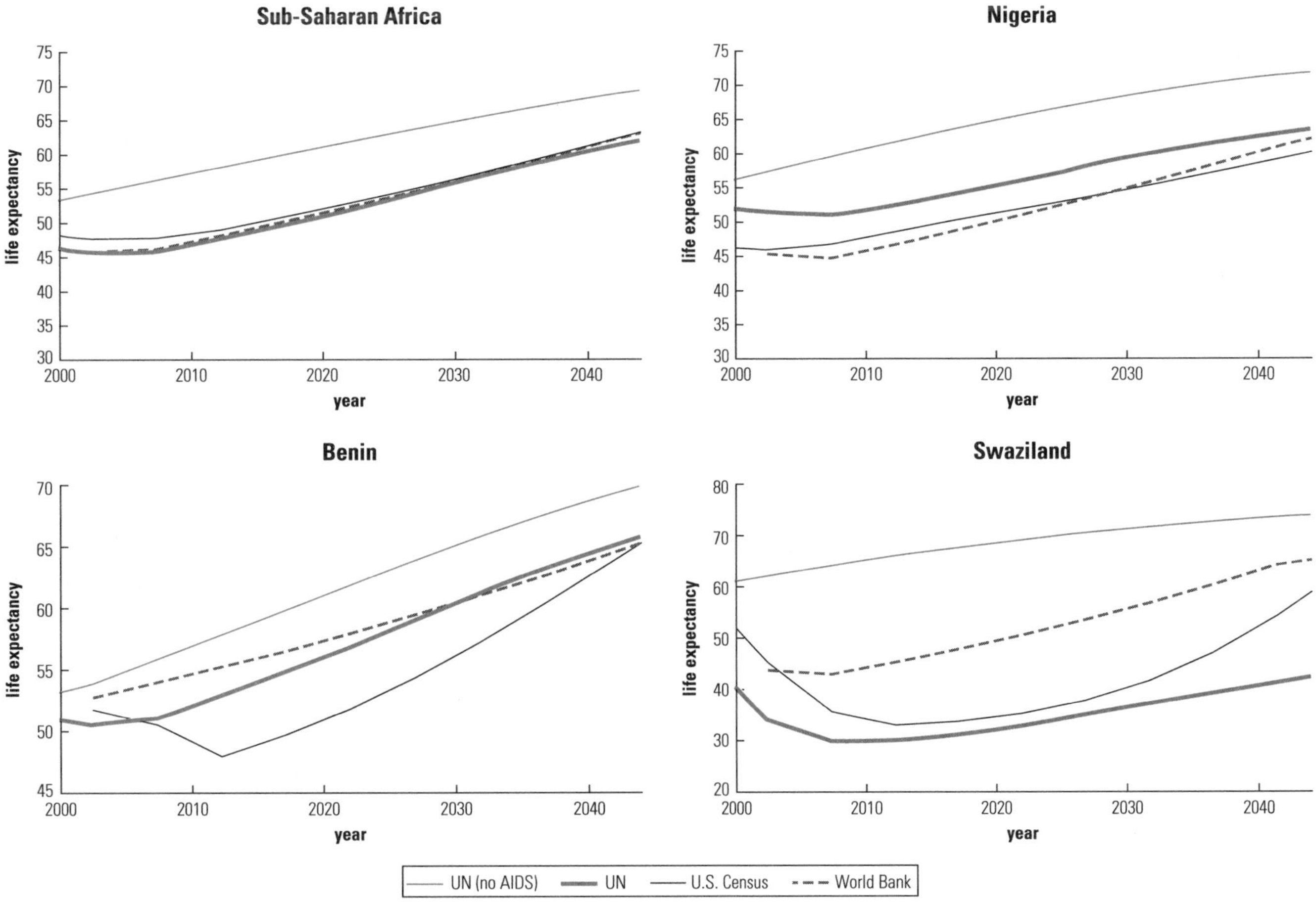

Sources: Stanecki 2004; United Nations 2004; World Bank 2004.

Figure 6.6 HIV Prevalence and Maximum Loss in Life Expectancy in Alternative Projections

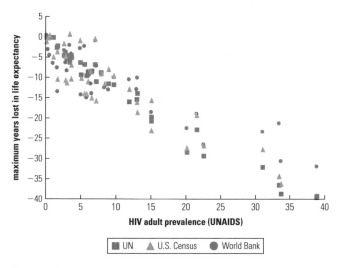

Sources: Calculated from Stanecki 2004, United Nations 2004, and World Bank 2004.

projects a substantial fall in life expectancy, unlike the other two agencies. For Swaziland, the decline in projected life expectancy up to about 2010–15 is greatest for the UN, which has it falling to 30 years. The decline is smallest for the World Bank, for which the minimum, in 2005–10, is 43 years. Subsequent trends for Swaziland are also quite different: the UN projects a long, slow recovery; the World Bank sees a quick, rapid recovery; and the Census Bureau finds a delayed but accelerating recovery.

How far life expectancy falls depends on current estimates of HIV prevalence. Figure 6.6 shows the maximum fall in life expectancy by country, when each set of projections is contrasted with the no-AIDS scenario. In the UN projection, a country loses four years of life expectancy when HIV prevalence is 2.5 percent among adults, and a little more than one additional year of life expectancy for every 1 percentage point rise in HIV prevalence.[2] The U.S. Census Bureau projects a similar result (when the comparison is made to the UN no-AIDS scenario), and the World Bank projects a somewhat less serious effect, particularly at high HIV levels. The greatest effect on life expectancy is most often seen in the period 2015–20. For the UN, the period may be five years earlier or later, but for the Census Bureau, there is less temporal variation. For the World Bank, however, the period of maximum deficit is 2005–10, and this is fairly constant across countries.

The crude death rate is affected similarly. The maximum increase in the rate is about 7 per 1,000 people when HIV prevalence is 2.5 percent, rising to 25 per 1,000 when HIV prevalence is 35 percent. The greatest increase in the crude

death rate tends to be a few years earlier than the greatest loss in life expectancy.

The decline in life expectancy affects women more than men. Worldwide, in the period 2000–05, women had a 4.3 year advantage in life expectancy. In Sub-Saharan Africa, their advantage would have been 3.1 years without AIDS and would have stayed essentially constant up to 2050 (in the no-AIDS scenario). Because of AIDS, their advantage has fallen to 1.9 years, according to the UN projection, and will fall further to 0.6 years for most of the period 2010–25, before recovering slowly, to barely more than 1.5 years by 2050. The Census Bureau shows less of a change, with the female advantage at 2.2 years in 2000–05, falling under two years during 2005–15, and recovering more quickly to about four years by 2050. (The World Bank does not provide these data.)

Country by country, projected trends in the female advantage can look strikingly different (figure 6.7). Although there are some commonalities in country patterns, the UN and the Census Bureau appear to disagree about many aspects of these trends: what the female advantage is initially, when and how steeply it declines, and if and when it begins to increase again. The Census Bureau generally assumes an earlier decline in the female advantage than the UN but a somewhat shallower decline at lower HIV prevalence levels. In both sets of projections, the female advantage falls by a year for every 4 to 5 percentage point increase in initial HIV prevalence. This can turn the female advantage into a disadvantage.

Where HIV prevalence reaches 20 percent or more, female life expectancy usually falls, at some point in the projection, at least two years below male life expectancy. Most of these countries are in southern Africa, or in the slightly broader Southern African Development Community (SADC). The UN always shows some recovery by 50 years, although in the worst case, Botswana, the female disadvantage, at 4.5 years, is still extreme at the end of this period. The Census Bureau, in contrast, shows either a quick and substantial recovery, as is shown in figure 6.7 for Zimbabwe, or an apparently unarrested fall, as for Namibia, where the female disadvantage exceeds seven years by 2050. Long-term trends, particularly where HIV prevalence is high, are a particular area of disagreement.

The changes in life expectancy, and in the female advantage, are the result, of course, of rising adult mortality. The estimates of adult mortality ($_{45}q_{15}$) used in the projections are available only for the UN. These show the substantial rise in mortality over projected trends without AIDS, as well

Figure 6.7 Female Advantage in Life Expectancy, Sub-Saharan Africa and Three Selected Countries

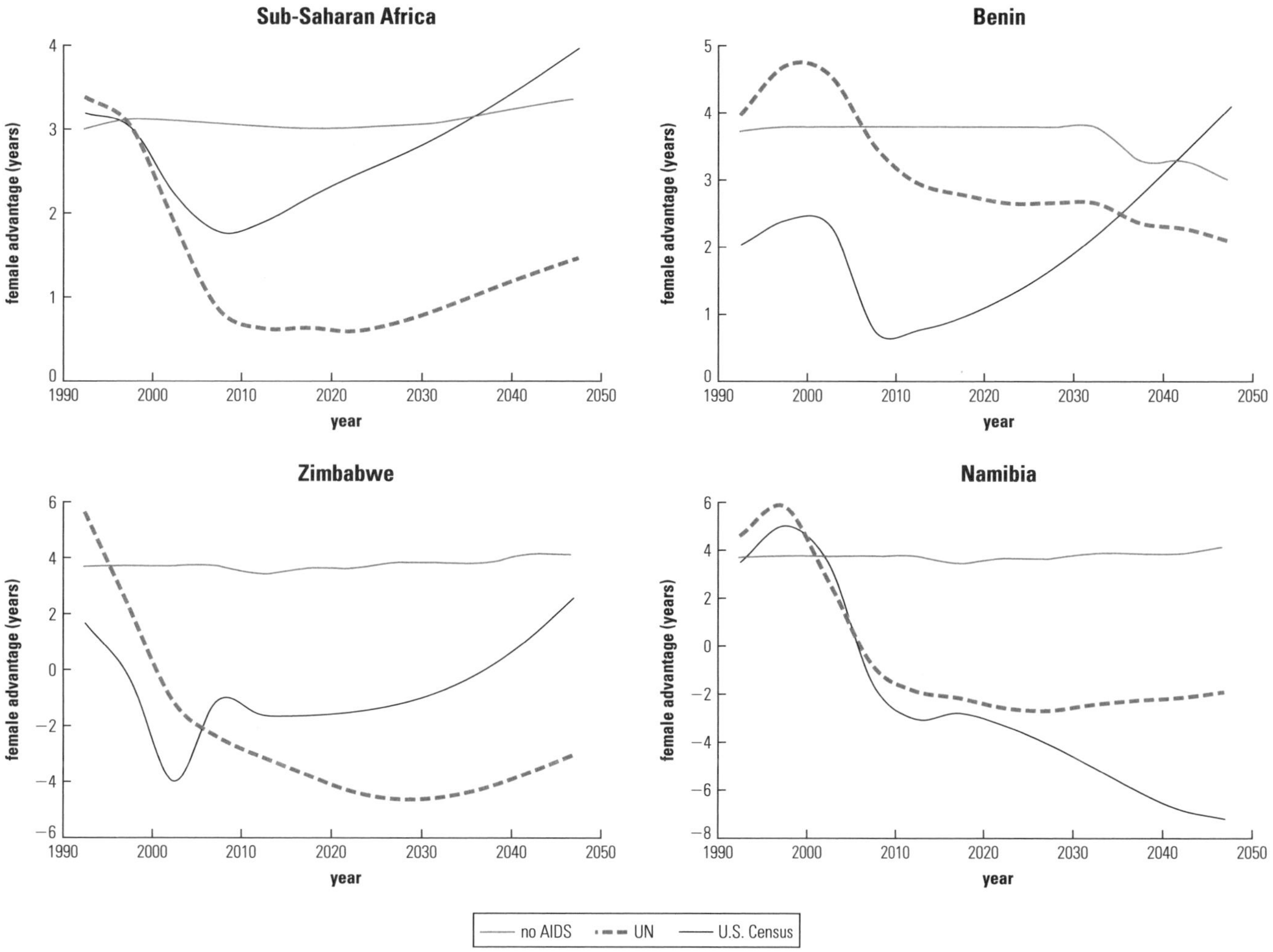

Sources: Calculated from Stanecki 2004 and United Nations 2004.

as the way female adult mortality catches up with and, in severe cases, passes male mortality (figure 6.8). The increases in the risk of death between ages 15 and 60, relative to the situation without an AIDS epidemic, can be substantial. If HIV prevalence in 2001 is 10 percent, the maximum increase in risk over the following two decades is, on average from a quadratic regression, 29 percentage points for males and 34 percentage points for females. If HIV prevalence is 30 percent, the increase in risk is 65 percentage points for males, 75 percentage points for females.

Population by Sex and Age

The shrinking (and occasionally disappearing) female advantage in life expectancy is projected to alter the sex ratio, although for national populations the effect is not large. For a handful of southern African or SADC countries,

the sex ratio may rise 10 to 20 percentage points in the UN projection and slightly more in the Census Bureau projection. As a result, the highest sex ratio in these projections would be about 120 males per 100 females. This is not unprecedented. In 2000, five countries—all in the Persian Gulf and none particularly affected by AIDS—had higher ratios, up to 190 males per 100 females. National sex ratios approaching 120 could be destabilizing, depending on the flexibility, or lack of it, of particular cultures.

At specific ages, sex ratios may become more extreme. Figure 6.9 illustrates the situation for Zimbabwe, one of the countries most affected by AIDS mortality. Over decades, the imbalance between males and females resulting from higher female AIDS mortality produces a hump in the sex ratio, which, in this case, reaches about 230 in the year 2030 for those age 50 to 54 years. This hump, as it rises, gradually moves toward older and older ages and eventually begins to

Figure 6.8 Adult Mortality ($_{45}q_{15}$) by Sex in UN Projections, Sub-Saharan Africa and Lesotho

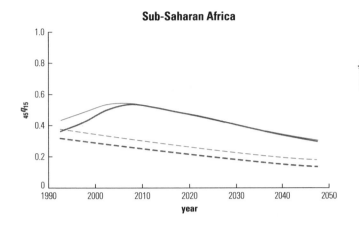

Sub-Saharan Africa

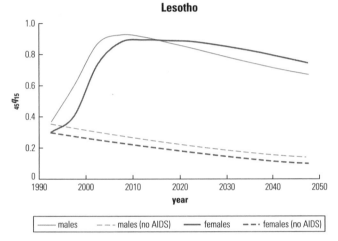

Lesotho

| | males | – – – | males (no AIDS) | —— | females | – – · | females (no AIDS) |

Source: United Nations 2004.

Figure 6.9 Sex Ratios by Age from UN Projections, Zimbabwe

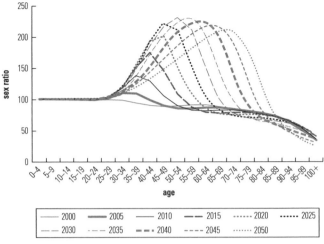

| | 2000 | | 2005 | | 2010 | | 2015 | | 2020 | | 2025 |
| | 2030 | | 2035 | | 2040 | | 2045 | | 2050 |

Source: United Nations 2004.

demographic transition—toward lower dependency, a stalled fertility decline is at least as effective an impediment.

Initial Assumptions

Is it possible to sort out the differences in projections and come to some reasonable conclusions about the likely demographic impact of AIDS? There is no way to determine in advance which forecasts will be most accurate in the decades to come. The only useful approach to assessing the relative adequacy of the different projections, therefore, would be to look at their methodology, especially the way they model the effects of HIV/AIDS. These models, however, are quite complex, not completely transparent, and beyond the scope of this chapter to critique in detail. We therefore settle for examining some of the initial assumptions that go into these projections, particularly assumptions about adult mortality and HIV prevalence. These two sets of parameters undergird projections of AIDS impact.

For the World Bank projections, calculations of adult mortality can be made from the WHO life tables for 2000 (Lopez et al. 2002). Similar calculations can be made from UN survivorship ratios; for 2000, we average estimates for the periods 1995–2000 and 2000–05. (Similar data are not available from the Census Bureau.) UN figures are plotted against WHO figures by country in figure 6.11.

The UN and WHO adult mortality estimates generally agree. On average, UN estimates are only 1 percent lower than WHO estimates. (The differences may be slightly greater at high mortality levels.) Figure 6.11 also shows, however, another set of estimates of adult mortality, derived by Timaeus and Jasseh (2004) from sibling histories and

subside. Having almost two-and-a-half males for every female at older ages is unusual, but whether it is a serious issue depends on the culture.

Where age patterns are involved, the dependency ratio might be a particular concern. A low dependency ratio, implying a relatively large workforce, could be an economic advantage, but AIDS impedes progress toward a lower ratio by increasing adult mortality more than infant and child mortality. How great the effect is, though, is difficult to tell. In the countries most severely affected by AIDS, the dependency ratio might rise from 50 or 60 dependents per 100 adults of working age to 70 or 80 dependents. Comparison of the UN projection with the no-AIDS scenario suggests such a rise for various countries in southern Africa. However, the exact level of the dependency ratio will be heavily influenced by future fertility, about which there appears to be little consensus (figure 6.10). The apparent effect of AIDS is easily swallowed up by differences in assumed fertility trends. Although AIDS does delay the movement—typical in the

Figure 6.10 Dependency Ratio, Sub-Saharan Africa and Three Selected Countries

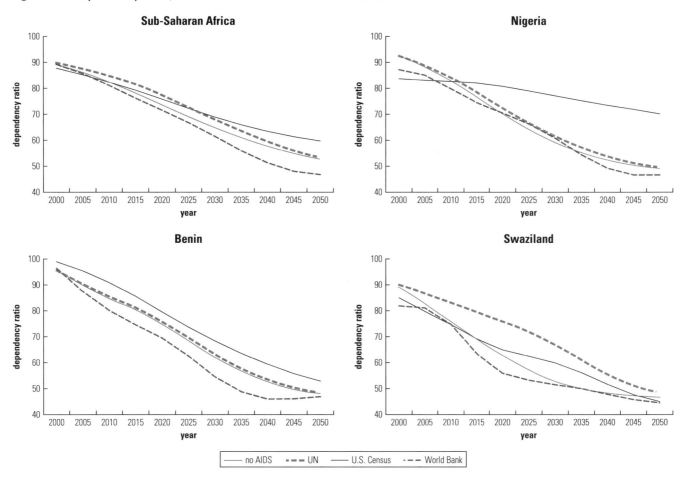

Sources: Stanecki 2004; United Nations 2004; World Bank 2004.

incorporating recent Demographic and Health Surveys (DHS) data. These estimates, which cover seven countries, appear consistently lower than those from the WHO and the UN. (The only exception is for Zimbabwe, where the WHO estimate, but not the UN estimate, is slightly lower.) The gap appears to be substantial. The probability of dying between ages 15 and 60, averaged without weighting across the seven countries, is between 51 and 57 percent in the WHO and UN estimates (depending on which estimates and which sex is involved). The averages for Timaeus and Jasseh's estimates, in contrast, are 44 percent for males and 34 percent for females.

Somewhat more countries can be compared for 1995, for which year Timaeus and Jasseh (2004) cover 20 countries. These estimates are mostly well below the UN estimates for 1995 (estimated as the average for 1990–95 and 1995–2000). The average probability of dying between ages 15 and 60 across the 20 countries is 36 percent for males and 29 percent for females, according to Timaeus and Jasseh (2004). According to the UN, the respective averages are 50 percent for males and 42 percent for females.

The Timaeus and Jasseh (2004) estimates cannot be considered an entirely reliable standard because of the limited data on which they are based and the assumptions necessary in their calculation, such as the assumption of a common age pattern of mortality increase across countries (see also chapter 4 in this volume). Nevertheless, the consistently lower levels of adult mortality they determine may suggest some overstatement in the UN and WHO mortality estimates, which could be tied to an overestimation in modeling of the mortality impact of AIDS.

Without getting into the intricacies of these models, we can look at the estimates of HIV prevalence with which the modeling starts. These are generally UNAIDS estimates for 2001. The UN estimates, as noted earlier, begin with these estimates but may be adjusted in order to fit the prevalence trend. The Census Bureau maintains the database that UNAIDS uses in making its estimates and reports similar figures, at least for countries for which it has estimates. The source of the WHO estimates is not specified but is presumably the same.

Figure 6.11 Consistency among Alternative Estimates of Current Adult Mortality ($_{45}q_{15}$)

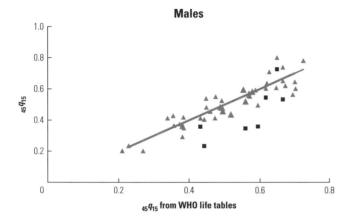

Males

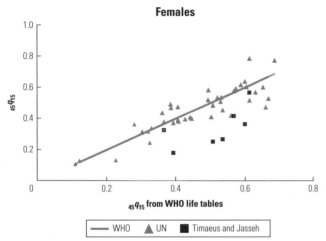

Females

— WHO   ▲ UN   ■ Timaeus and Jasseh

Sources: Timaeus and Jasseh 2004; United Nations 2004; Lopez et al. 2002.

Figure 6.12 HIV Prevalence in 2001 and 2003

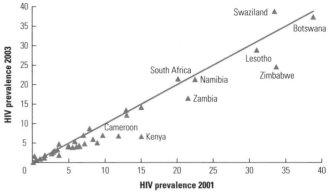

Source: UNAIDS 2002, 2004.

A problem with each of these projections is the 2001 UNAIDS estimates themselves. In 2004, UNAIDS (2004) revised these estimates, changing almost twice as many downward as upward. The changes were sometimes large. UNAIDS (2002) had previously reported "low" and "high" estimates to bracket their main estimates for 2001. In 10 cases, the new estimates were lower than the previous "low" estimates. In only two cases were they higher than the previous "high" estimates. The adjustments may have been made to ensure consistency with new estimates for 2003. These were generally lower than the earlier 2001 estimates, which might have suggested epidemics on the decline. Instead, by lowering 2001 estimates, UNAIDS can speak of "stabilization" in HIV prevalence in the region, which it attributes to a balance between deaths and new infections.

Figure 6.12 compares UNAIDS estimates of HIV prevalence in 2003 with the earlier estimates for 2001 (UNAIDS 2002, 2004). Among the reductions, 15 countries have 2003 rates that are at least 1.5 percentage points lower than the earlier 2001 estimates, three of them at least 5 percentage

points lower. Among the increases, only one country (Swaziland) has a 2003 rate at least 1.5 points higher than in 2001. Between 1999 and 2001, in contrast, increases and decreases in prevalence were more balanced, with increases being slightly more likely and somewhat larger.

If the epidemics are indeed at a plateau or past their peak, that may be uncomfortable for the agency projections. The Census Bureau projections are inconsistent with this idea, since they assume that peak prevalence is not reached until 2010. Whether the UN projections are consistent with plateauing epidemics is not clear. The UN reports that peak incidence for the epidemics—not peak prevalence—was reached on average about 1994, which could be consistent with some decline in prevalence by 2001. Country by country, however, there is no relationship between an earlier assumed incidence peak for the UN and the amount of apparent prevalence decline in the UNAIDS estimates. Only the World Bank projections, which effectively assume that AIDS-related mortality is already in decline, would be consistent with the interpretation of epidemics in at least early decline in the region.

The correction of 2001 HIV prevalence rates is also uncomfortable for projections, which relied on the earlier rates. The correction seems to have some basis. Table 6.2 compares UNAIDS estimates with estimates from DHS data for five countries. Based mainly on antenatal clinic reports, the earlier UNAIDS estimates were typically higher than the DHS estimates. Among these countries, rather high rates for Kenya and Zambia were brought into the range of the DHS estimates, and rates for the other three countries were also lowered.

The survey estimates are meant to cover the adult population more comprehensively than sentinel surveillance systems based on special populations, especially pregnant women. Survey estimates do have their own problems, such

Table 6.2 Estimates of HIV Prevalence among Adults Age 15 to 49, 2001–03
(percent)

Country, by prevalence	UNAIDS			Demographic and Health Surveys		
	2001	2001 (rev.)	2003	Year	Female	Male
Zambia	21.5	16.7	16.5	2001–02	17.8	12.9
Kenya	15.0	8.0	6.7	2003	8.7	4.6
Burkina Faso	6.5	4.2	4.2	2003	1.8	1.9
Ghana	3.0	3.1	3.1	2003	2.7	1.6
Mali	1.7	1.9	1.9	2001	2.0	1.3

Sources: Initial 2001 estimate from UNAIDS 2002; revised 2001 estimate and 2003 estimate from UNAIDS 2004.

as nonresponse, for which adjustments are attempted. The survey reports suggest one important reason why earlier UNAIDS estimates could have been too high. In four out of five cases, male prevalence is clearly lower than female prevalence. The exception, in Burkina Faso, occurs at a low prevalence level. This is in keeping with the typical pattern expected in primarily heterosexual epidemics, where male infections are initially more frequent than female infections, but the reverse eventually becomes the case. Given that UNAIDS applies rates for pregnant women to the population as a whole, earlier overestimates are certainly plausible, particularly at higher HIV prevalence levels. Further downward adjustments in prevalence may be needed as more surveys become available. They will, of course, come too late for the current set of population projections, all of which—if this interpretation is correct—start out from too-high levels of HIV prevalence and therefore AIDS deaths.

Revised Projections

These projections may be revised, in later rounds, to allow for slightly lower current adult mortality overall and, particularly in the most affected countries, either lower or declining HIV prevalence levels, if further research confirms either to be the case. Pending such revision, precise conclusions about the demographic impact of AIDS in the region cannot safely be drawn. The revisions to the projections might have to be substantial in some cases. For Kenya, for instance, the UNAIDS estimate of HIV prevalence for 2001 was 15.0, and the current set of projections depend on this estimate. The 2003 estimate fell to 6.7, consistent with DHS results. The 2001 estimate implies that the maximum reduction in life expectancy—relative to the no-AIDS scenario—would be 17.7 years, using the equation in note 2. The 2003 estimate implies a maximum reduction half as large, at 8.7 years.

To get a further, although only preliminary, idea of how projections might change in the most affected countries,

we draw on projections recently prepared for the Central Statistical Offices (CSOs) in Zambia and Botswana (Bulatao 2003a, 2003b). The Zambia projection adopts HIV prevalence estimates from the 2001–02 DHS rather than from UNAIDS. The DHS data suggest that HIV prevalence among all adult women is only 75 percent of that among pregnant women, and that male prevalence is still lower. These assumptions are adopted for the neighboring country of Botswana, for which DHS data are not available. Botswana, with a relatively good health system for the region, has monitored the proportion of males infected, based on clients at counseling and testing centers. The proportion of males infected is, indeed, lower than that for women. Surveillance data on the age distribution of both men and women infected in Botswana also match quite closely the distributions in the Zambia DHS.[3]

Other procedures for these CSO projections follow World Bank methodology. However, in place of WHO life tables incorporating AIDS mortality, Coale-Demeny (1983) life tables without AIDS are used, so that AIDS mortality can be specifically modeled. The modeling follows the usual procedures, involving calculations of HIV incidence from prevalence and estimation of subsequent deaths, relying on procedures previously described (Bulatao and Bos 1992) but with curves fit to prevalence trends rather than specific calculations, from sexual behavior, of transmission probabilities.

The Zambia projection begins with a 1980 census, in order to incorporate the effects of an epidemic initially recognized about 1984, and progresses to 2025. The Botswana projection begins with a 1981 census and goes to 2031. The assumed total fertility trends were constructed from census and survey data, some of them only locally available, but are generally in the range of those that the UN, the Census Bureau, and the World Bank assume for the country.

Figure 6.13 compares the projected population with the previous projections. The effect of AIDS still seems to be

Figure 6.13 Alternative Population Projections, Zambia and Botswana
(thousands)

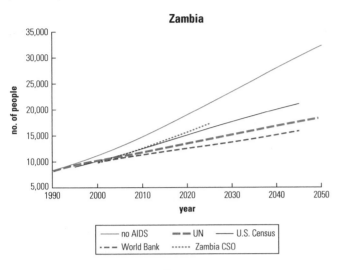

Zambia

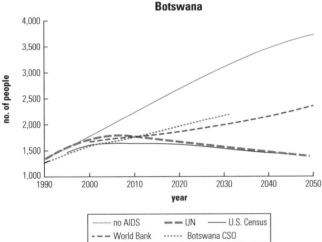

Botswana

Sources: Stanecki 2004; United Nations 2004; World Bank 2004; Bulatao 2003a, 2003b.

Figure 6.14 Alternative Projections of Life Expectancy in Zambia and Botswana

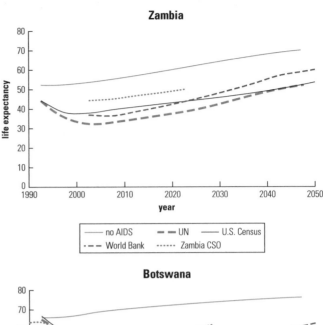

Zambia

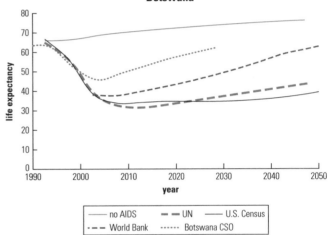

Botswana

Sources: Stanecki 2004; United Nations 2004; World Bank 2004; Bulatao 2003a, 2003b.

large, relative to the UN no-AIDS scenario, but for both countries, these CSO projections give higher population figures than those from the international agencies. Which of the preceding projections the CSO projections are closest to is determined more by fertility assumptions than the modeling of the AIDS effect, since the World Bank has the highest fertility trend for Botswana and the Census Bureau for Zambia. By 2025, the CSO projections give a Zambia population 6 to 32 percent larger than the other projections, but still almost 20 percent below that in the no-AIDS scenario. For Botswana at the same date, the CSO projection is 10 to 30 percent higher than the others but almost 30 percent below the no-AIDS scenario. Like the World Bank, but unlike the UN and the Census Bureau, the CSO projections show no population decline.

If we look instead at projected life expectancy (figure 6.14), the differences from the other projections stand out as sharply. For Zambia, the CSO projection shows levels 5 to 10 years higher than the other projections for the period 2000–25, although still about 10 years short of what the no-AIDS scenario shows. For Botswana, all three agency projections show a similar decline up to about 2000, followed by rapid divergence. The CSO projection shows no further decline beyond 2001–06, so that about 2025 life expectancy is 15 to 25 years higher than in the other projections, although almost 15 years below the no-AIDS scenario. Adjusting projections to incorporate somewhat lower survey estimates of HIV prevalence could therefore have a substantial effect. In these severely affected countries, it reduces the deficit in life expectancy for 2025 by anywhere from one-third to two-thirds.

CONCLUSION

The demographic impact of AIDS in Sub-Saharan Africa is substantial, but its precise dimensions remain largely a matter of conjecture. Sophisticated models of the course of HIV/AIDS epidemics have been developed and linked with population projection approaches that have proved relatively reliable in the past (National Research Council 2000). However, these projection models have used inadequate data on mortality and HIV/AIDS.

The regional projections, part of the global work done by three agencies, the UN Population Division, the U.S. Census Bureau, and the World Bank, show the population of Sub-Saharan Africa falling below what it would be without AIDS, by 11 to 13 percent by 2020 and by anywhere from 10 to 25 percent by 2050. For individual countries, the population shortfall is projected as high as 34 to 48 percent by 2020 and 48 to 68 percent by 2050. That there will be a shortfall relative to what it would have been had HIV/AIDS not invaded the region is certain. That it will be of these dimensions is not. Each of the projections of countries affected by HIV/AIDS starts with UNAIDS estimates for HIV prevalence in 2001, some of which were clearly overestimates. For how many this is true cannot yet be told.

Between 2002 and 2004, UNAIDS generally revised downward its estimates for 2001 adult HIV prevalence in Sub-Saharan Africa. DHS data show sharply lower estimates of adult prevalence in three countries, and UNAIDS made matching adjustments for two (and somewhat smaller adjustments for the rest). For countries where HIV prevalence is high, initial overestimates could have been due to the practice of generalizing prevalence estimates for pregnant women to the adult population. Prevalence among males tends to be lower than among females, particularly at higher levels.

Unfortunately, the population projections available rely on the earlier estimates of HIV prevalence. This could lead to overstated base adult mortality, as well as to an overstated future trend in AIDS deaths. Comparing projections that rely on survey-based HIV estimates suggests that, in severely affected countries, the reduction in population due to AIDS may be only 50 to 75 percent of what the agency projections show and that life expectancy may be reduced, at the maximum, by a third to two-thirds of what agency projections show.

If the agency projections are not, at present, a reliable guide to future populations in areas affected by HIV/AIDS, they nevertheless illustrate patterns of demographic impact. The effect on population does appear larger when countries are strongly affected by HIV/AIDS. However, even in these cases, AIDS is not necessarily the dominant factor in future population trends nor the main source of uncertainty about them. Fertility is at least as important. Differing judgments about future fertility trends can produce at least as great variation in future population as the variation between situations with and without an AIDS epidemic.

Fertility itself is affected by HIV/AIDS. Younger women are more likely to be infected than older women, but their eventual deaths leave gaps in the age structure that persist into and become increasingly evident at older ages. Crude birth rates actually rise slightly as a result, because younger, more fertile women continue to be replenished in the age structure. Unfortunately, this compositional effect is the only effect on fertility that can be seen in current projections. Biological and behavioral mechanisms that may lead to lower fertility are insufficiently understood to be modeled across countries.

The effect of HIV/AIDS on mortality, the primary mechanism by which it affects population growth in agency projections, appears substantial but may be overblown. Life expectancy is projected to fall a maximum of one year below its expected path for every one percentage point increase in initial HIV prevalence. With UNAIDS adjusting its estimates of HIV prevalence downward, life expectancy should probably be expected not to decline as much. For Kenya, for example, UNAIDS reduced its estimate of 2001 HIV prevalence from 15 to 8 percent. The projections show maximum loss in years of life ranging from 15 to 21 years, but a smaller loss of 8 to 14 years would seem more likely.

Given that the HIV/AIDS epidemics in Sub-Saharan Africa are mainly heterosexual, the rise in mortality affects women more than men. The female advantage in life expectancy will shrink and could turn into a female disadvantage. This effect too depends on levels of HIV prevalence, and the projections may overstate the change. Effects on the sex ratio, as well as on age structure, are more substantial at high HIV prevalence levels, but even in these cases they do not appear to produce patterns more extreme than those seen in other populations.

Each agency projection will undoubtedly be revised in the future to take adjusted HIV prevalence levels into account. How they came to adopt HIV prevalence levels that were too high is an interesting question. The agencies devote some effort to ensuring that they use the best possible estimates of current fertility and mortality. Perhaps they have not spent as much effort carefully considering the accuracy of input data on HIV/AIDS and have been insufficiently critical of UNAIDS reports. Even with the adjustments made to previous HIV prevalence estimates, there remain some that probably deserve closer scrutiny.

There also remain other challenges to future rounds of these projections. Although data on HIV prevalence are gradually improving, what path the epidemics will take on the downslope remains conjectural. How therapies and vaccines may help, what behavior changes can be anticipated, and what the implications for infections and deaths will be are matters about which little if any empirical information can be adduced. In this area projections are, at best, educated guesses.

Another challenge will be managing the complexity of the methodology to project AIDS mortality. Complexity need not itself be a problem, but where it disguises a poverty of data and lends an inappropriate air of authoritativeness to results while concealing the calculations on which they are based, it can easily mislead. Projections need to convince not only with sophisticated models but also with a good appreciation of historical patterns and trends. More transparency would probably make it easier not just to detect the weaknesses of the projections but also to better appreciate what they actually contribute.

NOTES

1. If P_t is the projected population to time t and P_t^* is the projected population with which it is being compared, then $P_t/P_t^* = P_0/P_0^* \, e^{(b-b^*)t} \, e^{(-d+d^*)t} \, e^{(m-m^*)t}$, where P_0 is the base population for the projection and b, d, and m represent crude birth, death, and net migration rates. Bulatao (2001) uses a similar decomposition in assessing projection accuracy.

2. The equation, derived from the UN projection, is: Loss in $e_0 = -1.5 - 1.08 \times$ HIV adult prevalence in percent in 2001 ($R^2 = 0.97$).

3. Preliminary results from the 2004 Botswana AIDS Impact Survey II, conducted after these projections were completed, appear to confirm the need to use substantially lower adult HIV prevalence levels in projections. They show adult HIV prevalence at 25.3 percent, well below the 37.3 percent that UNAIDS reports.

REFERENCES

Ahmad, O. B., A. D. Lopez, and M. Inoue. 2000. "The Decline in Trends in Child Mortality: A Reappraisal." *Bulletin of the World Health Organization* 78 (10): 1175–91.

Bos, E., M. T. Vu, E. Massiah, and R. A. Bulatao. 1994. *World Population Projections, 1994–95 Edition: Estimates and Projections with Related Demographic Statistics.* Baltimore: Johns Hopkins University Press.

Bulatao, R. A. 2001. "Visible and Invisible Sources of Errors in World Population Projections." Paper presented at the annual meeting of the Population Association of America, Washington, DC, March.

———. 2003a. "Population Projections for Botswana up to 2031." Paper prepared for the Central Statistical Office, Gaborone, Botswana.

———. 2003b. "Population Projections for Zambia, 2000–2025." Paper prepared for the Central Statistical Office, Lusaka, Zambia.

Bulatao, R. A., and E. Bos. 1992. "Projecting the Demographic Impact of AIDS." Policy Research Working Paper 941, World Bank, Washington, DC.

Coale, A. J., and P. Demeny, with B. Vaughn. 1983. *Regional Model Life Tables and Stable Populations.* 2nd ed. New York: Academic Press.

Lopez, A. D., O. B. Ahman, M. Guillot, B. D. Ferguson, J. A. Salomon, and C. J. L. Murray. 2002. *World Mortality in 2000: Life Tables for 191 Countries.* Geneva: WHO.

Lopez, A. D., J. Salomon, O. Ahman, C. J. L. Murray, and D. Mafat. 2001. "Life Tables for 191 Countries: Data, Methods and Results." Global Program on Evidence for Health Policy, Discussion Paper 9, WHO, Geneva.

McDevitt, T. M. 1999. *World Population Profile: 1998.* Report WP/98. Washington, DC: U.S. Census Bureau.

Murray, C. J. L., O. B. Ahmad, A. D. Lopez, and J. Salomon. 2000. "WHO System of Model Life Tables." Global Program on Evidence for Health Policy, Discussion Paper 8, WHO, Geneva.

National Research Council. 2000. *Beyond Six Billion: Forecasting the World's Population.* Washington, DC: National Academy Press.

Salomon, J. A., E. E. Gakidou, and C. J. L. Murray. 1999. "Methods for Modelling the HIV/AIDS Epidemic in Sub-Saharan Africa." Global Program on Evidence for Health Policy, Discussion Paper 3, WHO, Geneva.

Stanecki, K. A. 2004. *The AIDS Pandemic in the 21st Century.* U.S. Census Bureau, International Population Reports WP02-2. Washington, DC: U.S. Government Printing Office.

Stanley, E. A., S. T. Seitz, P. O. Way, P. D. Johnson, and T. F. Curry. 1991. "The IwgAIDS Model for the Heterosexual Spread of HIV and the Demographic Impacts of the AIDS Epidemic." In *The AIDS Epidemic and Its Demographic Consequences.* New York: United Nations.

Timaeus, I. M., and M. Jasseh. 2004. "Adult Mortality in Sub-Saharan Africa: Evidence from Demographic and Health Surveys." *Demography* 41 (4): 757–72.

UNAIDS. 2000. *Report on the Global HIV/AIDS Epidemic–June 2000.* Geneva: UNAIDS.

———. 2002. *Report on the Global HIV/AIDS Epidemic 2002.* Geneva: UNAIDS.

———. 2004. *Report on the Global AIDS Epidemic, July 2004.* Geneva: UNAIDS.

UNAIDS Reference Group on Estimates, Modelling and Projections. 2002. "Improved Methods and Assumptions for Estimation of the HIV/AIDS Epidemic and Its Impact: Recommendations of the UNAIDS Reference Group on Estimates, Modelling and Projections." *AIDS* 16: W1–14.

United Nations. 1998. *World Population Prospects: The 1998 Revision.* New York: United Nations.

———. 2003a. *World Population Prospects: The 2002 Revision.* Vol. 1: *Comprehensive Tables.* New York: United Nations.

———. 2003b. *World Population Prospects: The 2002 Revision.* Vol. 2: *Sex and Age Distribution of the World Population.* New York: United Nations.

———. 2004. *World Population Prospects: The 2002 Revision.* Vol. 3: *Analytical Report.* New York: United Nations.

World Bank. 2004. *World Development Indicators 2004.* Washington, DC: World Bank.

Zaba, B., and S. Gregson. 1998. "Measuring the Impact of HIV on Fertility in Africa." *AIDS* 12 (Suppl. 1): S41–50.

Chapter 7

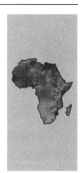

Levels and Patterns of Mortality at INDEPTH Demographic Surveillance Systems

Osman A. Sankoh, Pierre Ngom, Samuel J. Clark, Don de Savigny, and Fred Binka

Empirical, longitudinal, population-based data on mortality in Africa have, until recently, been unavailable. This critical information gap for Sub-Saharan Africa became even more evident as an impediment to our understanding of health and disease in Africa with the arrival of a major new cause of rapidly increasing mortality in the form of HIV/AIDS. At about the same time, during the 1990s, many large-scale mortality intervention trials were conducted at the community level, principally for understanding the efficacy of new interventions such as vitamin A supplementation, and the use of insecticide-treated mosquito nets for malaria control (Alonso et al. 1991; Binka et al. 1996; Nevill et al. 1996; Ross et al. 1995). All these trials used demographic surveillance systems (DSSs) to measure the impact of mortality. These successful mortality intervention trial efforts focused renewed attention on the usefulness of DSSs for illuminating the fundamental age, sex, and cause structure of mortality in resource-constrained settings in Africa. The malaria intervention trials themselves forced a complete reconsideration of the previously underestimated role of malaria as a direct and indirect cause of mortality in Africa (Breman, Egan, and Keusch 2002). More and more DSS sites

established for these trials have continued to operate long after the end of the original trials and have proved increasingly useful for both researchers and policy makers (Armstrong et al. 1999; de Savigny et al. 1999; Tanzania Ministry of Health 1997).

Accurate data on mortality conditions in Africa are still scarce. Until recently, the main tool for bridging this gap was the use of indirect demographic estimation techniques and model age-specific mortality schedules produced by Brass and colleagues (1973), Coale and Demeny (1966), and the United Nations Department of International Economic and Social Affairs (1982). The Brass relational system is based on empirical data collected in West Africa during the middle of the twentieth century. In contrast, neither the Coale and Demeny nor the UN model life table systems use significant amounts of data collected from Africa. Moreover, all three of the systems are based on 30- to 50-year-old data. Given the dramatic demographic changes that have affected Africa in the past 20 to 30 years and the fact that two of the systems are based largely on data collected from other regions of the world, whereas the third is based on data from only one region of Africa, it may be problematic to use them in the current African context. No doubt, the World Fertility Survey (WFS) and the Demographic and Health Surveys (DHSs) have remedied the above situation in part by increasing our knowledge of the level, trends, and differentials in infant and child mortality in the developing world. Also, since independence, several African countries have undertaken national censuses, but mortality data from these sources are often plagued with underreporting and need, therefore, to be adjusted using hypotheses that are not always realistic.

Much of the developing world is not adequately covered by accurate vital registration systems, leading to a substantial lack of direct empirical data describing mortality. Because planning must still be undertaken, information on mortality is inferred through interpolation or extrapolation from existing commonly observed age patterns of mortality—the so-called model life tables. These model age patterns of mortality are used to substitute, extend, or fill in where observed mortality data are missing and are often key ingredients in methods used to estimate demographic indicators from sparse data. Underlying epidemiological profiles are inferred based on those that are known to underlie the existing model of mortality patterns that most closely match the observed data. The closest-fitting model patterns are then used, among other things, to estimate levels of child mortality and create population projections.

DSSs bridge the data gap that exists in resource-constrained countries. A DSS refers to a methodological approach for monitoring a registered, dynamic cohort of the total population of a geographically confined area. Typical DSS populations monitored include at least 60,000 individuals per site. This is usually sufficient to provide adequate sample sizes to monitor trends in all-cause mortality and the most common cause-specific mortality, by sex and age group. Members of the dynamic DSS cohort are registered as such during an initial census. New members enter the cohort either by system-registered births or in-migrations, and members exit either by system-registered deaths or by out-migration. Causes of death are determined for all deaths by verbal autopsy. Continuous cycles of reenumeration maintain an accurate person-time denominator and help identify numerator events such as pregnancies, births, deaths, and migration. These cycles of reenumeration typically take place three to four times per year in order to optimize the chance to identify pregnancies and thus determine outcomes of pregnancy. In addition to the routine data capture performed by specialist teams of enumerators and supervisors, larger numbers of community key-informants continuously notify the system of birth or death events for immediate follow-up. Only events occurring to registered households and members are linked to the database for analysis. Sophisticated field operational logistics and linked data quality control and computing systems support this routine DSS surveillance (MacLeod, Phillips, and Binka 1995; Phillips, MacLeod, and Pence 2000). DSS sites can generate accurate population structures, person-years at risk, mortality rates, cause-specific mortality rates, proportional mortality, fertility rates, and rates of internal and external migrations. In addition, because of the intensity of household survey frequency, DSS sites commonly document a large array of contextual information on household structures, dependency, occupation, education, access to and use of services, as well as socioeconomic status. A typical DSS produces more than 100 health- and poverty-monitoring indicators annually on each household. Details of DSS concepts and methods are provided by INDEPTH Network (2002).

On the completeness and reliability of data produced by DSS, Korenromp and colleagues (2003) wrote in their review paper, "For Africa, with an increasing number of sites that monitor cause-specific mortality at a population level by means of standard methods under the INDEPTH network, DSS may at present form one of the more complete data sources." And WHO/UNICEF (2003, 20) conclude in their *Africa Malaria Report—2003* that "[a]t present, the most reliable data on trends in malaria death in children under 5 years of age is obtained from demographic surveillance systems (DSS)."

In 1998 a large number of DSS sites formed an international network called the INDEPTH Network. Details of the sites, their locations, the populations they follow, and basic demographic outputs of each site are available on the Internet (www.indepth-network.net) and in INDEPTH Network (2002). The central purpose of the INDEPTH Network is to facilitate cross-site analyses of comparable data across broader geographic areas with more diverse circumstances in order to answer questions that cannot be answered within individual sites. Comparative mortality and mortality patterns are an obvious first endeavor of such a network, and these are provided in this chapter. By the efforts of the members of the INDEPTH Network, for the first time schedules of mortality in Africa and empirical data on age standardization and on age and sex structure are available. This network is the source of the analyses presented in this chapter.

Standardized mortality rates were computed based on the new INDEPTH Network standard population that for the first time is derived from empirical data. The INDEPTH standard population typifies the true structure of the young population in Sub-Saharan Africa. The chapter then presents basic life table indicators for INDEPTH sites, based on their age-specific mortality rates over the 1995–99 period. Seven new mortality patterns are developed from more than 4.2 million person-years of observation at the African INDEPTH sites. These patterns are demonstrated to be substantially different from conventionally used model mortality patterns applied to Africa.

LEVELS OF MORTALITY AT INDEPTH NETWORK SITES

The data used in this chapter come from 17 DSS sites in Sub-Saharan Africa for which information on mortality was available for at least a full year from 1995 to 1999 (table 7.1).

The overall average length of the observation period for the contributing sites is four years. The data yield a total of 3,979,155 person-years of exposure, during which 55,356

deaths occurred. An average of about 17 percent of the person-years exposed were lived at ages younger than five years, and an average of 39 percent of the deaths also occurred between birth and age five. The crude death rate for both sexes combined ranges from a low of 7 per 1,000 in Agincourt, South Africa, to 39 per 1,000 in Bandim, Guinea-Bissau.

Overall Mortality

The crude death rate and the expectation of life at birth are the two indicators used in this section to examine overall levels of mortality at the INDEPTH sites. In order to remove the influence of each site's age structure and to make the comparison of the crude death rates more reasonable, it is necessary to standardize such rates. To do this, there are several widely used standard age distributions, including Segi's world standard and World Health Organization (WHO) standard age distributions (Estève, Benhamou, and Raymond 1994). Both of these standards reflect populations with relatively low fertility and mortality. Consequently, they give significant weight to the middle years of life. All the INDEPTH sites record information from relatively young

Table 7.1 Summary of Mortality Data from INDEPTH Sites, 1995–99

Site	Country	Reporting period	Duration of period	Observed deaths	Observed person-years	Crude death rate	Deaths under age 5 (%)	Person-years under age 5 (%)
Agincourt	South Africa	1995–99	5	1,738	304,530	7.11	15.54	13.79
Bandafassi	Senegal	1995–99	5	901	41,286	33.57	53.16	19.86
Bandim	Guinea-Bissau	1995–97	3	1,830	64,434	38.65	56.01	27.69
Butajira	Ethiopia	1995–96	2	834	72,873	19.20	41.49	16.94
Dar es Salaam	Tanzania	1994/95–1998/99a	5	4,515	354,041	21.75	27.44	13.87
Farefenni	The Gambia	1995–99	5	1,201	81,872	21.23	45.05	17.12
Gwembe	Zambia	1991–95	5	576	37,089	26.89	59.72	19.37
Hai	Tanzania	1994/95–1998/99a	5	8,106	746,864	16.09	23.14	14.30
Ifakara	Tanzania	1997–99	3	1,812	159,639	20.28	41.17	16.23
Manhica	Mozambique	1998–99	2	973	67,344	20.97	35.66	17.06
Mlomp	Senegal	1995–99	5	374	37,051	13.75	20.59	10.80
Morogoro	Tanzania	1994/95–1998/99a	5	9,548	538,286	30.01	29.03	13.01
Navrongo	Ghana	1995–99	5	11,278	691,679	27.72	34.46	14.10
Niakhar	Senegal	1995–98	4	1,993	116,133	24.30	51.03	18.05
Nouna	Burkina Faso	1995–98	4	1,650	117,156	17.00	40.48	18.24
Oubritenga	Burkina Faso	1995–98	4	6,967	478,315	24.83	49.63	17.40
Rufiji	Tanzania	1999	1	1,060	70,563	33.96	35.47	16.32
Total or average			4	55,356	3,979,155	23.37	38.77	16.71

Source: INDEPTH Network 2002.

a. Reporting in mid-year to mid-year annual periods resulted in a five-year reporting period from July 15, 1994, to July 15, 1998.

populations with comparatively high fertility and high mortality. Under those conditions, there are proportionally more young people in the population, giving it a "younger" age distribution. When the Segi or WHO standard age distributions are applied to the INDEPTH data, they give too much weight to the relatively high mortality rates prevailing at middle and older ages and too little weight to mortality at younger ages. Consequently, the absolute level of the age-standardized crude death rates produced with those standards significantly overestimates the true level of mortality at the INDEPTH Network sites.

To address this problem and create age-standardized crude death rates that more accurately reflect the true level of mortality at the INDEPTH sites, we have constructed the INDEPTH standard age distribution. An average age distribution is constructed for each site over the period 1995–99 by taking the weighted average of the person-years of exposure in each age group across all the years for which data are reported. The weight for each year is the total number of person-years reported for all ages during that year. The INDEPTH standard age distribution is calculated by taking the weighted average of the individual site average age distributions in each age group. In this case the weights are the total number of person-years in each of the individual site average age distributions. In figure 7.1, the younger age distribution of the INDEPTH standard, which is typical of developing countries, is contrasted with the much older population structures of the Segi and WHO standards.

Figure 7.1 Standard Population Age Structure from INDEPTH, Segi, and WHO

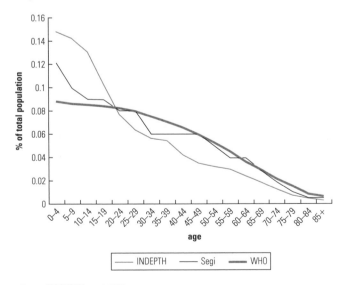

Source: INDEPTH Network 2002.

Table 7.2 displays the crude death rate for each site and the age-standardized crude death rates calculated using both the INDEPTH and Segi standard age distributions along with the values for the expectation of life at birth.

The INDEPTH Network standardized crude death rates range from 7 to 33 per 1,000 for males and 5 to 27 per 1,000 for females, revealing a wide range of mortality at the INDEPTH sites. The figures for the expectation of life at birth vary in a relationship that is loosely inverse to the values of the crude death rate (figure 7.2), and they cover a similarly wide range of from 66 to 36 years for males and 74 to 40 years for females. The data from Bandim are anomalous and reflect some unresolved questions concerning the manner in which they were collected and reported.

There is some geographic clustering. Together at the low end of the spectrum are three rural sites from Tanzania (Hai, Ifakara, and Rufiji) and one site in Senegal (Mlomp). In the middle of the pack are three sites in West Africa: Farefenni, Nouna, and Oubritenga. At the high end there is a mixture of sites from West, East, and southern Africa. The absolute level of mortality varies considerably over space; sites located close to each other have similar levels of mortality, but all major regions of Africa show a wide range of mortality levels.

For the most part the sex differentials are relatively small but are generally in favor of females, as expected. Two of the sites in southern Africa—Agincourt, in South Africa, and Manhica, in Mozambique—have significant male migration and register more substantial sex differentials, which stand out in contrast to the rest of the sites. Bandim, West Africa, also records a substantial sex differential, but as noted above there may be a methodological explanation for this.

Infant and Child Mortality

The measures of child mortality displayed in table 7.3 are the life table probabilities of dying in a specified age group: $_1q_0$ for ages zero to one year, $_4q_1$ for ages one to five years, and $_5q_0$ for ages zero to five years. The conventional infant mortality rate—the ratio of the number of deaths below one year of age and the number of births for a given period—is also included.

As shown in figure 7.3, there is a wide range in the level of child mortality. The probability that a newborn dies before reaching its fifth birthday ranges from 32 per 1,000 to 255 per 1,000 for males and 34 per 1,000 to 217 per 1,000 for females. The Agincourt site in South Africa records a comparatively low level of child mortality. Another cluster,

Table 7.2 Crude Death Rates and Expectation of Life at Birth
(per thousand)

Site	Male				Female			
	CDR	ASCDR$_I$	ASCDR$_S$	e_0	CDR	ASCDR$_I$	ASCDR$_S$	e_0
Agincourt	5.93	7.42	9.43	66.12	4.65	4.90	5.90	74.38
Mlomp	10.35	10.80	12.51	60.46	9.83	8.59	9.68	64.78
Hai	12.33	11.56	13.49	56.26	9.49	8.65	9.74	62.80
Rufiji	14.67	12.19	13.57	53.40	15.35	12.61	13.28	52.18
Ifakara	11.70	12.45	13.98	55.73	11.01	11.37	12.28	58.22
Butajira	11.65	12.50	13.79	55.81	11.25	12.44	13.50	56.68
Nouna	13.74	13.62	14.46	54.20	14.42	14.41	15.71	53.06
Oubritenga	15.68	14.93	15.95	51.63	13.58	13.05	13.53	55.08
Farefenni	16.24	15.84	17.47	50.83	13.17	13.56	14.08	55.05
Dar es Salaam	12.84	17.15	20.52	50.32	12.66	16.45	19.42	49.76
Niakhar	18.45	17.45	18.26	48.80	15.89	14.40	14.81	53.59
Manhica	17.00	17.50	20.11	47.47	12.41	11.36	12.60	58.12
Navrongo	17.66	18.07	20.42	47.22	15.10	15.82	17.66	51.39
Gwembe	18.69	19.27	21.89	47.32	16.82	17.95	19.67	53.66
Morogoro	18.70	19.27	21.90	44.44	16.82	17.95	19.67	46.11
Bandafassi	23.49	20.62	21.62	44.74	20.36	18.30	18.71	47.54
Bandim	31.35	32.86	38.63	35.86	25.65	27.48	31.42	38.91

Source: INDEPTH Network 2002.
Note: CDR = crude death rate; ASCDR = age-standardized crude death rate; I = standardized with INDEPTH Standard Age Structure; S = standardized with Segi Standard Age Structure; e_0 = expectation of life at birth.

Figure 7.2 Crude Death Rate and Expectation of Life at Birth

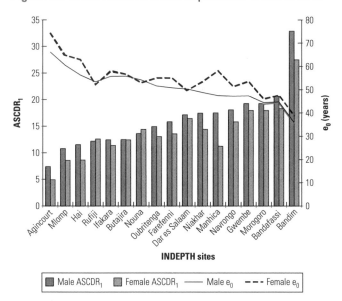

Source: INDEPTH Network 2002.
Note: ASCDR$_1$ = age-standardized crude death rate, INDEPTH Standard Age Structure; e_0 = expectation of life at birth.

composed of Mlomp in Senegal and Hai in Tanzania, reports low levels of child mortality but not nearly as low as that of the South Africa site. The next higher cluster is composed of sites from various regions of Africa including Dar es Salaam, Tanzania; Butajira, Ethiopia; Ifakara, Tanzania; Nouna, Burkina Faso; and Manhica, Mozambique. Following after that with $_5q_0$ close to 175 per 1,000 for males and females are Farefenni, The Gambia; Rufiji, Tanzania; Navrongo, Ghana; Gwembe, Zambia; Morogoro, Tanzania; and Oubritenga, Burkina Faso. The three remaining sites—Niakhar, Senegal; Bandim, Guinea-Bissau; and Bandafassi, Senegal—all have substantially higher values of $_5q_0$ closer to 225 per 1,000. There is a wide range in the level of child mortality, but except at the lowest and highest levels, there does not appear to be any geographical clustering. The lowest levels are definitely found in South Africa, whereas the highest levels are reported from West Africa.

Table 7.3 also displays the ratio of $_1q_0$ to $_4q_1$ in order to elucidate the changing risk of death faced by children before and after their first birthday.[1] This ratio reveals that children in Rufiji who survive to age one face a probability of death that is improved by nearly a factor of four, whereas children

Table 7.3 Infant and Child Mortality
(per thousand)

Site	IMR	Male				Female			
		$_1q_0$	$_4q_1$	$_5q_0$	$_1q_0/_4q_1$	$_1q_0$	$_4q_1$	$_5q_0$	$_1q_0/_4q_1$
Agincourt	16.93	15.06	17.52	32.32	0.86	16.63	17.35	33.69	0.96
Mlomp	45.18	48.24	42.61	88.80	1.13	49.42	51.74	98.60	0.96
Hai	67.13	66.78	26.73	91.73	2.50	56.54	26.68	81.71	2.12
Dar es Salaam	71.13	66.38	50.86	113.86	1.30	67.20	52.49	116.16	1.28
Butajira	67.82	65.62	57.73	119.56	1.14	71.09	62.20	128.87	1.14
Ifakara	93.22	76.12	52.23	124.37	1.46	86.09	50.27	132.03	1.71
Nouna	40.85	34.31	107.53	138.15	0.32	42.71	106.82	144.97	0.40
Manhica	72.65	85.75	68.91	148.75	1.24	59.37	60.41	116.19	0.98
Farefenni	74.65	68.04	110.47	171.00	0.62	66.46	109.12	168.32	0.61
Rufiji	—	91.0	46.4	133.2	1.96	110.0	35.1	141.6	3.13
Navrongo	109.59	106.58	83.54	181.21	1.28	102.96	73.23	168.65	1.41
Gwembe	—	105.24	87.26	183.32	1.21	111.94	78.78	181.90	1.42
Morogoro	116.73	105.24	87.26	183.32	1.21	111.94	78.78	181.90	1.42
Oubritenga	96.49	102.25	95.97	188.41	1.07	91.88	104.84	187.09	0.88
Niakhar	—	89.80	146.84	223.45	0.61	72.16	129.14	191.98	0.56
Bandim	—	112.37	129.78	227.57	0.87	101.52	128.31	216.80	0.79
Bandafassi	124.88	138.60	134.59	254.54	1.03	116.43	114.29	217.42	1.02

Source: INDEPTH Network 2002.
Note: IMR = infant mortality ratio; — = not available.

Figure 7.3 Child Mortality: Probability of Dying between Birth and Age Five ($_5q_0$)

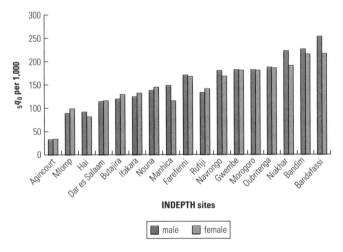

INDEPTH sites

■ male ■ female

Source: INDEPTH Network 2002.

in Bandafassi face a nearly constant probability of dying throughout the first five years of life.

Differences in child mortality according to sex are relatively small and do not appear to consistently favor one sex over the other. Interestingly this pattern is broken by four sites—Manhica, Mozambique; Rufiji, Tanzania; Niakhar, Senegal; and Bandafassi, Senegal—where there is a clear difference favoring females, except in Rufiji, where males are favored.

Adult Mortality

Values for the probability that persons who survive to their twentieth birthday will survive to their fiftieth birthday, that is, $_{30}q_{20}$, are displayed in table 7.4 along with values of $_5q_0$ and the ratio of $_5q_0$ to $_{30}q_{20}$.[2] There are wide variations in the levels of adult mortality from 159 per 1,000 to 501 per 1,000 for males and 112 per 1,000 to 421 per 1,000 for females. A number of sites record substantial differences in adult mortality between the sexes—Agincourt, South Africa; Hai, Tanzania; Manhica, Mozambique; Mlomp, Senegal; and Navrongo, Ghana, in particular. There also exists the opposite differential, wherein female mortality rates exceed male rates, at two sites: Rufiji, Tanzania; and Dar es Salaam, Tanzania. The human immunodeficiency virus and acquired immune deficiency syndrome (HIV/AIDS) and maternal mortality may explain these patterns.

For the first time, Agincourt in South Africa does not define the low end of the range. There also does not appear

Table 7.4 Adult Mortality and Child and Adult Mortality Ratio
(per thousand)

Site	Male			Female		
	$5q_0$	$30q_{20}$	$5q_0/30q_{20}$	$5q_0$	$30q_{20}$	$5q_0/30q_{20}$
Mlomp	88.80	159.03	0.56	98.60	111.51	0.88
Niakhar	223.45	165.25	1.35	191.98	141.86	1.35
Agincourt	32.32	196.35	0.16	33.69	100.77	0.33
Nouna	138.15	199.93	0.69	144.97	184.51	0.79
Farefenni	171.00	205.13	0.83	168.32	149.88	1.12
Oubritenga	188.41	210.62	0.89	187.09	157.60	1.19
Bandafassi	254.54	226.27	1.12	217.42	200.42	1.08
Butajira	119.56	227.19	0.53	128.87	193.86	0.66
Rufiji	133.2	234.77	0.57	141.6	268.42	0.53
Ifakara	124.37	240.09	0.52	132.03	185.07	0.71
Navrongo	181.21	298.01	0.61	168.65	188.86	0.89
Hai	91.73	304.77	0.30	81.71	229.38	0.36
Dar es Salaam	113.86	331.46	0.34	116.16	369.74	0.31
Manhica	148.75	382.13	0.39	116.19	197.39	0.59
Gwembe	183.32	408.82	0.45	181.90	372.81	0.49
Morogoro	183.32	409.03	0.45	181.90	372.81	0.49
Bandim	227.57	500.75	0.45	216.80	421.42	0.51

Source: INDEPTH Network 2002.

to be any substantial geographical clustering of similar risk of adult mortality within the region. The cluster of moderate risk includes sites from all major regions of Sub-Saharan Africa as does the high risk cluster.

The relationship between child and adult mortality reveals two distinct groups: sites in West Africa and those in the rest of Africa. Some of the West African sites clearly record levels of child mortality that are high relative to the corresponding levels of adult mortality. In the West African sites of Bandafassi, Senegal; Farefenni, The Gambia; Oubritenga, Burkina Faso; and Niakhar, Senegal, this is the result of unusually high child mortality coupled with substantial adult mortality.

INDEPTH NETWORK MORTALITY PATTERNS

This section summarizes the method used to identify the seven INDEPTH patterns of mortality. For a full description of the process, see INDEPTH Network 2002, chap. 7. Key considerations in identifying common underlying patterns (empirical regularities) are the filtering out of small, unimportant, and potentially random variation; the reduction of

the dimensionality of the data to as few dimensions as possible; and the provision of a common reference to which all of the observed patterns can be compared.

Principal Components

The principal components technique is used to identify 15 age components that together are able to represent all but a negligible amount of the variation in age patterns of mortality among the 70 male and female site periods. In fact, the first four of these components represent the vast majority of the variation in the original data. When recombined with the appropriate weights the components are able to represent all the observed age patterns of mortality in the INDEPTH database, and furthermore, by choosing different weights any arbitrary age pattern of mortality can be represented to within a negligible error.

The first four principal components address all three of the key considerations important to identifying common underlying patterns: by dropping the other components much of the small-magnitude, random noise is eliminated; the dimensionality of the data is reduced to four weights instead of 18 age groups; and the four principal components provide a common reference against which all the observed patterns can be compared. The task then becomes how to identify similar observed patterns.

Clustering

The aim of cluster analysis is to identify groups of similar objects. The objects are usually described by a vector of numbers representing measurements of some attributes of the objects. In this case, the vectors each contain four coefficients representing the weights on the first four principal components that are necessary to reproduce a given observed mortality pattern.[3] The hierarchical clustering algorithm is used to identify five clusters of similar mortality patterns for males and seven for females. Because the seven female patterns are quite different from one another and because the male patterns corresponding to the two additional female patterns are grouped together in the male clusters, the seven female clusters are chosen as the final clusters of observed mortality patterns.

Once the clusters are identified the person-year weighted average of the individual age patterns in each cluster is calculated to yield the characteristic age pattern of mortality for each cluster.

The Seven INDEPTH Mortality Patterns

The seven commonly observed age patterns of mortality emerging from the INDEPTH data are sufficiently different from the existing model life tables (INDEPTH Network 2002) to qualify as *new* mortality patterns; and because almost all the data on which they are based come from Africa, they are African patterns appropriate for use in Africa. The natural log–transformed, $\ln(_nq_x)$, values are displayed in figure 7.4.

Underlying epidemiological profiles underpinning each pattern are still being identified. The INDEPTH Network is actively engaged in gathering and analyzing information on cause of death corresponding to the raw mortality rates presented here. Once that work is complete, it will be possible to identify the specific causes of death contributing to each pattern. However, until that time we must speculate and infer from what is known about the regional distribution of major causes of death in Africa.

The following discussion of the patterns has largely been excerpted from chapter 7 of *Population, Health, and Survival at INDEPTH Sites* (INDEPTH Network 2002).

Pattern 1. The first pattern is similar to the Coale-Demeny North and UN Latin American model life table age patterns of mortality (INDEPTH Network 2002). There is no indication that HIV/AIDS affects pattern 1, and the male and female age patterns are similar with the exception of a bulge in the female pattern during the reproductive years, presumably caused by maternal mortality. Pattern 1 is primarily derived from sites in West Africa over the entire period covered by the INDEPTH Network data set. HIV/AIDS has not yet become as significant a problem in West Africa as it is in central and southern Africa, so a large impact of AIDS in the data from West Africa is not expected. It is worth noting that child mortality between the ages of one and nine is significant and substantially elevated above the most similar existing models. This is in keeping with the fact that malaria is a significant cause of death in West Africa, and it has a large impact on those ages.

Pattern 2. The INDEPTH Network pattern 2 is derived largely from Asian data and for that reason is not discussed here; see INDEPTH Network 2002 for a discussion of pattern 2.

Pattern 3. The sites contributing to pattern 3 are almost exclusively located in southern Africa and East Africa, South Africa and Tanzania in particular. This pattern obviously contains some influence of HIV/AIDS but not nearly to the degree observed in pattern 5. The South African data come from the Agincourt site (INDEPTH Network 2002), where mortality is extraordinarily low compared with the other INDEPTH sites in Africa, and where HIV/AIDS is recognized but does not yet affect the population in the catastrophic sense that it does in other parts of southern and East Africa. The remainder of the data come from the Dar es Salaam site, where the impact of HIV/AIDS appears to be greater. This pattern is most similar to the UN Far East pattern of mortality, corresponding to the low infant and child mortality compared with mortality at older ages (INDEPTH Network 2002). A noteworthy feature of this pattern is that infant and child mortality does not appear to be substantially elevated, as might be expected when HIV/AIDS is an important contributor to mortality. Timaeus (1998) suggests that the strong secular decrease in child mortality that has been observed in many settings in Africa during the latter half of the twentieth century may largely cancel out the increase in child mortality brought about by HIV to yield approximately unchanging child mortality, rather than the

Figure 7.4 INDEPTH Mortality Patterns 1–7, $\ln(_nq_x)$

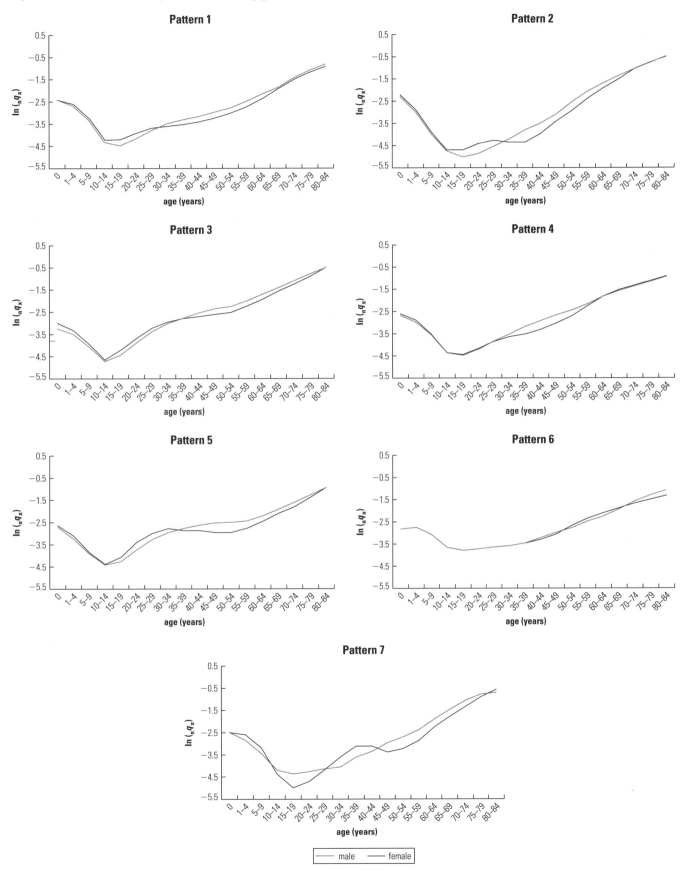

increase that might be expected when HIV is having such an easily observed impact on adult mortality.

Pattern 4. Pattern 4 is a variation on pattern 1 with the important difference manifested in the 35 to 69 age range. At all other ages, patterns 1 and 4 are negligibly different except that infant and child mortality in pattern 4 is consistently slightly lower than pattern 1. But between ages 35 and, roughly, 69 pattern 4 reveals significantly higher mortality than pattern 1. This pattern is most similar to the UN general pattern for females and UN Latin American pattern for males (INDEPTH Network 2002). As was the case with pattern 1, most of the data contributing to pattern 4 comes from West Africa.

Pattern 5. The HIV/AIDS pattern of mortality is most clearly visible in pattern 5. The data contributing to pattern 5 are derived from the three Tanzanian sites run by the Adult Morbidity and Mortality Project (AMMP) in Dar es Salaam, Hai, and Morogoro (INDEPTH Network 2002). There is a striking bulge in the mortality of males between the ages of 20 and 54 and for females between the ages of 15 and 49. The female bulge is significantly narrower and more pronounced, corresponding to the earlier infection of the female population and within a tighter age range than the male population. This pattern is not particularly similar to any of the existing model patterns, but it is most closely matched with the UN General (female) and Latin American (male) model patterns (INDEPTH Network 2002). Pattern 5 differs from pattern 3 mainly in the shape of the HIV/AIDS impact. The effect is more diffuse with age in pattern 3, meaning that mortality is elevated through a broader age range, the magnitude of the elevation is more consistent, and the differences between the sexes are less apparent. Pattern 3 is derived largely from the Dar es Salaam data, and this may reflect the fact that the epidemic is more mature in Dar es Salaam and has consequently had enough time to infect a wider age range of people of both sexes. As with pattern 3, it is worth noting that infant and child mortality do not appear to be substantially affected in a manner comparable to adult mortality.

Pattern 6. Pattern 6 is one of the two additional patterns identified in the female data. It is an interesting pattern that reveals high mortality of children and teenagers and comparatively low mortality of infants and adults of all ages. This pattern is exhibited by sites in northeastern Africa and West Africa, with most of the data coming from Ethiopia.

Without additional information, it is not possible to speculate on what may be producing this unique pattern. The male pattern is most similar to the Coale-Demeny North model pattern, and the female pattern is closest to the Coale-Demeny West model, both of which embody high mortality in the same age ranges (INDEPTH Network 2002). They deviate from those patterns in that infant mortality is substantially less than would be found in either model pattern, and child and adolescent mortality is significantly higher: this might be called the "Super North" pattern.

Pattern 7. Pattern 7 is the other additional pattern identified in the female data, and it, too, is interesting. It is derived from two sites located in central and West Africa. The reason it was identified in the female data is obvious; there is a substantial bulge in the female age pattern between ages 25 and 44. This pattern comes mainly from one small site in Zambia, so it is probably not worth extensive interpretation. The corresponding male pattern is similar to pattern 6, and both are similar to the Coale-Demeny North model pattern (INDEPTH Network 2002). The North model pattern contains relatively high child and teenage mortality coupled with comparatively low mortality at older ages. This is consistent with the fact that malaria is an important contributor to mortality in both sites.

CONCLUSION

In their 1996 review of demographic models, Coale and Trussell (1996) describe the identification of "empirical regularities" as one of the central motifs of demographic modeling. Their term accurately describes the formulation of model mortality schedules and hints strongly at the limits of their usefulness. Because there are no general, reliable, theory-driven models of the individual risk of death, we must rely on commonly observed patterns to guide us— *empirical regularities.* Because these are simply commonly observed patterns, however, we must be careful not to inappropriately overinterpret them or substitute them for a thorough understanding of the mechanisms underlying the risks of death that lead to each pattern. Beyond being the first step in understanding these mechanisms, identifying underlying empirical regularities in age patterns of mortality is still a useful exercise in its own right.

With fertility and to a lesser degree migration, mortality shapes the size and age composition of a population and is consequently of great interest to policy makers who must adequately plan for the future of a population. Mortality is one of the most valuable indicators of the health of a population and, as such, is of critical importance to those who manage health care infrastructures. As a sensitive indicator of where a population is and where it will be in the near future, knowledge of mortality is a vital component of population planning and management.

Existing systems of model life tables include systems developed by the Population Branch of the United Nations Department of Social Affairs (1955) in the early 1950s, by Coale and Demeny (1966) in the early 1960s, by Ledermann and Breas (1959) in the late 1950s, by Brass (1971) in the late 1960s, and finally by the UN again in the early 1980s (United Nations Department of International Economic and Social Affairs 1982). Only two are in common use today; the Coale and Demeny system and the 1982 UN set. However, neither of these systems was formulated with anything more than trivial data from Africa: apart from the West pattern that appears to contain a small amount of data from the white population of South Africa, none of the Coale and Demeny patterns is based on data from Africa; and apart from a small amount of data from Tunisia, neither are the recent UN patterns.

The lack of empirical data from Africa underlying either of the commonly used model mortality systems is a significant problem for demographers working in Africa, as Preston, Heuveline, and Guillot (2001) eloquently state: "A limitation, common to all the systems discussed so far [excluding the 1982 UN models], is that their empirical basis consists almost exclusively of the experience of developed countries. Most applications of model life tables, however, are addressed to developing countries with incomplete data."

Making this problem worse is the dissimilarity of the epidemiological profile of large parts of Africa to that of the developed world; it is clear that malaria and HIV are primarily to blame. Both increase overall levels of mortality and may affect certain age groups disproportionately. The significant endemic prevalence of these two diseases is responsible for vast excesses in mortality in some of the harder hit age groups; malaria for young children and HIV for children and young-to-middle-aged adults.

It is clear that the existing model mortality patterns are not appropriate for use in Africa, given that they were not built using data from Africa and that there is good reason to believe that the mortality profile of Africa is different from other parts of the world. Until now, however, there has been

no alternative. It is to begin addressing this need that the INDEPTH Network has compiled a database of primarily African empirical mortality data and has begun to identify common age patterns of mortality described by those data (INDEPTH Network 2002).

DSS site data are sometimes challenged as being unrepresentative (Lopez et al. 2000) of surrounding constituencies due to the history of clinical and community-based intervention trials that are conducted in such populations from time to time. However, there is little evidence that the mortality patterns in trial sites are markedly different from those prevailing in similar settings nearby, where trials have not been conducted. The reason for the paucity of evidence is that most trials are conducted on a subset of the population, and they target a specific cause of mortality. Usually the interventions do not continue after the trial, unless they are adopted as broad implementation policy (for example, insecticide-treated nets), whereby the nontrial areas are, within a few years, at the same level of coverage for the intervention. We must also appreciate that our health system interventions have relatively weak modulating effects on population mortality compared with secular trends in socioeconomic circumstances and environmental forces. We should recognize that the modest population size of a DSS site does not constitute a major flaw, however, as even sites monitoring small-sized populations can produce robust measures of age-specific mortality when data are aggregated over a period of several years. Moreover, data collected over long periods of time from the same population living in the same area can reveal important age-specific trends in the risk of death. Furthermore, when data from a number of widely dispersed sites are brought together, they provide both a geographically and temporally representative measure of mortality conditions. At present, only DSS sites provide data that can be used to depict the temporal and geographical contours of mortality patterns in Africa.

NOTES

1. $_1q_0$ represents the probability of dying before age one for newborns; $_4q_1$ represents the probability of dying before age five for those who survive to age one. In general, $_nq_x$ is the probability of dying between the ages of x and $x + n$ for those who survive to age x.

2. $_5q_0$ represents the probability of dying before age five for newborns.

3. See INDEPTH Network 2002 for a discussion of why the age pattern and level of mortality are orthogonal in the principal components model. This allows the clustering technique to identify clusters based on age pattern only, regardless of the level of mortality; essentially the principal components model controls for level.

REFERENCES

Alonso, P. L., S. W. Lindsay, J. R. Armstrong, M. Conteh, A. G. Hill, P. H. David, G. Fegan et al. 1991. "The Effect of Insecticide-Treated Bed Nets on Mortality of Gambian Children." *Lancet* 337: 1499–502.

Armstrong Schellenberg, J. R., S. Abdulla, H. Minja, R. Nathan, O. Mukasa, T. Marchant, H. Mponda et al. 1999. "KINET: A Social Marketing Programme of Treated Nets and Net Treatment for Malaria Control in Tanzania, with Evaluation of Child Health and Long-Term Survival." *Transactions of the Royal Society of Tropical Medicine and Hygiene* 93: 225–31.

Binka, F. N., A. Kubaje, M. Adjuik, L. A. Williams, C. Lengeler, G. H. Maude, G. E. Armah et al. 1996. "Impact of Permethrin Impregnated Bednets on Child Mortality in Kassena-Nankana District, Ghana: A Randomized Controlled Trial." *Tropical Medicine and International Health* 1 (2): 147–54.

Brass, W. 1971. "On the Scale of Morality." In *Biological Aspects of Demography*, ed. W. Brass. London: Taylor and Francis.

Brass, W., A. J. Coale, P. Demeny, D. F. Heisel, F. Lorimer, A. Romaniuk, and E. van de Walle. 1973. *The Demography of Tropical Africa*. Princeton, NJ: Princeton University Press.

Breman, J. G., A. Egan, G. T. Keusch. 2002. "The Intolerable Burden of Malaria: A New Look at the Numbers." *American Journal of Tropical Medicine and Hygiene* 64 (1, 2): iv–vii.

Coale, A., and P. Demeny. 1966. *Regional Model Life Tables and Stable Populations*. Princeton, NJ: Princeton University Press.

Coale, A., and J. Trussell. 1996. "The Development and Use of Demographic Models." *Population Studies* 50 (3): 469–84.

de Savigny, D., P. Setel, H. Kasale, D. Whiting, G. Reid, H. M. Kitange, C. Mbuya, L. Mgalula, H. Machibya, and P. Kilima. 1999. *Linking Demographic Surveillance and Health Service Needs—the AMMP/ TEHIP Experience in Tanzania*. Dar es Salaam.

Estève, J., E. Benhamou, and L. Raymond. 1994. *Statistical Methods in Cancer Research*. Vol. 4, *Descriptive Epidemiology*. Lyons: IARC.

INDEPTH Network. 2002. *Population, Health and Survival at INDEPTH Sites*. Vol. 1 of Population and Health in Developing Countries. Ottawa: International Development Research Centre.

Korenromp, E. L., B. G. Williams, E. Gouws, C. Dye, and R. W. Snow. 2003. "Measurement of Trends in Childhood Malaria Mortality in Africa: An Assessment of Progress Toward Targets Based on Verbal Autopsy." *Lancet* 3: 349–58.

Ledermann, S., and J. Breas. 1959. "Les dimension de la mortalité." *Population* 14 (4): 637–82.

Lopez, A., J. H. Salomon, O. B. Ahmad, C. J. L. Murray, and D. Mafat. 2000. "Life Tables for 191 Countries: Data, Methods, Results." GPE Discussion Paper 9, WHO, Geneva.

MacLeod, B., J. F. Phillips, and F. Binka. 1995. *Analysis of Longitudinal Data from the HRS*. New York: Population Council.

Nevill C. G., E. S. Some, V. O. Mung'ala, W. Mutemi, L. New, K. Marsh, C. Lengeler, and R. W. Snow. 1996. "Insecticide-Treated Bednets Reduce Mortality and Severe Morbidity from Malaria among Children on the Kenyan Coast." *Tropical Medicine and International Health* 1 (2): 139–280.

Phillips, J. F., B. MacLeod, and B. Pence. 2000. "The Household Registration System: Computer Software for Rapid Dissemination of Demographic Surveillance Systems." *Demographic Research* 2(6).

Preston, S. H., P. Heuveline, and M. Guillot. 2001. "Modeling Age Patterns of Vital Events." In *Demography: Measuring and Modeling Population Processes*, 191–210. Oxford: Blackwell.

Ross D. A., B. R. Kirkwood, F. N. Binka, P. Arthur, N. Dollimore, S. S. Morris, R. P. Shier, J. O. Gyapong, and P. G. Smith. 1995. "Child Morbidity and Mortality Following Vitamin A Supplementation in Ghana: Time Since Dosing, Number of Doses, and Time of Year." *American Journal of Public Health* 85 (9): 1246–51.

Tanzania Ministry of Health. 1997. "Policy Implications of Adult Morbidity and Mortality—End of Phase 1 Report." In *Adult Morbidity and Mortality Project*. Dar es Salaam: Government of Tanzania.

Timaeus, I. M. 1998. "Impact of the HIV Epidemic on Mortality in Sub-Saharan Africa: Evidence from National Surveys and Censuses." *AIDS* 12 (Suppl. 1): S15–27.

United Nations Department of Social Affairs. 1955. *Age and Sex Patterns of Mortality: Model Life Tables for Underdeveloped Countries*. New York: United Nations.

United Nations Department of International Economic and Social Affairs. 1982. *Model Life Tables for Developing Countries*. Population Studies 77. New York: United Nations.

WHO/UNICEF (World Health Organization/United Nations Children's Fund). 2003. *The Africa Malaria Report—2003*. Geneva: WHO and UNICEF.

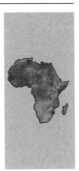

Chapter **8**

Trends and Issues in Child Undernutrition

Todd Benson and Meera Shekar

Child undernutrition remains one of Africa's most fundamental challenges for improved human development. Because the time and capacities of caregivers are limited, far too many children on the continent are unable to access and effectively use at all times the food and health services they need for a healthy life. An estimated 200 million people on the continent, both children and adults, are undernourished, their numbers having increased by almost 20 percent since the early 1990s (FAO 2003). This undernutrition starts early in life—more than a third of African children under the age of five are stunted in their growth and must face a range of physical and cognitive challenges not faced by their better-nourished peers. Malnutrition underlies 55 percent of all deaths of children under five years of age globally (Pelletier et al. 1994), and undernutrition is the major risk factor for over 28 percent of all deaths in Africa—some 2.9 million deaths annually (Ezzati et al. 2003). Further, Pelletier and Frongillo (2003) have shown that had countries in Sub-Saharan Africa reduced undernutrition rates over the period 1975–95 at the same modest rates as other regions of the world, the region would have experienced declines in under-five mortality rates 28 percent lower than those currently achieved. Childhood and maternal undernutrition is the primary risk factor contributing to almost 30 percent of the estimated annual burden of disease on the continent (table 8.1). The continuing human costs of undernutrition for individual Africans as measured by its contribution to high mortality and morbidity and unrealized human potential are enormous, and the aggregate costs at the national level impose a heavy burden on efforts to foster sustained economic growth and improved human development.

It is important to recognize the links between undernutrition, poverty, and, at the aggregate level, broad economic growth and national development. A necessary component for the success of new initiatives in Africa against poverty must be a sharp reduction in the current high levels of undernutrition. Broad-based economic growth is necessary to increase incomes and consumption and thereby to reduce poverty. Economic growth can primarily be achieved through enhanced economic productivity. Enhanced productivity comes about through broad improvements in the intellectual, physical, and technical capacity of the population. The potential intellectual, physical, and technical

Table 8.1 Percentage of Total Estimated Annual Burden of Disease in Africa Attributed to Major Risk Factors

Childhood and maternal undernutrition	*29.5*
Underweight	18.0
Iron deficiency	2.9
Vitamin A deficiency	4.7
Zinc deficiency	3.9
Other nutrition-related risks	*3.0*
High blood pressure	1.3
High cholesterol	0.6
High body-mass index (BMI)	0.4
Low fruit and vegetable intake	0.4
Physical inactivity	0.3
Sexual and reproductive health risks	*20.1*
Unsafe sex	19.4
Lack of contraception	0.8
Environmental risks	*10.1*
Unsafe water, sanitation, and hygiene	5.3
Indoor smoke from solid fuels	3.5
Other	1.1
Occupational risks	*0.7*
Addictive substances	*2.9*

Source: Ezzati et al. 2003.
Note: Percentage of total estimated annual burden of disease is the share of disability-adjusted life years (DALYs) lost attributed to major risk factors. Total estimated DALYs lost annually in Africa is 349,513,000.

capacity of the population is dependent on improved nutrition, particularly for young children and women in their childbearing years. Similarly, the effective use of such capacity is dependent on a properly nourished population in which individuals are living healthy and active lives and are able to creatively contribute to their own and the nation's economic well-being.

Malnutrition in any stage of childhood affects schooling and, thus, the lifetime earnings potential of the child. Malnutrition affects educational outcomes, including a reduced capacity to learn (as a result of early cognitive deficits or lowered current attention spans) and fewer total years of schooling. In Zimbabwe, stunting, via its association with a 7-month delay in school completion and a 0.7-year loss in grade attainment, has been shown to reduce lifetime income by 7 to 12 percent (Alderman, Hoddinott, and Kinsey 2003). In general, in low-income agricultural countries, the physical impairment associated with malnutrition is estimated to cost 2 to 3 percent of gross domestic product (GDP) per year, even without considering the long-term productivity losses associated with developmental and

cognitive impairment (Horton 1999). Iron deficiency in adults has been estimated to decrease productivity between 5 and 17 percent, depending on the nature of the work performed (Horton 1999). Data from 10 developing countries have shown that the median loss in reduced work capacity associated with anemia in adults is equivalent to 0.6 percent of GDP, whereas an additional 3.4 percent of GDP is lost as a result of the effects on cognitive development attributable to anemia in children (Horton and Ross 2003). The impact of iodine deficiency diseases on cognitive development alone has been associated with productivity losses totaling approximately 10 percent of GDP (Horton 1999).

It is only when Africans have improved nutrition security that we will begin to see sustained progress toward the achievement of the aspirations laid out in the Millennium Development Goals (MDG), in the plans under the New Partnership for Africa's Development (NEPAD), and in the many national poverty reduction strategies.

WHAT CAUSES UNDERNUTRITION?

The United Nations Children's Fund (UNICEF) conceptual framework of the determinants of the nutritional status of children shown in figure 8.1 presents a generalized understanding of how undernutrition is the outcome of specific development problems related directly to the dietary intake and the health status of the individual. The quality of these immediate determinants, in turn, is determined by the underlying food security status of the household in which a child resides. However, of equal importance is the availability of health services and a healthy environment and the quality of care the child receives—that is, whether the available dietary resources for good nutrition are used effectively through appropriate caring practices. Sustained healthy and active life is only possible when these underlying determinants—food, health, and care—are each maximized. None of these is sufficient in itself, but all are necessary for good child growth.

The degree to which these three underlying determinants are expressed positively or negatively is a question of resources. These resources include the availability of food but extend much further to include the physical and economic access that a child or his or her caregiver has to that food, the caregiver's knowledge of how to use available food and to properly care for the child, the caregiver's own health status, and the control the caregiver has over resources within the household that might be used to nourish the child. Finally, the level of access to information on and services for

Figure 8.1 The UNICEF Conceptual Framework of the Determinants of Nutritional Status

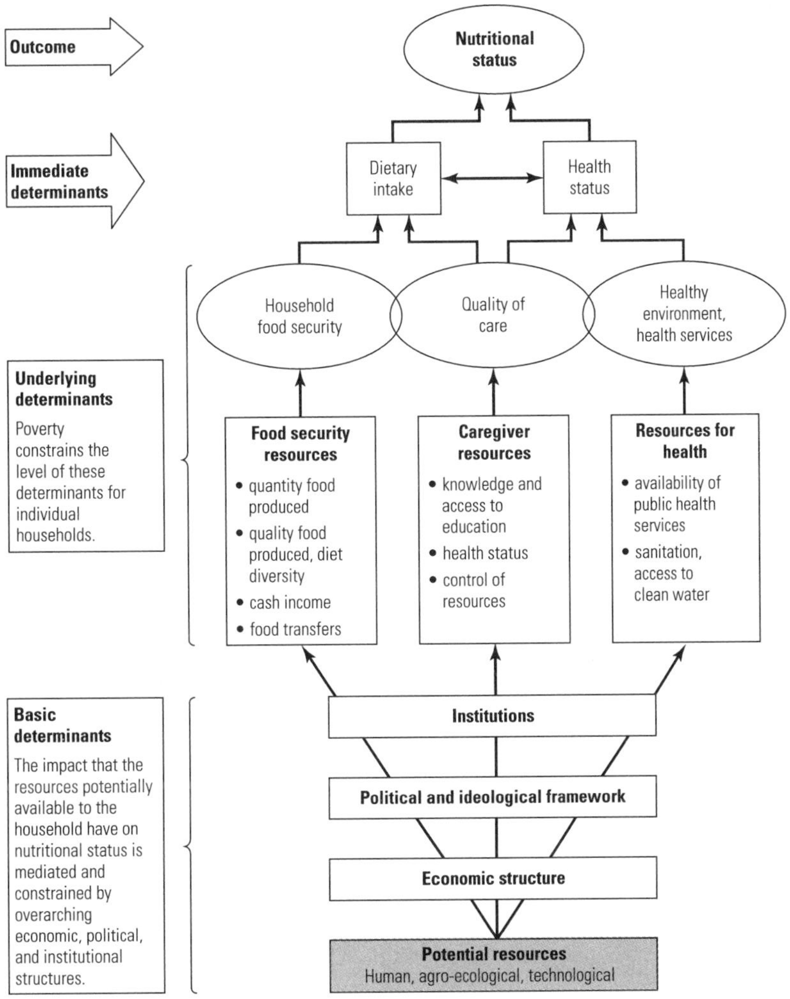

Sources: Jonsson 1993; Smith and Haddad 2000; and UNICEF 1990.

maintaining health, whether preventive and curative health services are available, and the presence or absence of a healthy environment with clean water, adequate sanitation, and proper shelter all contribute equally to determining the nutritional status of a child.

When the distribution of resources within society is central to accounting for why some are undernourished and others are not, the framework moves from the realm of the individual and household to the political. The framework links the availability of nutrition resources to a set of basic determinants, which are themselves a function of how society is organized in regard to economic structure, political and ideological expectations, and the institutions through which activities within society are regulated, social values are met, and potential resources are converted into actual resources. Consequently, this conceptual framework identifies undernutrition as a subject for political debate and an issue of immediate concern to any national development strategies.

Finally, it is important to recognize from this framework that a household or nation being food secure is not in itself sufficient to ensure the good nutritional status of children and others within that household or nation. It is possible to have poor nutritional outcomes without being food insecure. *Food security* is concerned with physical and economic access to food of sufficient quality and quantity. However, one may have reliable access to the components of a healthy diet, but because of poor health or care (such as poor infant-feeding practices), ignorance, or personal preferences, one may not be able or may choose not to use the nutrients to which one has access. In parallel to food security, one can speak of nutrition security. *Nutrition security* is achieved for a household when secure access to food is coupled with a sanitary environment, adequate health services, and knowledgeable care.

INDICATORS OF CHILD UNDERNUTRITION: OUTCOMES AND INPUTS

In this section, measures of child undernutrition and of its determinants—the outcomes and inputs, respectively, to the process determining nutritional status—are presented as a foundation for the discussion on the current status and trends in these measures in Sub-Saharan Africa.

Outcome Indicators

Table 8.2 provides a summary of the principal measures of both individual and aggregate nutritional status. Of these, the most commonly employed are the anthropometric measures of child nutritional status—stunting, underweight, and wasting. Children with abnormally low growth are identified by comparison with the growth characteristics of children of a similar age, disaggregated by sex, in a standard, nutritionally secure population. Children whose growth is more than two standard deviations (Z-scores) below the mean physical characteristics for the nutritionally secure reference population are considered undernourished.[1]

Of the other indicators of aggregate nutritional status, infant and under-five mortality and low birthweight prevalence are important proxy measures of nutrition security. Low birthweight reflects fetal growth retardation due to the poor health and nutrition of the mother and also serves as an indicator of risk of infant mortality and future poor health. From a life cycle perspective on nutrition and the intergenerational transmission of poverty within society, as presented in figure 8.2, low birthweight is a critical measure.

Table 8.2 Indicators of Nutritional Status

Indicator	How collected	Comments
Low height-for-age, "stunting"	Height (or length) measurements of children 6 to 60 months or 6 to 36 months in age. Children with abnormally low growth are identified by comparison to physical characteristics of children of similar age, disaggregated by sex, in a standard, nutritionally secure population.	Indicative of long-term nutritional status of children. Best measure of cumulative growth retardation.
Low weight-for-age, "underweight"	Weight measurements of children 6 to 60 months or 6 to 36 months in age. Analysis similar to that above.	Nonspecific indicator of overall undernutrition—measures a combination of chronic and acute undernutrition.
Low weight-for-height, "wasting"	Weight and height measurements of children 6 to 60 months or 6 to 36 months in age. Analysis similar to that above.	Measures acute child undernutrition. Indicative of sharp short-term fluctuations in nutritional status. Most useful in emergencies where severity of the nutritional crisis is being assessed or short-term progress in nutritional status is being monitored.
Mid-upper arm circumference	Distance around the mid-upper arm. Standard threshold values used to determine whether a child is at risk.	Used in emergencies in contexts similar to where the wasting measure would be used.
Body mass index	Computed as weight (in kg) divided by height (in meters) squared. Standard threshold values used to determine whether an individual is underweight or overweight.	Indicator of nutritional status in adults and older children. Only indicator commonly used to assess both short- and long-term nutritional status of adults, usually women of childbearing age. Used for assessing the prevalence of both underweight and overweight individuals in a population.
Micronutrient deficiency	Based on biochemical analysis (laboratory, some field tests) or symptomatic diagnosis of deficiency-related disease—night blindness (vitamin A), goiter (iodine), anemia (iron).	Difficult to collect on a large scale. Biochemical measures require access to analytical laboratory facilities. For some micronutrients, most notably zinc, biochemical measures of nutrient deficiency are not available and clinical diagnosis is not possible.
Infant mortality (under one year) and under-five mortality rates	Census, Demographic and Health Surveys.	Proxy measures of aggregate nutritional status. Integrated measure of risks to child survival, among which poor nutritional status is a major factor.
Low birthweight prevalence	Proportion of babies born weighing less than 2,500 g. Collected from health statistics.	Low birthweight reflects fetal growth retardation due to the poor health and nutrition of the mother. However, also serves as an indicator of risk of infant mortality and future poor health. Predicts, less precisely, economic and broad human potential of the child. From a life cycle perspective on nutrition and the intergenerational transmission of poverty within society (see figure 8.2), low birthweight is a critical measure.

Source: Compiled by authors.

Figure 8.2 The Burden of Undernutrition through the Life Cycle and across Generations

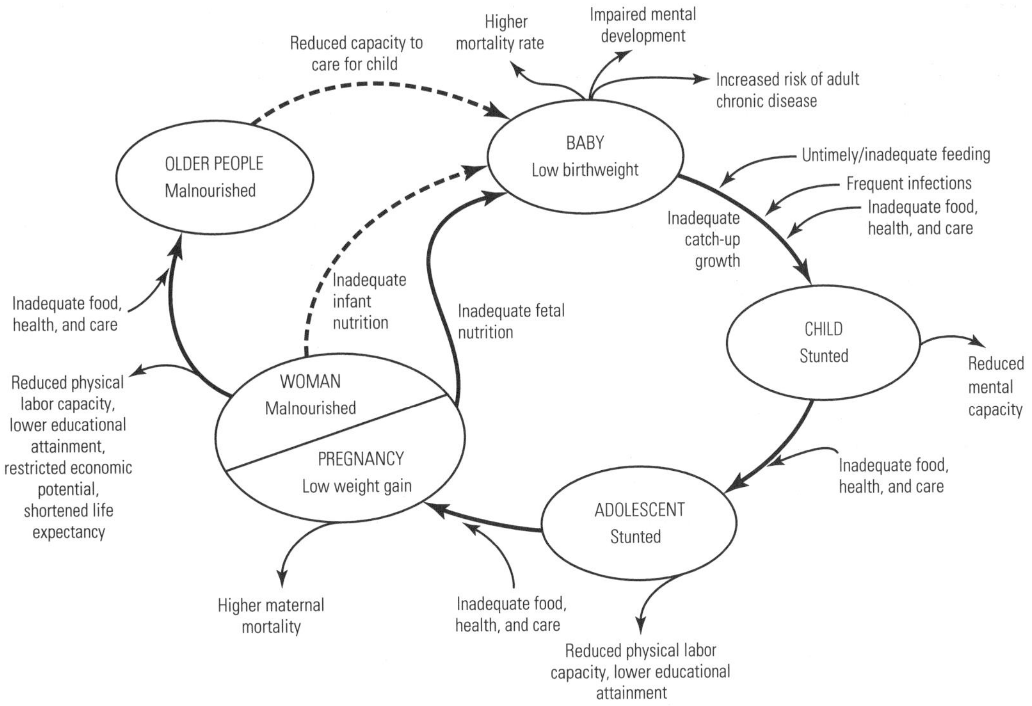

Higher
mortality rate

Impaired mental
development

Reduced capacity to
care for child

Increased risk of adult
chronic disease

OLDER PEOPLE
Malnourished

BABY
Low birthweight

Untimely/inadequate feeding
Frequent infections
Inadequate food,
health, and care

Inadequate
catch-up
growth

Inadequate food,
health, and care

Inadequate
infant
nutrition

Inadequate fetal
nutrition

CHILD
Stunted

Reduced
mental
capacity

Reduced physical
labor capacity,
lower educational
attainment,
restricted economic
potential,
shortened life
expectancy

WOMAN
Malnourished

PREGNANCY
Low weight gain

Inadequate food,
health, and care

ADOLESCENT
Stunted

Higher maternal
mortality

Inadequate food,
health, and care

Reduced physical labor
capacity, lower educational
attainment

Source: Adapted from SCN 2000.

Finally, measures of micronutrient deficiency are critical for assessing undernutrition in Africa. The burden of disease attributed to micronutrient deficiencies is often referred to as "hidden hunger": The clear link between a lack of sufficient food to eat and a poor physical state that one sees with a lack of carbohydrate, protein, and fat in the diet is not as readily seen when considering micronutrient deficiency. Subclinical levels of deficiency can have serious and irreparable consequences on health, mortality, and economic productivity. There are four principal micronutrient deficiencies of public health concern in Africa—vitamin A, iron, zinc, and iodine. Table 8.3 shows their principal sources and the health effects of deficiency.

Input Indicators

The three underlying determinants of child undernutrition are household food security; quality of care; resources for health, including access to health services; and a healthy environment (figure 8.1). These three inputs to the process determine nutritional outcomes both for individuals and for populations as a whole. It is important to recognize that balance is required across these factors if undernutrition is to be sustainably reduced.

Food availability, access to food, and diet quality are various dimensions of food security that can be measured.

Among the most common measures of access to food at the national level is the Food and Agriculture Organization of the United Nations (FAO) undernourishment measure, which takes into account food availability from production and trade and, using the distribution of consumption levels across the population, estimates what proportion of the population is unable to meet its daily energy requirements. Similar assessments can be made using detailed household consumption surveys. Dietary quality assessments can be made using information from both commodity-disaggregated national food balance sheets and household surveys. Although these estimates are by nature imprecise, and there are many valid critiques of them, in the absence of better indicators they are used extensively to monitor food security status.

Direct measurement of quality of care is more problematic, requiring the use of proxy measures. Female education and literacy levels are important elements in this regard. There is considerable evidence that the nutritional status of children varies directly with the level of education of their parents, and in particular, their mothers. Women who have more education are better able to understand important nutritional care practices and to follow them with the children in their care. An additional contribution to nutritional care is the availability of public health services, particularly for prenatal care and infant health and growth monitoring.

Table 8.3 Effects of Deficiency of Micronutrients and Principal Dietary Sources

Micronutrient	Principal dietary sources[a]	Health effects of deficiency
Vitamin A	Breast milk, liver, egg yolk, milk and dairy products, green leafy vegetables (esp. kale, amaranth, sweet potato, cowpea, and cassava leaves), yellow- and orange-colored fruits and vegetables (carrots, pumpkin, mango, papaya, oranges), orange-fleshed sweet potato, red palm oil.	In deficient populations, improvements in vitamin A status are associated with a 23 percent overall reduction in mortality among under-five children. Night blindness, the first stage in a set of increasingly severe eye problems (xerophthalmia) that leads to corneal ulcers and to blindness. Impaired resistance to infection.
Iron	Liver, meat, poultry, fish, cereals (esp. whole grain), nuts, beans, and green leafy vegetables. Also commercially produced iron-fortified foods.	Anemia, especially in women and children. Fatigue, with adverse effects on learning, productivity, and earnings. Pregnancy complications, maternal mortality, premature birth, and low birthweight. In children, significant loss of cognitive abilities as well as decreased physical activity and reduced resistance to disease. Significant impact on school enrollment and adult productivity.
Zinc	Animal and fish products, beans, and other legumes.	Low birthweight and poor growth, reduced resistance to infectious diseases, increased incidence of stillbirths, and possibly impaired cognitive development.
Iodine	Underlying cause of iodine deficiency is a deficiency of iodine in the local soil on which vegetation grows, animals graze, and crops are cultivated. This results in a shortage of iodine in local foodstuffs. Iodine fortification is the principal source of iodine, usually through iodized salt.	Mental retardation and stunted growth among children—"cretinism." Goiter is a symptom of iodine deficiency, which in itself may pose social, economic, and physiological burdens on the individual. Improvements in iodine status are linked to a 13-point improvement in IQ among children. Iodine deficiency is linked to reduced economic productivity.

Source: Compiled by authors.

a. Humans generally are less able to absorb and utilize the vitamin A, iron, and zinc that come from plant foods than those that come from animal and fish sources.

Although the availability of such services is an important measure in itself, measures of the degree to which caregivers adopt proper nutritional care practices—breastfeeding, other child-feeding practices, and health-seeking behavior, in particular—can also be generated using Demographic and Health Surveys (DHS). Finally, proxy measures for the relative control that women are able to exercise over their own and their household's income and other resources have also been shown analytically to be significantly correlated with the nutritional status of children in the household (Smith et al. 2003). The more control women have over such resources, the more likely it is that those resources will be used to provide proper nutritional care to children in the household.

A broad range of measures can be used to assess the degree to which good nutrition is assured by available health services and a healthy environment. These include access to health facilities and health professionals, the burden of disease that health systems must bear, immunization coverage, the percentage of mothers receiving prenatal care, the use of safe drinking water and sanitation facilities, and so on.

Finally, general and household welfare measures—income, assets, and poverty—are also important in accounting for the nutritional status of children. Within the conceptual framework, these cut across the underlying determinants considered in the previous paragraphs—for example, increased income will increase access to food, to health care, and to child care resources—and emerge, in part, from the basic determinants beneath the underlying determinants of the framework. Moreover, as was noted earlier, improved nutrition is itself an important determinant of economic growth and improved welfare—the relationship between these welfare measures and child nutritional status is neither linear nor one way. Nevertheless, they are important, relatively nonspecific inputs into the nutritional process.

Data Sources

The principal data sources for nutritional outcome indicators for Sub-Saharan Africa come from DHS surveys carried out by national statistical offices. These surveys also contain considerable information on nutritional caring practices. The World Health Organization (WHO) has compiled child undernutrition data from these and other surveys into a global database on child growth and malnutrition (WHO 2003). Other data sources for nutrition-related indicators include national population and agricultural censuses for demographic and agricultural production information, household economic surveys for welfare and consumption measures, and facilities surveys for access to social services.

STATUS AND TRENDS IN CHILD UNDERNUTRITION

Although poor nutrition and hunger affects all ages, the long-term development and welfare implications are especially important for young children because most undernutrition happens in the womb or in the first two years of life. Much of this early damage—both physical growth and brain development—is irreversible (SCN 2004, p. 40). Moreover, as the nutritional status of these children when in the womb is an important determinant of their developmental potential, maternal undernutrition is of equal concern. Figure 8.2 shows how undernutrition can be perpetuated across generations from mother to child in a spiral of poverty and despair. Consequently, sustainably enhancing the nutritional status of young children and their mothers is the key intervention in breaking this cycle to enable each succeeding generation to aspire to an increasingly healthy life.

In most of Sub-Saharan Africa increased levels of undernutrition are strongly associated with the age of the child. The decline in nutritional status from birth is astonishingly swift as newborns in many African households face a challenging health environment and, in many cases, receive suboptimal feeding, that is, lack of exclusive breastfeeding and inappropriate or untimely complementary feeding. Although the average nutritional status of newborns in these countries is similar to that of the well-nourished reference population, by about the age of 12 to 15 months about half of the children are underweight (weight-for-age Z-score less than −2.0) with very little improvement thereafter. This growth retardation experienced in the first year of life is very difficult to overcome in the later years of childhood.

Globally, progress is being made in reducing undernutrition. The prevalence of child undernutrition has declined significantly over the past 25 years. Rates of stunting (low height-for-age) among children age six months to five years in all developing countries dropped almost 20 percentage points from 49 to 30 percent between 1980 and 2000, whereas underweight (low weight for age) rates dropped from 38 to 25 percent (de Onis et al. 2004). Taken as a whole, however, Africa is an unfortunate exception to these trends. Over the period 1980 to 2000, stunting rates declined by less than 4 percentage points in Africa, so that, with population growth, the actual number of stunted children actually increased by more than 12 million to 48.5 million. Both relative and absolute numbers of underweight children in Africa increased over the same period.

National and broader regional patterns can be seen in the map portraying the national prevalence of stunted children

Figure 8.3 Prevalence of Stunting in Children Age 6 to 60 Months, by Country
(percent)

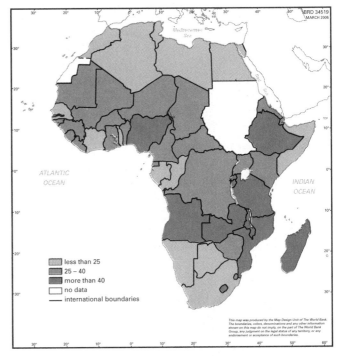

Source: Data from UNICEF 2003.

in figure 8.3. In contrast to North Africa, where child undernutrition appears to be addressed relatively effectively, in Sub-Saharan Africa the pattern is less encouraging and somewhat more complex. Coastal West Africa, central Africa, and southern Africa have lower rates of stunting. Landlocked countries and others with a large proportion of their population in the interior tend to have higher rates. General perceptions that developed in the 1980s of poorly nourished populations in the Sahel and Ethiopia remain relatively accurate today. The grouping of countries with the highest prevalence of stunting, however, is found in southern and eastern Africa, reflecting a complex set of challenges that include civil conflict, economic downturns due to macroeconomic mismanagement or commodity price shocks, and droughts and floods, or the legacies of such events.

The prevalence of undernutrition can also be assessed at a subnational level. Using data from a range of DHS surveys, the Center for International Earth Science Information Network (CIESIN) developed a series of maps describing the prevalence of undernutrition at this scale across the continent. Two of these are shown in figure 8.4. The map on the left of the figure is comparable in form to the map shown in figure 8.3 but shows underweight prevalence, instead of stunting, and subnational spatial units. The map on the

Figure 8.4 Subnational Estimates of the Prevalence of Underweight Preschool Children and Area Density of Underweight Children

a. Percentage of underweight children **b. Population density of underweight children per square kilometer**

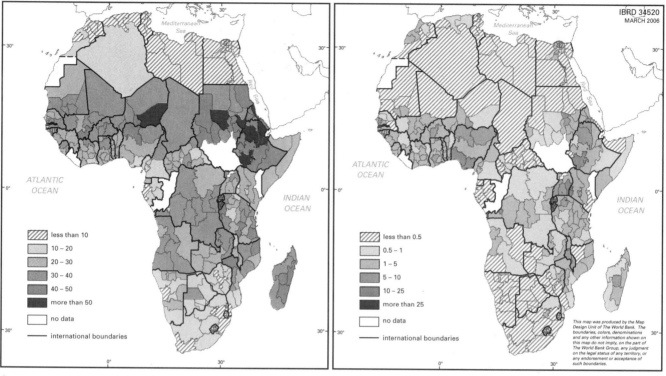

Source: Data from CIESIN 2004.

right provides a different perspective on undernutrition. By taking into account the area density of the population from which the estimates of underweight are being made, the map provides an indication of the spatial intensity of the problem of underweight children—"hotspots" of undernutrition. In this light, although problematic across much of subtropical Africa, the map shows undernutrition hotspots in a handful of areas, including coastal and northern Nigeria, upland Ethiopia, the Lake Victoria basin, southern Malawi, and central Mozambique. It is important to note that in many of these hunger hotspots, food production is not the limiting factor. One such example is the Iringa region in Tanzania, where over 70 percent of the children are stunted in their growth, even though it is a food basket for Tanzania.

Place of residence—rural or urban—can yield another important evaluation of the spatial pattern of child undernutrition in Africa. Figure 8.5 shows stunting prevalence for children under five, disaggregated by urban or rural residence. In all 17 countries, undernourished children are more prevalent in rural areas than in urban centers. Although food is produced on farms in rural areas, this does not mean that rural children are better nourished. Equally

important, safe water and adequate sanitation, health services, and the information needed by mothers or other caregivers to provide children with effective care are relatively less accessible in rural areas. It is not correct, however, to argue that undernourished children are primarily a rural phenomenon. In most of the countries examined in figure 8.5, at least one out of five urban preschoolers is stunted.

Child undernutrition in Africa can also be examined from the dimensions of the gender and the age of the child. In contrast to South Asia, for example, differences in the prevalence of child undernutrition according to gender are not strong. In Sub-Saharan Africa, the tendency is for boys to have a somewhat higher probability of being undernourished than girls (Svedberg 1990). For example, in an assessment of stunting rates for children age 6 to 36 months in 28 African countries during the period 1987 to 2002, the average difference in stunting rates between boys and girls was 2.6 percentage points, with stunting rates being higher among boys in all but four of these countries.

Yet another interesting dimension of undernutrition in Sub-Saharan Africa is reflected in figure 8.6, which shows that although undernutrition rates in these countries are higher among the poorer households, rates remain relatively

Figure 8.5 Stunting Prevalence among Preschoolers, by Urban or Rural Residence, Selected Countries

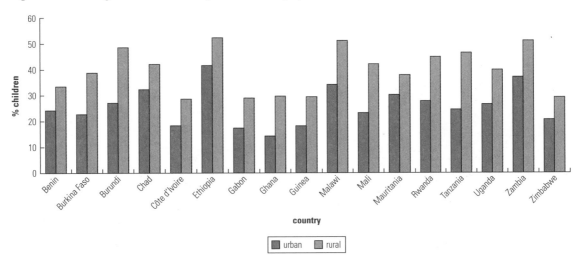

Source: Data from ORC/Macro 2004, DHS survey.

Figure 8.6 Prevalence of Underweight Preschool Children by Wealth Quintile, Selected Countries

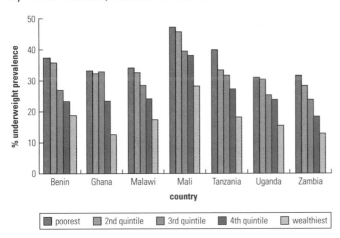

Source: Data from Gwatkin et al. 2003.

high among the nonpoor. In many countries in the region, more than 15 percent of the children in the highest wealth quintile are underweight. Given the significant proportion of nonpoor children that are undernourished, we should recognize that improved household welfare in itself is not sufficient to eliminate undernutrition. The higher level of nutritional resources available to wealthier households must be used effectively through proper care if undernutrition is to be eliminated in such households.

Progress has been made in Africa over the past 15 years in addressing micronutrient deficiency diseases. Although these problems are serious, clinical solutions are relatively inexpensive to implement—salt iodization, fortification of commonly consumed commercial foods, and supplemental

doses of vitamin A and iron for women and children. The simplest and most sustainable way to eliminate micronutrient deficiencies is to make sure that individuals and households know the importance of a balanced diet and have access to what is required to consume such diets. However, in spite of the progress made in combating this "hidden hunger," many Africans still consume insufficient amounts of the relatively small quantities of these nutrients that they require or, due to poor health, are unable to use effectively that which they do consume and continue to suffer from micronutrient deficiencies. High levels of anemia result in serious cognitive and productivity losses, reducing the ability of women to work and provide adequate care for their children and making pregnancy and childbirth much more risky for them than would otherwise be the case. Between 15,000 and 20,000 African women die each year owing to severe iron deficiency anemia. The high prevalence of goiter in school-age children points to hundreds of thousands of children in Africa who have lowered intellectual capacity as a result of iodine deficiency. Vitamin A deficiencies in children are common across the continent, reducing their ability to resist infection and contributing to the deaths of more than half a million African children annually (UNICEF and MI 2004).

Child undernutrition is closely correlated with under-five mortality. For the countries south of the Sahara, most recent estimates of under-five mortality are about 170 deaths in the first five years of life for every 1,000 live births (UNICEF 2003). Figure 8.7b shows that, although many countries are making progress in reducing child deaths, some countries are failing to maintain effective past efforts and are

Figure 8.7 Under-Five Mortality Rates and Progress Being Made in Reducing Under-Five Mortality, by Country

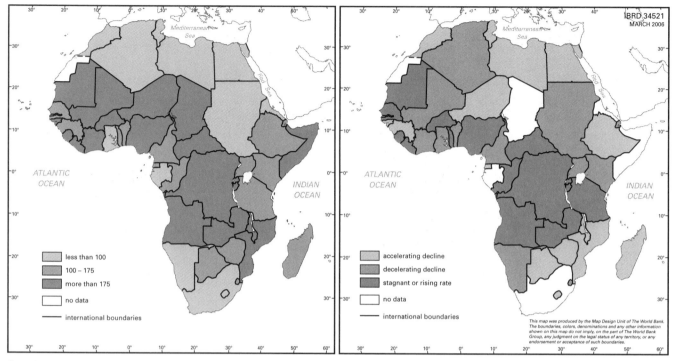

a. Under-five mortality rate, 2002

b. Progress in reducing under-five mortality, 1960–2002

Source: Data from UNICEF 2003.

Note: a. Under-five mortality is the number of deaths in the first five years of life per 1,000 live births. b. Progress in reducing under-five mortality is shown as a comparison of the annual rate of reduction in under-five mortality during 1990–2002 with that during 1960–90.

experiencing a decline in the rate of progress against under-five mortality. In spite of the high levels of under-five mortality in Africa, only a handful of African countries show accelerating declines in levels of under-five mortality. The scatter plot in figure 8.8 demonstrates the intertwining of nutritional and health concerns and highlights the scope of the linked problems of undernutrition and consequent under-five mortality in Sub-Saharan Africa. If one uses an underweight prevalence of 20 percent and an under-five mortality rate of 50 per 1,000 live births (bold gridlines in figure 8.8) as thresholds above which these issues should be seen as critical public health problems requiring urgent action, under-five mortality remains a pressing issue in all countries, and in more than two-thirds, undernutrition is a critical concern.

As noted, approximately 55 percent of all child deaths in developing countries can be attributed in part to undernutrition through its exacerbation of the effects of disease on a child's health (Pelletier et al. 1994). For example, 61 percent of diarrhea deaths and 57 percent of malaria deaths would not occur if it were not for the underlying undernutrition. Even mildly underweight children have nearly double the risk of death of their well-nourished counterparts. This risk increases to five- to eightfold in moderately to severely

Figure 8.8 Scatter Plot of National Under-Five Mortality and Underweight Prevalence Rates

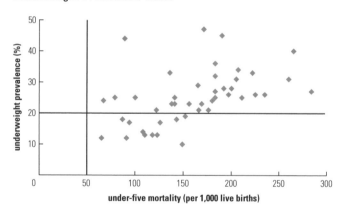

Source: Data from UNICEF 2003.

Note: **Countries with underweight prevalence below 20 percent:** Botswana, Rep. of Congo, Djibouti, Equatorial Guinea, Gabon, Gambia, Lesotho, São Tomé and Principe, South Africa, Sudan, Swaziland, Zimbabwe.

Countries with underweight prevalence above 20 percent (serious public health concern): Angola, Benin, Burkina Faso, Burundi, Cameroon, Central African Republic, Chad, Comoros, Dem. Rep. of Congo, Côte d'Ivoire, Eritrea, Ethiopia, Ghana, Guinea, Guinea-Bissau, Kenya, Liberia, Madagascar, Malawi, Mali, Mauritania, Mozambique, Namibia, Niger, Nigeria, Rwanda, Senegal, Sierra Leone, Somalia, Tanzania, Togo, Uganda, Zambia.

underweight children (Black, Morris, and Bryce 2003). Further, as noted earlier, Pelletier and Frongillo (2003) have shown that had the countries of Sub-Saharan Africa reduced undernutrition rates during 1975 to 1995 at the same

Figure 8.9 Daily Dietary Energy Supply Available and Food Production Index, by Country

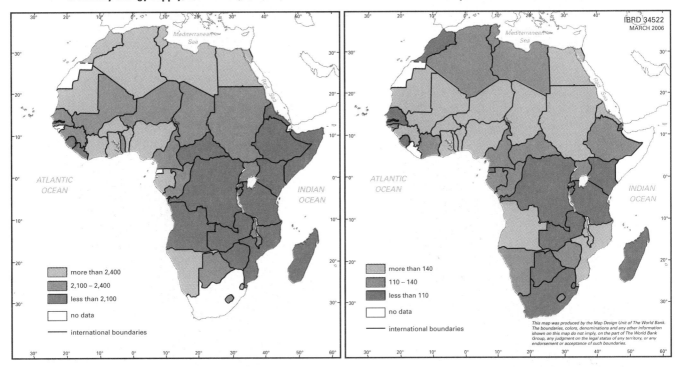

a. Dietary energy supply, 1999–2001 (calories)

b. Food production index, 1998–2000

Source: Dietary energy data from FAO 2003; food production data from World Bank 2003.

Note: a. Dietary energy supply (kcals/capita/day) was computed from total food production and food imports and exports.   b. 100 = aggregate value of national food crop production in 1989–91.

modest rates as other regions of the world, the region would have experienced under-five mortality rates 28 percent lower than those achieved.

What Accounts for the Patterns of Undernutrition Observed?

Two-thirds of Africans reside in rural areas, with the majority engaged in crop and livestock production for both their own use and market sale. Higher production on their own farm or from their own herds enhances the food security for such households. For food purchasers, higher production generally means lower food prices and access to a greater quantity of food in the market for a given income level. Elsewhere around the globe other underlying determinants of nutritional status, such as women's education and its impact on the quality of care provided or the availability of health resources, are of greater importance, but in Africa the relatively low food availability has been shown to be among the most important underlying determinants of the high levels of child undernutrition (Smith and Haddad 2000, p. 84). Nevertheless, as mentioned earlier, many regions of Africa that are notable for their relatively high level of food production also suffer from high levels of undernutrition.

The two maps in figure 8.9 provide some indication of current availability of food in Africa based on total dietary supply (from food balance sheet data) and an index of food production. The trends are not encouraging. A moribund food crop sector is found in combination with insufficient food in quite a few countries, particularly in eastern and central Africa. In such countries, it is likely that many rural households are unable to produce as much food as they require from their own land and cannot afford to go to the market to make up any deficiencies. Chronic food insecurity results. Any future negative shock to a household's well-being likely will propel it into deepening undernutrition and ill health.

Since most undernutrition happens in the first two years of age, when food security is less of an issue than are caring practices, such as exclusive breastfeeding and appropriate complementary feeding (and whether women have enough time within their household and other economic duties to provide such care), caring practices play a key role in undernutrition in Sub-Saharan Africa. Moreover, the high undernutrition rates found among the nonpoor suggest that even when access to food is not constrained and caring practices might be expected to be relatively good, other factors, such as an unhygienic environment or poor health services, also may underlie poor nutrition outcomes.

Figure 8.10 Access to Safe Water and Adequate Sanitation, by Country

a. Percentage of rural population with access to safe drinking water, 2000

b. Percentage of population with adequate sanitation, 2000

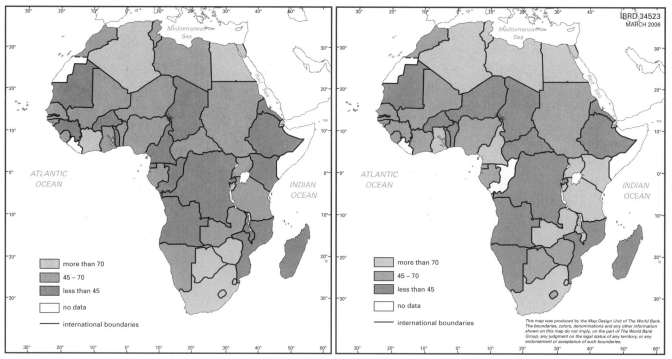

Source: UNDP 2003.

Figure 8.10 shows current progress in Africa in improving public health by providing clean water and adequate sanitation. Although several countries have made admirable strides in ensuring that their citizens live in a hygienic environment, most countries must continue their efforts. By comparing these maps with those in figure 8.9, one can identify several countries—Benin and Namibia, among others—where one should find reasonable access to food but where improved water and sanitation is clearly needed if sustainable reductions in child undernutrition are to be achieved.

Closely linked to a hygienic environment is the health status of the population more generally. Individuals suffering from illness are unable to properly use the nutrients in the food to which they have access. Consequently, lack of access to health services—both preventive and curative—is a central cause of undernutrition. A broad range of indicators can be used to assess this factor in Africa. In figure 8.11 two indicators of access to health care—number of doctors per 100,000 people and percentage of pregnant women receiving prenatal health care—are presented, together with a map showing the prevalence of human immunodeficiency virus (HIV) infection, an important challenge to African health care systems. Figure 8.11a, which shows the number of medical doctors per 100,000 persons, largely reflects the

pattern of wealth across the continent. Access to doctors and secondary and tertiary medical care facilities is as much a question of resources as it is of medical need. Poorer countries tend to have fewer doctors per capita. The map of prenatal care, however, is arguably the more useful for our purposes here. Prenatal care services are mainly provided as a component of primary health care programs. These programs are also the a principal means of providing direct nutrition services to the population. Indeed, an important component of prenatal care is proper nutrition to prevent low birthweight. Overall, the picture across Africa concerning the provision of these health care services is encouraging. Still, although there is room for expansion—large numbers of pregnant women still are receiving no attention—and likely the quality of the care provided can be enhanced, a foundation upon which to build is in place in many countries.

Over the past two decades, HIV infection has added an almost overwhelming additional burden to Africa's health care services. As shown in figure 8.11c, countries in southern and eastern Africa are currently facing the most severe levels of infection, but all countries must put in place mechanisms to effectively control the disease and care for those infected. Existing health services are and will be extremely stretched, and without significant additional resources, the

Figure 8.11 Health Services, by Country

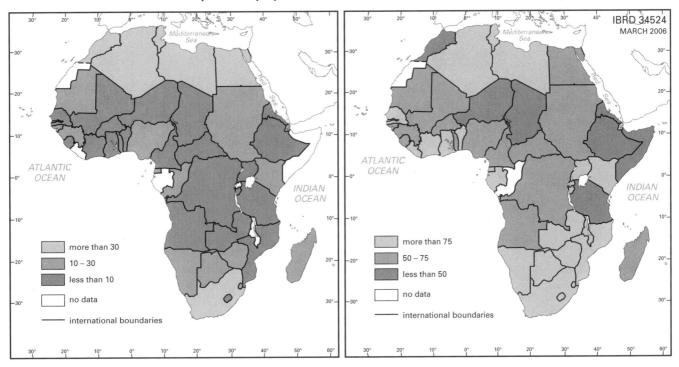

a. Number of medical doctors per 100,000 people

more than 30
10 – 30
less than 10
no data
international boundaries

ATLANTIC OCEAN

INDIAN OCEAN

b. Percentage of mothers receiving prenatal care

IBRD 34524
MARCH 2006

more than 75
50 – 75
less than 50
no data
international boundaries

ATLANTIC OCEAN

INDIAN OCEAN

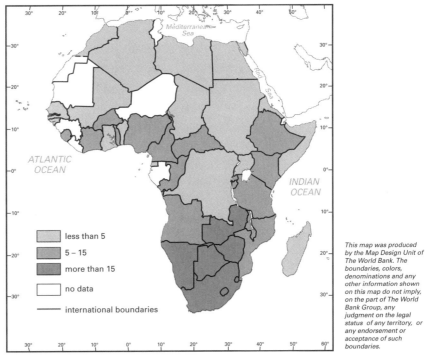

c. Prevalence of HIV-infected adults, age 15–49 years, end-2001 (percent)

less than 5
5 – 15
more than 15
no data
international boundaries

ATLANTIC OCEAN

INDIAN OCEAN

This map was produced by the Map Design Unit of The World Bank. The boundaries, colors, denominations and any other information shown on this map do not imply, on the part of The World Bank Group, any judgment on the legal status of any territory, or any endorsement or acceptance of such boundaries.

Sources: Data on medical doctors from UNDP 2003; data on prenatal care and HIV-infected adults from UNICEF 2003.

overall quality of service provision, including nutrition-oriented services, will suffer. Moreover, HIV has exacerbating effects on undernutrition far beyond its impact on health services. HIV infection reduces household food production both now and in the future, restricts the access to available food and necessary health care that the household had before a member or members became infected with HIV, and lowers the quality of nutritional care received

Figure 8.12 Female Adult Literacy Rates and Girls' Net Primary Enrollment Rates, by Country

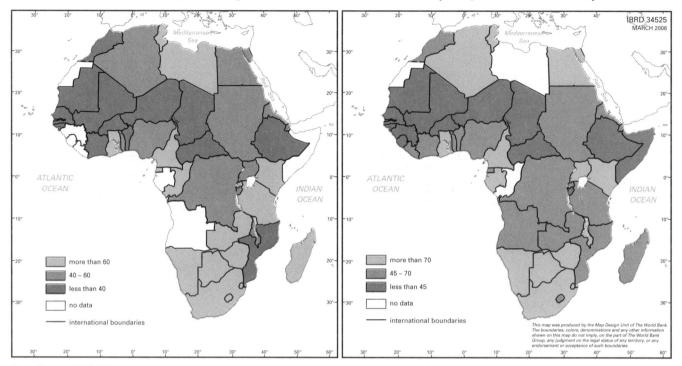

a. Adult female literacy rate, 2001 (percent)

Legend:
- more than 60
- 40 – 60
- less than 40
- no data
- international boundaries

b. Girls' net primary school enrollment rate (percent)

IBRD 34525
MARCH 2006

Legend:
- more than 70
- 45 – 70
- less than 45
- no data
- international boundaries

This map was produced by the Map Design Unit of The World Bank. The boundaries, colors, denominations and any other information shown on this map do not imply, on the part of The World Bank Group, any judgment on the legal status of any territory, or any endorsement or acceptance of such boundaries.

Source: Data from UNDP 2003.

Note: a. Adult female = 15 years and older.   b. Enrollments are of girls of primary school age attending primary school.

by children and others dependent on individuals infected with the virus.

The final underlying determinant of child nutritional status to consider is that of the quality of care children receive. It was highlighted earlier that an important proxy for this determinant is the educational attainment and literacy levels of women, as mothers with more education are more knowledgeable about the care their children need. Two measures of this are provided in figure 8.12. The first, female adult literacy, reflects past broad knowledge building. The second, the net enrollment rate for girls in primary school, reflects the degree to which knowledge, both general and more nutrition-focused knowledge, is being gained to enhance the nutritional status of future generations. Where one finds low literacy and low enrollment of girls in school, one should also expect relatively higher levels of undernutrition now and in the future, all things being equal.

The patterns seen across Sub-Saharan Africa are mixed. Encouraging levels for both measures are seen in many countries of eastern and central Africa. If the educational curriculum in these countries provides basic nutritional and child care principles, we should expect that poor-quality care will not be a critical factor contributing to undernutrition. Many children in the Sahelian countries in particular,

however, cannot be expected to enjoy nutrition security, in part because of the lower-quality care they receive from their relatively less-well-educated mothers. In spite of the increases in food production shown for the countries of the Sahel in figure 8.9, without knowledgeable care, sustained reduction in child undernutrition there cannot be ensured.

Similarly, we can also examine actual child care practices, in particular whether mothers practice exclusive breastfeeding in the first four to six months of life of their children. Exclusive breastfeeding limits the exposure of children to disease while providing all the nutrients an infant requires for normal growth. As presented in figure 8.13, a mixed picture is seen on the degree to which exclusive breastfeeding is practiced across the countries in Sub-Saharan Africa. Certainly the fact that so many infants in Sub-Saharan Africa are not exclusively breastfed in their early infancy accounts for a significant portion of the high levels of undernutrition and under-five mortality observed in the region, as well as for the speed with which infants become undernourished after birth.

Finally, economic growth, income, and poverty levels provide important insights into understanding the levels of undernutrition seen in Sub-Saharan Africa. With little

Figure 8.13 Proportion of Infants Receiving Only Breast Milk in the First Year of Life, Selected Countries

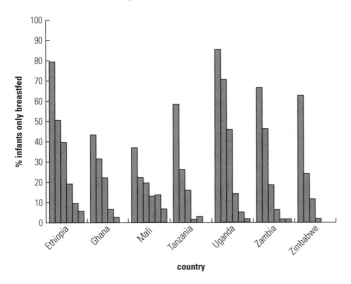

Source: Data from ORC/Macro 2004, DHS survey.

Note: Each bar represents a two-month interval during the first year of life. Missing bars indicate that no infants were being exclusively breastfed in those age ranges (e.g., 9 to 10 months, 11 to 12 months).

growth, the various African economies are generating little additional wealth.

Consequently, income levels remain stagnant and purchasing power will likely decline. The low GDP per capita and the meager existence experienced by significant segments of the population in Sub-Saharan Africa, are unlikely to change for some time to come. The impact of this on levels of undernutrition is obvious. Stagnant incomes imply no increased access to the food required for a healthy diet. Necessary public services for improved child nutrition—public and curative health services, educational systems, support to agriculture, and infrastructure for marketing and trade—will receive insufficient resources. The prospects are gloomy for sharp reductions in child undernutrition within the context of stagnant economies and pervasive poverty.

DISCUSSION

The conceptual framework of child undernutrition presented in figure 8.1 highlights the multisectoral nature of the nutrition problem. It is usually not possible to point to a single factor to account for high levels of undernutrition. However, the high levels of undernutrition seen in those nations in Africa that have experienced conflict and the absence of an effective central government in recent years is not surprising. Burundi, the Democratic Republic of Congo, Liberia, Somalia, and Sierra Leone, when assessed based on those nutritional measures for which data exist, are consis-

tently ranked among the worst on the continent. Conflict exacerbates poverty and poor governance. These governments have been unable to provide basic public goods, which results in a consequent lack of access to food, care, health services, and a healthy environment for their citizens. Although in several of these countries, encouraging signs have been seen since the early years of the twenty-first century, it will take several years of such positive trends before children in these countries can be brought up in conditions that will result in their enjoying a healthy and active life.

It is more challenging to account for why most countries in Africa are exhibiting only poor to fair progress in ensuring the nutritional well-being of their children. The majority of Africans live in these countries. Assessing their performance in light of the various factors that determine child undernutrition in order to judge what changes they might make can only be done case by case.

In those countries in which food availability is deficient, food production must be enhanced at the same time as trade policies must be reexamined to allow a more reliable supply of food from the global market. Other countries may exhibit quite high levels of food available at an aggregate level but still have crippling rates of undernutrition. In these countries, attention should be directed to issues of access to food (the distribution of resources and consumption levels across society and within households) and to the context within which the food is used (sanitation, health services, level of knowledgeable care, and the broad range of related issues outlined earlier). Where HIV rates are high, the links between HIV and nutrition must be addressed. Moreover, the quality of policy making and the effective and responsible implementation of those policies are important basic determinants of the degree to which undernutrition is effectively addressed in any country in Africa, as elsewhere.

Actions Needed to Eliminate Undernutrition

The challenge of child undernutrition in Africa is immense. Of all the developing regions of the world, it is only in Sub-Saharan Africa that large increases in the number of undernourished are anticipated—worse, in some regions of the continent increases in the prevalence of undernourished children are also expected. These patterns are further exacerbated by the continuing spread of HIV infection. Recent patterns of action by governments in Africa and their development partners in addressing undernutrition must be changed if the realization of these grim projections is to be avoided. It is quite evident that efforts to date are not sufficient to meet the challenge.

National governments must lead several aspects of the effort to improve child nutrition. They have a responsibility to establish the conditions and institutions necessary to enable children and their caregivers to access the basic requirements for improved nutrition outcomes.

- Sustained and broadly based economic growth is needed. To end hunger in Sub-Saharan Africa by 2050, it is estimated that the region must attain an annual 3.5 percent average growth rate in per capita GDP (Runge et al. 2003). In the past decade, however, only half a dozen countries had growth rates above 2.5 percent.

  Although it has been shown that income growth will improve nutrition, the process is relatively slow. Consequently, we cannot expect that income growth alone will be sufficient to improve nutrition outcomes at the rates that are required to achieve one of the targets of the first Millennium Development Goal of cutting the prevalence of underweight children in half by 2015. Studies for Tanzania show that even under an optimistic scenario of 5.0 percent per capita GDP growth and using a 0.51 elasticity between income and nutrition outcomes, income growth alone will take up to 2026 to achieve the MDG. For this MDG target to be achieved in Tanzania through income growth alone, a per capita growth of 5.0 percent and an elasticity of 0.85 would be needed, a scenario that is totally unrealistic for any country in Africa. With more realistic income growth estimates, the potential for achieving the MDG are even further in the time horizon. However, the results of simulations undertaken for Kagera region in Tanzania that are presented in table 8.4 show that if income growth is combined with direct nutrition interventions, the chances of achieving the MDG become real.

- Significant increases in the resources allocated to preventive public health interventions directed to young children and their mothers are necessary. Since the window of opportunity for nutrition interventions is small, these efforts must be directed during this brief time—from the mother's pregnancy through the child's first two years of life. In addition, basic preventive and curative health services need to be made more available to enable young children in Africa to cope better with the heavy disease burdens they face—a disease burden that can be seen as both an outcome and a cause of their poor nutritional status.

  The health sector is usually responsible for coordinating and leading direct nutrition intervention programs. Such interventions, particularly those that address micronutrient undernutrition and broad child survival concerns, have proved effective and efficient in improving the nutritional status of, in particular, preschool children and women of childbearing age. In assessing how best to address undernutrition, it is crucial not to underestimate the impact of such direct nutritional interventions. These programs are important investments for improved human welfare and economic productivity.

  Their benefits can be seen most dramatically in efforts to reduce the prevalence of low birthweight babies. Behrman, Alderman, and Hoddinott (2004) present the results of a cost-benefit analysis of programs of various sorts that seek to improve fetal nutrition and increase infant birthweight—prenatal care, in the broadest sense. The direct costs of the programs that they examined ranged from US$14 to US$100 per low birthweight birth averted. They calculated the present discounted value of the benefits that accrue from averting a low birthweight birth to amount to more than US$550. The benefits from

Table 8.4 Projected Impact of Economic Growth and Direct Large-Scale Nutrition Intervention Programs on Stunting and Poverty, Kagera Region, Tanzania, 2015
(percent)

Projected per capita income growth (1993–2015)	Reduction in income poverty	Reduction in prevalence of stunted children			
		No large-scale nutrition intervention	Intervention covering 10% of population	Intervention covering 50% of population	Intervention covering all of population
0.0	0	0	2	22	49
1.0	44	5	8	28	*54*
2.0	*67*	11	14	32	*58*
3.0	*84*	17	17	36	*61*

Source: Alderman et al. 2005.

Note: Italicized values meet the MDG targets. Other factors contributing to reduced malnutrition include non-farm income greater than 25 percent of total income: 2 percent; passable roads throughout the year in every village: 5 percent; additional year of education to every father: 8 percent.

improved fetal nutrition accrue from a range of sources, including reduced costs of health care and productivity gains from the increased physical and mental abilities of the child through his or her life. The most important of these benefits is simply from the increased economic productivity potential of the child. Through such interventions, the health sector has played an important role in the gains that have been achieved in addressing undernutrition for human development in Sub-Saharan Africa. However, these efforts must be duplicated many times over to successfully fight child undernutrition.

- In addressing child undernutrition in Sub-Saharan Africa, agriculture cannot be ignored. Growth in food supplies has the dual effect of increasing the income of the farming household and reducing the prices households must pay to acquire food in the marketplace, both of which contribute to better nutrition.

- Education is a critical input to good nutritional status, particularly for girls. The nutrition education messages that need to be learned are relatively simple—the components of a balanced diet and information on how locally available foods can be used to build balanced diets, the value of exclusive breastfeeding and appropriate and timely complementary feeding for infants, the importance of prenatal care and regular monitoring of child growth, sanitation and maintaining a healthy environment, and the control of infant and childhood illnesses, in particular.

  Although it is not an obvious element of nutrition strategies, ensuring that girls are able to go to school and attain their full educational potential is a critical component of any longer-term effort to enhance nutrition in Africa.

- A close link exists between successful improvements in child nutrition and increasing women's social access to resources they can use to improve care and increase the diversity and quantity of food provided the children under their care. Consequently, improving the level of equity between men and women is good for child nutrition.

- Regarding institutional and policy issues, it is important to consider the particular characteristics of nutrition as a subject for policy making and program implementation by national government institutions. Nutrition is usually neglected in the formulation of government and sectoral policies and strategies and in the allocation of government resources. As already emphasized, addressing child undernutrition requires action across sectors. With no one sectoral ministry responsible for nutrition and, consequently, no strong sectoral advocates responsible

for seeing that attention is paid, human resources are made available, or adequate funds are allocated to nutrition, it can easily be ignored or addressed only in an uncoordinated, piecemeal fashion. However, the issue of improving child nutrition is not unique in this regard. Although the cross-sectoral barriers to effectively addressing undernutrition may be particularly salient, most development issues ultimately require coordinated cross-sectoral action. Such coordination is fostered by political leaders exercising political will. Child undernutrition is a high-priority development challenge in most African countries. Individual sectors can make important contributions to facilitating the access of households to what they require to ensure the nutrition of their children. Ultimately, however, the responsibility for implementing activities across sectors lies with the political leaders. These leaders must be champions for improving nutrition within their countries, and this commitment must be sustained over time.

Scale and Commitment

Ultimately, the outcome of all efforts to improve child nutrition must be realized at the level of the individual child. As is clear from the UNICEF framework on the determinants of nutritional status, however, many, if not most, of the determinants of nutritional status operate on much broader geographic scales than that of the individual. What does this imply for policy making and planning, resource allocation, and program implementation to reduce food and nutrition insecurity?

Several issues must be kept in mind. First, at the broader scales, heterogeneity exists in the key constraints to improved child nutrition. Consequently, although broad strategies to enhance child nutrition can be developed, these strategies must be context specific in their implementation.

Second, and emerging in part from the first point, efforts aimed at sustainably reducing child undernutrition that involve strong central government planning and control are unlikely to succeed, especially in Sub-Saharan Africa, where decentralization is taking root. Locally conceived and implemented action is the primary manner in which the barriers and constraints to such security can be removed. The role of the central government should be much broader and looser, consisting of giving broad general direction to local efforts and facilitating those efforts by allocating resources, providing needed expertise, offering institutional support, and the like. Although many African countries face severe capacity constraints at local levels, such a locally derived approach to address undernutrition should serve as the model for such efforts.

Finally, policy making and program planning have always been guided by those whose voices are heard within the policy-making arena. Over the past 10 years, democratic political frameworks have increased in number across Sub-Saharan Africa. The possible increase in attention paid to the "will of the people" and the new political calculations required of politicians within these new competitive systems may either improve the attention given to or draw attention away from nutritional considerations in policy making. Consequently, community-level political leaders and others who seek government support for nutrition-related interventions are unlikely to succeed without strategically engaging in the political processes of which they are a part.

Increasing attention to significantly reduce child undernutrition requires dedicated efforts to gain more commitment at all policy levels—decentralized, national, and global—and as an issue of broad public concern. To compete successfully within a democratic political arena, the issue must be communicated effectively and understood widely, its significance for the welfare of all members of society recognized, and action catalyzed around proposed solutions. Dedicated and sustained commitment is required. Ultimately, the effort should be to seek to establish the political will and commitment to devote the necessary resources to reduce child undernutrition. Although these children have a basic human right to be properly nourished, efforts to make sure that they are must still be evaluated and find support within the arena of politics.

Policies and Resources Needed to Support These Actions

If we agree that policy, when developed in a democratic and transparent manner, defines the common good and serves as a statement of how government will prioritize its actions and its expenditures, then eliminating child undernutrition must be central to government policies across Africa. Although the broad trends in the prevalence of stunting are slightly downward, the aggregate continental trend is not reflected consistently at the individual country level as economic, food, and social sector policies change or are not given consistent support, conflict shatters any progress that has been made, or emergency food crises are not effectively managed. Clarity in purpose and proper allocation of resources in line with appropriate policies is a necessary element in any efforts to sharply reduce undernutrition. Thus, it is critical that the poverty reduction strategy papers

that many African nations have developed in the past five years and that serve as master development plans for many are explicit on the importance of investing in nutrition to reduce poverty and generate sustained economic growth.

Similarly, for governments in Africa to address problems of undernutrition effectively, cross-sectoral action is required. It is unlikely that sustainable reductions in the number of African children who are undernourished will be achieved if undernutrition is seen as a problem for the health sector or the agricultural sector alone to address. Sectoral plans and strategies should be oriented toward objectives that result in improved nutrition, along with their other long-standing objectives. Advocates for improved nutrition must engage in the higher-level policy processes guiding the revisions of the poverty reduction strategy papers and sectoral strategy documents. The key message should be that the arrow of cause and effect between improved child nutrition and income and broader and sustained economic growth runs both ways. Just as income growth enhances nutrition, healthy, active, well-nourished children are an important precondition for sustained future growth in income. Nutrition concerns must be among the primary components of such strategies.

Moreover, regional and global policy initiatives can be drawn upon in support of advocacy for improved nutrition. Increasing food supplies and reducing hunger are central objectives of the Comprehensive Africa Agriculture Development Programme of the New Partnership for Africa's Development (NEPAD 2002). Although nutrition security requires more than increased food supplies, this NEPAD initiative does commit African governments to addressing undernutrition.

The Millennium Development Goals also imply the need for strong resource allocations to reducing child undernutrition. The prevalence of underweight children is one of the indicators being used to track progress toward attaining the MDG target of halving between 1990 and 2015 the proportion of people who suffer from hunger. Recent assessments show that only 6 of the almost 50 countries in Sub-Saharan Africa will meet this target. In 13 countries, prevalence rates in 2015 relative to 1990 are expected to have increased (Chhabra and Rokx 2004). The trends in the prevalence of underweight children, shown in figure 8.14, points to just how large the gap from the goal will be if current patterns are maintained in all regions of Sub-Saharan Africa. Clearly, current levels of attention to undernutrition among children are grossly inadequate. The commitment to allocate resources to attain the MDGs was made by African governments in the support they gave the United Nations

Figure 8.14 Effect of Economic Growth on Attaining the Millennium Development Goal of Reducing the Prevalence of Underweight Preschool Children, Tanzania

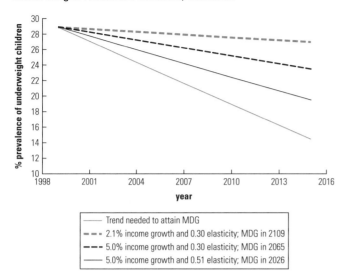

Legend:
— Trend needed to attain MDG
--- 2.1% income growth and 0.30 elasticity; MDG in 2109
--- 5.0% income growth and 0.30 elasticity; MDG in 2065
— 5.0% income growth and 0.51 elasticity; MDG in 2026

Source: Data from World Bank 2006.

Note: Income growth is per capita. The elasticity indicates the magnitude of the effect of income growth on the reduction in underweight prevalence.

Millennium Declaration of 2000. Promoters of improved nutrition in Africa must now hold the governments accountable to their pledge.

Similarly, budgetary allocations by central governments should reflect the importance that improved nutrition has for the welfare of all people and the immense economic benefits it provides for relatively little cost. In this regard, the donor funding that supports the vast majority of direct nutrition programs in Sub-Saharan Africa should be viewed as a secondary resource to complement government's own. African governments should make expenditure on nutrition programs a core element of their annual budgets.

All African countries can eliminate child undernutrition. What is needed is commitment to this goal, identification of the right mix of strategies, dedicated efforts to marshal the human, institutional, and material resources necessary for the task, followed by the application of the political will to undertake the actions at a scale necessary to achieve it.

NOTE

1. The three measures indicate different nutritional processes. Children who are wasted have suffered acute nutritional deprivation in the recent past, such as occurs during famine. In contrast, stunted children have experienced cumulative retardation in their physical growth due to any of a range of factors, diet-related or otherwise. The nutritional processes experienced by underweight children are nonspecific, possibly resulting both from chronic and from acute undernutrition. The prevalence of

underweight children is one of the indicators being used to track progress toward attaining the target of halving between 1990 and 2015 the proportion of people who suffer from hunger under the first MDG of eradicating extreme poverty and hunger.

REFERENCES

Alderman, H., J. Hoddinott, and B. Kinsey. 2003. "Long-Term Consequences of Early Childhood Malnutrition." Food Consumption and Nutrition Division Discussion Paper 168, International Food Policy Research Institute, Washington, DC.

Alderman, H., H. Hoogeveen, and C. Rossi. 2005. "Reducing Child Malnutrition in Tanzania—Combined Effects of Income Growth and Program Interventions." Policy Research Working Paper 3567, World Bank, Washington, DC.

Behrman, J. R., H. Alderman, and J. Hoddinott. 2004. "Hunger and Malnutrition." Paper for the Copenhagen Consensus: Challenges and Opportunities series. Photocopy of January draft, University of Pennsylvania, Philadelphia.

Black, R. E., S. S. Morris, and J. Bryce. 2003. "Where and Why Are 10 Million Children Dying Every Year?" *Lancet* 361: 2226–34.

Chhabra, R., and C. Rokx. 2004. "The Nutrition MDG Indicator—Interpreting Progress." Health, Nutrition, and Population Discussion Paper, World Bank, Washington, DC.

CIESIN (Center for International Earth Science Information Network). 2004. "Sub-National Estimates of Underweight Prevalence in Africa." Maps. Earth Institute of Columbia University, New York.

de Onis, M., M. Blössner, E. Borghi, R. Morris, and E. A. Frongillo. 2004. "Methodology for Estimating Regional and Global Trends of Child Malnutrition." *International Journal of Epidemiology* 33 (6): 1260–70.

Ezzati, M., A. D. Lopez, A. Rodgers, S. Vander Hoorn, C. J. L. Murray, and the Comparative Risk Assessment Collaborating Group. 2003. "Selected Major Risk Factors and Global and Regional Burden of Disease." *Lancet* 360: 1347–60.

FAO (Food and Agriculture Organization [of the United Nations]). 2003. *The State of Food Insecurity in the World, 2003.* Rome: FAO.

Gwatkin, D. R., S. Rutstein, K. Johnson, R. B. Pande, and A. Wagstaff. 2003. *Initial Country-Level Information about Socio-Economic Differences in Health, Nutrition, and Population.* 2 vols. Washington, DC: World Bank. Online analytical results: http://devdata.worldbank.org/hnpstats/.

Horton, S. 1999. "Opportunities for Investments in Nutrition in Low-Income Asia." In *Investing in Child Nutrition in Asia*, ed. J. Hunt and M. G. Quibria, 246–73. Asian Development Nutrition and Development Series 1. Manila: Asian Development Bank.

Horton, S., and J. Ross. 2003. "The Economics of Iron Deficiency." *Food Policy* 28: 51–75.

Jonsson, U. 1993. "Integrating Political and Economic Factors within Nutrition-Related Policy Research: An Economic Perspective." In *The Political Economy of Food and Nutrition Policies*, ed. P. Pinstrup-Andersen, 193–205. Baltimore: Johns Hopkins University Press.

NEPAD (New Partnership for Africa's Development). 2002. Comprehensive Africa Agriculture Development Programme. Rome: FAO.

ORC/Macro. 2004. "Demographic and Health Surveys STATcompiler." DHS data extraction tool. http://www.measuredhs.com/start.cfm.

Pelletier, D. L., and E. A. Frongillo Jr. 2003. "Changes in Child Survival Are Strongly Associated with Changes in Malnutrition in Developing Countries." *Journal of Nutrition* 133: 107–19.

Pelletier, D. L., E. A. Frongillo Jr., D. G. Schroeder, and J.-P. Habicht. 1994. "A Methodology for Estimating the Contribution of Malnutrition to

Child Mortality in Developing Countries." *Journal of Nutrition* 124 (Suppl. 10): 2106S–122S.

Runge, C. F., B. Senauer, P. G. Pardey, and M. W. Rosegrant. 2003. *Ending Hunger in Our Lifetime: Food Security and Globalization.*" Baltimore: Johns Hopkins University Press.

SCN (United Nations Standing Committee on Nutrition). 2000. *Fourth Report on the World Nutrition Situation.* Geneva: SCN in collaboration with International Food Policy Research Institute.

———. 2004. *Fifth Report on the World Nutrition Situation: Nutrition for Improved Development Outcomes.* Geneva: SCN.

Smith, L. C., and L. Haddad. 2000. *Explaining Child Malnutrition in Developing Countries: A Cross-Country Analysis.* Research Report 111. Washington, DC: International Food Policy Research Institute.

Smith, L. C., U. Ramakrishnan, A. Ndiaye, L. Haddad, and R. Martorell. 2003. *The Importance of Women's Status for Child Nutrition in Developing Countries.* Research Report 131. Washington, DC: International Food Policy Research Institute.

Svedberg, P. 1990. "Undernutrition in Sub-Saharan Africa: Is There a Gender Bias?" *Journal of Development Studies* 26 (3): 469–86.

UNICEF (United Nations Children's Fund). 1990. *Strategy for Improved Nutrition of Children and Women in Developing Countries.* A UNICEF policy review. New York: UNICEF.

———. 2003. "The State of the World's Children 2003." Database. http://www.unicef.org/sowc03.

UNICEF and MI (Micronutrient Initiative). 2004. "Vitamin and Mineral Deficiency: A Global Damage Assessment Report." http://www.micronutrient.org/reports/default.asp.

UNDP (United Nations Development Programme). 2003. "Human Development Indicators 2003." Database. New York: UNDP. http://hdr.undp.org/

WHO (World Health Organization). 2003. "Global Database on Child Growth and Malnutrition." Online database. Geneva. http://www.who.int/nutgrowthdb.

World Bank. 2003. "The 2003 World Development Indicators CD-ROM." Washington DC: Development Data Group, World Bank.

———. 2006. *Repositioning Nutrition as Central to Development: A Strategy for Large-Scale Action.* Washington, DC: World Bank.

Chapter 9

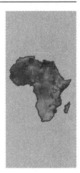

Diarrheal Diseases

Cynthia Boschi-Pinto, Claudio F. Lanata, Walter Mendoza, and Demissie Habte

Of the estimated total 10.6 million deaths among children younger than five years of age worldwide, 42 percent occur in the World Health Organization (WHO) African region (Bryce et al. 2005). Although mortality rates among these children have declined globally from 146 per 1,000 in 1970 to 79 per 1,000 in 2003 (WHO 2005), the situation in Africa is strikingly different. As compared with other regions of the world, the African region shows the smallest reductions in mortality rates and the most marked slowing down trend (figure 9.1). The under-five mortality rate in the African region is seven times higher than that in the European region. In 1980 this difference was equal to 4.3 times (WHO 2005).

During the 1990s, the decline of under-five mortality rates in 29 countries of the world stagnated, and in 14 countries rates went down but then increased again. Most of these countries are from the African region (WHO 2005). A factor that may contribute to this situation is the human immunodeficiency virus/acquired immune deficiency syndrome (HIV/AIDS) epidemic in the region, but an underlying weakness of the implementation capacity of the health system is also likely to blame (Walker, Schwartländer, and Bryce 2002).

Similarly to all-cause mortality, global estimates of the number of deaths due to diarrhea have shown a steady decline, from 4.6 million in the 1980s (Snyder and Merson 1982) to 3.3 million in the 1990s (Bern et al. 1992) to 2.5 million in the year 2000 (Kosek, Bern, and Guerrant 2003). However, diarrheal diseases continue to be an important cause of morbidity and mortality worldwide, and despite all advances in health technology, improved management, and increased use of oral rehydration therapy (ORT) in the past decades, they remain among the five major killers of children under five years of age.

In contrast to mortality trends, morbidity due to diarrhea has not shown a parallel decline, and global estimates remain between two and three episodes of diarrhea per child under five per year. Kosek, Bern, and Guerrant (2003) estimated a global median incidence of diarrhea to be 3.2 episodes per child-year in the year 2000, similar to those found in previous reviews by Snyder and Merson (1982) and by Bern and colleagues (1992) as well as to those reported in the first edition of *Disease Control Priorities in Developing Countries* (Jamison et al. 1993).

Figure 9.1 Slowing Progress in Child Mortality
(per 1,000 births)

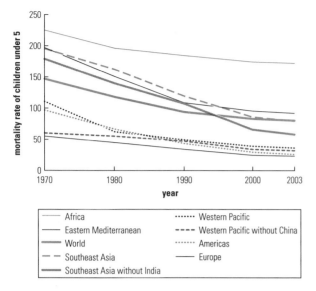

Legend:
— Africa
— Eastern Mediterranean
— World
- - Southeast Asia
— Southeast Asia without India
···· Western Pacific
- - - Western Pacific without China
···· Americas
— Europe

Source: Adapted from WHO 2005.

This chapter reviews available information published since the 1980s on the morbidity and mortality burden of diarrheal diseases in children under five years of age in the WHO African region.

METHODS

Reliable and comparable estimates of morbidity and mortality are difficult to obtain because of variations in methodology, failure to standardize case definitions of diarrhea, and seasonal nature of the disease, among other factors. Nevertheless, such estimates, mainly based on the available studies in the literature, are provided here.

HIV infection has added considerably to the burden of diarrheal diseases among adults and children. This is of particular importance in African countries that show high HIV prevalence. However, the scarcity of data makes it difficult to quantify comorbidity and its contribution to the mortality burden. Because of the probable influence of HIV/AIDS, especially in the mortality due to diarrheal disease, we have followed the WHO's division of the African region into two subregions, which takes into account mortality levels: the AFR D subregion (high child and high adult mortality) and the AFR E subregion (high child and very high adult mortality). Stratum E includes the countries in Sub-Saharan Africa where HIV/AIDS has had a substantial impact (Mathers et al. 2002). Specific estimates have been provided

for each subregion whenever available data permitted. Countries included in each subregion are listed in appendix table 9A.1.

DATA SOURCES AND LITERATURE REVIEW: MORBIDITY

The usual sources of diarrhea morbidity data are either national surveys, such as Demographic and Health Surveys (DHSs) and the United Nations Children's Fund (UNICEF) Multiple Indicator Cluster Surveys (MICS, conducted from 1996 to 2000; http://www.childinfo.org/MICS2/Gj99306k. htm, accessed April 12, 2003), or the published literature.

The main limitation of using currently available national survey data to estimate diarrhea morbidity is the cross-sectional nature of data collection. The information obtained from these surveys is of diarrhea prevalence in the two weeks previous to the survey, which does not account for seasonality. Therefore, data are not comparable either across sites or over time. Moreover, there is a potential for important recall bias in such morbidity surveys (Boerma et al. 1991; Snow et al. 1993). Some of the major limitations of longitudinal studies are lack of representativeness, possible site bias, low frequency of surveillance visits, and recall bias.

Most reviews carried out so far (Bern et al. 1992; Kosek, Bern, and Guerrant 2003; Snyder and Merson 1982) have relied on published studies to estimate the incidence or prevalence of diarrheal disease. Some of the limitations of this type of study are the small number of data points and the lack of representativeness, given the specific sites where most studies are carried out.

The most recent morbidity review (Kosek, Bern, and Guerrant 2003) included five prospective studies from African countries, carried out between 1987 and 1990: two studies were from the AFR D subregion (Guinea-Bissau and Nigeria) and three from the AFR E subregion (Democratic Republic of Congo, Kenya, and Zimbabwe). These studies are listed in appendix table 9A.2.

DATA SOURCES AND LITERATURE REVIEW: MORTALITY

Nationally representative surveys such as the DHS do not usually report causes of death, but the number of diarrhea-associated deaths can be obtained from either vital statistics registration systems or from special study populations.

From each of these sources, the proportion of deaths attributed to diarrhea can be estimated as well as diarrhea mortality rates. However, the representativeness and accuracy of the data vary according to the type of source and various study design features.

The main limitations of vital registration systems are underreporting of the number of deaths and miscoding of the causes of death. Most of the limitations described for the use of longitudinal studies for estimating morbidity also apply to mortality estimation, such as lack of representativeness, possible site bias, and misclassification of the causes of death.

The only countries in the African region for which there is some reported vital registration (VR) coverage are Mauritius, South Africa, and Zimbabwe. The coverage for Mauritius was reported to be 100 percent in the year 2000. Only 1.4 percent of all deaths among children under five were due to diarrhea in this country. The latest information available for South Africa and Zimbabwe (1996 and 1990, respectively) reported estimated coverage rates of less than 50 percent (http://www.who.int/whosis/mort/table4). Therefore, in the African region, most information on cause-specific mortality relies on special studies available in the literature.

The studies included in our review were identified by a systematic search of the scientific literature published since 1980, performed through the WHO's library on Medline/Pubmed using the following terms: Africa, mortality, different spellings of "diarrhea," and all terms combined. No restriction was placed on publication language. The reference sections of these studies were then reviewed to identify additional studies.

The review performed by Kirkwood (1991) for the previous edition of *Disease and Mortality in Sub-Saharan Africa* included data from cross-sectional studies and from national diarrhea programs. In the current review we have considered only longitudinal studies. Inclusion criteria were the following: studies carried out in countries from Sub-Saharan Africa, studies published from 1980 on, studies containing diarrhea-specific mortality data, studies containing a minimum of 25 total deaths, community-based studies with at least one year of follow-up, and a follow-up time multiple of 12 months to minimize seasonal effects.

Twenty-four studies were identified that met the above criteria and were therefore included in this review (appendix table 9A.3). They were carried out in 15 (33 percent) of the 46 countries of the African region: seven were carried out in countries from AFR D, and eight from AFR E. Figure 9.2

Figure 9.2 Sites with Available Under-Five Diarrhea Mortality Data

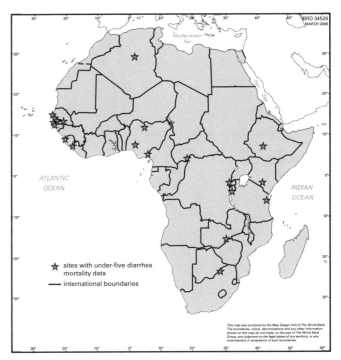

Source: Authors.

illustrates the countries and the sites in each country for which studies were available.

The 24 longitudinal studies identified in the current literature represent an important increase in information when compared with the 7 available studies included in the previous review (Kirkwood 1991). There has been more than a threefold increase in the available literature of longitudinal studies reporting diarrhea mortality in Sub-Saharan Africa. This increase in the number of publications from Sub-Saharan Africa resulted in a doubled number of African countries for which diarrhea mortality data were available, thus adding to the precision of the current estimates.

DATA SOURCE AND LITERATURE REVIEW: ETIOLOGY

Similarly to what was described for morbidity and mortality estimates, the main data source to estimate diarrheal etiology is the published literature. We conducted a search of papers published since 1990, using Medline/Pubmed; the terms used were as follows: Africa, Sub-Saharan Africa, diarrhea, etiology, epidemiology, and children. Different spellings as well as combinations of terms were also

Table 9.1 Median Estimates of Episodes of Diarrhea per Child per Year in the African Region, by Age Group

Review	Age group					
	0–5 months	6–11 months	1 year	2 years	3 years	4 years
Snyder and Merson 1982	2.6	4.3	2.3	1.0	0.7	0.4
Bern et al. 1992	2.7	4.5	2.4	2.7	1.9	1.7
Kosek, Bern, and Guerrant 2003	2.5	4.1	2.9[a]	2.2[a]	—	—

Source: Authors.
Note: — = not available.
a. Only one observation available.

considered. In addition, we considered keywords for specific etiologies known to cause diarrhea in children. Articles published in languages other than English, Spanish, Portuguese, Italian, and French that did not have an English abstract were not included. Further sources were identified from cross-references, consultation with experts in the field, and use of the "related articles" link in PubMed.

We used the following inclusion criteria: studies carried out at community level, among outpatient and inpatient health services; studies that covered at least 12 months of surveillance; and studies in which one or more causes of diarrhea were identified through the use of standard laboratory procedures. Exclusion criteria were studies reporting diarrhea outbreaks, studies carried out among children with HIV/AIDS, studies reporting nosocomial infections, and studies carried out in day-care centers.

Thirty-four studies were identified that met the above criteria, covering 12 African countries, 6 from each of the two African subregions. These are listed in appendix table 9A.4.

REVIEWS AND ESTIMATIONS

In the 1980s Snyder and Merson (1982) reviewed 24 published studies in order to estimate morbidity and mortality from diarrheal disease. Three of these studies, carried out in the African region (Ethiopia, Kenya, and Nigeria), reported the annual number of episodes of diarrhea per child by age group.

In an attempt to update these estimates, Bern and colleagues (1992) reviewed articles published between 1980 and 1990. There were seven studies available for the African regions, covering three countries: The Gambia, Ghana, and Nigeria.

Kosek, Bern, and Guerrant (2003) included four studies from the African region in their review, which had been carried out in the Democratic Republic of Congo, Guinea-Bissau, Kenya, Nigeria, and Zimbabwe (appendix table 9A.2).

Table 9.1 summarizes the results from these studies. Unlike mortality, estimates of morbidity due to diarrhea do not show a decline over time, according to the reviews carried out. Estimates remain consistent for all age groups for which data are available. However, the number of observations, varying from three to five, is low for all three studies, and the uncertainty that prevails because of this low number and the different sites where the studies were carried out should be taken into account when interpreting these data.

Because some of the mortality studies were carried out in more than one country or more than one point in time, they provided a total of 27 data points to be included in the analysis. More than 50 percent of these 27 data points showed proportions of diarrhea mortality between 12 percent and 17 percent; 19 out of the 27 data points (70 percent) had proportions between 12 percent and 19 percent; and only 8 data points provided proportions greater than 20 percent. Because of the skewness of the frequency distributions, we chose to use medians rather than means to calculate diarrhea proportional mortality for each African subregion.

We have used two different approaches to estimate the numbers and proportions of diarrhea deaths for Sub-Saharan Africa in the year 2000: calculation of simple medians for each African subregion and extrapolation from the regression of medians of diarrhea proportional mortality against time.

Simple Medians of Diarrhea Proportional Mortality

As a first approach to estimating the number of deaths due to diarrhea among children younger than five years of age in the African region for the year 2000, we applied the median of the proportions of diarrhea deaths to the total number of deaths among children under five in each of the two African subregions. These medians were similar for the two subregions: 17.7 percent (interquartile intervals [IQI] 12.7–24.5 percent) in AFR D and 17.6 percent (IQI 12.9–19.3 percent) in AFR E. The WHO estimates that approximately 4.3 million children under five died in Africa in the year 2000: 2.0 million in AFR D and 2.3 million in AFR E (WHO, unpublished data). Applying the proportion of diarrhea deaths estimated to have occurred among children under five in Sub-Saharan Africa in the year 2000 to the total number of deaths in these children in that same year yields an approximate total of 760,000 diarrheal deaths.

Proportions over Time

It has been suggested that at least for some countries diarrhea mortality has been declining over the past years, mostly due to the spread of ORT use (Baltazar, Nadera, and Victora 2002; Miller and Hirschhorn 1995; Victora et al. 1996; Victora et al. 2000). We thus examined the medians of the proportions for studies carried out in Sub-Saharan Africa in different time periods.

Because there were only two observations in the late 1970s, we disregarded data from this time period and examined the following time periods: 1980–84, 1985–89, and 1990–94. Figure 9.3 shows that there were virtually no changes in diarrhea proportional mortality ($\beta = -0.055$) in the African region over the years 1980–95. Indeed, the medians of the proportion of diarrhea deaths were equal to 16.6 percent in the early 1980s, 17.7 percent in the late 1980s, and 16.1 percent in the early 1990s. If the situation remains the same and no major changes have occurred during more recent years, for which no data were available, the proportion of diarrhea deaths in the year 2000 could be estimated to be equal to 16.2 percent. This corresponds to an estimated total of 700,000 deaths, similar to the estimate obtained with the simple median calculation.

Figure 9.3 Medians of Diarrheal Proportional Mortality among Children under Five in the African Region, 1980–95

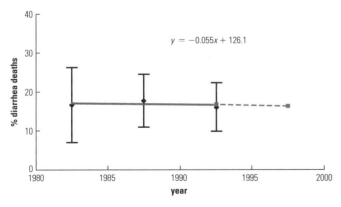

Source: Authors, from studies listed in appendix table 9A.3.
Note: – – – = extrapolation.

Figure 9.4 Medians of Diarrheal Proportional Mortality among Children under Five in the African Region and Other Developing Regions, 1980–95

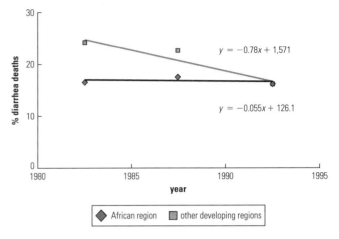

Source: Authors, from studies listed in appendix table 9A.3.

When comparing the median data points observed in the African region with those from other developing regions of the world (figure 9.4), we note that although there was a steep decline in the proportions of diarrhea mortality in the other regions ($\beta = -0.78$), virtually no decline was observed in Sub-Saharan Africa. These observations correspond to an approximately 33 percent decline in the proportion of diarrheal deaths between 1980 and 1995 in the other developing regions of the world and basically no changes in the African region.

Comparison of Estimates from Recent Reviews of the Burden of Diarrhea Mortality

Kosek, Bern, and Guerrant (2003) recently reviewed 30 studies from all developing regions of the world that had available data on diarrhea proportional mortality for children under five years of age and that were published in the 1990s. Ten of these studies were from the African region and covered seven different countries (five from AFR D and two from AFR E). The medians of the diarrhea proportional mortality were 23.2 percent in AFR D and 14.2 percent in AFR E. By applying these medians to the total number of deaths among children under five estimated by the WHO in each of the two subregions in the year 2000, estimates of 454,000 deaths for AFR D and 329,000 deaths for AFR E were obtained. These correspond to a total 783,000 deaths for the whole region.

Morris, Black, and Tomaskovic (2003) have also recently reviewed the literature on causes of death among children under five and used a metaregression model with some selected covariates to estimate the proportional distribution

Table 9.2 Estimated Number and Proportion of Deaths Due to Diarrhea among Children under Five
(thousands)

Approaches	AFR D (no.)	AFR D (%)	AFR E (no.)	AFR E (%)	African region (no.)	African region (%)
Median of proportions	354	17.7	405	17.6	759	—
Regression on time	—	—	—	—	700	16.2
Kosek, Bern, and Guerrant 2003	454	23.2	329	14.2	783	—
Morris, Black, and Tomaskovic 2003	—	—	—	—	935	21.9
WHO 2005	—	—	—	—	741	17.0

Source: Authors, from studies listed in chapter and in appendix table 9A.3.
Note: — = not available.

of under-five deaths by cause in Sub-Saharan Africa and South Asia. The authors predicted that 21.9 percent (95 percent CI, 15.5–28.2 percent) of all deaths of children up to four years of age in Sub-Saharan Africa in the year 2000 were due to diarrhea, corresponding to a total of 935,000 deaths attributable to diarrhea.

Table 9.2 summarizes the estimates obtained from the main approaches used in this review and from the recent work performed by Kosek, Bern, and Guerrant (2003) and Morris, Black, and Tomaskovic (2003) as well as from the WHO's most recent mean estimates for the period 2000–03 (WHO 2005). Given the uncertainty of the estimates due to the scarcity and limited representativeness of data, a reasonable and plausible range for the numbers and proportions of deaths due to diarrhea among children under five in Africa can be provided by summarizing different approaches from various methodologies and their respective results. The two estimates provided for AFR D were 354,000 (18 percent) and 454,000 deaths (23 percent) and those provided for AFR E were 329,000 (14 percent) and 405,000 deaths (18 percent). By reviewing the five available estimates for the total African region, we might conclude that approximately 750,000 deaths that occurred among children under five in the year 2000 were due to diarrhea, with a range of estimates that varied between 700,000 (WHO 2005) and 935,000 deaths (Morris, Black, and Tomaskovic 2003). Our estimates are similar to the 741,000 deaths estimated by WHO for the African region, and recently published in *The World Health Report* (WHO 2005).

Our estimates of deaths from diarrhea among children in Sub-Saharan Africa relied on published epidemiological studies using mostly verbal autopsy methods and thus have limitations inherent in the type of data used, such as lack of representativeness and site bias, observations over time, misclassification of the causes of death, and comparability of data from different studies.

The locations of these studies were rarely representative of the entire country population, as they were usually conducted in populations that are either easy to access or have atypical mortality rates. Furthermore, using studies from a few countries to predict distributions for many countries or a region would require empirical external validation, which we were not able to perform because of the unavailability of other sources of data, such as vital registration data for Sub-Saharan Africa or nationally representative surveys that included causes of death. However, we have tried to stratify countries according to their mortality patterns, especially in what concerns mortality due to HIV/AIDS, to minimize discrepancies between them. Although the observations over time should be interpreted with caution because of the different sites where the studies were conducted, this problem was minimized by including a reasonable number of studies from different sites for each of the three time periods under observation, which should provide an average of the distribution of mortality in these sites. Also, it should be kept in mind that these estimates were summarized as *one single observation over time* for all of Sub-Saharan Africa, based on a few sites from some countries (figure 9.2). As countries often vary widely in many important socioeconomic and health aspects, summarizing data across countries of a region may obscure important differences.

Some studies of childhood deaths in developing countries have shown that causes of death established using verbal autopsy methods are not always consistent with diagnoses based on more complete clinical data (Kalter, Gray, and Black 1990; Mobley et al. 1996; Snow et al. 1992). However, the estimates of the cause-specific mortality fraction (proportions of deaths attributable to one cause) resulting from verbal autopsy studies may not necessarily be inaccurate, if misclassification is random.

Finally, the studies reviewed used different case definitions of diarrhea as a cause of death and different methods for assigning them, both of which limit their comparability. Any review that attempts to compile and summarize data from the published literature, especially those data that use both standard and nonstandard verbal autopsy as the means of ascertaining cause of death, faces these limitations. However, the thorough literature search and the restrictive inclusion criteria used in this review, such as population-based studies with follow-up time a multiple of 12 months and studies with at least 25 total deaths, ensured that the studies used for the current estimates consisted of the most valid information available.

Enteropathogens, such as rotavirus, entero-adherent pathogenic *Escherichia coli* (EAEC), and enterotoxigenic *Escherichia coli* (ETEC), have been identified as important pathogens in diarrheal diseases, and rotavirus, which causes severe complications of diarrhea, has been found to be the most prominent cause of death in the world (Bern and Glass 1994; Bishop 1994; Haffejee 1995).

The severity of the etiological agent can be assessed by the setting in which it was most frequently isolated (community, inpatients, or outpatients). Less severe agents would be more frequently found in community settings, whereas more severe ones should be more common in either outpatients or (mainly) inpatients. Median proportions of diarrheal episodes attributable to each major cause of diarrhea from community studies could therefore be applied to estimates of diarrhea morbidity to obtain episodes of diarrheal diseases by cause, and median proportions from inpatient studies could be applied to estimates of diarrhea mortality to calculate the number of diarrheal deaths by etiology.

Table 9.3 Available Etiology Data, by Country and Study Setting

Countries	Community studies	Inpatient studies	Outpatient studies	Total
AFR D				
Cameroon	—	—	1	1
Gambia, The	1	—	—	1
Ghana	1	—	1	2
Guinea-Bissau	4	—	—	4
Madagascar	—	1	—	1
Nigeria	—	—	8	8
AFR E				
Central African Republic	3	—	—	3
Ethiopia	—	—	1	1
Kenya	1	1	3	5
South Africa	1	3	1	5
Zambia	—	1	—	1
Zimbabwe	—	—	1	1

Source: Authors.
Note: — = not available. See appendix table 9A.4 for the studies included.

However, because of the scarcity of data available for the African region we did not pursue these calculations.

The studies included in the estimates of etiology by setting are listed in more detail in appendix table 9A.4. Table 9.3 shows the countries for which data on etiology were available by setting (community, inpatients, or outpatients).

Tables 9.4 and 9.5 present the estimated median of the proportions of etiological agents identified and corresponding IQI by study site for subregions AFR D and AFR E,

Table 9.4 Median of the Proportions of Etiological Agents among Children under Five in the AFR D Subregion, by Study Site

Etiological agents	Community Median	Community (IQ range)	Inpatient Median	Inpatient (IQ range)	Outpatient Median	Outpatient (IQ range)
Salmonella	2.3	(2.0–2.6)	1.3	(1–13.3)	—	—
Shigella sp.	14.5	(1.5–27.5)	1.7	(1.1–8.8)	—	—
Campylobacter	5.9	(3.1–8.7)	17.7	(7.7–30.5)	—	—
V. cholerae	0.6	(0.6–0.6)	1.9	(1.9–1.9)	—	—
ETEC	8.5	(4.6–12.4)	1.2	(0.5–1.8)	—	—
EAEC	4.2	(3.8–4.6)	21.4	(1.2–24.0)	—	—
Rotavirus	6.2	(3.5–24.9)	19.6	(16.3–33.0)	12.3	(12.3–12.3)
Giardia	15.1	(14.7–18.2)	—	—	—	—
Cryptosporidium	6.5	(5.7–7.7)	—	—	—	—
E. hystolitica	4.1	(0.0–7.0)	—	—	—	—
Coinfection	15.8	(4.8–34.6)	—	—	—	—
Unknown	16.4	—	32.8	—	11.4	—

Source: Authors, from studies listed in appendix table 9A.4.
Note: — = not available.

Table 9.5 Median of the Proportions of Etiological Agents among Children under Five in the AFR E Subregion, by Study Site

Etiological agents	Community Median	Community (IQ range)	Inpatient Median	Inpatient (IQ range)	Outpatient Median	Outpatient (IQ range)
Salmonella	1.9	(0.6–1.9)	7.4	(7.4–7.4)	2.5	(1.4–3.6)
Shigella sp.	2.9	(2.0–3.8)	6.5	(6.5–6.5)	4.8	(3.6–6.0)
Campylobacter	11.3	(3.5–11.7)	10.1	(4.8–15.3)	3.8	(2.2–5.3)
V. cholerae	0.3	(0.3–0.3)	0.5	(0.5–0.5)	—	—
ETEC	1.9	(1.6–3.1)	4.9	(4.9–4.9)	—	—
EAEC	8.8	(8.6–9.7)	8.8	(8.8–8.8)	21.6	(15.6–27.6)
Rotavirus	9.8	(6.3–15.5)	23.5	(19.3–31.1)	24.3	(20.8–32.3)
Giardia	6.4	(0.9–10.0)	4.9	(4.9–4.9)	—	—
Cryptosporidium	2.5	(2.5–2.5)	—	—	—	—
E. hystolitica	3.3	(0.3–6.3)	7.8	(7.8–7.8)	—	—
Coinfection	7.0	(7.0–7.0)	—	—	—	—
Unknown	43.0	—	23.9	—	27.6	—

Source: Authors, from studies listed in appendix table 9A.3.
Note: — = not available.

respectively. In our review, *Giardia lamblia* was more frequently isolated among children with diarrhea in the community studies, whereas EAEC was mainly seen among outpatients. Rotavirus was the etiological agent most frequently isolated in both inpatient and outpatient health services. Therefore, it is likely that rotavirus is the leading cause of mortality due to diarrhea in Africa, as has been observed in other parts of the world. Coinfection of various agents was reported in 16 percent and 7 percent of community-level studies in AFR D and AFR E, respectively. Because our review did not include publications of diarrhea outbreaks, the magnitude of *Vibrio cholerae,* and *Shigella dysenteriae* type 1 is underrepresented in this review.

Our estimates of the distribution of diarrhea etiology among children in Sub-Saharan Africa relied on published epidemiological studies. The same limitations reported for the morbidity and mortality estimates therefore apply to these etiological estimates. Moreover, very few studies were identified through the literature search for the African region, and of those, not all have attempted to identify the whole set of etiological agents.

THE ROLE OF RISK FACTORS FOR DIARRHEAL DISEASE IN THE AFRICAN REGION

Broadly recognized risk factors for diarrheal diseases include little or no access to safe water and sanitation, as well as poor hygiene and feces disposal practices at home

(Daniels et al. 1990; Haggerty et al. 1994; LaFond 1995; MacDougall and McGahey 2003). These and many other factors, such as poor housing and crowding, are intrinsically associated with poverty. Furthermore, poverty usually limits access to health care and restricts appropriate and balanced diets. Inequities in exposure and resistance add up to inequities in coverage of available preventive interventions, access to an appropriate health provider, and care, making poor children more likely to become sick than the better-off children (Victora et al. 2003).

Some studies have identified a few family characteristics as protective factors. These are monogamy of the father, defined residential area (Vaahtera et al. 2000), having a private kitchen, and being cared for by the mother (Oni, Schumann, and Oke 1991). These factors are of special importance in Sub-Saharan Africa, where the AIDS epidemic has led to an unprecedented number of orphans (about 12 million by the end of 2001) that is likely to more than double during this decade (Dabis and Ekpini 2002).

A WHO report on global water supply provides worrisome figures of current and future scenarios for Africa (WHO 2000). Of all the regions in the world, the African region was the only one showing a decline in the proportion of the population that had access to sanitation between 1990 and the year 2000 (figure 9.5).

Approximately 50 percent (300 million individuals) of the African population have no access to safe water, and 66 percent (400 million individuals) lack access to hygienic sanitation. It is expected that by the year 2020 these figures will rise to 400 million and 500 million, respectively.

Figure 9.5 Change in Sanitation Coverage by Region, 1990–2000

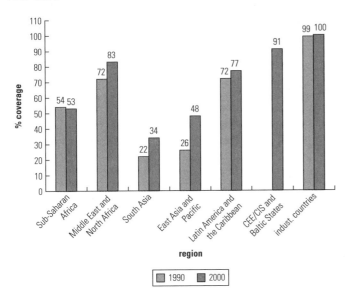

Source: WHO 2000.

Note: CEE = Central and Eastern Europe; CIS = Commonwealth of Independent States; no data available for 1990.

Table 9.6 gives data on feces disposal practices at home in urban and rural regions of four African countries. Such practices have provided the rationale for more preventive interventions and are likely to explain the higher prevalence of diarrheal disease in rural areas. As in most developing regions of the world, African countries' poorest populations live in rural areas. Table 9.7 presents the medians of the prevalence of diarrheal disease according to urban and rural areas.

SOME ADDITIONAL COMMENTS

There is an increasing concern that gender disparities might influence the distribution of ill-health and treatment, particularly in under-five girls. Some evidence suggests that girls in developing countries are prone to higher mortality

and poorer nutritional status than boys (Helen Keller International 1994; Sundary 1986). In Sub-Saharan Africa, few prospective studies lasting at least one year report sex differences at the community level (Perch et al. 2001). Some prospective studies conducted in health facilities on outpatients (Gomwalk et al. 1993; Gomwalk, Gosham, and Umoh 1990) and inpatients (Mpabalwani et al. 1995; Steele et al. 1998) show that boys are more likely than girls to be taken to the facility because of diarrhea (boy-girl ratios are 2 to 1 and 4 to 1, respectively). However, nationally representative studies, such as the DHSs, conducted from 1987 to 2001 in several Sub-Saharan African countries show no significant sex differences for health care–seeking behavior and treatment received, whether it is given at home or at a health facility. Findings are summarized in table 9.8.

The African region has been a target of diarrheal epidemic outbreaks for several decades. One of the most dramatic manifestations of these outbreaks occurred in July 1994 among Rwandan refugees in Goma, Democratic Republic of Congo (formerly Zaire), when almost 50,000 refugees died during a diarrhea epidemic.

The African region has replaced the Indian subcontinent as the new home of *V. cholerae*. The seventh cholera pandemic that originated in Asia reached Africa in the early 1970s. In 2001 there were more than 170,000 reported cases of cholera, which represented 94 percent of the globally reported cases. From these, 2,590 people died. Nearly all countries in Sub-Saharan Africa now regularly report cases of cholera. Table 9.9 shows the reported number of cases and deaths from cholera in the world and in the African region between 1996 and 2001. These figures, however, need to be interpreted with caution, since countries that have endemic cholera appear not to have notified the WHO of any cases of cholera.

Early reports of *Vibrio parahaemolyticus* in gastroenteritis cases in Africa (Utsalo, Eko, and Antia-Obong 1991)

Table 9.6 Feces Disposal Practices at Home, by Urban and Rural Residences in Four African Countries
(percent)

| Country (year of DHS) | Urban | | | | | Rural | | | | |
	Child uses toilet	Throw in toilet/ latrine	Bury in the yard	Throw outside the dwelling	Throw outside the yard	Child uses toilet	Throw in toilet/ latrine	Bury in the yard	Throw outside the dwelling	Throw outside the yard
Benin (2002)	4.5	35.9	—	22.6	6.8	1.2	6.2	—	39.1	32.4
Malawi (2000)	8.2	80.3	0.5	0.5	9.6	7.5	69.8	3.2	2.7	7
Uganda (2000/2001)	13.5	75.7	1	3.9	—	7.5	60.5	6	8.5	10.4
Zimbabwe (1999)	26.2	52.6	5.5	0.3	13.9	7.4	37.6	24.4	4.5	16.4

Source: Data from Demographic and Health Surveys 1987–2002.

Note: — = not available.

Table 9.7 Prevalence (Median) of Diarrheal Disease, the Two Weeks before Survey, by Urban and Rural Site of Residence in AFR D and AFR E
(percent)

African subregion	Urban	Rural
AFR D	17.3	20.2
AFR E	14.9	19.1
African region	16.7	20.1

Source: Data from Demographic and Health Surveys 1987–2002.

have been confirmed to be associated with the O3:K6 pandemic strain (Ansaruzzaman et al. 2004; Chowdhury et al. 2000), documenting the extension of this pandemic into the region. *S. dysenteriae* serotype 1 has also been documented to cause outbreaks of dysenteric diarrhea in several African countries (Birmingham et al. 1997; Guerin et al. 2003; Malakooti et al. 1997), including in refugee camps (Paquet et al. 1995). These organisms are important causes of morbidity and mortality in diarrhea outbreaks among stable communities and more so in displaced populations or those affected by catastrophic events. The widespread use of antibiotics across all regions has increased the prevalence of antibiotic resistance in most bacterial enteropathogens, increasing the risk in the region of an outbreak of *S. dysenteriae* serotype 1 with multiresistant strains.

THE ROLE OF INTERVENTIONS TO CONTROL DIARRHEAL DISEASES

There is sufficient evidence that several interventions are effective in the prevention and treatment of diarrheal diseases (Jones et al. 2003). These interventions are exclusive breastfeeding, complementary feeding, safe water, good sanitation and hygiene, zinc and vitamin A supplementation, ORT, and antibiotics for dysentery. It is estimated that these interventions could prevent 22 percent of deaths due to diarrhea (Jones et al. 2003). Most of these interventions are feasible for implementation in low-income countries such as those in the African region; however, the capacity to deliver these important interventions effectively should be strengthened (Bryce et al. 2003). The availability of safe and effective rotavirus vaccines (Ruiz-Palacios et al. 2006; Vesikari et al. 2006), introduced in several countries in Latin America in 2005 are likely to complement these interventions, if effectively delivered. However, the stability of diarrhea rates observed in all reviews done since the 1980s shows that despite the reduction of diarrhea mortality, most likely through better case management, very little has been done to prevent the transmission of diarrheal diseases. The progress toward better water and sanitation observed in other regions has not yielded a reduction of diarrhea morbidity, suggesting

Table 9.8 Children under Five Taken to Health Facilities or Receiving Treatment for Diarrheal Disease in the Two Weeks before Survey, by Sex
(percent)

	Taken to health facility	Using antibiotics	RHS at home	Using home remedy/other	Receiving ORS packet	Receiving increased fluids	Receiving no treatment
Boys	28.8	14.1	13.7	39.9	25.6	36.0	17.4
Girls	29.2	11.8	12.1	38.2	25.2	37.6	17.3

Source: Data from Demographic and Health Surveys 1987–2001.
Note: RHS = recommended home solutions; ORS = oral rehydration salt.

Table 9.9 Cases and Deaths Due to *V. cholerae* Reported to WHO, 1996–2001

	1996	1997	1998	1999	2000	2001
World						
Total no. of cases	143,349	147,425	293,121	254,310	137,071	184,311
Total no. of deaths	6,689	6,274	10,586	9,175	4,908	2,728
Case-fatality rate (%)	4.7	4.3	3.6	3.6	3.6	1.5
African region						
Total no. of cases	108,535	118,349	211,748	206,746	118,932	173,359
Total no. of deaths	6,216	5,853	9,856	8,728	4,610	2,590
Case-fatality rate (%)	5.7	4.9	4.1	4.2	3.9	1.5

Source: League of Nations 1996–2002.

that poor hygiene practices (Yeager et al. 1999) and the ingestion of contaminated food (Lanata 2003) may be the most important factors and where preventive interventions, like handwashing (Curtis and Cairncross 2003), should be promoted.

CONCLUSION

Despite data limitations in estimating accurate numbers of diarrhea cases and deaths, it becomes clear from the results of this and other reviews that diarrheal disease remains an important cause of morbidity and mortality among children under five years of age in the African region. As opposed to the declining trends in the proportion of diarrhea mortality in other developing regions of the world, virtually no decline has been observed in the African region since the early 1980s. Diarrheal diseases remain one of the major killers of children under five, being responsible for about 750,000 of a total of 4.3 million deaths of African children up to four years of age.

More important than the precision in the numbers and in the exact contribution of each pathogen to diarrhea morbidity and mortality are the patterns and trends shown in this review. The fact that almost 40 percent of all diarrhea deaths in children under five worldwide occur in the African region is striking. The diarrhea mortality burden among children under five in Sub-Saharan Africa reveals the persistent magnitude of this preventable and treatable disease in the region.

The efficacy of existing interventions to prevent or treat diarrheal diseases and to thereby reduce diarrhea mortality has been proved. Large reductions in child mortality could be achieved with their implementation. Therefore, careful planning and evaluation of interventions to control cases and deaths due to diarrhea will be important if under-five mortality is to be reduced and goal four of the Millennium Development Goals—to reduce under-five mortality by two-thirds by 2015, from the base year 1990 (United Nations 2000)—is to be achieved in the African region.

APPENDIX

Table 9A.1 Regional Reporting Categories for Global Burden of Disease 2000: WHO African Subregions

WHO region	Mortality stratum	WHO Member States
AFR	D	Algeria, Angola, Benin, Burkina Faso, Cameroon, Cape Verde, Chad, Comoros, Equatorial Guinea, Gabon, The Gambia, Ghana, Guinea, Guinea-Bissau, Liberia, Madagascar, Mali, Mauritania, Mauritius, Niger, Nigeria, São Tomé and Principe, Senegal, Seychelles, Sierra Leone, Togo
AFR	E	Botswana, Burundi, Central African Republic, Republic of Congo, Côte d'Ivoire, Democratic Republic of Congo, Eritrea, Ethiopia, Kenya, Lesotho, Malawi, Mozambique, Namibia, Rwanda, South Africa, Swaziland, Uganda, Tanzania, Zambia, Zimbabwe

Source: WHO 2002.

Table 9A.2 Main Characteristics of the Studies Included in the Morbidity Review

Authors and year of publication	Region and country	Study period	N	No. of diarrhea episodes per child-year, by age group
	AFR D			
Oni, Schumann, and Oke 1991	Nigeria	1989–90	351	3.3 episodes (0–5 months) 4.1 episodes (6–11 months) 2.9 episodes (1 year) 2.2 episodes (2 years)
Mølbak et al. 1997	Guinea-Bissau	1987–90	1,314	10.4 episodes (0–4 years)
	AFR E			
Mirza et al. 1997	Kenya	1989–90	920	3.5 episodes (0–3 years)
Manun'ebo et al. 1994	Dem. Rep. of Congo	1987–88	1,914	6.3 episodes (0–4 years)
Moy et al. 1991	Zimbabwe	1987–88	204	1.8 episodes (0–5 months) 4.8 episodes (6–11 months)

Source: Adapted from Kosek, Bern, and Guerrant 2003.

Table 9A.3 Main Characteristics of the Studies Included in the Mortality Review

Authors and year of publication	Region and country	Mid-year of study[a]	No. of deaths	Under-five mortality rate[b]	% diarrhea deaths
	AFR D				
Bendib, Dekkar, and Lamdjadani 1993	Algeria	1987	1,502	—	8.1
De Francisco et al. 1993	Gambia, The	1989	856	34.5	18.0
Greenwood et al. 1987	Gambia, The	1982	184	72.1	13.6[c]
Greenwood et al. 1990	Gambia, The	1983	76	70.2	15.8
Greenwood et al. 1990	Gambia, The	1985	187	58.6	26.7
Jaffar et al. 1997	Gambia, The	1991	3,776	98.9	8.4
Mølbak et al. 1992	Guinea-Bissau	1988	153	55.6	30.7
Becker, Diop, and Thornton 1993	Liberia	1984	—	100.0	13.7[c]
Becker, Diop, and Thornton 1993	Liberia	1987	—	79.0	12.1[c]
Bradley and Gilles 1984	Nigeria	1978	151	—	24.5
Ekanem, Asindi, and Okoi 1994	Nigeria	1991	314	—	12.1
Jinadu et al. 1991	Nigeria	1990	120	62.2	32.5
Fontaine et al. 1984	Senegal	1983	42	21.6	26.2
Pison et al. 1993	Senegal	1987	75	17.3	20.3
Victora et al. 1993	Senegal	1986	1,517	63.1	35.0
Amin 1996	Sierra Leone	1990	559	33.0	12.7
Hodges and Williams 1998	Sierra Leone	1989	4,264	—	17.7
	AFR E				
Delacollette and Barutwanayo 1993	Burundi	1990	160	41.9	19.4
Georges et al. 1987	Central African Republic	1983	188	28.5	19.1
Delacollette et al. 1989	Congo, Dem. Rep. of	1986	358	69.0	8.4
Shamebo et al. 1991	Ethiopia	1988	436	49.0	8.4
Omondi-Odhiambo, Ginneken, and Voorhoeve 1990	Kenya	1977	338	—	19.5
Kahn et al. 1999	South Africa	1994	216	—	20.4
Mtango and Neuvians 1986	Tanzania	1984	325	40.1	16.9
Mtango and Neuvians 1986	Tanzania	1985	347	35.0	12.7
Mtango et al. 1992	Tanzania	1987	610	30.8	13.3
Watts, Ng'andu, and Wray 1990	Zambia	—	26	—	18.2[c]

Source: Data from sources in table.

Note: — = not available.

a. Some studies did not report mid-year of study and those have been either informed by contacting authors or approximately estimated from other available information in the study.

b. Under-five mortality rate is the number of total under-five deaths per 1,000 children per year (obtained either directly from the study or calculated from data available in the study).

c. Proportions corrected or adjusted to age group 0–59 months.

Table 9A.4 Main Characteristics of the Studies Included in the Etiology Review

Authors and year of publication	Region and country	Study setting
	AFR D	
Koulla-Shiro, Loe, and Ekoe 1995	Cameroon	Outpatient
Rowland et al. 1985	Gambia, The	Community
Armah et al. 1994	Ghana	Outpatient
Nakano et al. 1990	Ghana	Community
Fisher et al. 2000	Guinea-Bissau	Community
Mølbak 1990	Guinea-Bissau	Community
Mølbak et al. 1994	Guinea-Bissau	Community
Perch et al. 2001	Guinea-Bissau	Community
Cassel-Beraud, Michel, and Garbarg-Chenon 1993	Madagascar	Inpatient
Akinyemi et al. 1998	Nigeria	Outpatient
Audu et al. 2002	Nigeria	Outpatient
Gomwalk, Gosham, and Umoh 1990	Nigeria	Outpatient
Gomwalk et al. 1993	Nigeria	Outpatient
Obi et al. 1997	Nigeria	Outpatient
Okeke et al. 2000	Nigeria	Outpatient
Pennap et al. 2002	Nigeria	Outpatient
Pennap et al. 2000	Nigeria	Outpatient
	AFR E	
Georges-Courbot et al. 1987	Central African Republic	Community
Georges-Courbot et al. 1990	Central African Republic	Community
Georges-Courbot et al. 1988	Central African Republic	Community
Gedlu and Aseffa 1996	Ethiopia	Outpatient
Chunge et al. 1989	Kenya	Community
Mutanda et al. 1986	Kenya	Outpatient
Mutanda et al. 1985	Kenya	Inpatient
Nakata et al. 1999	Kenya	Outpatient
Saidi et al. 1997	Kenya	Outpatient
Griffiths, Steele, and Alexander 1992	South Africa	Inpatient
Mnisi, Williams, and Steele 1992	South Africa	Inpatient
Sebata and Steele 2001	South Africa	Outpatient
Steele et al. 1998	South Africa	Inpatient
Steele et al. 1988	South Africa	Inpatient
Mpabalwani et al. 1995	Zambia	Inpatient
Tswana et al. 1990	Zimbabwe	Outpatient

Source: Information from sources in table.

REFERENCES

Akinyemi, K. O., A. O. Oyefolu, B. Opere, V. A. Otunba-Payne, and A. O. Oworu. 1998. "*Escherichia Coli* in Patients with Acute Gastroenteritis in Lagos, Nigeria." *East African Medical Journal* 75: 512–15.

Amin, R. 1996. "Immunization Coverage and Child Mortality in Two Rural Districts of Sierra Leone." *Social Science and Medicine* 42: 1599–1604.

Ansaruzzaman, M., N. A. Bhuiyan, G. B. Nair, D. A. Sack, M. Lucas, J. L. Deen, J. Ampuero, and C. L. Chaignat. 2004. The Mozambique Cholera Vaccine Demonstration Project Coordination Group. "Cholera in Mozambique, Variant of *Vibrio cholerae*." *Emerging Infectious Diseases* 10: 2057–59.

Armah, G. E., J. A. A. Mingle, A. K. Dodoo, A. Anyanful, R. Antwi, J. Commey, and F. K. Nkrumah. 1994. "Seasonality of Rotavirus Infections in Ghana." *Annals of Tropical Paediatrics* 14: 223–30.

Audu, R., S. A. Omilabu, M. de Beer, I. Peenze, and A. D. Steele. 2002. "Diversity of Human Rotavirus VP6, VP7, and VP4 in Lagos State, Nigeria." *Journal of Health, Population, and Nutrition* 20: 59–64.

Baltazar, J. C., D. P. Nadera, and C. G. Victora. 2002. "Evaluation of the National Control of Diarrhoeal Disease Programme in the Philippines, 1980–93." *Bulletin of the World Health Organization* 80: 637–43.

Becker, S. R., F. Diop, and J. N. Thornton. 1993. "Infant and Child Mortality Estimates in Two Counties of Liberia; Results of a Survey in 1988 and Trends Since 1984." *International Journal of Epidemiology* 22 (Suppl. 1): S56–63.

Bendib, A., N. Dekkar, and N. Lamdjadani. 1993. "Facteurs associés à la mortalité juvénile, infantile et néonatale. Résultats d'une enquête nationale en Algérie." *Archives Françaises de Pediatrie* 50: 741–47.

Bern, C., and R. I. Glass. 1994. "Impact of Diarrheal Diseases Worldwide." In *Viral Infections of the Gastrointestinal Tract*, 2nd ed., ed. A. Z. Kapikian. New York: Marcel Dekker.

Bern, C., J. Martines, I. de Zoysa, and R. I. Glass. 1992. "The Magnitude of the Global Problem of Diarrhoeal Disease: A Ten-Year Update." *Bulletin of the World Health Organization* 70: 705–14.

Birmingham, M. E., L. A. Lee, M. Ntakibirora, F. Bizimana, and M. S. Deming. 1997. "A Household Survey of Dysentery in Burundi: Implications for the Current Pandemic in Sub-Saharan Africa." *Bulletin of the World Health Organization* 75: 45–53.

Bishop, R. 1994. "Natural History of Human Rotavirus Infection." In *Viral Infections of the Gastrointestinal Tract*, 2nd ed., ed. A. Z. Kapikian. New York: Marcel Dekker.

Boerma, J. T., R. E. Black, A. E. Sommerfelt, S. O. Rustein, and G. T. Bicego. 1991. "Accuracy and Completeness of Mothers' Recall of Diarrhoea Occurrence in Pre-School Children in Demographic and Health Surveys." *International Journal of Epidemiology* 20: 1073–80.

Bradley, A. K., and H. M. Gilles. 1984. "Pointers to Causes of Death in the Malumfashi Area, Northern Nigeria." *Annals of Tropical Medicine and Parasitology* 78: 265–71.

Bryce, J., C. Boschi-Pinto, K. Shibuya, R. E. Black, and the Child Health Epidemiology Reference Group. 2005. "WHO Estimates of the Causes of Death in Children." *Lancet* 365: 1147–52.

Bryce, J., S. el Arifeen, G. Pariyo, C. Lanata, D. Gwatkin, and J. P. Habicht. 2003. Multi-Country Evaluation of IMCI Study Group. "Reducing Child Mortality: Can Public Health Deliver?" *Lancet* 362: 159–64.

Cassel-Beraud, A. M., P. Michel, and A. Garbarg-Chenon. 1993. "Epidemiological Study of Infantile Rotavirus Diarrhea in Tananarive (Madagascar)." *Journal of Diarrhoeal Diseases Research* 11: 82–87.

Chowdhury, N. R., S. Chakraborty, T. Ramamurthy, M. Nishibuchi, S. Yamasaki, Y. Takeda, and G. B. Nair. 2000. "Molecular Evidence of Clonal *Vibrio Parahaemolyticus* Pandemic Strains." *Emerging Infectious Diseases* 6: 631–36.

Chunge, R. N., I. A. Wamola, S. N. Kinoti, J. Muttunga, L. N. Mutanda, N. Nagelkerke, L. Muthami, E. Muniu, J. M. Simwa, P. N. Karumba, and P. Kabiru. 1989. "Mixed Infections in Childhood Diarrhoea: Results of a Community Study in Kiambu District, Kenya." *East African Medical Journal* 66: 715–23.

Curtis, V., and S. Cairncross. 2003. "Effect of Washing Hands with Soap on Diarrhoea Risk in the Community: A Systematic Review." *Lancet Infectious Diseases* 3: 275–81.

Dabis, F., and E. R. Ekpini. 2002. "HIV-1/AIDS and Maternal and Child Health in Africa." *Lancet* 359: 2097–104.

Daniels, D. L., S. N. Cousens, L. N. Makoae, and R. G. Feachem. 1990. "A Case-Control Study of the Impact of Improved Sanitation on Diarrhea Morbidity in Lesotho." *Bulletin of the World Health Organization* 68: 455–63.

De Francisco, A., A. J. Hall, J. R. Schellenberg, A. M. Greenwood, and B. M. Greenwood. 1993. "The Pattern of Infant and Childhood Mortality in Upper River Division, The Gambia." *Annals of Tropical Paediatrics* 13: 345–52.

Delacollette, C., and M. Barutwanayo. 1993. "Mortalité et morbidité aux jeunes âges dans une région à paludisme hyperendémique stable, commune de Nyanza-Lac, Imbo Sud, Burundi." *Bulletin de la Societé de Pathologie Exotique* 86: 373–79.

Delacollette, C., P. Van der Stuyft, K. Molima, C. Delacollette-Lebrun, and M. Wery. 1989. "Étude de la mortalité globale et de la mortalité liée au paludisme dans le Kivu montagneux, Zaire." *Revue d' Epidémiologie et de Santé Publique* 37: 161–66.

Ekanem, E. E., A. A. Asindi, and O. U. Okoi. 1994. "Community-Based Surveillance of Paediatric Deaths in Cross River State, Nigeria." *Tropical and Geographical Medicine* 46: 305–8.

Fisher, T. K., H. Steinsland, K. Mølbak, R. Ca, J. R. Gentsch, P. Valentiner-Branth, P. Aaby, and H. Sommerfelt. 2000. "Genotype Profiles of Rotavirus Strains from Children in a Suburban Community in Guinea-Bissau, Western Africa." *Journal of Clinical Microbiology* 38: 264–67.

Fontaine, O., B. Diop, J. P. Beau, A. Briend, and M. Ndiaye. 1984. "La diarrhée infantile au Senegal." *Médecine Tropicale: Revue du Corps de Santé Colonial* 44: 27–31.

Gedlu, E., and A. Aseffa. 1996. "*Campylobacter Enteritis* among Children in North-West Ethiopia: A 1-Year Prospective Study." *Annals of Tropical Paediatrics* 16: 207–12.

Georges, M. C., C. Roure, R. V. Tauxe, D. M. Y. Meunier, M. Merlin, J. Testa, C. Baya, J. Limbassa, and A. J. Georges. 1987. "Diarrheal Morbidity and Mortality in Children in the Central African Republic." *American Journal of Tropical Medicine and Hygiene* 36: 598–602.

Georges-Courbot, M. C., A. M. Beraud-Cassel, I. Gouandjika, and A. J. Georges. 1987. "Prospective Study of Enteric *Campylobacter* Infections in Children from Birth to Six Months in the Central African Republic." *Journal of Clinical Microbiology* 25: 836–39.

Georges-Coubot, M. C., A. M. Cassel-Beraud, I. Gouandjika, J. Monges, and A. J. Georges. 1990. "A Cohort Study of Enteric Campylobacter Infection in Children from Birth to Two Years in Bangui (Central African Republic)." *Transactions of the Royal Society of Tropical Medicine and Hygiene* 84: 122–25.

Georges-Courbot, M. C., J. Monges, A. M. Beraud-Cassel, I. Gouandjika, and A. J. Georges. 1988. "Prospective Longitudinal Study of Rotavirus Infections in Children from Birth to Two Years of Age in Central Africa." *Annales de l'Institut Pasteur. Virology* 139: 421–28.

Gomwalk, N. E., L. T. Gosham, and U. J. Umoh. 1990. "Rotavirus Gastroenteritis in Pediatric Diarrhea in Jos, Nigeria." *Journal of Tropical Pediatrics* 36: 52–55.

Gomwalk, N. E., U. J. Umoh, L. T. Gosham, and A. A. Ahmad. 1993. "Influence of Climatic Factors on Rotavirus Infection among Children with Acute Gastroenteritis in Zaria, Northern Nigeria." *Journal of Tropical Pediatrics* 39: 293–97.

Greenwood, B. M., A. K. Bradley, P. Byass, A. M. Greenwood, A. Menon, R. W. Snow, R. J. Hayes, and A. B. Hatib-N'Jie. 1990. "Evaluation of a Primary Health Care Programme in The Gambia. II. Its Impact on Mortality and Morbidity in Young Children." *Journal of Tropical Medicine and Hygiene* 93: 87–97.

Greenwood, B. M., A. M. Greenwood, S. Bradley, S. Tulloch, R. Hayes, and F. S. J. Oldfield. 1987. "Deaths in Infancy and Early Childhood in a Well-Vaccinated, Rural, West African Population." *Annals of Tropical Paediatrics* 7: 91–99.

Griffiths, F. H., A. D. Steele, and J. J. Alexander. 1992. "The Molecular Epidemiology of Rotavirus-Associated Gastro-Enteritis in the Transkei, Southern Africa." *Annals of Tropical Paediatrics* 12: 259–64.

Guerin, P. J., C. Brasher, E. Baron, D. Mic, F. Grimont, M. Ryan, P. Aavitsland, and D. Legros. 2003. "Shigella Dysenteriae Serotype 1 in West Africa: Intervention Strategy for an Outbreak in Sierra Leone." *Lancet* 362: 705–6.

Haffejee, I. E. 1995. "The Epidemiology of Rotavirus Infections: A Global Perspective." *Journal of Pediatric Gastroenterology and Nutrition* 20: 275–86.

Haggerty, P. A., K. Muladi, B. R. Kirkwood, A. Ashworth, and M. Manunebo. 1994. "Community-Based Hygiene Education to Reduce Diarrhoeal Disease in Rural Zaire: Impact of the Intervention on Diarrhoeal Morbidity." *International Journal of Epidemiolology* 23: 1050–59.

Helen Keller International. 1994. "Summary Report on the Nutritional Impact of Sex-biased Behavior." Nutritional Surveillance Project, Dhaka, Bangladesh.

Hodges, M., and R. A. M. Williams. 1998. "Registered Infant and Under-Five Deaths in Freetown, Siera Leone from 1987–1991 and a Comparison with 1969–1979." *West African Journal of Medicine* 17: 95–98.

Jaffar, S., A. Leach, A. M. Greenwood, A. Jepson, O. Muller, M. O. C. Ota, K. Bojang, S. Obaro, and B. M. Greenwood. 1997. "Changes in the Pattern of Infant and Childhood Mortality in Upper River Division, The Gambia, from 1989 to 1993." *Tropical Medicine & International Health* 2: 28–37.

Jamison, D. T., H. W. Mosley, A. R. Measham, and J. L. Bobadilla. 1993. *Disease Control Priorities in Developing Countries*. New York: Oxford University Press.

Jinadu, M. K., S. O. Olusi, J. I. Agun, and A. K. Fabiyi. 1991. "Childhood Diarrhea in Rural Nigeria. I. Studies on Prevalence, Mortality and Socio-Environmental Factors." *Journal of Diarrhoeal Diseases Research* 9: 323–27.

Jones, G., R. W. Steketee, R. E. Black, Z. A. Bhutta, S. S. Morris, and the Bellagio Child Survival Study. 2003. "How Many Child Deaths Can We Prevent This Year?" *Lancet* 362: 65–71.

Kahn, K., S. M. Tollman, M. Garenne, J. S. Gear. 1999. "Who Dies from What? Determining Cause of Death in South Africa's Rural North-East." *Tropical Medicine & International Health* 4: 433–41.

Kalter, H. D., R. H. Gray, and R. E. Black. 1990. "Validation of Postmortem Interviews to Ascertain Selected Causes of Death in Children." *International Journal of Epidemiology* 19: 380–86.

Kirkwood, B. 1991. "Diarrhea." In *Disease and Mortality in Sub-Saharan Africa*, ed. R. G. Feachem and D. T. Jamison, 134–57. New York: Oxford University Press.

Kosek, M., C. Bern, and R. Guerrant. 2003. "The Global Burden of Diarrheal Disease, As Estimated from Studies Published Between 1992 and 2000." *Bulletin of the World Health Organization* 81: 197–204.

Koulla-Shiro, S., C. Loe, and T. Ekoe. 1995. "Prevalence of *Campylobacter* Enteritis in Children from Yaounde (Cameroon)." *Central African Journal of Medicine* 4: 91–94.

LaFond, A. K. 1995. "A Review of Sanitation Program Evaluation in Developing Countries." Activity Report 5, Environmental Health Project, Arlington, VA.

Lanata, C. F. 2003. "Studies of Food Hygiene and Diarrhoeal Disease." *International Journal of Environmental Health Research* 13: S175–83.

League of Nations, Health Section of the Secretariat. 1996–2002. Weekly Epidemiological Record, vols 71–77. http://www.who.int/wer/archives/en/

MacDougall, J., and C. McGahey. 2003. "Three Community-Based Environmental Sanitation and Hygiene Projects Conducted in the Democratic Republic of Congo." Activity Report 119, USAID, New York.

Malakooti, M. A., J. Alaii, G. D. Shanks, and P. A. Phillips-Howard. 1997. "Epidemic Dysentery in Western Kenya." *Transactions of the Royal Society of Tropical Medicine and Hygiene* 91: 541–43.

Manun'ebo, M. N., P. A. Haggerty, M. Kalengaie, A. Ashworth, and B. R. Kirkwood. 1994. "Influence of Demographic, Socioeconomic and Environmental Variables on Childhood Diarrhea in a Rural Area of Zaire." *Journal of Tropical Medicine and Hygiene* 97 (1): 31–38.

Mathers, C. D., C. Stein, D. Ma Fat, C. Rao, M. Inoue, N. Tomijima, C. Bernard, A. Lopez, and C. J. L. Murray. 2002. "Global Burden of Disease 2000: Version 2 Methods and Results." Global Programme on Evidence for Health Policy Discussion Paper 50, WHO, Geneva.

Miller, P., and N. Hirschhorn. 1995. "The Effect of a National Control of Diarrheal Diseases Program on Mortality: The Case of Egypt." *Social Science and Medicine* 40: S1–30.

Mirza, N. M., L. E. Caulfield, R. E. Black, and W. M. Macharia. 1997. "Risk Factors for Diarrheal Duration." *American Journal of Epidemiology* 146 (9): 776–85.

Mnisi, Y. N., M. M. Williams, and A. D. Steele. 1992. "Subgroup and Serotype Epidemiology of Human Rotaviruses Recovered at Ga-Rankuwa, Southern Africa." *Central African Journal of Medicine* 38: 221–25.

Mobley, C. C., J. T. Boerma, S. Titus, B. Lohrke, K. Shangula, and R. E. Black. 1996. "Validation Study of a Verbal Autopsy Method for Causes of Childhood Mortality in Namibia." *Journal of Tropical Pediatrics* 42: 365–69.

Mølbak, K., P. Aaby, L. Ingholt, N. Hojlyng, A. Gottschau, and H. Andersen. 1992. "Persistent and Acute Diarrhea as the Leading Causes of Child Mortality in Urban Guinea-Bissau." *Transactions of the Royal Society of Tropical Medicine and Hygiene* 86: 216–20.

Mølbak, K., N. Hojlyng, L. Ingholt, A. P. Da Silva, S. Jepsen, and P. Aaby. 1990. "An Epidemic Outbreak of Cryptosporidiosis: A Prospective Community Study from Guinea Bissau." *Pediatric Infectious Disease Journal* 9: 566–70.

Mølbak, K., H. Jensen, L. Ingholt, and P. Aaby. 1997. "Risk Factors for Diarrheal Disease Incidence in Early Childhood: A Community Cohort Study from Guinea-Bissau." *American Journal of Epidemiology* 146: 273–82.

Mølbak, K., N. Wested, N. Hojlyng, F. Scheutz, A. Gottschau, P. Aaby, and A. P. J. da Silva. 1994. "The Etiology of Early Childhood Diarrhea: A Community Study from Guinea-Bissau." *Journal of Infectious Disease* 169: 581–87.

Morris, S. S., R. E. Black, and L. Tomaskovic. 2003. "Predicting the Distribution of Under-Five Deaths by Cause in Countries without Adequate Vital Registration Systems." *International Journal of Epidemiology* 32: 1041–51.

Moy, R. J., I. W. Booth, R. G. Choto, and A. S. McNeish. 1991. "Recurrent and Persistent Diarrhea in a Rural Zimbabwean Community: A Prospective Study." *Journal of Tropical Pediatrics* 37: 293–99.

Mpabalwani, M., H. Oshitani, F. Kasolo, K. Mizuta, N. Luo, N. Matsubayashi, G. Bhat, H. Suzuki, and Y. Numazaki. 1995. "Rotavirus Gastro-Enteritis in Hospitalized Children with Acute Diarrhea in Zambia." *Annals of Tropical Paediatrics* 15: 39–43.

Mtango, F. D. E., and D. Neuvians. 1986. "Acute Respiratory Infections in Children under Five Years. Control Project in Bagamoyo District, Tanzania." *Transactions of the Royal Society of Tropical Medicine and Hygiene* 80: 851–58.

Mtango, F. D. E., D. Neuvians, C. V. Broome, A. W. Hightower, and A. Pio. 1992. "Risk Factors for Deaths in Children under 5 Years Old in Bangamoyo District, Tanzania." *Tropical Medicine and Parasitology* 43: 229–33.

Mutanda, L. N., W. Gemert, S. K. Kangethe, and R. Juma. 1986. "Seasonal Pattern of Some Causative Agents of Childhood Diarrhoea in Nairobi." *East African Medical Journal* 63: 373–81.

Mutanda, L. N., S. K. Kangethe, R. Juma, E. O. Lichenga, and C. Gathecha. 1985. "Aetiology of Diarrhoea in Malnourished Children at Kenyatta National Hospital." *East African Medical Journal* 62: 835–42.

Nakano, T., F. N. Binka, E. A. Afari, D. Agbodaze, M. E. Aryeetey, J. A. A. Mingle, H. Kamiya, and M. Sakurai. 1990. "Survey of Enteropathogenic Agents in Children with and without Diarrhoea in Ghana." *Journal of Tropical Medicine and Hygiene* 93: 408–12.

Nakata, S., Z. Gatheru, S. Ukae, N. Adachi, N. Kobayashi, S. Honma, J. Muli, J. Nyangao, E. Kiplagat, P. M. Tukei, and S. Chiba. 1999. "Epidemiological Study of the G Serotype Distribution of Group A Rotavirus in Kenya from 1991 to 1994." *Journal of Medical Virology* 58: 296–303.

Obi, C. L., A. O. Coker, J. Epoke, and R. N. Ndip. 1997. "Enteric Bacterial Pathogens in Stools of Residents of Urban and Rural Regions in Nigeria: A Comparison of Patients with and without Diarrhoea and Controls without Diarrhoea." *Journal of Diarrhoeal Diseases Research* 15: 241–47.

Okeke, I. N., A. Lamikanra, H. Steinrück, and J. K. Kaper. 2000. "Characterization of *Escherichia Coli* Strains from Cases of Childhood Diarrhea in Provincial Southwestern Nigeria." *Journal of Clinical Microbiology* 38: 7–12.

Omondi-Odhiambo, J., K. Ginneken, and A. M. Voorhoeve. 1990. "Mortality by Cause of Death in a Rural Area of Machakos District, Kenya in 1975–78." *Journal of Biosocial Science* 22: 63–75.

Oni, G. A., D. A. Schumann, and E. A. Oke. 1991. "Diarrheal Disease Morbidity, Risk Factors and Treatments in a Low Socioeconomic Area of Ilorin, Kwara State, Nigeria." *Journal of Diarrhoeal Diseases Research* 9: 250–57.

Paquet, C., P. Leborgne, A. Sasse, and F. Varaine. 1995. "An Outbreak of Shigella Dysenteriae Type 1 Dysentery in a Refugee Camp in Rwanda." *Santé* 5: 181–84.

Pennap, G., C. T. Pager, I. Peenze, M. C. de Beer, J. K. P. Kwaga, W. N. Ogalla, J. U. Umoh, and A. D. Steele. 2002. "Epidemiology of Astrovirus Infection in Zaria, Nigeria." *Journal of Tropical Pediatrics* 48: 98–101.

Pennap, G., I. Peenze, M. de Beer, C. T. Pager, J. K. P. Kwaga, W. N. Ogalla, J. U. Umoh, and D. Steele. 2000. "VP6 Subgroup and VP7 Serotype of Human Rotavirus in Zaria, Northern Nigeria." *Journal of Tropical Pediatrics* 46: 344–47.

Perch, M., M. S. Sodemann Jakobsen, P. Vallentiner-Branth, H. Steinland, T. K. Fisher, L. D. Duarte, P. Aaby, and K. Mølbak. 2001. "Seven Years' Experience with *Cryptosporidium parvum* in Guinea-Bissau, West Africa." *Annals of Tropical Paediatrics* 21: 313–18.

Pison, G., J. F. Trape, M. Lefebvre, and C. Enel. 1993 "Rapid Decline in Child Mortality in a Rural Area of Senegal." *International Journal of Epidemiology* 22 (1): 72–80.

Rowland, S. G. J., N. Lloyd-Evans, K. Williams, and M. G. M. Rowland. 1985. "The Etiology of Diarrhea Studied in the Community in Young Urban Gambian Children." *Journal of Diarrhoeal Diseases Research* 3: 7–13.

Ruiz-Palacios, G. M., I. Perez-Schael, R. Velazquez, H. Abate, T. Breuer, S. A. Costa-Clemens, B. Cheuvart, et al. 2006. "Safety and Efficacy of an Attenuated Vaccine against Severe Rotavirus Gastroenteritis." *New England Journal of Medicine* 354: 11–22.

Saidi, S. M., Y. Iijima, W. K. Sang, A. K. Mwangudza, J. O. Oundo, K. Taga, M. Aihara, K. Nagayama, H. Yamamoto, P. G. Waiyaki, and T. Honda. 1997. "Epidemiological Study on Infectious Diarrhoeal Diseases in Children in a Coastal Rural Area of Kenya." *Microbiology and Immunology* 41: 773–78.

Sebata, T., and D. Steele. 2001. "Atypical Rotavirus Identified from Young Children with Diarrhea in South Africa." *Journal of Health, Population, and Nutrition* 19: 199–203.

Shamebo, D., L. Muhe, A. Sandstrom, and S. Wall. 1991. "The Butajira Rural Health Project in Ethiopia: Mortality Pattern of the Under Fives." *Journal of Tropical Pediatrics* 37: 254–61.

Snow, R. W., J. R. Armstrong, D. Forster, M. T. Winstanley, V. M. Marsh, C. R. Newton, I. Mwangi, P. A. Winstanley, and K. Marsh. 1992. "Childhood Deaths in Africa: Uses and Limitations of Verbal Autopsies." *Lancet* 340: 351–55.

Snow, R. W., I. Bast de Azevedo, D. Forster, S. Mwankuyse, G. Bomu, G. Kassiga, C. Nyamawi, T. Teuscher, and K. Marsh. 1993. "Maternal Recall of Symptoms Associated with Childhood Deaths in Rural East Africa." *International Journal of Epidemiology* 22: 677–83.

Snyder, J. D., and M. H. Merson. 1982. "The Magnitude of the Global Problem of Acute Diarrheal Disease: A Review of Active Surveillance Data." *Bulletin of the World Health Organization* 60: 605–13.

Steele, A. D., H. R. Basetse, N. R. Blacklow, and J. E. Herrmann. 1998. "Astrovirus Infection in South Africa: A Pilot Study." *Annals of Tropical Paediatrics* 18: 315–19.

Steele, A. D., A. Geyer, J. J. Alexander, H. H. Crewe-Brown, and P. J. Fripp. 1988. "Enteropathogens Isolated from Children with Gastro-Enteritis at Ga-Rankuwa Hospital, South Africa." *Annals of Tropical Paediatrics* 8: 262–67.

Sundary, R. 1986. "Health Implications of Sex Discrimination in Childhood: A Review Paper and an Annotated Bibliography." WHO/UNICEF/FHE 86.2, WHO, Geneva.

Tswana, S. A., P. H. Jorgensen, R. W. Halliwell, R. Kapaata, and S. R. Moyo. 1990. "The Incidence of Rotavirus Infection in Children from Two Selected Study Areas in Zimbabwe." *Central African Journal of Medicine* 36: 241–46.

United Nations. 2000. United Nations Millennium Declaration. General Assembly resolution 55/2, United Nations, New York. http://www.un.org/millennium/declaration/ares552e.pdf.

Utsalo, S. J., F. O. Eko, and O. E. Antia-Obong. 1991. "Cholera and *Vibrio parahaemolyticus* Diarrhoea Endemicity in Calabar, Nigeria." *West African Journal of Medicine* 10: 175–80.

Vaahtera, M., T. Kulmala, K. Maleta, T. Cullinan, M.-L. Salin, and P. Ashorn. 2000. "Epidemiology and Predictors of Infant Morbidity in Rural Malawi." *Paediatric and Perinatal Epidemiology* 14: 363–71.

Vesikari, T., D. O. Matson, P. Dennehy, P. Van Damme, M. Santosham, Z. Rodriguez, M. J. Dallas, et al. 2006. "Safety and Efficacy of a Pentavalent Human-Bovine (WC3) Reassortant Rotavirus Vaccine." *New England Journal of Medicine* 354: 23–33.

Victora, C. G., J. Bryce, O. Fontaine, and R. Monasch. 2000. "Reducing Deaths from Diarrhea Through Oral Rehydration Therapy." *Bulletin of the World Health Organization* 78: 1246–55.

Victora, C. G., S. R. Huttly, S. C. Fuchs, F. C. Barros, M. Garenne, O. Leroy, O. Fontaine, J. P. Beau, V. Fauveau, and H. R. Chowdury. 1993. "International Differences in Clinical Patterns of Diarrheal Deaths: A Comparison of Children from Brazil, Senegal, Bangladesh, and India." *Journal of Diarrhoeal Diseases Research* 11 (1): 25–29.

Victora, C. G., M. T. Olinto, F. C. Barros, and L. C. Nobre. 1996. "Falling Diarrhea Mortality in Northeastern Brazil: Did ORT Play a Role?" *Health Policy and Planning* 11: 132–41.

Victora, C. G., A. Wagstaff, J. A. Schellenberg, D. Gwatkin, M. Claeson, and J.-P. Habicht. 2003. "Applying an Equity Lens to Child Health Mortality: More of the Same Is Not Enough." *Lancet* 362: 233–41.

Walker, N., B. Schwartländer, and J. Bryce. 2002. "Meeting International Goals in Child Survival and HIV/AIDS." *Lancet* 360: 284–89.

Watts, T., N. Ng'andu, and J. Wray. 1990. "Children in an Urban Township in Zambia. A Prospective Study of Children during Their First Year of Life." *Journal of Tropical Pediatrics* 36: 287–93.

WHO (World Health Organization). 2000. *WHO-UNICEF-WSSCC Global Water Supply and Sanitation Assessment 2000 Report.* Geneva: WHO.

———. 2002. *The World Health Report 2002: Reducing Risks, Promoting Healthy Life.* Geneva, WHO.

———. 2005. "Mothers and Children Matter—So Does Their Health." In *The World Health Report 2005—Make Every Mother and Child Count.* Geneva: WHO.

Yeager, B. A., S. R. Huttly, R. Bartolini, M. Rojas, and C. F. Lanata. 1999. "Defecation Practices of Young Children in a Peruvian Shanty Town." *Social Science and Medicine* 49: 531–41.

Chapter 10

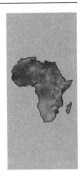

Developmental Disabilities

Geoff Solarsh and Karen J. Hofman

Developmental Disabilities are disorders of the developing nervous system that manifest during infancy or childhood as developmental delay or as limitations of function in one or multiple domains, including cognition, motor performance, vision, hearing and speech, and behavior. Because of the variable nature, extent, and timing of the disorders in the developing nervous system their clinical expression varies enormously from one individual to another, both in severity and in relative effect on the different areas of function. Because developmental disabilities are a composite of a large number of different health conditions, primary and secondary prevention strategies vary for each of the component conditions, whereas tertiary prevention strategies, which address later effects on capacities in broad areas of function, are largely shared across disorders. These disabilities are likely to continue indefinitely and to result in substantial limitations on many life activities, such as affected individuals' ability to care for themselves, express and receive language, learn, be mobile, and live independent and economically self-sufficient lives.

MEDICAL AND SOCIAL MODELS OF DISABILITY

The definition just given has its origins in the *medical model* of disability, which views disability as a problem of the person, directly caused by disease, trauma, or other health condition and requiring individual medical care from health or rehabilitation professionals. Management of the disability is aimed at cure or, more realistically, at producing personal adjustment or behavior change by the individual in response to the disability. In contrast, the *social model* sees the issue mainly as a socially created problem attributable to environmental and contextual factors, such as lack of awareness or social stigma in the broader society and deficient social policies and legislation. These factors together create an environment for people with disabilities that limits activity and restricts participation. In the medical model intervention usually means the prevention and early treatment of health conditions in the individual (primary and secondary prevention), whereas in the social model it means the promotion of functional capacity and the achievement of full

Figure 10.1 Relationship between Impairment, Disability, and Handicap (ICIDH)

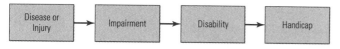

Source: WHO 1980.

Figure 10.2 Relationship between Body Functions, Activities, and Participation (ICF)

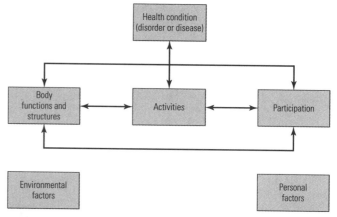

Source: Authors.

participation in the physical and social environment (tertiary prevention). In this chapter an attempt is made to integrate these perspectives.

The International Classification of Functioning

In 1980 the World Health Organization (WHO) published the *International Classification of Impairments, Disabilities and Handicaps* (WHO 1980) as a companion classification to the *International Classification of Diseases* to document the consequences of congenital or acquired illnesses with nonfatal outcomes (figure 10.1). These consequences were evident in *impairments*, defined as abnormalities of body or organ structures and functions; *disabilities*, defined as reduction of a person's ability to perform basic and everyday tasks; and *handicaps*, defined as a person's disadvantage in fulfilling social roles. This framework suggested a hierarchical and linear relation between these three dimensions that entailed a problem-solving sequence in which interventions at one level have the potential to modify succeeding elements (Fryers 1992).

Two of the most important criticisms of this classification that are particularly relevant for this review are its failure to adequately cover disabilities affecting children and its limited utility for public health applications. A closely related criticism has been its failure to take into account the pervasive role of the environment in exacerbating or reducing the nature and extent of disablement.

In its revised *International Classification of Functioning, Disability and Health* the WHO (2001) has sought to address some of these criticisms and, in particular, to unify the apparent polarities in the medical and social models of disability (figure 10.2). In the *International Classification of Functioning* a person's functioning and disability is conceived as a dynamic interaction between health conditions (diseases, disorders, injuries, and trauma) and the effect of contextual and environmental factors in limiting activity and restricting participation.

The Effect of Poverty

In developing countries serious developmental disabilities represent only a proportion of the poor developmental

outcomes of children and young adults. The neurological and developmental deficits that have their primary origin in adverse social and environmental conditions, such as poverty, poor nutrition, and social deprivation, during the critical years of early brain growth and development usually present later in childhood as cognitive impairments and poor performance at school. This group of at-risk infants and children is likely to exceed by many times the number of children with readily identifiable developmental disabilities. Because the contribution of this group to the burden of developmental disabilities is difficult to measure and the interventions are more closely linked to broad community development and poverty alleviation strategies, they will not be considered, except in passing, in this chapter. This in no way implies that they have any less a priority in policies and programs that address developmental disabilities in low-income countries.

THE CHANGING BURDEN OF DISEASE IN CHILDHOOD

Developmental disabilities and their prevention have not had much prominence on the public health agenda in developing countries over the past three or four decades. Steady shifts in the patterns of mortality and morbidity over this period are now beginning to challenge these traditional public health priorities.

The Health Transition

Infant and child mortality has steadily declined in Sub-Saharan Africa countries during the second half of the twentieth century (Ahmad, Lopez, and Inoue 2000; Hill et al.

1999) along with an accompanying fall in fertility (Cleland, Onuoha, and Timaeus 1994; Cohen 1993). This is a result of a complex process of social and economic change in these countries coupled with sustained implementation of family planning programs (United Nations Population Division 1998) and primary health care interventions (Fauveau et al. 1990; Grant 1992; Velema et al. 1991) that specifically target preventable diseases in infancy and childhood.

This "demographic and epidemiological transition" has occurred at varying rates in different African countries. Infant mortality trends during the health transition in developed countries have shown large absolute decreases in postneonatal mortality accompanied by increases in the proportional contribution of neonatal mortality to overall infant mortality (MacFarlane and Mugford 1984). These shifts in the ratio of neonatal to postneonatal mortality have also occurred in countries in Sub-Saharan Africa with the lowest infant mortality rates. Neonatal mortality now accounts for 45 percent of all infant deaths in South Africa (SADHS 1998, 7). These demographic changes suggest that a higher priority should be given to programs that address perinatal conditions. They also signify a need to move away from an exclusive preoccupation with child survival strategies to those that aim to improve the quality of survival in the 92 to 95 percent of children now surviving beyond five years in many African countries. Pointing to pregnancy and the neonatal period targets high-risk groups not only for residual infant mortality but also for developmental disabilities, because many of the most important causes of these disabilities are addressed by interventions during this period.

The Impact of HIV

Arguments for the assignment of a higher priority to research and programs that address developmental disabilities in low-income countries are regularly based on evidence for the health transition in these countries. These transitions, however, are generally uneven both between and within countries, and this is particularly true of the African subcontinent. The "unfinished agenda" of infectious diseases and malnutrition continues to make a variable contribution to postneonatal mortality and morbidity in the different countries and their subpopulations, depending on social, economic, and political conditions and the coverage and quality of primary health care services. Many African countries are now reporting rising postneonatal mortality with patterns of disease often indistinguishable from those in the previous decade (Ahmad et al. 2000), and in many cases, the increase is attributed to the human immunodeficiency virus (HIV) epidemic (Nicoll et al. 1994; United Nations Population Division 1999). Recent evidence suggests that the proportion of under-five mortality attributable to HIV and the acquired immune deficiency syndrome (AIDS) in Sub-Saharan Africa is quite variable (0.1 to 42.4 percent) and that it is highest in some of the countries with the steepest reductions in postneonatal mortality in the past two decades (Walker, Schwartlander, and Bryce 2002).

These data suggest that programs to tackle developmental disabilities may have a greater claim on national resources in some Sub-Saharan Africa countries than in others during this complex health transition. But even in countries with high under-five mortality and HIV seroprevalence rates, 8 or 9 out of every 10 children will survive beyond five years. Many of them will continue to be at risk for developmental disabilities because of preventable biological factors and the lack of services and programs to identify, treat, and ameliorate the impact of these disabilities. Additionally, as will be discussed later, children with HIV infection may be at special risk for developmental disabilities.

Measuring the Burden of Developmental Disabilities

Developmental disabilities, because of their early onset and lifelong requirement for support and care, impose enormous social and economic burdens on affected individuals, their families, and their communities. Calculation of the loss of disability-adjusted life years (DALYs) is now the method widely used to capture and compare the combined effect on the global burden of disease (GBD) of premature mortality and decreased functional capacity resulting from designated health conditions (Murray 1994). An important obstacle to the measurement of the burden of developmental disabilities in low-income countries is the lack of good quality prevalence data. An additional concern stems from the characteristics and applications of the measurement itself.

In burden-of-disease calculations the years of life lost for each death are estimated and assigned a relative value based on the age at death (age weighting). Age weighting is intended to reflect differential productivity of an individual at different stages of his or her life cycle and, thereby, assigns a different social value to lives lived at different ages. A year lived at age 2 counts for only 20 percent of a year lived at 25, when the age-weighting function is at a maximum. The effect of this is to reduce the DALYs lost by premature death of children with developmental disabilities and to potentially lower the relative importance of these conditions in decisions about resource allocations (Anand and Hanson 1997).

To measure the additional contribution of disability, the number of years of healthy life lost is estimated by multiplying the expected duration of the condition (to remission or death) by a disability weighting (0–1). Disability weighting does not take into account the way that individual and social resources can compensate for the level of disability experienced. The failure to factor in these compensatory mechanisms distorts burden-of-death estimates and undervalues the therapeutic and rehabilitation benefits offered by rehabilitation professionals and programs (Jelsma, De Weerdt, and De Kock 2002).

Developmental disabilities incorporate many different disease entities with their different causes; time of onset; natural histories; amenability to primary, secondary, and tertiary prevention; and the relative risk of premature mortality and functional limitation. Since the burden-of-disease methodology is based on calculations for individual disease entities, each of these would need to be addressed separately in order to arrive at a burden-of-disease estimate for developmental disabilities as a whole. Without this information, more pressing and immediate issues, such as HIV/AIDS and malaria, will dominate the health agenda and displace developmental disabilities from consideration for resource allocation.

PREVALENCE AND INCIDENCE

In low-income countries estimates of the frequency of developmental disabilities invariably come from cross-sectional surveys, which measure *prevalence*, or the number of existing cases in the population. Although data on *incidence,* or the number of newly occurring cases, provide a better measure of true frequency in populations, repeat assessments of the same children over shorter periods of time are not cost-effective in most low-income countries.

Two-Phase Childhood Disability Surveys

The best available standard for the measurement of the prevalence of developmental disabilities in population-based surveys is the two-phase survey method, which has been validated in many different population settings in the developing world (Durkin et al. 1994; Thorburn, Desai, and Davidson 1992; Zaman et al. 1990). The first phase consists of a survey of all households in a drawn sample or target population in which all children are screened using the "ten questions" questionnaire. In the second phase all children screening positive and a random 10 percent

sample of those screening negative undergo a detailed medical and psychological examination from which an etiological diagnosis is made and disability rated (none, mild, moderate, and severe) in each of the following areas: gross motor, fine motor, vision, hearing, cognition, speech, and seizures.

Two-phase surveys of this kind have been shown to have a high sensitivity but a low positive predictive value. They are, therefore, ideally suited to serve as screening instruments but completely inappropriate as case-finding tools for epidemiological studies or as the basis for referring children with disabilities for rehabilitation services. Using the ten-question screen as the only basis for determining prevalence of disabilities has been shown to overestimate prevalence by up to 300 percent (Durkin, Hasan, and Hasan 1995).

Many clinical researchers have set the ethical requirement that all children screening positive in a target population should be included in the second phase so that they can be referred to medical and rehabilitation services. Although no similar imperative applies to those screening negative, the inclusion of negatives is necessary (thus the minimal sample of 10 percent) because, using this method, the prevalence estimate for the total population is obtained as a weighted average of the rates in those screening positive versus those screening negative (Shrout and Newman 1989).

Disability Prevalence Data in Sub-Saharan Africa

Reliable data based on the criteria set above on the prevalence of developmental disabilities is scarce in the African subcontinent. An initial Medline search was combined with a search of two major specialist disability journals, *Disability and Rehabilitation* and *The International Journal of Rehabilitation Research,* for the years 1995 to 2004 and a detailed review of all peer-reviewed publications within which the two-phase methodology is employed to measure the prevalence of developmental disabilities in developing countries. In the relatively few studies identified in Sub-Saharan Africa, not a single one fulfilled the methodological criteria laid out above for two-phase disability studies.

Most of the identified studies were conducted in South Africa. The prevalence rates for all categories of developmental disability in these studies varied from 11 to 60 per 1,000 children (Cornielje et al. 1993; Couper 2002; Irlam 1996; Katzenellenbogen et al. 1995; Schneider 1997). Although two-phase surveys were used in most studies, the phase 1 screening questionnaires were not standardized in all cases and were not validated for use in African populations in any of the studies (table 10.1).

Table 10.1 Prevalence of Disability in Sub-Saharan Africa

Year	Country	Author(s)	Methods	Overall prevalence	Cognition	Motor	Vision	Speech, hearing	Behavior	Epilepsy
					(per 1,000 target population)					
1987	Zambia	Stein, Belmont, and Durkin 1987	2-phase survey TQ questionnaire Medical exam 3–9 years	—	35.0 (total) 30.0 (mild) 5.0 (severe)	—	—	—	—	—
1992	South Africa, Gelukspan	Cornielje et al. 1993	2-phase survey No medical exam 5–37 months	11.0 (no severity rating)	—	—	—	—	—	—
1995	South Africa, Western Cape	Katzenellen-bogen et al. 1995	2-phase survey No medical exam All ages	44.0 (moderate to severe)	—	—	—	—	—	—
1995	South Africa KwaZulu	Irlam 1996	2-phase survey TQ questionnaire No medical exam 2–19 years	16.9 (no severity rating)	—	—	—	—	—	—
1997	South Africa	Schneider 1997	1-phase survey Questionnaire All ages	16.0 (1–5 years) 32.0 (6–10 years) 45.0 (11–15 years)	—	—	—	—	—	—
2000	South Africa Bushbuckridge	Christianson et al. 2002	2-phase survey TQ questionnaire Medical exam 2–9 years	—	35.5 (total) 29.1 (mild) 6.4 (severe)	—	—	—	—	7.3
2002	South Africa KwaZulu	Couper 2002	2-phase survey TQ questionnaire No medical exam 0–10 years	60.0	—	28.0	2.0	24.0 (speech) 20.0 (hearing)	37	4.0

Source: Authors.
Note: TQ = ten questions; — = not available.

A more serious limitation is the variation in the methods or content of the evaluation in the second phase. These clinical assessments were not standardized, and they varied from repeat questionnaires by fieldworkers to assessments by rehabilitation assistants, rehabilitation professionals, and neurodevelopmental pediatricians. Additionally, for valid calculations of prevalence in two-phase studies a 10 percent sample of individuals screening negative should be included in the second phase. This did not occur in any of the cited studies, nor was it always clear from the description of the methods how prevalence rates were derived. A final concern is the lack of a standardized approach in most studies to the grading of severity of disability. Since it is clear from carefully conducted studies elsewhere that the ratio between severe and mild disabilities may be very high, comparisons between studies that include children of differing severity may lead to erroneous conclusions about the true size and nature of the problem in different areas.

A tabulation of some of the two-phase studies conducted elsewhere in the developing world is provided as table 10.2 for comparison and similarly shows wide variations in prevalence rates for all categories of disability in childhood from different studies (Durkin et al. 1994; Durkin, Hasan, and Hasan 1995; Islam, Durkin, and Zaman 1993; Milaat et al. 2001; Natale et al. 1992; Tamrat et al. 2001; Zaman et al. 1990). The studies in Bangladesh, Jamaica, and Pakistan that provided the range in prevalence of from 8.1 to 31.0 per 1,000 children were based on identical and established methodologies, used the same set of instruments, and relied on identical rating systems for severity. These rates in all likelihood reflect true differences in the prevalence of developmental disabilities in these three countries and provide a strong platform on which to begin to look at types, determinants, and causes of disability and on which to build a rational approach to intervention.

Table 10.2 Prevalence of Disability in Other Developing Countries

Year	Country	Author(s)	Methods	Overall prevalence	Cognition	Motor	Vision	Speech, hearing	Learning	Epilepsy
				(per 1,000 target population)						
1990	Bangladesh	Zaman et al. 1990	2-phase survey TQ questionnaire Medical exam 2–9 years	16.0 (moderate to severe)	—	—	—	—	—	—
1992	India	Natale et al. 1992	1-phase survey TQ questionnaire 2–9 years	172.0 (poorer) 82 (richer)	—	—	—	—	—	—
1993	Bangladesh	Islam, Durkin, and Zaman 1993	2-phase survey TQ questionnaire Medical exam 2–9 years	—	5.9 (severe)	—	—	—	—	—
1994	Bangladesh			8.1 (moderate to severe)	—	—	—	—	—	—
	Jamaica	Durkin et al. 1994	2-phase survey TQ questionnaire Medical exam 2–9 years	19.8 (moderate to severe)	—	—	—	—	—	—
	Pakistan			31.0 (moderate to severe)	—	—	—	—	—	—
1995	Pakistan	Durkin, Hasan, and Hasan 1995	2-phase survey TQ questionnaire Medical exam 2–9 years	44.3	19.0 (severe)	19.5	15.0	5.2 (hearing)	—	5.0
2001	Saudi Arab	Milaat et al. 2001	1-phase survey TQ questionnaire 0–15 years	36.7 (no severity rating)	—	—	—	—	—	—
2001	Ethiopia	Tamrat et al. 2001	1-phase survey TQ questionnaire 5–14 years	31 (no severity rating)	—	—	—	—	—	—

Source: Authors.
Note: TQ = ten questions; — = not available.

Cognitive Disabilities

Population-based prevalence data on cognitive disabilities are sparse in developing countries, and what little is available comes mainly from outside Sub-Saharan Africa. *Severe mental retardation* (MR), defined as a decreased general intelligence quotient of less than or equal to 55, accompanied by significant limitations in adaptive capability, is consistently found to be in the range of 3 to 5 per 1,000 persons in developed countries. In the few available studies from low-income countries, rates are significantly higher and range from 6 per 1,000 and 22 per 1,000 for severe MR and 14.5 per 1,000 and 65.3 per 1,000 for mild MR in Bangladesh (Islam, Durkin, and Zaman 1993) and Pakistan (Durkin, Hasan, and Hasan 1998), respectively. The only equivalent figures from well-designed population-based

disability surveys come from Zambia (Stein, Belmont, and Durkin 1987), where rates of 5 per 1,000 were recorded for severe MR and 30 per 1,000 for mild MR, and in a recent study from rural South Africa (Christianson et al. 2002), where similar rates of 6.4 per 1,000 were noted for severe MR and 29.1 per 1,000 for mild MR. These figures are a little lower than suggested averages for severe MR in developing countries (9.3 per 1,000) but similar to suggested averages for mild MR (29.8 per 1,000; Roeleveld, Zielhuis, and Gabreels 1997). The failure to ascertain a specific biological cause in many of these children suggests that many cognitive disabilities may have their origins in maternal and infant malnutrition and impoverished environments, which have pervasive adverse effects on growth and psychological development.

Motor Disabilities

No methodologically sound studies could be found that reported population-based prevalence estimates for motor disabilities or its subtypes in Sub-Saharan Africa. One report, which lacked a detailed second-phase medical evaluation and did not include children screening negative, set the prevalence at 28 per 1,000 in a rural South African district (Couper 2002). A comparative rate of 19.5 per 1,000 for severe motor disabilities and 52.5 per 1,000 for mild motor disabilities was reported from Pakistan. There is a clear and immediate need for studies to document independent prevalence rates for motor disabilities, given its common association with severe cognitive disabilities and the observation from studies elsewhere that it is an important and common functional limitation in children with developmental disabilities (Durkin, Hasan, and Hasan 1995).

Vision Disabilities

There are estimated to be 1.5 million blind children worldwide (WHO 1992). The prevalence of blindness in children in European countries varies from 0.2 to 0.4 per 1,000 children and in African countries from 0.5 to 1.1 per 1,000 (Gilbert et al. 1999). Several studies have estimated that as much as 47 percent of blindness or severe visual impairment in developing countries is preventable or curable (Adeoye 1996; Nwosu 1998; Silver et al. 1995). Data from studies done in schools for the blind in East, central, and West African countries show that the most common causes of blindness in children are acquired diseases, such as vitamin A deficiency (29 percent) and measles (27 percent) (Gilbert et al. 1993; Gilbert et al. 1995).

Quite variable rates might be expected in countries at different stages in the health transition. A recent study on the prevalence of blindness in South African schools for the blind supports this view (O'Sullivan, Gilbert, and Foster 1997). An overall estimate of blindness prevalence was 0.35 to 0.6 per 1,000 children. Although 39 percent of causes of blindness or severe visual impairment were found to be preventable, only 5 percent of the affected children had conditions amenable to primary preventive measures, such as vitamin A deficiency or measles. Almost a quarter of the children (23 percent) had inherited conditions, intrauterine infections, or retinopathy of prematurity; the majority of these problems were potentially preventable through genetic counseling and improved antenatal and neonatal care. The remaining 11 percent needed sophisticated surgery for such conditions as cataracts of unknown origin and glaucoma.

Hearing Disabilities

Estimates of hearing loss and profound deafness in developed countries are on the order of 1 per 1,000, compared with 1.4 to 4.0 in developing countries. The WHO estimates that there are 120 million people worldwide with hearing impairment, and 78 million of those affected are in developing countries (WHO 1995b). As in other domains, there are few prevalence data on hearing disabilities in Sub-Saharan Africa. Where data are available, it is often difficult to separate methodological limitations from true differences in prevalence between these studies (WHO 1995b). Reported rates of profound hearing loss range from 2.1 per 1,000 (sensorineural loss) in Swaziland (Swart et al. 1995) to 4.0 per 1,000 in Sierra Leone (Seely et al. 1995; see table 10.3). Chronic otitis media has been demonstrated to be the most frequent cause of hearing impairment in many developing countries (Smith et al. 1996). Estimates suggest that as much as 50 to 66 percent of all hearing impairment in the developing world is preventable (Smith and Hatcher 1992).

Table 10.3 Prevalence of Hearing Disability in Sub-Saharan Africa

Year	Country	Author(s)	Methods	Hearing disability (per 1,000 target population)
1985	The Gambia	McPherson and Holborow 1985	Schoolchildren	2.7 (severe to profound)
1987	Tanzania	Manni and Lema 1987	Schoolchildren	3.5 (severe to profound)
1995	Sierra Leone	Seely et al. 1995	Population-based survey (5–15 years)	4.0 (profound)
1995	Kenya	Hatcher et al. 1995	Schoolchildren	2.4 (profound)
1995	Swaziland	Swart et al. 1995	Schoolchildren (class 1)	2.1 (sensorineural loss)

Source: Authors.

Learning Disabilities

A learning disability is traditionally defined as a disorder in one or more of the basic psychological processes involved in understanding or in using language, spoken or written, resulting in an imperfect ability to listen, think, speak, read, write, spell, or do mathematical calculations. The definition specifically excludes learning problems that are primarily the result of visual, hearing, or motor disabilities and those resulting from mental retardation or emotional disturbance. In Sub-Saharan Africa it may be difficult to distinguish between traditional learning disabilities and the consequences of adverse social and environmental conditions.

No studies could be found that described the prevalence of learning disabilities in Sub-Saharan Africa. A Cape Town study in a population not typical of most of the rest of the subcontinent found that the origin of 45 percent of learning disabilities was prenatal, 17 percent was perinatal, 9 percent was postnatal, and about 25 percent was unknown (Molteno and Lachman 1996). The distribution between these etiological categories varied by ethnic group; children from white and mixed race families had relatively high prenatal contributions (55 percent) compared with children from black African families (23 percent). These relative contributions were reversed in the perinatal category; black African children contributed 37 percent, and children from mixed race groups, 8 percent. Similar distributions were found in an earlier Zimbabwean study but with a much higher proportion being of unknown cause (Axton and Levy 1974). Forty percent of all cases were considered to be preventable. Many of the children in these studies had other major disabilities, including motor, cognitive, and sensory deficits, raising doubts as to whether they fit the traditional definition for this disorder.

As developing countries go through the health transition, it seems likely that learning disabilities will become an increasingly important concern as the countries begin to make more qualitative investments in the future human potential and productivity of their populations. In a country like South Africa, where economic development and rapid political change have coincided, the great demand for access to educational opportunities has highlighted the learning deficits and, in some cases, the disabilities of many children.

DETERMINANTS AND RISK FACTORS

Developmental disabilities have a wide range of origins, occurring from the time of conception through an extended period of rapid brain growth and development during pregnancy, infancy, and childhood. They may have their early beginnings in the genetic makeup of the parents, in the nutritional status of the mother throughout her life cycle, in maternal health conditions and environmental exposure during pregnancy, or in an early or abnormal birth process. They may be the consequence of adaptation difficulties soon after birth; infections, poor nutrition, and injuries in infancy and childhood; or the complex and pervasive effects of adverse social and environmental conditions in impoverished communities (figure 10.3). These factors may act singly or in combination and may make contributions of varying magnitude, depending on background infant and under-five mortality rates, the quality of health services, and special risk factors that may apply in individual locations or subpopulations. These factors may also vary in their amenability to intervention.

An understanding of these factors and their population-attributable risk is a critical preamble to the development of strategies for primary and secondary prevention. This section highlights risk factors for developmental disabilities for which evidence exists from Sub-Saharan Africa or other developing countries of high prevalence or public health and economic impacts, or both, and viable, if unrealized, potential for prevention.

Congenital Disorders

Congenital disorders are defined here as any potentially disabling condition arising before birth and including those caused by environmental, genetic, and unknown factors, whether they are evident at birth or become manifest later in life. It does not include congenital infections or nutritional factors influencing intrauterine growth, which will be discussed later.

The frequency of congenital disorders is best described in terms of birth prevalence, that is, affected births per 1,000 in the absence of a prevention program. Since there are no prevalence data from developing countries, projections are based on data from developed countries; adjustments are made for regional differences in the prevalence of hemoglobin disorders (WHO 1994), glucose-6-phosphate dehydrogenase deficiency (Luzzato and Mehta 1989), and the effect of customary consanguineous marriage (Alwan and Modell 1997), all of which have their greatest burden in less-developed parts of the world (table 10.4). The estimated rate of 61 per 1,000 in Sub-Saharan Africa, which approximates or exceeds infant mortality in some Sub-Saharan African countries, is inflated by the inclusion of fetal losses,

Figure 10.3 Research Steps in the Development of Public Health Interventions

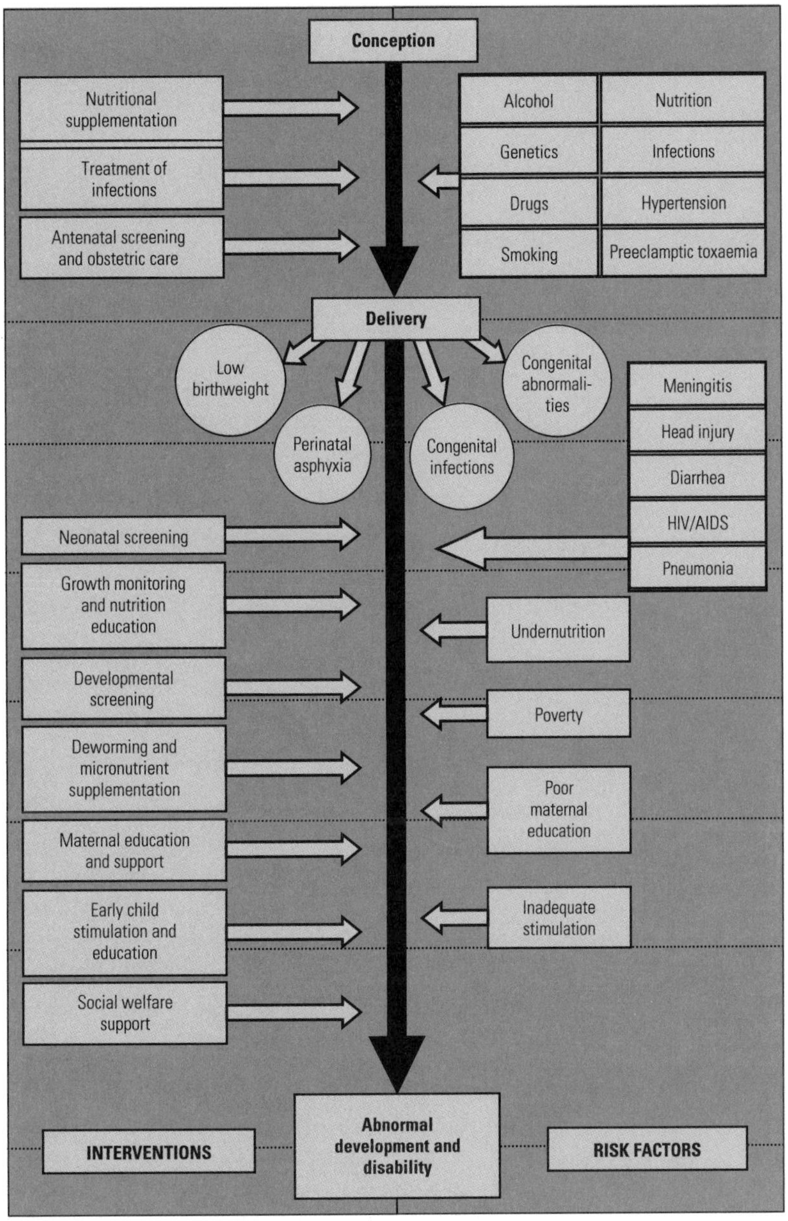

Source: Authors.

Table 10.4 Estimated Birth Prevalence of Infants with Serious Congenital Disorders, by WHO Region

WHO region	Population (millions) 1996	Births per year (millions) 1996	Congenital malformations per 1,000	Chromosomal disorders per 1,000	Single gene disorders per 1,000	Total congenital disorders per 1,000	Annual affected live births
Eastern Mediterranean	506	18.1	35.7	4.3	27.3	69.0	1,237,225
African	540	23.0	30.8	4.4	25.0	61.0	1,412,427
South East Asian	1,401	38.2	31.0	3.9	14.7	51.0	1,946,606
European	867	10.8	31.3	3.7	12.4	49.0	522,832
American	782	16.2	30.9	3.8	11.9	48.0	774,235
Western Pacific	1,650	31.3	30.6	3.5	11.4	47.0	1,464,067
Total	5,746	137.6	31.5	3.9	16.8	53.0	7,357,392

Source: WHO 1999.

but it does provide some indication of the increasing contribution of congenital disorders to burden of disease and disability as infant mortality rates fall (WHO 1999).

In West Africa 2 to 3 percent of all children have a serious hemoglobinopathy (sickle-cell anemia, thalassemia) (Adeoye 1973; Obama et al. 1994). These children are at risk for nervous system complications, the frequency of which may be as high as 12.8 percent. Complications of sickle-cell disease in children include mental changes, cerebrovascular accidents, cranial nerve palsies, dural sinus thrombosis, and increased susceptibility to meningitis, especially salmonella and pneumococcal meningitis. A recent study in the United States revealed that 33 percent of children observed with sickle-cell disease had mild mental retardation (Steen et al. 1999).

Down syndrome has until quite recently been regarded as rare in black African populations. Reports of a birth prevalence of 1.16 (Adeyokunnu 1982) and 2.09 (Venter et al. 1995) per 1,000 from Nigeria and South Africa, respectively, suggest that it may be more common than previously thought. These figures may also underrepresent the true prevalence, because evidence suggests that the syndrome in some of these children may go unrecognized or undeclared in rural black communities (Christianson and Kromberg 1996). The prevalence is likely to be higher in Sub-Saharan Africa countries that have high fertility rates, where effective family planning programs and prenatal screening programs are often lacking and where 11 to 15 percent of births occur to mothers over the age of 35 years (Drugan et al. 1999).

The reported incidence of neural tube defects varies from country to country, from region to region within the same country, and from time to time (Windham and Edmonds 1982). A reported prevalence for neural tube defects of 7 per 1,000 children in Nigeria may have overestimated the incidence, because the study was based at a tertiary referral hospital (Windham and Edmonds 1982). The only available population-based estimate of 3.35 per 1,000 comes from a previously cited study in rural South Africa.

Although consanguineous marriages are considered to be an important cause of congenital abnormalities in many parts of the world, having particularly high prevalence in parts of South Asia, the Middle East, and North Africa, the contribution of such marriages to the burden of developmental disabilities appears to be relatively small in most parts of Sub-Saharan Africa. It has been extrapolated from the birth incidence of single gene disorders in developed countries that the equivalent birth incidence in Sub-Saharan Africa is likely to be on the order of 25 per 1,000 (table 10.4). The collective impact is significant, but none of the individual disorders is a public health problem with sufficiently high population-attributable risk to currently merit targeted intervention.

Perinatal and Neonatal Conditions

Perinatal events, such as preterm delivery, low birthweight, intrauterine growth retardation (IUGR), and birth asphyxia or injury, are commonly associated with an elevated risk of early neonatal death and, in those who survive, of impaired physical, sensory, or mental development in infancy and childhood. Many factors, acting singly or in combination, contribute to the elevated frequency of these events in low-income countries. These include the effect on the growing and developing fetus of maternal macro- and micronutrient deficiencies before and during pregnancy; the direct and indirect effects of maternal systemic and genital tract infections, such as syphilis, rubella, cytomegalovirus, and malaria; and the neurological effects of low blood glucose, hypoxia, bilirubin toxicity, and acquired infections in the first few days of life. Many of these risks may be aggravated or ameliorated, depending on the availability and quality of antenatal, delivery, and postnatal services.

In areas in which maternal and neonatal services are poor and birth asphyxia is an important cause of developmental disabilities, operational research to develop and evaluate alternative approaches to the delivery of these services should be a first priority. In settings in which adequate maternal and neonatal services are available, research is urgently needed on the etiology and prevention of adverse perinatal outcomes, such as low birthweight, preterm birth, and IUGR; on the causal pathways between these factors and developmental disabilities; and on the differential impact of their prevention on the prevalence of neurodevelopmental disabilities in low-income countries. In undertaking this research it will be important to define IUGR and its subtypes (Goldenberg et al. 1989); distinguish between IUGR and its antecedents, many of which are independent risk factors for poor neurodevelopmental outcome (Breart and Poisson-Salomon 1988); control for poor social and environmental conditions that operate postnatally and that may modify neurodevelopmental outcomes (Breart and Poisson-Salomon 1988); select a set of outcomes that are sufficiently prevalent, well defined, and stable over time so that they can be measured with precision at defined time points; and use reasonable sample sizes.

INFECTION

Numerous prenatal, perinatal, and postnatal infections can damage the developing nervous system or sensory pathways and cause long-term disabilities in children and young adults. The relative contribution of these infections to the burden of developmental disabilities is likely to vary from country to country, influenced by overall infant mortality, postneonatal contribution to infant mortality, and regional differences in the distribution of the infections known to be associated with neurological sequelae during these different periods in the early life cycle.

Congenital Rubella

Congenital rubella is a major global cause of preventable hearing impairment, blindness, and intellectual disability. Mathematical modeling has yielded a global disease burden estimate for congenital rubella syndrome (CRS) of 110,000 to 300,000 new cases per year (Cutts and Vynnycky 1999). The incidence of CRS has been variably set at 0.5 to 2.2 per 1,000 live births in developing countries during epidemics, which occur every four to seven years (Cutts et al. 1997). Although many developed countries have set elimination goals, only 28 percent of developing countries routinely vaccinate against rubella (Robertson et al. 1997). No countries in Sub-Saharan Africa include rubella in their national immunization program, and rubella serology, which is essential for surveillance, is unavailable in much of the subcontinent (Robertson 2000).

It is recommended that countries wishing to undertake prevention programs for CRS should either mount vaccination programs for adolescent girls or women of reproductive age or offer universal vaccination in infancy as part of routine childhood immunizations, accompanied by serological surveillance of women of reproductive age. These programs should be undertaken only if the current expanded programs of immunization are already achieving coverage of 80 percent or more. Coverage of less than 80 percent may result in reduced transmission in childhood but leave a large number of women susceptible when they reach reproductive age. A recent cost-benefit analysis of universal rubella vaccination indicates economic benefits comparable to *Haemophilus influenzae* type B (Hib) and hepatitis B virus (HBV) vaccines (Hinman et al. 2002).

Congenital Syphilis

Congenital syphilis is a common and important cause of diverse clinical manifestations in the newborn infant that include deafness, interstitial keratitis, and mental retardation. It is largely preventable through screening and adequate treatment in pregnancy of the 4 to 15 percent of women known to be affected in Sub-Saharan Africa (Schulz, Cates, and O'Mara 1987).

In spite of the availability of an established and highly cost-effective intervention, it was found, in a recent survey of 22 countries in Sub-Saharan Africa, that only 38 percent of women attending antenatal clinics were being screened and treated for syphilis (Gloyd, Chai, and Mercer 2001). It has been roughly estimated that every year up to 600,000 opportunities are missed to reduce adverse fetal and infant outcomes in Sub-Saharan Africa. Although reductions in fetal wastage and neonatal mortality may be the main benefits, more effective antenatal treatment will also reduce defined risks for developmental disabilities in these children.

Other congenital infections such as cytomegalovirus, toxoplasmosis, and herpes infections are also responsible for important neurological sequelae, but because they occur less frequently and are less amenable to primary or secondary prevention, they are given less weight in this review.

HIV Infection

HIV infection is known to have an adverse effect on the developing central nervous system and could potentially make a substantial contribution to the burden of developmental disabilities in populations with high HIV seroprevalence. HIV infection causes damage to the central nervous system through direct cytopathic effects such as occurs in HIV-associated encephalopathy (Brustle et al. 1992), or as a result of vasculopathy or immune-mediated factors. Secondary complications of immunodeficiency, such as opportunistic infections, malignancy, and intracranial hemorrhage, may lead to brain damage. Thrombocytopenia, from direct damage to the bone marrow or as an indirect consequence of opportunistic infections, predisposes HIV-infected children to intracranial hemorrhages and strokes (Mueller 1994). These children are also at higher risk for opportunistic infections of the central nervous system, such as toxoplasmosis or cryptococcal meningitis (Aylward et al. 1992; Mueller 1994), although such infections occur less frequently in children than in adults. Neurological problems in HIV-infected children have been described with varying frequency from different parts of the world. In a natural history study from South Africa, neurological abnormalities were found in approximately 50 percent of children followed to 18 months of age (Bobat et al. 1998). In Rwanda,

15 to 40 percent of HIV-infected infants were found to have abnormalities by 6 months of age (Msellati et al. 1993).

The developmental trajectory of such infected children is confounded by maternal, social, and biological risk factors during pregnancy and early childhood. Maternal substance and drug abuse, more common in HIV-infected women, is known to have an independent adverse effect on brain growth and neurodevelopmental outcome. Low birthweight and prematurity, poverty, protein calorie malnutrition, and micronutrient deficiencies, more frequently seen in HIV-infected children, particularly in developing countries, may similarly compromise early child development (Brouwers et al. 1996). Children who are persistently ill lose a sense of mastery motivation and hence fail to practice new development skills, especially during the first two years of life (Trad et al. 1994). Maternal-child interaction is affected as HIV disease progresses and as maternal emotional availability decreases, resulting in irregular attachment. The observation has been made that HIV-uninfected children of HIV-positive mothers are also at higher risk for cognitive academic and language delays than the general population (Condini et al. 1991). This may be similarly mediated through the social, economic, and environmental consequences of the infection on other household members (Faithfull 1997; Kotchik 1997; Miles et al. 1997).

Malaria

Malaria is the leading cause of childhood mortality and morbidity in large tracts of the subcontinent. Because cerebral malaria is a well-known and not infrequent complication and may result in neurological sequelae in survivors, malaria has the potential to make a significant contribution to the burden of developmental disabilities in Sub-Saharan Africa.

The neuropathology of cerebral malaria stems from a series of complex mechanisms, which may operate independently or in combination to adversely affect the developing brain. These include hypoglycemia, multiple seizures, reduced cerebral perfusion associated with raised intracranial pressure, hypoxia associated with microvascular obstruction, and tissue damage following induction of cytokine cascades (Marsh 1995). The sequelae reported in order of frequency were hemiplegia or hemiparesis, speech disorders, blindness, hearing impairment, cerebral palsy, and epilepsy. Because children often have multiple neurological sequelae it is not possible to disaggregate these data to provide absolute rates for each type of sequelae.

In a pooled analysis from five recent studies with similar definitions of cerebral malaria and comparable methodologies and diagnostic criteria, a neurological sequelae rate in survivors of 16 percent was reported (Snow et al. 1999). A range in reported incidence of neurological sequelae from 9 percent (Molyneux et al. 1989) to 23 percent (van Hensbroek et al. 1997) reflects differences in what are considered to be significant deficits on discharge and those that resolve over subsequent periods of observation. The overall rate of persisting neurological sequelae in studies that lasted at least six months was 5.6 percent and provides a better estimate of true incidence. Assuming that only children with cerebral malaria who reach hospitals are likely to survive, that even these children have a case-fatality rate of 16.7 percent, and that only 5.6 percent of survivors have persistent neurological sequelae after six months, it has been estimated that the annual risk of neurological sequelae for cerebral malaria is 0.03 per 1,000 in children zero to four years of age and 0.006 per 1,000 in children five to nine years of age (van Hensbroek et al. 1997). This amounts to 2,443 and 402 annual neurological sequelae events in these two age groups, respectively. Because the underlying assumptions for these estimates are quite conservative, it is likely that the burden of sequelae is higher than the figure presented. These assumptions, if correct, also suggest that primary prevention of malaria may have differential impact on malaria-specific mortality and disability.

Bacterial Meningitis

A recent survey of mostly hospital-based epidemiological studies throughout Sub-Saharan Africa provides an initial basis for calculating incidence rates for bacterial meningitis and its most common pathogens in the subcontinent (Peltola 2001). These studies also provide important information on overall and pathogen-specific case-fatality and neurological sequelae rates in African children.

In the absence of prospective population-based studies, the few incidence data available for all causes of bacterial meningitis permit a tentative estimate of annual incidence at about 25 per 100,000, or 180,000 cases for the subcontinent as a whole. On the basis of published epidemiological and laboratory data, 50 percent of cases can be assumed to be caused by Hib, giving an estimate of about 90,000 cases of Hib meningitis per year. Because the vast majority of cases occurred in children under the age of five years, the incidence in this age group is estimated to be 74 cases per 100,000. This calculation tallies quite well with data in the same age group from five African countries. Annual incidence rates of

Hib meningitis (per 100,000 children under the age of five years) was 72 in Senegal (Cadoz, Denis, and Mar 1981), 62 in Burkina Faso (Tall et al. 1994), 60 in The Gambia (Bijlmer and van Alphen 1992), 53 in Niger (Campagne et al. 1999), and 51 among black children in South Africa (Hussey et al. 1994). Although meningococcal meningitis predominates in the meningitis belt, it has its greatest impact on adults, and overall, Hib and *Streptococcus pneumoniae* predominate as causes of meningitis in young children in the subcontinent as a whole.

On the basis of data from several studies evaluating neurological sequelae of bacterial meningitis according to etiology, it is estimated that about 40 percent of those surviving Hib meningitis, 50 percent of those surviving pneumococcal meningitis, and 10 percent of those surviving meningococcal meningitis had long-term sequelae.

Measles

For the vast majority of children with measles infection the main risk is death rather than nonintact survival. A notable exception, as has been mentioned earlier, is the occurrence of blindness in measles survivors, which has been cited as one of the most important preventable causes of blindness in the populations of Sub-Saharan Africa. Measles immunization has long been accepted as one of the most cost-effective interventions in child health. The main challenge will be to replicate more widely the high vaccination coverage and virtual elimination of measles that has been achieved in many countries on the subcontinent.

Tetanus

Neonatal tetanus (NNT) remains an important cause of infant mortality in Sub-Saharan Africa, where it has been estimated that 150,000 neonates suffer from NNT each year (Galazka and Gasse 1995). The full extent of the problem may be much larger than this, and the WHO has suggested that in some areas as many as 95 percent of cases may go unrecognized (WHO 1997). Since high case-fatality rates of up to 90 percent have been reported for NNT, the main end point of interest in most studies has been neonatal death rather than neurological sequelae. In early studies it was thought that no permanent neurological damage occurred in survivors of NNT (Gadoth et al. 1981; Sharma et al. 1976). However, frequent uncontrolled spasms associated with prolonged apnea and drops in oxygen saturation may lead to hypoxic brain damage. Later long-term studies from India and Turkey have suggested that 13 to 37.5 percent of

survivors had significant impairments (Anlar, Yalaz, and Dizmen 1989; Gadoth et al. 1981). In a recent study in Kenya significant reductions in head circumference were noted in NNT survivors (Barlow et al. 2001). These children also had more problems with hand-eye coordination, lower developmental scores, more mild neurological abnormalities, and more frequently reported behavioral problems.

The main intervention to prevent NNT is the provision of three doses of tetanus toxoid (TT) to women in their first pregnancy and a single booster dose in each of the subsequent pregnancies, in addition to following safe hygienic practices at birth and in the postnatal period. In a global end-of-decade assessment of TT coverage, 71.3 percent of pregnant women were reported to have received at least two doses of TT in their previous pregnancy (UNICEF 1999). It has been shown in tetanus seroprevalence surveys in Sub-Saharan Africa that estimates of TT coverage significantly under measure protection against NNT (Deming et al. 2002) and that many countries may be approaching World Summit of Children year 2000 goals of 90 percent TT coverage. This is reflected in a dramatic decline in the number of clinical cases in some parts of the subcontinent (Jeena, Wesley, and Coovadia 1999).

Given that vaccination coverage is reasonably high and serological protection even higher, and that high mortality rates in unvaccinated populations result in high neonatal mortality, we speculate that NNT makes a very modest contribution to burdens of developmental disability in Sub-Saharan Africa as a whole. It may represent a more significant problem in selected countries, where the main thrust must be to improve TT coverage.

NUTRITION

There is now evidence linking many nutritional deficiencies to deficits in cognition, motor performance, and behavior. There is substantial evidence that protein-energy malnutrition and deficiencies in iron and iodine, all of which have been and continue to be prevalent in parts of Sub-Saharan Africa, are associated with long-term deficits in cognition and school performance. However, this relationship is complex and affected by the severity and duration of the deficiency, the stage of the child's development, the coexistence of other biological conditions, and a number of sociocultural factors. It is difficult to establish that the association is causal, as there have been few randomized controlled treatment trials with long-term follow-up. The evidence for an association between common nutrient deficiencies in

Sub-Saharan Africa and later development is briefly reviewed below.

Iodine Deficiency

Iodine deficiency has multiple and serious adverse effects, including impaired cognitive function, and it is considered to be the leading cause of preventable mental retardation and brain damage worldwide. A 1999 review of data on the status of iodine deficiency disorders (IDD) demonstrated that IDD is a public health problem in 44 out of 46 countries in Sub-Saharan Africa and that an estimated 295 million people living in these countries are potentially at risk for iodine deficiency (WHO, UNICEF, and ICCIDD 1999). Its well-known effect on mental development has played an important role in mobilizing political, public health, and nutritional activists in support of national and international prevention programs. Efforts at prevention and control focus mainly on the iodization of salt, and as a result of concerted public health prevention efforts, salt iodization was reported, by 1999, to have reached 63 percent of households in Sub-Saharan Africa. In a recent study of seven African countries one year following the introduction of salt iodization, increases in median urinary iodine to above levels considered to constitute iodine deficiency was observed in all countries (Delange, de Benoist, and Alnwick 1999). Progress toward the elimination of IDD through universal salt iodization, with its anticipated impact on cognitive impairment, appears to be one of the most significant successes in the field of noncommunicable diseases. However, the challenge still remains to ensure that salt iodization reaches all populations. Recent studies in South Africa and Lesotho showed that, in spite of compulsory iodization of salt, iodine deficiency remains a significant problem in primary school children in more remote areas of the country (Sebotsa et al. 2003; van Stuijvenberg et al. 1999).

Vitamin A Deficiency

Vitamin A is an essential micronutrient for normal growth, for normal functioning of the visual system, for the maintenance of normal epithelial integrity and immune function, and for normal reproduction. Consequently, vitamin A deficiency (VAD) results in increased severity of certain infections and an increased risk of disease and death in young children. More severe vitamin A depletion leads to night blindness, which can evolve to irreversible partial or total blindness if the depletion continues (Sommer and West 1996; WHO 1996). Evidence for the contribution of VAD to the burden of visual impairment in Sub-Saharan Africa is the main interest in this review and has been presented earlier. There is evidence to suggest that there has been a decrease in clinical VAD (ACC/SCN 1997), manifest as eye lesions, largely as a result of more effective vitamin A supplementation programs in many developing countries, including Sub-Saharan Africa. However, recent estimates for clinical VAD and subclinical VAD still range between 2.8 million and 3.3 million and 140 million to 251 million preschool children, respectively (UNICEF and Tulane University 1998; WHO 1995a). It, therefore, continues to be a major public health problem for which there are relatively simple and cost-effective interventions.

Iron Deficiency

The WHO has estimated that about 40 percent of the world's population suffer from anemia and that a substantial proportion of that burden is attributable to iron deficiency. There is a particularly high prevalence of anemia in pregnant women (50 percent), children in the first two years of life (40 percent), and schoolchildren (40 percent) (WHO 2000). With regard to preschool children, anemia prevalence is the highest in Africa (42 to 53 percent) and Asia of all WHO regions (WHO 1998). An association between hemoglobin concentration and psychomotor performance has been demonstrated at all stages of life. Although there is a good biological basis for claiming that a deficiency of iron might impair mental and motor development, an Expert Group, in weighing up the available evidence (Idjradinata and Pollitt 1993), concluded that only anemia, and not iron deficiency without anemia, impairs the behavior and development of infants (Draper 1997). There now appears to be sufficient evidence to show that iron supplementation of anemic children over two years of age improves development but that this effect is less conclusive in children under the age of two years (Grantham-McGregor and Ani 2001).

Poverty and Protein-Energy Malnutrition

Although there is evidence that the levels of protein-energy malnutrition (PEM) in Sub-Saharan populations have improved and the spectrum of these deficiencies has changed over the past 30 to 40 years, there is still a substantial burden of PEM in many populations in the subregion. For many reasons it has been difficult to establish a causal relationship between undernutrition and behavioral and cognitive development in these children. The main classification of malnutrition used in these studies defines a mixture of clinical signs that are a product of coexistent infections and many other deficiencies, such as zinc, magnesium, copper, and iron, as well as protein and energy, each of which may have an independent and different effect on developmental outcomes (Grantham-McGregor 1995). Malnourished children usually come from families who suffer from numerous disadvantages. These include poor social, economic, and environmental living conditions and unstable family units with large numbers of closely spaced children. The parents are often unwell, poorly nourished, and depressed; young with low intelligence and levels of education; either unemployed or in low-skilled occupations; and likely to have low social and media contacts. Few toys or books can be found in the homes of these families, and parents participate little in play activities; thus there is little stimulation.

The best evidence for a causal effect of undernutrition on cognition and behavior is likely to come from randomized controlled trials. It has been considered unethical to conduct randomized controlled trials to study the effects of malnutrition on behavior and development. It has therefore been necessary to rely on less satisfactory epidemiological study designs, such as case-control studies, which have been unable to control for the wide-ranging nature of these children's disadvantages.

There is also some uncertainty about whether cognitive impairment is an inevitable consequence of severe early malnutrition and what form it is likely to take. Animal experimentation initially suggested that early malnutrition significantly reduced brain growth and left it permanently smaller in size (Winick and Noble 1966). More recent work has shown that many of these dramatic anatomic alterations are reversible. It also shows that parallel alterations in neurotransmitter and receptor characteristics are evident, resulting in subtler neurodevelopmental deficits in motivation, emotional reactivity, and cognitive flexibility rather than in frank reductions in intelligence (Levitsky and Strupp 1995).

In spite of all these limitations and uncertainties evidence suggests that previously malnourished children show a deficit in tests of cognitive function or intelligence. This effect is particularly strong if the undernutrition is chronic and if they return to poor environments. The effect is less clear in children exposed to acute episodes of malnutrition who do not return to impoverished social conditions

(Grantham-McGregor 1995). In unraveling the complex relationship between malnutrition and cognition, several questions remain unanswered—these include questions about the duration of the cognitive deficits, the specific types of cognitive functions that are affected, the relative effect of malnutrition at different points in early childhood, whether complete recovery can occur following placement in enriched environments, and the relative contribution of individual nutrients to cognitive deficits.

ENVIRONMENTAL TOXINS

Alcohol

Fetal alcohol syndrome is the most common single preventable cause of mental retardation worldwide (Viljoen 1999), and the overall rate for the developed world, where the vast majority of prevalence studies have been based, has been placed at 0.97 per 1,000 children (Abel 1995). It has its highest rates in subgroups of the population characterized by low socioeconomic status and confounded by race. For example, in American Indians and African Americans, rates of 8 per 1,000 children (May et al. 1983) and 2.29 per 1,000 have been found, considerably in excess of rates in the U.S. population as a whole.

The only published studies or reports on fetal alcohol syndrome in Sub-Saharan Africa are confined to a subgroup of the "coloured," or mixed race, community in the Western Cape of South Africa, where a prevalence rate of 40.5 to 46.4 per 1,000 children age five to nine years has recently been measured (May et al. 2000). This is the highest rate for fetal alcohol syndrome ever recorded anywhere in the world and appears to be attributable to very high alcohol intake in this South African subpopulation as a consequence of a special set of historical and social conditions.

The principal effect of alcohol teratogenicity is brain damage with consequent lowering of intelligence (mean intelligence quotient 65), behavioral abnormalities (attention deficit, hyperactivity, aggressiveness), and poor language assimilation. The syndrome also presents with a recognizable cluster of facial features and a maternal history of heavy alcohol intake in pregnancy, often imbibed in a pattern of binge drinking. There is no reason to believe that the overall prevalence in Sub-Saharan Africa is particularly high, but it may occur in other subpopulations with low socioeconomic status and histories of high alcohol intake. In these subpopulations, interventions to prevent or reduce alcohol ingestion should assume high priority.

Other Toxins

Other toxins, such as drugs, nicotine, and heavy metals, may result in cognitive and developmental deficits in young children. No information could be found on the prevalence of disabilities attributable to these toxins in Sub-Saharan Africa, although there is clear evidence of exposure to lead, for example, and every reason to expect that some contribution, albeit small, is made by these and other toxins to the burden of disabilities in this subregion.

ACCIDENTS AND INJURIES

For children in Africa who survive the first four years of life, head injury becomes the most likely cause of disability or death, and this remains true until the fourth decade of life (Kibel, Joubert, and Bradshaw 1990). Insofar as these accidents and injuries result in significant damage to the developing central nervous systems, they can be said to make a contribution to the burden of developmental disabilities in young children in the subcontinent. In 1990, DALY rates attributable to injuries and noncommunicable diseases, taken together, among children age five to fourteen years had already exceeded those attributable to infectious, perinatal, and nutritional conditions (Deen et al. 1999). DALY rates attributable to injuries were highest in Sub-Saharan Africa and India, were higher for boys than for girls and for children zero to four years than for children five to nine years of age. Road traffic accidents, falls, burns, and accidental poisoning are the most common categories of childhood accidents and unintentional injuries. The largest number of intentional injuries was caused by war. Hundreds of thousands of children are permanently disabled in Africa every year as a consequence of war injuries and poor trauma care (Bickler and Rode 2002). During 2000 a total of 11 major wars were being fought in Africa, involving 20 percent of the population on the subcontinent. It is estimated that 120,000 to 200,000 child soldiers age five to sixteen years are participating in such conflicts, some of whom sustain bullet and shrapnel wounds as well as burns and land mine injuries. No figures are available for intentional injuries, but these figures may significantly increase the total burden of injuries in some populations.

In a community-based survey of injury-related disability in Ghana, children zero to five and five to fourteen years of age accounted for 14 percent and 10 percent, respectively, of all disability in urban populations and 2.8 percent and 12.3 percent, respectively, of injuries in rural populations (Mock et al. 1999). The majority of these injuries in the zero to four age group were due to falls or burns in both urban and rural populations.

INTERVENTIONS

Given the large and continued contribution of infectious, perinatal, and nutritional conditions to under-five mortality in many parts of Sub-Saharan Africa, the goal and measure of success of most public child-health interventions in Sub-Saharan Africa continues to be an improvement in child survival. We argued earlier that since the majority of these children (90 to 95 percent) are likely to survive beyond early childhood, some consideration should be given to the reduction of developmental disabilities as a parallel end point for child health programs in the subcontinent. We also argued that given the increasing focus on pregnant women and neonates as the target groups for these interventions and shared causal pathways for mortality and disability in early childhood, these parallel end points, namely, reductions in mortality and developmental disabilities, make programmatic sense.

The effect of existing interventions that reduce child mortality on the prevalence and incidence of childhood disabilities is likely to be complex. In the absence of any data on this relationship in developing countries, it seems reasonable to speculate that effective primary prevention of many of the conditions covered in this review, such as vaccine-preventable diseases, is likely to have parallel effects in reducing burdens of both mortality and disability in Sub-Saharan Africa, although the extent of disability reduction may be quite modest. It has been suggested that this group of children in developing countries may have a disproportionately high mortality rate later in childhood as a consequence of ongoing limitations in their access to high-quality medical and social care (Durkin 2002).

Secondary prevention is likely to have, if anything, the opposite effect; intervention at the point where disease is already present may prevent death at the expense of nonintact survival. Interestingly, although cerebral palsy prevalence increased during the early 1970s and 1980s in developed countries (Bhushan, Paneth, and Kiely 1993; Stanley and Watson 1992), cerebral palsy rates in the 1980s and 1990s, presumably as a consequence of improvements in neonatal intensive care and increased survival of infants with antenatal and postnatal brain damage, have been either stable (Colver et al. 2000; Hagberg et al. 1996) or decreasing (Grether and Nelson 1997; O'Shea, Klinepeter, and

Dillard 1998; Topp, Uldall, and Langhoff-Roos 1997) as survival rates continue to increase. It has been suggested that changing rates of postnatal brain damage are the more likely explanation for the secular trends in cerebral palsy prevalence in developed countries over the last three decades (O'Shea 2002). These trends are confounded by variations in case definitions, ascertainment strategies, and study methods between studies and over time. These issues, particularly in the area of secondary prevention, will be equally if not more problematic for the measurement of trends in developmental disability prevalence in developing countries and particularly in Sub-Saharan Africa.

Primary Prevention

Population-based interventions aimed at primary prevention of diseases the risk of which is attributable to high population offer the most attractive approach to tackling developmental disabilities in Sub-Saharan Africa. A general conceptual framework that has been proposed to guide the development and evaluation of all public health interventions (de Zoysa et al. 1998) has potential applications for interventions in the field of developmental disabilities (figure 10.4).

The starting point in this framework is a detailed description of the prevalence, types, severity, and distribution of developmental disabilities in methodologically sound two-phase population-based surveys. The case for good descriptive epidemiological data on developmental disabilities in Sub-Saharan Africa has already been made. Given the expense and effort in mounting these surveys, these descriptions have often been combined in previous studies with the next steps in the research framework, namely, the determination of biological risk factors and social determinants for developmental disabilities. Together these data provide the necessary information to formulate potentially viable interventions and to set up efficacy trials to test them. Subsequent steps, of less immediate relevance to this chapter, involve the refinement of these interventions based on trial findings and their application and evaluation in "real-world" settings.

Secondary Prevention

Neonatal screening programs for congenital disorders, the identification of high-risk newborns for early multidisciplinary intervention programs, or screening in infancy for developmental delays at primary health care clinics have all been proposed as secondary prevention strategies to minimize the effect of neurological disorders once they have already occurred. In some Sub-Saharan countries, such as South Africa, that have high attendance for antenatal care, supervised deliveries, postnatal care, and "well-baby" services in the first year of life, these strategies provide the possibility of early intervention within established health facility networks at strategic points during the neonatal and postneonatal periods. Once screening has occurred, they permit definitive assessments and the institution of appropriate programs of management for identified children. The feasibility and relative benefit of these access strategies and early intervention programs need to be carefully weighed against primary and tertiary prevention in different population settings.

A full consideration of the available primary and secondary interventions and their relative cost-effectiveness is beyond the scope of this chapter. An exercise of this kind is under way and will be the subject of a chapter in a separate monograph (*Disease Control Priorities in Developing*

Figure 10.4 Causal Pathways for Developmental Disabilities

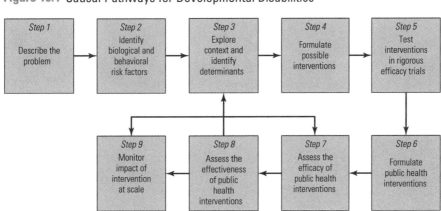

Source: De Zoysa et al. 1998.

Countries, 2nd ed.) Because tertiary prevention is concerned with ameliorating the impact of established developmental disabilities and has been an important, if not the main, thrust in Sub-Saharan Africa, it merits special attention.

Tertiary Prevention

Tertiary prevention programs are needed for all children with established disabilities and this is particularly true for Sub-Saharan Africa, where a large burden of established disability already exists as a result of past failures in primary and secondary prevention of the many conditions discussed earlier in this chapter. As the focus turns from mortality to disability as a public health end point, a better understanding is needed of the dynamic interplay between existing child survival strategies and interventions to specifically reduce or ameliorate developmental disabilities in developing countries, in general, and in Sub-Saharan Africa, in particular.

For the majority of countries in Sub-Saharan Africa, service provision to people with established disabilities will be the starting point and, for some time, the dominant approach in addressing the needs of people with developmental disabilities. The concern in these programs is less with underlying causes than with improvement of functional capacity of affected individuals and the enhancement of their participation in all aspects of community life. Their aim will be to combine direct and indirect therapeutic inputs by health and rehabilitation workers with support and training for families and caregivers and societal interventions to limit stigma and equalize opportunities in all walks of life. In all these processes people with disabilities and their immediate family members will be expected to take a leading role with support and guidance, but not direction, from health and rehabilitation professionals.

For health and rehabilitation professionals in developing countries faced with the large number of children and adults with established disability, tertiary prevention continues to remain an important priority. The failure to meet the rehabilitation needs of the majority of people with disabilities through existing services and growing concerns about the inherent limitations of institutional rehabilitation gave rise to an alternative approach to care for the disabled in developing countries, called community-based rehabilitation (CBR).

Community-Based Rehabilitation

The concept of CBR has been defined by the WHO as a community development strategy focusing on equalization of opportunities and social integration of people with disabilities (WHO, UNESCO, and ILO 1994). CBR activities are holistic in nature and, in attempting to integrate social and medical models of disability, include all or some of the following: awareness raising in communities; advocacy for the rights of people with disabilities; development of parents' and caregivers' groups; income generation; networking with educational, social, and employment authorities; and provision of rehabilitation and health services. The focal person in the CBR program is the person with disabilities, and the main goals, in addition to providing access to rehabilitation services, are to ensure that people with disabilities have rights to self-determination; enjoy the full benefits of family membership; are active and responsible community members; have equal access to education, skills training, work, and recreation; play a significant role in the CBR program itself; participate in organizations that cater to people with disabilities; and act as lobbyists for the disabled and their families.

CBR programs vary in their content, but most include some of the following services:

- a decentralized approach to service delivery with the primary focus and integration of these services at district level within established models of primary health care
- training and support for general-purpose mid-level rehabilitation workers who operate at household and community level
- screening and early identification of children with developmental disabilities
- home-based support and training for activities of daily living
- promotion of inclusive education in pre- and primary schools
- provision of vocational training at secondary schools
- referral to specialist rehabilitation services
- reorientation of the roles of rehabilitation professionals, where available, to support, train, and manage rehabilitation teams and CBR programs in addition to directly providing rehabilitation services.

Defining the sequence and level of input at each of these levels may vary from country to country and from program to program but will be facilitated in all cases by the existence of national health systems based on primary health care and national rehabilitation strategies at all tiers of the health system.

EVALUATION AND COST-BENEFIT ANALYSES

Research and evaluation has not been a prominent feature of the CBR movement. These programs occur in resource-constrained environments, where the need for service provision is preeminent and the necessary motivation, resources, and skills for research have often been lacking. However, many questions remain about CBR, and the field is criticized for having poor indicators with which to measure success (Wirz and Thomas 2002). Divergent views about the primary goals and end points of CBR programs have to some extent impeded the development of a clear set of indicators. Although some believe that standard end points, such as measures of functional improvement of specific disabilities, are required, others are more concerned with measuring shifts in attitudes of community members toward people with disabilities or the extent of inclusion of the disabled in institutional or community life. Those who see CBR as a community development activity are interested in the direct participation of people with disabilities in CBR program activities or income-generating activities as key measures of outcome. Most practitioners, however, see all of these outcomes as important. An approach to evaluation that integrates medical and social models is needed, and the recently revised WHO *International Classification of Functioning*, discussed earlier in this chapter, may provide useful and more standardized guidelines for future approaches of this kind.

A review of the literature confirms that there is a dearth of rigorous evaluations of CBR programs. This is probably as much a reflection of the lack of well-designed programs as it is of the lack of well-designed evaluations, because the two processes often go hand-in-hand. There appears to be an urgent need for the delineation of an evaluation framework that lays out the goals of CBR programs and clearly characterizes the possible inputs, outputs, and expected outcomes of these programs in order both to inform future program design and to guide subsequent program evaluation.

Given that tertiary prevention will continue to be an important intervention for developmental disabilities, irrespective of the successes of primary and secondary prevention, and that CBR programs are likely to continue to be the strategy of choice in developing countries, there is an urgent need for credible evaluations that show an advantageous cost-benefit relationship. Without this it will be increasingly difficult to obtain the ongoing support of policy makers and external funders for these programs.

CONCLUSION

There is an extreme dearth of good-quality data on the prevalence, types, and causes of developmental disabilities in Sub-Saharan Africa. Although a fair number of facility-based and population-based studies do provide some epidemiological descriptions of the conditions that together give rise to the childhood burden of disability, these data vary in quality and there is insufficient understanding of their relative and population-attributable risks for disability. This makes it difficult to quantify disability burdens for children on the subcontinent with accuracy and to intervene effectively in these conditions or to advocate on behalf of children with developmental disabilities. Studies are urgently needed that provide these data and, as the health transition deepens in certain countries, that focus on disability rather than mortality as an end point.

Developmental disabilities bring together clinicians from medical, nursing, and rehabilitation backgrounds; scientists with biomedical, population, and social science perspectives; and researchers, service providers, and people with disabilities with quite different worldviews. Together they must tackle this public health problem through balanced approaches to primary, secondary, and tertiary prevention.

The immediate challenge in countries with large competing health needs and severe resource constraints may be to "start at the end." Many underserved populations in these countries carry large and unaddressed burdens of established disabilities. The provision of services and programs that aim to improve the function of affected children and improve their participation in these societies is their right and our obligation, and this goal must be pursued in parallel with strategies to tackle primary and secondary prevention of the many conditions that contribute to the burden of disabilities in the subcontinent. The diverse and functional needs of these children in these constrained environments must be analyzed, and appropriate programs that realistically address these needs and constraints must be developed and carefully evaluated. For many children these needs, unlike their basic health needs, are simply not being met. Without demonstrating care for the affected, health workers may lack the credibility to advocate for prevention of disabilities in the unaffected.

REFERENCES

Abel, E. L. 1995. "An Update on Incidence of FAS: FAS Is Not an Equal Opportunity Birth Defect." *Neurotoxicology and Teratology* 17 (4): 437–43.

ACC/SCN (Administrative Committee on Coordination/Sub-committee on Nutrition). 1997. *Third Report on the World Nutrition Situation.* Geneva: ACC/SCN.

Adeoye, A. 1973. "Sickle-Cell Anaemia." *British Medical Journal* 2 (5861): 304.

———. 1996. "Survey of Blindness in Rural Communities of South-Western Nigeria." *Tropical Medicine and International Health* 1 (5): 672–76.

Adeyokunnu, A. A. 1982. "The Incidence of Down's Syndrome in Nigeria." *Journal of Medical Genetics* 19 (4): 277–79.

Ahmad, O. B., A. D. Lopez, and M. Inoue. 2000. "The Decline in Child Mortality: A Reappraisal." *Bulletin of the World Health Organization* 78 (10): 1175–91.

Alwan, A., and B. Modell. 1997. *Community Control of Genetic and Congenital Disorders.* EMRO Technical Publications Series 24. Geneva: WHO Regional Office for the Eastern Mediterranean.

Anand, S., and K. Hanson. 1997. "Disability-Adjusted Life Years: A Critical Review." *Journal of Health Economics* 16 (6): 685–702.

Anlar, B., K. Yalaz, and R. Dizmen. 1989. "Long-Term Prognosis after Neonatal Tetanus." *Developmental Medicine and Child Neurology* 31 (1): 76–80.

Axton, J. H., and L. F. Levy. 1974. "Mental Handicap in Rhodesian African Children." *Developmental Medicine and Child Neurology* 16 (3): 350–55.

Aylward, E. H., A. M. Butz, N. Hutton, M. L. Joyner, and J. W. Vogelhut. 1992. "Cognitive and Motor Development in Infants at Risk for Human Immunodeficiency Virus." *American Journal of Diseases in Children* 146 (2): 218–22.

Barlow, J. L., V. Mung'Ala-Odera, J. Gona, and C. R. Newton. 2001. "Brain Damage after Neonatal Tetanus in a Rural Kenyan Hospital." *Tropical Medicine and International Health* 6 (4): 305–8.

Bhushan, V., N. Paneth, and J. L. Kiely. 1993. "Impact of Improved Survival of Very Low Birth Weight Infants on Recent Secular Trends in the Prevalence of Cerebral Palsy." *Pediatrics* 91 (6): 1094–1100.

Bickler, S. W., and H. Rode. 2002. "Surgical Services for Children in Developing Countries." *Bulletin of the World Health Organization* 80 (10): 829–35.

Bijlmer, H. A., and L. van Alphen. 1992. "A Prospective, Population-Based Study of Haemophilus Influenzae Type B Meningitis in The Gambia and the Possible Consequences." *Journal of Infectious Diseases* 165 (Suppl. 1): S29–32.

Bobat, R., D. Moodley, A. Coutsoudis, H. Coovadia, and E. Gouws. 1998. "The Early Natural History of Vertically Transmitted HIV-1 Infection in African Children from Durban, South Africa." *Annals of Tropical Paediatrics* 18 (3): 187–96.

Breart, G., and A. S. Poisson-Salomon. 1988. "Intrauterine Growth Retardation and Mental Handicap: Epidemiological Evidence." *Baillieres Clinical Obstetrics and Gynaecology* 2 (1): 91–100.

Brouwers, P., C. Decarli, M. P. Heyes, H. A. Moss, P. L. Wolters, G. Tudor-Williams, L. A. Civitello, et al. 1996. "Neurobehavioral Manifestations of Symptomatic HIV-1 Disease in Children: Can Nutritional Factors Play a Role?" *Journal of Nutrition* 126 (Suppl. 10): 2651S–62S.

Brustle, O., H. Spiegel, S. L. Lieb, T. Finn, H. Stein, P. Kleihues, and O. D. Wiestler. 1992. "Distribution of Human Immunodeficiency Virus (HIV) in the CNS of Children with Severe HIV Encephalomyelopathy." *Acta Neuropathology (Berl)* 84 (1): 24–31.

Cadoz, M., F. Denis, and I. D. Mar. 1981. "An Epidemiological Study of Purulent Meningitis Cases Admitted to Hospital in Dakar, 1970–1979." *Bulletin of the World Health Organization* 59 (4): 575–84.

Campagne, G., A. Schuchat, S. Djibo, A. Ousseini, L. Cisse, and J. P. Chippaux. 1999. "Epidemiology of Bacterial Meningitis in Niamey, Niger, 1981–96." *Bulletin of the World Health Organization* 77 (6): 499–508.

Christianson, A. L., and J. G. Kromberg. 1996. "Maternal Non-Recognition of Down Syndrome in Black South African Infants." *Clinical Genetics* 49 (3): 141–44.

Christianson, A. L., M. E. Zwane, P. Manga, E. Rosen, A. Venter, D. Downs, and J. G. Kromberg. 2002. "Children with Intellectual Disability in Rural South Africa: Prevalence and Associated Disability." *Journal of Intellectual Disability Research* 46 (Part 2): 179–86.

Cleland, J., N. Onuoha, and I. Timaeus. 1994. "Fertility Change in Sub-Saharan Africa: A Review of the Evidence." In *The Onset of the Fertility Transition in Sub-Saharan Africa,* ed. T. Locoh and V. Hertrich. Liège: International Union for the Scientific Study of Population.

Cohen, B. 1993. "Fertility Levels, Differentials and Trends." In *Demographic Change in Sub-Saharan Africa,* ed. K. Foote, K. H. Hill, and L. G. Martin, 8–67. Washington DC: National Academy Press.

Colver, A. F., M. Gibson, E. N. Hey, S. N. Jarvis, P. C. Mackie, and S. Richmond. 2000. "Increasing Rates of Cerebral Palsy Across the Severity Spectrum, in North-east England 1964–1993. The North of England Collaborative Cerebral Palsy Survey." *Archives of Disease in Childhood. Fetal and Neonatal Edition* 83 (1): F7–F12.

Condini, A., G. Axia, C. Cattelan, M. R. D'Urso, A. M. Laverda, F. Viero, and F. Zacchello. 1991. "Development of Language in 18–30-Month-Old HIV-1-Infected but Not Ill Children." *AIDS* 5 (6): 735–39.

Cornielje, H., P. Ferrinho, D. Coetsee, and S. G. Reinach. 1993. "Development of a Community-based Rehabilitation Programme for a Poor Urban Area in South Africa. A Disability Prevalence Study." *Community Health Association of South Africa Journal* 14 (1): 26–32.

Couper, J. 2002. "Prevalence of Childhood Disability in Rural Kwazulu-Natal." *South African Medical Journal* 92 (7): 549–52.

Cutts, F. T., S. E. Robertson, J. L. Diaz-Ortega, and R. Samuel. 1997. "Control of Rubella and Congenital Rubella Syndrome (CRS) in Developing Countries. Part 1: Burden of Disease from CRS." *Bulletin of the World Health Organization* 75 (1): 55–68.

Cutts, F. T., and E. Vynnycky. 1999. "Modelling the Incidence of Congenital Rubella Syndrome in Developing Countries." *International Journal of Epidemiology* 28 (6): 1176–84.

de Zoysa, I., J. P. Habicht, G. Pelto, and J. Martines. 1998. "Research Steps in the Development and Evaluation of Public Health Interventions." *Bulletin of the World Health Organization* 76 (2): 127–33.

Deen, J. L., T. Vos, S. R. Huttly, and J. Tulloch. 1999. "Injuries and Noncommunicable Diseases: Emerging Health Problems of Children in Developing Countries." *Bulletin of the World Health Organization* 77 (6): 518–24.

Delange, F., B. de Benoist, and D. Alnwick. 1999. "Risks of Iodine-Induced Hyperthyroidism after Correction of Iodine Deficiency by Iodized Salt." *Thyroid* 9 (6): 545–56.

Deming, M. S., J. B. Roungou, M. Kristiansen, I. Heron, A. Yango, A. Guenengafo, and R. Ndamobissi. 2002. "Tetanus Toxoid Coverage as an Indicator of Serological Protection against Neonatal Tetanus." *Bulletin of the World Health Organization* 80 (9): 696–703.

Draper, A. 1997. *Child Development and Iron Deficiency: The Oxford Brief. Opportunities for Micronutrient Interventions Project and Partnership for Child Development.* Washington, DC: USAID.

Drugan, A., Y. Yaron, R. Zamir, S. A. Ebrahim, M. P. Johnson, and M. I. Evans. 1999. "Differential Effect of Advanced Maternal Age on Prenatal Diagnosis of Trisomies 13, 18, and 21." *Fetal Diagnosis and Therapy* 14 (3): 181–84.

Durkin, M. 2002. "The Epidemiology of Developmental Disabilities in Low-income Countries." *Mental Retardation and Developmental Disabilities Research Reviews* 8 (3): 206–11.

Durkin, M. S., L. L. Davidson, P. Desai, Z. M. Hasan, N. Khan, P. E. Shrout, M. J. Thorburn, et al. 1994. "Validity of the Ten Questions Screened for Childhood Disability: Results from Population-Based Studies in Bangladesh, Jamaica, and Pakistan." *Epidemiology* 5 (3): 283–89.

Durkin, M. S., Z. M. Hasan, and K. Z. Hasan. 1995. "The Ten Questions Screen for Childhood Disabilities: Its Uses and Limitations in Pakistan." *Journal of Epidemiology and Community Health* 49 (4): 431–36.

———. 1998. "Prevalence and Correlates of Mental Retardation among Children in Karachi, Pakistan." *American Journal of Epidemiology* 147 (3): 281–88.

Faithfull, J. 1997. "HIV-Positive and AIDS-Infected Women: Challenges and Difficulties of Mothering." *American Journal of Orthopsychiatry* 67 (1): 144–51.

Fauveau, V., B. Wojtyniak, J. Chakraboty, A. M. Sarder, and A. Briend. 1990. "The Effect of Maternal and Child Health and Family Planning Services on Mortality: Is Prevention Enough?" *British Medical Journal* 301 (6743): 103–7.

Fryers, T. 1992. "Epidemiology and Taxonomy in Mental Retardation." *Paediatric and Perinatal Epidemiology* 6 (2): 181–92.

Gadoth, N., R. Dagan, U. Sandbank, D. Levy, and S. W. Moses. 1981. "Permanent Tetraplegia as a Consequence of Tetanus Neonatorum. Evidence for Widespread Lower Motor Neuron Damage." *Journal of Neurological Sciences* 51 (2): 273–78.

Galazka, A., and F. Gasse. 1995. "The Present Status of Tetanus and Tetanus Vaccination." *Current Topics in Microbiology and Immunology* 195: 31–53.

Gilbert, C. E., L. Anderton, L. Dandona, and A. Foster. 1999. "Prevalence of Visual Impairment in Children: A Review of Available Data." *Ophthalmic Epidemiology* 6 (1): 73–82.

Gilbert, C. E., R. Canovas, M. Hagan, S. Rao, and A. Foster. 1993. "Causes of Childhood Blindness: Results from West Africa, South India and Chile." *Eye* 7 (Pt. 1): 184–88.

Gilbert, C. E., M. Wood, K. Waddel, and A. Foster. 1995. "Causes of Childhood Blindness in East Africa: Results in 491 Pupils Attending 17 Schools for the Blind in Malawi, Kenya, and Uganda." *Ophthalmic Epidemiology* 2 (2): 77–84.

Gloyd, S., S. Chai, and M. A. Mercer. 2001. "Antenatal Syphilis in Sub-Saharan Africa: Missed Opportunities for Mortality Reduction." *Health Policy and Planning* 16 (1): 29–34.

Goldenberg, R. L., G. R. Cutter, H. J. Hoffman, J. M. Foster, K. G. Nelson, and J. C. Hauth. 1989. "Intrauterine Growth Retardation: Standards for Diagnosis." *American Journal of Obstetrics and Gynecology* 161 (2): 271–77.

Grant, J. 1992. *State of the World's Children.* New York: UNICEF.

Grantham-McGregor, S. 1995. "A Review of Studies of the Effect of Severe Malnutrition on Mental Development." *Journal of Nutrition* 125 (Suppl. 8): 2233S–38S.

Grantham-McGregor, S., and C. Ani 2001. "A Review of Studies on the Effect of Iron Deficiency on Cognitive Development in Children." *Journal of Nutrition* 131 (2S–2): 649S–66S, discussion 666S–68S.

Grether, J. K., and K. B. Nelson. 1997. "Maternal Infection and Cerebral Palsy in Infants of Normal Birth Weight." *Journal of the American Medical Association* 278 (3): 207–11.

Hagberg, B., G. Hagberg, I. Olow, and L. van Wendt. 1996. "The Changing Panorama of Cerebral Palsy in Sweden. VII. Prevalence and Origin in the Birth Year Period 1987–1990." *Acta Paediatrica* 85 (8): 954–60.

Hatcher, J., A. Smith, I. Mackenzie, S. Thompson, I. Bal, I. Macharia, P. Mugwe, et al. 1995. "A Prevalence Study of Ear Problems in School Children in Kiambu District, Kenya, May 1992." *International Journal of Pediatric Otorhinolaryngology* 33 (3): 197–205.

Hill, K., R. Pande, M. Mahy, and G. Jones. 1999. *Trends in Child Mortality in the Developing World: 1966–1996.* New York: UNICEF.

Hinman, A. R., B. Irons, M. Lewis, and K. Kandola. 2002. "Economic Analyses of Rubella and Rubella Vaccines: A Global Review." *Bulletin of the World Health Organization* 80 (4): 264–70.

Hussey, G., J. Hitchcock, H. Schaaf, G. Coetzee, D. Hanslo, E. van Schalkwyk, J. Pitout, et al. 1994. "Epidemiology of Invasive Haemophilus Influenzae Infections in Cape Town, South Africa." *Annals of Tropical Paediatrics* 14 (2): 97–103.

Idjradinata, P., and E. Pollitt. 1993. "Reversal of Developmental Delays in Iron-Deficient Anaemic Infants Treated with Iron." *Lancet* 341 (8836): 1–4.

Irlam, J. 1996. "The Prevalence of Childhood Disability in a Rural Area of KwaZulu-Natal." Amatikulu Primary Health Care Training Centre, Durban.

Islam, S., M. S. Durkin, and S. S. Zaman. 1993. "Socioeconomic Status and the Prevalence of Mental Retardation in Bangladesh." *Mental Retardation* 31 (6): 412–17.

Jeena, P. M., A. G. Wesley, and H. M. Coovadia. 1999. "Admission Patterns and Outcomes in a Paediatric Intensive Care Unit in South Africa Over a 25-Year Period (1971–1995)." *Intensive Care Medicine* 25 (1): 88–94.

Jelsma, J., W. De Weerdt, and P. De Kock. 2002. "Disability Adjusted Life Years (DALYs) and Rehabilitation." *Disability and Rehabilitation* 24 (7): 378–82.

Katzenellenbogen, J., G. Joubert, K. Rendall, and T. Coetzee. 1995. "Methodological Issues in a Disablement Prevalence Study: Mitchells Plain, South Africa." *Disability and Rehabilitation* 17 (7): 350–57.

Kibel, S. M., G. Joubert, and D. Bradshaw. 1990. "Injury-Related Mortality in South African Children, 1981–1985." *South African Medical Journal* 78 (7): 398–403.

Kotchik, B. 1997. "The Impact of Maternal HIV Infection on Parenting in Inner-City African American Families." *Journal of Family Psychology* 11: 447–61.

Levitsky, D. A., and B. J. Strupp. 1995. "Malnutrition and the Brain: Changing Concepts, Changing Concerns." *Journal of Nutrition* 125 (Suppl. 8): 2212S–20S.

Luzzato, L., and A. Mehta 1989. "Glucose-6-Phosphate Dehydrogenase Deficiency." In *The Metabolic Basis of Inherited Disease*, 6th ed., ed. C. R. Scriver, A. L. Beaudet, W. S. Sly, and D. Valle. New York: McGraw-Hill.

MacFarlane, A., and M. Mugford. 1984. "Birth Counts." In *Statistics of Pregnancy and Childhood.* London: Her Majesty's Stationery Office.

Manni, J. J., and P. N. Lema. 1987. "Otitis Media in Dar es Salaam, Tanzania." *Journal of Laryngology and Otology* 101 (3): 222–28.

Marsh, K. 1995. "Neurological Sequelae of Cerebral Malaria." Paper presented at the WHO/TDR meeting, Geneva, December 4–8.

May, P. A., L. Brooke, J. P. Gossage, J. Croxford, C. Adnams, K. L. Jones, L. Robinson, et al. 2000. "Epidemiology of Fetal Alcohol Syndrome in a South African Community in the Western Cape Province." *American Journal of Public Health* 90 (12): 1905–12.

May, P. A., K. J. Hymbaugh, J. M. Aase, and J. M. Samet. 1983. "Epidemiology of Fetal Alcohol Syndrome among American Indians of the Southwest." *Social Biology* 30 (4): 374–87.

McPherson, B., and C. A. Holborow. 1985. "A Study of Deafness in West Africa: The Gambian Hearing Health Project." *International Journal of Pediatric Otorhinolaryngology* 10 (2): 115–35.

Milaat, W. A., T. M. Ghabrah, H. M. Al-Bar, B. A. Abalkhail, and M. N. Kordy. 2001. "Population-Based Survey of Childhood Disability in Eastern Jeddah Using the Ten Questions Tool." *Disability and Rehabilitation* 23 (5): 199–203.

Miles, M., P. Burchinal, D. Holditch-Davis, Y. Wasilewski, and B. Christian. 1997. "Personal, Family and Health-Related Correlates of Depressive Symptoms in Mothers with HIV." *Journal of Family Psychology* 11 (1): 23–34.

Mock, C. N., F. Abantanga, P. Cummings, and P. Koepsell. 1999. "Incidence and Outcome of Injury in Ghana: A Community-Based Survey." *Bulletin of the World Health Organization* 77 (12): 955–64.

Molteno, C., and P. Lachman. 1996. "The Aetiology of Learning Disability in Preschool Children with Special Reference to Preventability." *Annals of Tropical Paediatrics* 16 (2): 141–48.

Molyneux, M. E., T. E. Taylor, J. J. Wirima, and A. Borgstein. 1989. "Clinical Features and Prognostic Indicators in Paediatric Cerebral Malaria: A Study of 131 Comatose Malawian Children." *Quarterly Journal of Medicine* 71 (265): 441–59.

Msellati, P., P. Lepage, D. G. Hitimana, C. Van Goethem, P. Van de Perre, and F. Dabis. 1993. "Neurodevelopmental Testing of Children Born to Human Immunodeficiency Virus Type 1 Seropositive and Seronegative Mothers: A Prospective Cohort Study in Kigali, Rwanda." *Pediatrics* 92 (6): 843–48.

Mueller, B. 1994. "Hematological Problems and Their Management in Children with HIV Infection." In *Paediatric AIDS: The Challenge of HIV Infection in Infants, Children and Adolescents*, ed. Phillip Pizzo and Catherine Wilfert. Baltimore: Williams and Wilkins.

Murray, C. J. 1994. "Quantifying the Burden of Disease: The Technical Basis for Disability-Adjusted Life Years." *Bulletin of the World Health Organization* 72 (3): 429–45.

Natale, J. E., J. G. Joseph, R. Bergen, R. D. Thulasiraj, and L. Rahmathullah. 1992. "Prevalence of Childhood Disability in a Southern Indian City: Independent Effect of Small Differences in Social Status." *International Journal of Epidemiology* 21 (2): 367–72.

Nicoll, A., I. Timaeus, R. M. Kigadye, G. Walraven, and J. Killewo. 1994. "The Impact of HIV-1 Infection on Mortality in Children Under 5 Years of Age in Sub-Saharan Africa: A Demographic and Epidemiologic Analysis." *AIDS* 8 (7): 995–1005.

Nwosu, S. N. 1998. "Ocular Problems of Young Adults in Rural Nigeria." *International Ophthalmology* 22 (5): 259–63.

Obama, M. T., L. Dongmo, C. Nkemayim, J. Mbede, and P. Hagbe. 1994. "Stroke in Children in Yaounde, Cameroon." *Indian Pediatrics* 31 (7): 791–95.

O'Shea, T. M. 2002. "Cerebral Palsy in Very Preterm Infants: New Epidemiological Insights." *Mental Retardation and Developmental Disabilities Research Reviews* 8 (3): 135–45.

O'Shea, T. M., K. L. Klinepeter, and R. G. Dillard. 1998. "Prenatal Events and the Risk of Cerebral Palsy in Very Low Birth Weight Infants." *American Journal of Epidemiology* 147 (4): 362–69.

O'Sullivan, J., C. Gilbert, and A. Foster. 1997. "The Causes of Childhood Blindness in South Africa." *South African Medical Journal* 87 (12): 1691–95.

Peltola, H. 2001. "Burden of Meningitis and Other Severe Bacterial Infections of Children in Africa: Implications for Prevention." *Clinical Infectious Diseases* 32 (1): 64–75.

Robertson, S. 2000. "Background Document: Data on Rubella Vaccination Schedules." Report of a meeting on preventing CRS, WHO, Geneva, January 12–14.

Robertson, S. E., F. T. Cutts, R. Samuel, and J. L. Diaz-Ortega. 1997. "Control of Rubella and Congenital Rubella Syndrome (CRS) in Developing Countries. Part 2. Vaccination against Rubella." *Bulletin of the World Health Organization* 75 (1): 69–80.

Roeleveld, N., G. A. Zielhuis, and F. Gabreels. 1997. "The Prevalence of Mental Retardation: A Critical Review of Recent Literature." *Developmental Medicine and Child Neurology* 39 (2): 125–32.

SADHS (South African Demographic and Health Survey). 1998. *Child Health.* Tygerberg: South African Medical Research Council and Macro International.

Schneider, M. 1997. *We Also Count. The Extent of Moderate to Severe Reported Disabilities and the Nature of the Disability Experience in South Africa.* Pretoria: Community Agency for Social Enquiry.

Schulz, K. F., W. Cates Jr., and P. R. O'Mara. 1987. "Pregnancy Loss, Infant Death, and Suffering: Legacy of Syphilis and Gonorrhoea in Africa." *Genitourinary Medicine* 63 (5): 320–25.

Sebotsa, M. L., A. Dannhauser, P. L. Jooste, and G. Joubert. 2003. "Prevalence of Goitre and Urinary Iodine Status of Primary-School Children in Lesotho." *Bulletin of the World Health Organization* 81 (1): 28–34.

Seely, D. R., S. S. Gloyd, A. D. Wright, and S. J. Norton. 1995. "Hearing Loss Prevalence and Risk Factors among Sierra Leonean Children." *Archives of Otolaryngology and Head and Neck Surgery* 121 (8): 853–58.

Sharma, A., P. S. Dhatt, J. C. Lall, H. Singh, H. L. Gupta, and R. N. Sallan. 1976. "Neonatal Tetanus: A Developmental Follow-Up Study." *Indian Pediatrics* 13 (1): 51–54.

Shrout, P. E., and S. C. Newman. 1989. "Design of Two-Phase Prevalence Surveys of Rare Disorders." *Biometrics* 45 (2): 549–55.

Silver, J., C. E. Gilbert, P. Spoerer, and A. Foster. 1995. "Low Vision in East African Blind School Students: Need for Optical Low Vision Services." *British Journal of Ophthalmology* 79 (9): 814–20.

Smith, A., and J. Hatcher. 1992. "Preventing Deafness in Africa's Children." *African Health* 15 (1): 33–55.

Smith, A. W., J. Hatcher, I. J. McKenzie, S. Thompson, I. Bal, I. Macharia, and P. Mugwe. 1996. "Randomised Controlled Trial of Treatment of Chronic Suppurative Otitis Media in Kenyan Schoolchildren." *Lancet* 348 (9035): 1128–33.

Snow, R. W., M. Craig, U. Deichmann, and K. Marsh. 1999. "Estimating Mortality, Morbidity and Disability Due to Malaria among Africa's Non-Pregnant Population." *Bulletin of the World Health Organization* 77 (8): 624–40.

Sommer, A., and K. P. West. 1996. *Vitamin A Deficiency: Health, Survival and Vision.* New York: Oxford University Press.

Stanley, F. J., and L. Watson. 1992. "Trends in Perinatal Mortality and Cerebral Palsy in Western Australia, 1967 to 1985." *British Medical Journal* 304 (6843): 1658–63.

Steen, R. G., X. Xiong, R. K. Mulhem, J. W. Langston, and W. C. Wang. 1999. "Subtle Brain Abnormalities in Children with Sickle Cell Disease: Relationship to Blood Hematocrit." *Annals of Neurology* 45 (3): 279–86.

Stein, Z., L. Belmont, and M. Durkin. 1987. "Mild Mental Retardation and Severe Mental Retardation Compared: Experiences in Eight Less Developed Countries." *Upsala Journal of Medical Sciences* (Suppl. 44): 89–96.

Swart, S. M., R. Lemmer, J. N. Parbhoo, and C. A. Prescott. 1995. "A Survey of Ear and Hearing Disorders amongst a Representative Sample of Grade 1 Schoolchildren in Swaziland." *International Journal of Pediatric Otorhinolaryngology* 32 (1): 23–34.

Tall, F., A. Elola, F. Vincent-Ballereau, and T. Prazuck. 1994. "Anti-Haemophilus Influenzae B (Hib) Natural Immunity in Children in Burkina Faso." *Archives of Pediatrics* 1 (2): 143–46.

Tamrat, G., Y. Kebede, S. Alemu, and J. Moore. 2001. "The Prevalence and Characteristics of Physical and Sensory Disabilities in Northern Ethiopia." *Disability and Rehabilitation* 23 (17): 799–804.

Thorburn, M. J., P. Desai, and L. L. Davidson. 1992. "Categories, Classes and Criteria in Childhood Disability—Experience from a Survey in Jamaica." *Disability and Rehabilitation* 14 (3): 122–32.

Topp, M., P. Uldall, and J. Langhoff-Roos. 1997. "Trend in Cerebral Palsy Birth Prevalence in Eastern Denmark: Birth Period 1979–86." *Paediatric and Perinatal Epidemiology* 11 (4): 451–60.

Trad, P. V., M. Kentros, G. E. Solomon, and E. R. Greenblatt. 1994. "Assessment and Psychotherapeutic Intervention for an HIV-Infected Preschool Child." *Journal of the American Academy of Child and Adolescent Psychiatry* 33 (9): 1338–45.

UNICEF (United Nations Children's Fund). 1999. *Evaluation of Multiple Indicator Cluster Surveys.* New York: UNICEF.

UNICEF (United Nations Children's Fund) and Tulane University. 1998. "Progress in Controlling Vitamin A Deficiency." *Micronutrient Initiative.* Ottawa: UNICEF.

United Nations Population Division. 1998. *World Contraceptive Use.* New York: United Nations.

———. 1999. *The Demographic Impact of HIV/AIDS.* Report of the Technical Meeting. New York: United Nations.

van Hensbroek, M., A. Palmer, S. Jaffar, G. Schneider, and D. Kwiatkowski. 1997. "Residual Neurologic Sequelae After Childhood Cerebral Malaria." *Journal of Pediatrics* 131 (1 Part 1): 125–29.

van Stuijvenberg, M. E., J. D. Kvalsvig, M. Faber, M. Kruger, D. G. Kenoyer, and A. J. Banade. 1999. "Effect of Iron-, Iodine-, and Beta-Carotene-Fortified Biscuits on the Micronutrient Status of Primary School Children: A Randomized Controlled Trial." *American Journal of Clinical Nutrition* 69 (3): 497–503.

Velema, J. P., E. M. Alihonou, T. Gandaho, and F. H. Hounye. 1991. "Childhood Mortality among Users and Non-Users Of Primary Health Care in a Rural West African Community." *International Journal of Epidemiology* 20 (2): 474–79.

Venter, P. A., A. L. Christianson, C. M. Hutamo, M. P. Makhura, and G. S. Gericke. 1995. "Congenital Anomalies in Rural Black South African Neonates—A Silent Epidemic?" *South African Medical Journal* 85 (1): 15–20.

Viljoen, D. 1999. "Fetal Alcohol Syndrome." *South African Medical Journal* 89 (9): 958–60.

Walker, N., B. Schwartlander, and J. Bryce. 2002. "Meeting International Goals in Child Survival and HIV/AIDS." *Lancet* 360 (9329): 284–89.

WHO (World Health Organization). 1980. *International Classification of Impairments, Disabilities and Handicaps.* Geneva: WHO.

———. 1992. *Prevention of Childhood Blindness.* Geneva: WHO.

———. 1994. *Guidelines for Control of Haemoglobin Disorders.* WHO/HDP/HB/GL/94.1. Geneva: WHO.

———. 1995a. "Global Prevalence of Vitamin A Deficiency. Micronutrient Deficiency Information System." WHO/NUT/95.3. Working Paper 2, WHO, Geneva.

———. 1995b. "Prevention of Hearing Impairment: Resolution of the 8th World Health Assembly, 48.9." WHO, Geneva.

———. 1996. *Indicators for Assessing Vitamin A Deficiency and Their Application in Monitoring and Evaluating Intervention Programmes.* WHO/NUT/96.10. Geneva: WHO.

———. 1997. *Neonatal Tetanus—Progress towards the Global Elimination of Neonatal Tetanus, 1990–1997.* Geneva: WHO.

———. 1998. Global Database on Anaemia. Geneva, WHO.

———. 1999. "Approaches for Control of Congenital Disorders and Disability in Primary Health Care." Report of a WHO Meeting Held in Cairo December 6–8. WHO, Geneva.

———. 2000. *Malnutrition, the Global Picture.* Geneva: WHO.

———. 2001. *International Classification of Functioning, Disability and Health.* Geneva: WHO.

WHO, UNESCO (United Nations Educational, Scientific, and Cultural Organization), and ILO (International Labour Office). 1994. "Community-Based Rehabilitation for and with People with Disabilities." Joint Position Paper, WHO, Geneva.

WHO, UNICEF (United Nations Children's Fund), and ICCIDD (International Council for Control of Iodine Deficiency Disorders). 1999. *Progress towards the Elimination of Iodine Deficiency Disorders.* WHO/NHD/99.4. Geneva: WHO.

Windham, G. C., and L. D. Edmonds. 1982. "Current Trends in the Incidence of Neural Tube Defects." *Pediatrics* 70 (3): 333–37.

Winick, M., and A. Noble. 1966. "Cellular Response in Rats during Malnutrition at Various Ages." *Journal of Nutrition* 89 (3): 300–06.

Wirz, S., and M. Thomas. 2002. "Evaluation of Community-Based Rehabilitation Programmes: A Search for Appropriate Indicators." *International Journal of Rehabilitation Research* 25 (3): 163–71.

Zaman, S. S., N. Z. Khan, S. Islam, S. Banu, S. Dixit, P. Shrout, and M. Durkin. 1990. "Validity of the 'Ten Questions' for Screening Serious Childhood Disability: Results from Urban Bangladesh." *International Journal of Epidemiology* 19 (3): 613–20.

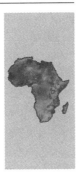

Chapter 11

Acute Respiratory Infections

Shabir A. Madhi and Keith P. Klugman

Acute respiratory infections (ARI), particularly lower respiratory tract infections (LRTI), are the leading cause of death among children under five years of age and are estimated to be responsible for between 1.9 million and 2.2 million childhood deaths globally. Forty-two percent of these ARI-associated deaths occur in Africa (Williams 2002). Despite its importance in regard to morbidity as well as childhood mortality, the epidemiology and pathogenesis of LRTI, particularly in Africa, remains understudied and consequently underappreciated. Although structured management programs coordinated by the World Health Organization (WHO) made some strides during the 1980s and early 1990s toward reducing childhood mortality from LRTI (Sazawal and Black 2003; WHO 1990), the HIV epidemic in many countries of Sub-Saharan Africa has reversed many of these gains (Walker, Schwartlander, and Bryce 2002). The reduction of morbidity and mortality in Sub-Saharan Africa requires a multifaceted approach that includes addressing risk factors associated with increased susceptibility to LRTI among children. These factors include lack of access to basic amenities, such as adequate housing, electricity, and running tap water. Availability of these amenities would help to reduce exposure to such risk factors as indoor smoke

pollution and overcrowding in households. Reducing these risk factors may take some time, but recent advances in medical science hold promise in regard to preventing morbidity and possibly mortality from the most common perceived causes of severe LRTI—those due to bacteria, such as *Haemophilus influenzae* type b (Hib) and *Streptococcus pneumoniae* (Cutts et al. 2005; Klugman et al. 2003; Mulholland et al. 1997). Despite these advances, the challenge remains to address the inequity in health care accessibility and affordability of new-generation vaccines that have been found to be effective in preventing disease caused by these bacteria in developed and developing countries. Furthermore, a priority for most countries in Sub-Saharan Africa in dealing with the reversal of gains that occurred during the late 1980s and early 1990s is to work to prevent the transmission of HIV to children through effective HIV mother-to-child transmission prevention programs.

THE EPIDEMIOLOGY OF ARI AND LRTI

Despite the recognition of LRTI as the leading cause of childhood mortality in Sub-Saharan Africa (Williams 2002), data on the epidemiology of LRTI in these countries are sparse. The most recent community- and hospital-based longitudinal studies aimed at measuring the burden of LRTI in African countries were conducted during the mid-1980s (Bale 1990; Selwyn 1990), prior to the HIV epidemic that has engulfed most of these countries (Asamoah-Odel et al. 2003). These studies were supported as part of an effort by the Board of Science and Technology for International Development (BOSTID) of the U.S. National Research Council to define the burden of LRTI among developing countries (Bale 1990; Selwyn 1990). Based on an estimate of ARI, it was concluded that approximately 4 million deaths from ARI occurred annually (Leowski 1986). In addition to the African studies sponsored by BOSTID, namely, rural Kenya and urban Nigeria (Oyejide and Osinusi 1990; Wafula et al. 1990), the only other areas from which there are reliable estimates of the burden of LRTI are rural areas in The Gambia and Ghana (Afari 1991; Campbell et al. 1989).

The literature published between 1966 and 2000 on the incidence of LRTI (including that in Sub-Saharan Africa) has recently been reviewed by Rudan and colleagues, who estimated the median incidence of LRTI in developing countries at 44 episodes per 100 child-years, equal to approximately 150.7 million new cases each year, 7 to 13 percent of which were severe enough to warrant hospitalization (Rudan et al. 2004). They estimate that there were approximately 33.7 million cases of LRTI annually in African children, with an incidence rate of 31 to 33 per 100 child-years, which was higher than the overall average for all developing countries (23 per 100 child-years) (Rudan et al. 2004). These estimates were, however, exclusive of the impact that the HIV epidemic may have had on the incidence of LRTI. Rudan and colleagues (2004) also found that the burden of LRTI, albeit from studies outside of Africa, was greatest among children less than one year old, and, relative to an incidence of 1.0 in the first year of life, the mean ratios for the subsequent four years of life were 0.58 (year 2), 0.48 (year 3), 0.31 (year 4), and 0.19 (year 5).

Although the few published studies allow an analysis of the burden of LRTI mainly during the mid-1980s and early 1990s, a major pitfall in the studies was the differences in the methodology, not only of diagnostic tests, but also of the clinical definitions used in the studies, all of which may have a bearing on the measured incidence rates as well as the described etiology of LRTI. Although the studies sponsored by BOSTID aimed at reducing the differences in methodology between studies, the wide range of the incidence of LRTI (0.4–8.1 per 100 child-weeks) between the studies,

despite a similar incidence rate of ARI (12.7–16.1 per 100 child-weeks) in most studies, except the study from Thailand (Selwyn 1990), suggest widely varying risk factors, which may have predisposed the children to progression from upper respiratory tract infections to LRTI. Another possibility is that there remain significant differences in the study methodology, including the implementation of different study definitions between the studies. This underlines the importance of recent initiatives by the WHO to standardize the definition of pneumonia so that comparisons may be made between bacterial conjugate vaccines efficacy trials on the burden of LRTI in developing countries (Black et al. 2002; Cherian et al. 2005; Cutts et al. 2005; Klugman et al. 2003; Mulholland et al. 1997).

The study in Kenya suggested that, in addition to the high burden of ARI and LRTI among children, on average, ARI accounted for their illness 21.7 percent of the time and LRTI 0.4 percent of the time (Selwyn 1990). Studies from other non-African developing countries suggest that the burden of disease may be even greater elsewhere, with children being affected for 40 to 60 percent and 14 percent of the year with ARI and LRTI, respectively (Black et al. 1982; Selwyn 1990). The prolonged morbidity associated with ARI, in addition to being associated with mortality, may also affect the physical, emotional, and intellectual development of the child. This situation is further compounded by the finding that the rates of ARI are greatest during the initial years of life (about 7.5 to 8 episodes per year among infants versus about 4 to 6 episodes per year among children 48 to 59 months of age; Selwyn 1990). Furthermore, the proportion of time that children are affected by an ARI ranged from about one-third of the year among infants to less than 20 percent of the time among older children (Oyejide and Osinusi 1990; Wafula et al. 1990). The study from Nigeria also documented the benefits of measles immunization on the incidence of LRTI, showing that children vaccinated for measles had a 2.8-fold reduction in the incidence of LRTI (Oyejide and Osinusi 1990).

The only longitudinal burden-of-disease study in Africa to have defined the incidence of radiologically confirmed pneumonia was performed in The Gambia (Campbell et al. 1989). In that study the incidence of LRTI was 45 per 100 child-years, and 35.5 percent of episodes were associated with radiologically confirmed pneumonia. Another cross-sectional study done in the Central African Republic also found that, although radiologically confirmed pneumonia was present in only 41 percent of children hospitalized for LRTI, the presence on chest radiograph of the involvement of three or more lobes was associated with a 4.6-fold greater risk of death than that of a single lobe (Demers et al. 2000). The overall mortality rate from LRTI among children in developing countries based on the longitudinal studies reviewed by Rudan and colleagues (2004) ranged from 6.6 to 14.1 percent.

The high burden of LRTI among developing countries is partly related to the increased exposure of children in these countries to those poverty-linked risk factors that predispose them to developing LRTI. In a multivariate analysis of data from various studies, Rudan and colleagues (forthcoming) identified the risk factors most consistently associated with LRTI as malnutrition (relative risk [RR] 1.8), low birthweight (less than 2,500 grams at birth, RR 1.4), lack of exclusive breastfeeding in the first four months of life (RR 1.3), overcrowding in the household (more than five people in the household, RR 1.2), and lack of measles immunization (RR 0.7). It was estimated that these risk factors were prevalent among 27.4 percent, 14.7 percent, 54.1 percent, 80.3 percent, and 52.5 percent, respectively, of the world's 523 million children age zero to four years. Additional poverty-related factors that predispose to LRTI include domestic smoke and air pollution (Anderson 1978; Sofoluwe 1968). Consequently, it can be extrapolated that a significant burden of LRTI among children in the developing world is avoidable by addressing factors associated with poverty and lower socioeconomic development.

THE IMPACT OF THE HIV EPIDEMIC ON THE EPIDEMIOLOGY OF LRTI

A further limitation of the published longitudinal studies is that they were conducted at an early stage or even prior to the HIV epidemic. This is particularly pertinent when considering that in some centers more than 80 percent of deaths from LRTI occur among children infected with the human immunodeficiency virus (HIV), despite only 4 to 6 percent of children in the general pediatric population being so infected (Madhi, Petersen, Madhi, Khoolsal, et al. 2000; Zwi, Pettifor, and Soderlund 1999). Although a few studies have looked at differences in the etiology of LRTI between HIV-infected and HIV-uninfected children, only one published study has described the impact that the HIV epidemic has had on the relative burden of LRTI among children in Africa. This study was limited to hospital-based surveillance and underestimates the overall burden of LRTI. Nevertheless, the study emphasized that despite only an estimated 4.5 percent of children in the study population being HIV infected, these children accounted for 45 percent of all LRTI-associated hospitalizations (Madhi, Petersen, Madhi, Khoolsal, et al. 2000).

Although there are no longitudinal studies from Sub-Saharan Africa, including surveillance at the community–health care level, of the incidence of LRTI among HIV-infected children, data from developed countries illustrate the heightened burden of LRTI among HIV-infected children. In a recent review of 3,331 children infected with HIV-1 who participated in several different clinical trials, the incidence rate of any clinically or radiologically diagnosed pneumonia was estimated to be 11.1 (95 percent confidence interval [CI], 10.3–12.0) per 100 child-years (Dankner, Lindsey, and Levin 2001). The trials included children who were on one to three antiretroviral drugs, excluding protease inhibitors. The mean age of children in this study was 39 months; the oldest subject was 20.9 years of age (Dankner, Lindsey, and Levin 2001). In an earlier cohort study evaluating the efficacy of intravenous immunoglobulin prophylaxis, performed among HIV-infected children in the United States, the incidence of LRTI was estimated to be 24 per 100 child-years (Mofenson et al. 1998). This was sevenfold greater than historical incidence rates of 3 to 4.2 per 100 child-years observed among preschool children in the United States and Finland prior to the HIV-1 epidemic (Foy et al. 1973; Murphy et al. 1981). Mofenson and colleagues (1998) described the increased burden of LRTI among HIV-infected children but underestimated the true burden of disease in young children, since the mean age of children recruited into the study (40 months) was greater than the ages (less than 18 months of age) when HIV-infected and HIV-uninfected children are most susceptible to developing and dying of pneumonia (Chintu et al. 1995; Langston et al. 2001; Mofenson et al. 1998; Pillay et al. 2001; Selwyn 1990). During the course of the study by Mofenson and colleagues (1998), pneumonia was second (12 percent) only to upper respiratory tract infections as a cause of bacterial infections among HIV-infected children. Thirty-seven percent of the children with acute pneumonia had multiple episodes of pneumonia, which was also a risk factor for mortality (odds ratio [OR], 2.1; 95 percent CI, 1.3–3.4).

Data from South Africa indicated that the incidence of hospitalization for LRTI among nearly 20,000 placebo recipients (who all received Hib conjugate vaccine) participating in a pneumococcal conjugate vaccine trial, of whom an estimated 6.04 percent were infected with HIV-1, was approximately 6.6 times greater among HIV-infected children (16.7 cases per 100 child-years) than HIV-uninfected children (2.6 cases per 100 child-years) (Madhi et al. 2005). Although the incidence rates observed for HIV-infected children were less than the rate observed by Mofenson and colleagues (1998) among HIV-infected children in the United States (24 per 100 child-years), the data from South Africa included only children who were hospitalized for LRTI as opposed to children who were hospitalized for LRTI and ARI and those who were outpatients in the United States. Although differences in the age of children are also important, these data may illustrate the increased burden of LRTI among African HIV-infected children compared with HIV-infected children in industrial countries.

Williams (2002) recently reviewed the estimates of childhood deaths due to ARI mainly based on published data prior to the current HIV epidemic. It was estimated that globally ARI causes 1.9 million (95 percent CI, 1.6 million to 2.2 million) deaths annually of children under five, 794,000 (40 percent) of which occur in Africa (Williams 2002). The proportion of deaths attributable to ARI was found to be related to the under-five childhood mortality rate of the countries. In countries where the under-five childhood mortality rate is 50 per 1,000, as in most of Sub-Saharan Africa (UNICEF 1996, pp. 90–98), ARI is estimated to be responsible for 23 percent of deaths, compared with only 15 percent of deaths in countries where the under-five mortality rate is 10 per 1,000 per year (Williams 2002). The lower contribution of ARI as a cause of childhood deaths as under-five mortality rates improve was further characterized by trends in under-five mortality among black South Africans that were observed between the 1960s and 1980s (Von Schirnding, Yach, and Klein 1991). In the indigenous South African population of black people from 1968 to 1973, a corrected estimate of 22.5 percent of the under-five mortality of 40 per 1,000 was attributed to ARI, compared with 1980–85, when, with an under-five mortality rate of 17.3 per 1,000, the proportion of deaths due to ARI decreased to 17.7 percent (Von Schirnding, Yach, and Klein 1991). Similarly, ARI was linked to a high proportion (21 to 24 percent) of deaths in other African countries, where the under-five mortality rate ranged between 35 and 63 per 1,000 children during the 1980s (de Francisco et al. 1993; Fantahun 1998; Greenwood et al. 1987; Mtango and Neuvians 1986; Williams 2002).

Much of the improvement in under-five mortality as well as the reduction in the proportion of deaths due to ARI that has been observed in other Sub-Saharan Africa countries, however, have possibly been reversed due to the impact that the HIV epidemic has had on childhood mortality in Sub-Saharan Africa since 1990 (Walker, Schwartlander, and Bryce 2002). In addition to the increased predisposition of HIV-infected children to bacterial- and viral-associated LRTI, HIV-infected children (13.1 percent) have also been found to have a 6.5 times greater (95 percent CI, 3.5–12.1) case-fatality rate than HIV-uninfected children (2.3 percent) even in a country with relatively good resources, such as South Africa (Madhi, Petersen, Madhi, Khoolsal, et al. 2000). Although the case-fatality rate for children with pneumococcal bacteremic pneumonia was similar among those infected with HIV (18 percent) compared with those uninfected (11 percent, $P = 0.18$), the overall higher case-fatality rate for LRTI among HIV-infected children may be explained by the poor outcome of African HIV-infected children who have *Pneumocystis carinii* pneumonia (PCP) (case-fatality rate 20 to 65 percent) (Graham et al. 2000; Madhi et al. 2002).

THE ETIOLOGY OF LRTI

Unfortunately, the sensitivity of current diagnostic tools in defining the etiology of LRTI is woefully suboptimal, particularly for diagnosing bacterial infections, even in the countries with the most resources, such as Finland and the United States (Heiskanen-Kosma et al. 1998; Wubbel et al. 1999). Among industrial countries, where the common respiratory viruses, particularly respiratory syncytial virus, are the dominant (40 to 50 percent of episodes) pathogens identified among children with LRTI, no etiological agent was identified among 30 to 40 percent of children with LRTI, despite the use of an array of advanced microbiological methods, including some that had not been validated against "gold standards" (Heiskanen-Kosma et al. 1998; Wubbel et al. 1999).

The case-management strategy of the WHO is based on the premise that bacteria are the leading cause of LRTI, especially as a cause of severe illness, among children in developing countries (WHO 1990). Nevertheless, most of the etiological studies performed in developing countries suggest that respiratory viruses are as important a cause of LRTI among these children as among those in developed countries (Forgie et al. 1991a, 1991b; Heiskanen-Kosma et al. 1998; Selwyn 1990; Wubbel et al. 1999).

The common respiratory viruses isolated among African infants hospitalized for LRTI in The Gambia include respiratory syncytial virus (37 percent), adenovirus (5 percent), parainfluenza virus (3 percent), rhinovirus (6 percent), and influenza virus (1 percent) (Forgie et al. 1991a, 1991b). Furthermore, more recently, a newly discovered respiratory virus named metapneumovirus (van den Hoogen et al. 2001) has also been identified as a cause of severe LRTI among 10 percent of HIV-uninfected and 3 percent of HIV-infected infants (Madhi et al. 2003). Bacteria were, however, proportionally as common and were identified in 30 percent of the infants, albeit using unvalidated diagnostic methods, with the dominant identified pathogens being *S. pneumoniae* (20 percent) and *H. influenzae* (11 percent) (Forgie et al. 1991a). Mixed bacterial-viral infections were identified among 15 percent of infants. Although 73 percent of infants had radiological evidence of pneumonia, only 28 percent had evidence of a lobar pneumonia(Forgie et al. 1991a). Among older children (one to four years of age) hospitalized with LRTI in The Gambia, identification of bacteria was relatively more common (75 percent) than identification of common respiratory viruses (40 percent) (Forgie et al. 1991b). Although *S. pneumoniae* (60.9 percent) and *H. influenzae* (13.8 percent) remained the most dominant bacterial isolates, other bacteria identified included *Staphylococcus aureus* and *Moraxella catarrhalis* (6.2 percent each) (Forgie et al. 1991b). These studies, similar to others from developing countries, including those that were sponsored by BOSTID, underpin the importance of respiratory syncytial virus as well as *S. pneumoniae, H. influenzae,* and viruses as the etiology of LRTI among children in developing countries (Selwyn 1990).

The spectrum of pathogens and proportional representation thereof appeared to be similar between children with moderate and severe LRTI in the BOSTID-sponsored studies (Selwyn 1990). The clinical relevance of distinguishing between respiratory viral and bacterial infections has, however, gained renewed interest with the recent observation that pneumococcal coinfections are prevalent in at least 30 to 40 percent of children with documented respiratory viral infections (Madhi, Klugman, and Pneumococcal Vaccine Trialist Group 2004).

Other factors that may affect the spectrum of bacteria that causes pneumonia include environmental factors and nutritional status (Adegbola et al. 1994; O'Dempsey et al. 1994). Gram-negative bacteria that include *Salmonella* and coliforms were found to be more common than *S. pneumoniae* and Hib as causes of LRTI during those rainy months of the year when malaria transmission is at its greatest in a malaria-endemic area in The Gambia (O'Dempsey et al. 1994).

Advances in preventing LRTI caused by *S. pneumoniae* and *H. influenzae* type b have refocused attention to measuring the burden of disease due to these pathogens in order to define the burden of LRTI that may be prevented through vaccination of children with the bacterial conjugate vaccines (Black et al. 2002; Klugman et al. 2003; Mulholland et al. 1997). Although fine needle aspiration of the lung is the gold standard for identifying bacterial infections of the lung, it only has a sensitivity of 70 percent and is limited to being performed mainly on children with clearly defined alveolar consolidation, accessible to aspiration (Vuori-Holopainen and Peltola 2001). Because of the empirical management of severe LRTI with antibiotics, the use of fine needle aspirates of the lung has waned (Vuori-Holopainen and Peltola 2001) but has recently received more attention as a diagnostic approach in Finland (Vuori-Holopainen et al. 2002).

The majority of studies that have used fine needle aspirates as a potential diagnostic modality have been performed in Africa (Vuori-Holopainen and Peltola 2001). The performance of lung aspirates is, however, associated with some risk (less than 2 percent), such as that of pneumothoraces and hemoptysis, which may preclude its use in clinical practice as well as in large-scale epidemiological studies (Vuori-Holopainen and Peltola 2001). Furthermore, the yield from lung aspirates may be operator dependent and could also be influenced by other factors, such as preceding exposure to antibiotics, age of the study participants, and the extent of lung infiltrate. This may, at least in part, explain why the yield ranged from 17 percent to 100 percent in various studies. On average, a bacterial pathogen from lung aspirates was isolated in 52 percent (17 to 77 percent) of cases, compared with a blood isolation rate of 25 percent (2 to 45 percent) in studies in which both procedures were done concurrently (Adegbola et al. 1994; Garcia de Olarte et al. 1971; George, Bai, and Cherian 1996; Rapkin 1975; Silverman et al. 1977; Vuori-Holopainen and Peltola 2001; Wall et al. 1986).

Table 11.1 illustrates those studies that included only children with pneumonia who had not received antibiotics prior to having had a fine needle aspirate performed. Except for a small study from South Africa, all the studies confirmed *S. pneumoniae* as the leading isolate among children with pneumonia, although there was a wide range of positive pneumococcal isolates (18 to 51 percent) among other studies performed in developing countries. A summary of lung aspirate studies performed in Africa has, however, suggested that *S. aureus* may also be an important cause of LRTI (20 percent of children) (Vuori-Holopainen et al. 2002; Mimica et al. 1971).

Table 11.1 Results of Lung Aspirations of Children Who Had Not Received Antibiotics and Not Mentioned Underlying Illness

Country	Age	No. of children	Percentage testing positive[a]	Pneumococcus	H. influenzae	S. aureus	E. coli	Other bacteria
USA	2 mos.–15 yrs.	27	22	50 (11)	0 (0)	0 (0)	0 (0)	50 (11)
South Africa	2 mos.–9 yrs.	29	17	20 (3)	40 (6)	0 (0)	0 (0)	40 (3)
Nigeria	4 mos.–8 yrs.	88	79	64 (51)	14 (11)	14 (11)	0 (0)	31 (39)
Zimbabwe	2 mos.–11 yrs.	40	33	54 (18)	23 (8)	31 (10)	0 (0)	0 (0)
Papua New Guinea	<10 yrs.	18	44	88 (39)	13 (6)	0 (0)	0 (0)	0 (0)

Sources: Data from Rapkin 1975 (United States); Prinsloo and Cicoria 1974 (South Africa); Silverman et al. (Nigeria) 1977; Ikeogu (Zimbabwe) 1998; and Riley et al. (Papua New Guinea) 1983.
Note: Numbers in parentheses are percentages.
a. Value indicated in the cells under bacteria is the proportion of all positive isolates and in parenthesis are the values as a percentage of all tests performed. More than one bacterium may have been isolated in some children.

Table 11.2 Estimated Incidence of Organism-Specific, Bacteremic, Community-Acquired Severe LRTI in HIV-1-Infected and HIV-1-Uninfected Children Age 2 to 24 Months

Organism	HIV-1-infected children (per 100,000)	HIV-1-uninfected children (per 100,000)	Relative risk; 95% CI; P value
Streptococcus pneumoniae	1,233	29	42.9; 20.7–90.2; $P < 10^{-5}$
Haemophilus influenzae type b	569	27	21.4; 9.4–48.4; $P < 10^{-5}$
Staphylococcus aureus	337	3	49.0; 15.4–156.0; $P < 10^{-5}$
Escherichia coli	474	10	97.9; 11.4–838.2; $P < 10^{-5}$
Salmonella species	95	7	13.4; 2.2–78.1; $P = 0.02$
Mycobacterium tuberculosis	1,470	65	22.5; 13.2–37.6; $P < 10^{-5}$

Source: Madhi, Petersen, Madhi, Khoolsal, et al. 2000.

Additionally, investigators in Chile and India reported that *S. aureus* was the dominant isolate (25 to 27 percent), whereas *S. pneumoniae* was isolated in only 2 to 5 percent of children, among whom 50 to 70 percent had received antibiotics prior to the performance of the lung aspirate (Mimica et al. 1971). In another report among children who were receiving antibiotics (77 percent) prior to the lung aspirate, *S. pneumoniae* was isolated more frequently than *S. aureus* (11 percent as opposed to 6 percent, respectively) (Prakash et al. 1996). Silverman and colleagues (1977) showed that although the yield of bacteria in Nigerian children with an ill-defined infiltrate (bronchopneumonia) was similar to that in children with lobar consolidation or empyema, the spectrum of isolates differed, with the yield of *S. pneumoniae* being 53.6 and 15.9 percent, respectively (Silverman et al. 1977). Similarly, Mimica and colleagues (1971) in Chile showed that although a bacterium was isolated in 28 percent compared with 45 percent of children with lobar consolidation and bronchopneumonia, respectively, the rates of isolation of *S. pneumoniae* were much lower among children with bronchopneumonia (1 percent versus 24 percent) (Mimica et al. 1971).

Data regarding the relative risk of bacterial pneumonia as well as common respiratory viral-associated LRTI among African HIV-infected children are few (Madhi, Petersen, Madhi, Khoolsal, et al. 2000; Madhi, Schoub, et al. 2000). Although many studies have investigated the etiology of LRTI among African HIV-infected children (Graham et al. 2000; Nathoo et al. 1996; Zar et al. 2001), only limited data exist regarding the pathogen-specific relative risk of LRTI among HIV-infected compared with uninfected children. Table 11.2 illustrates the heightened burden of pathogen-specific bacteremic pneumonia among HIV-infected as compared with HIV-uninfected children. Significantly, although a broader spectrum of bacteria is implicated in HIV-infected children—in particular, gram-negative pathogens—*S. pneumonia* and Hib remained the dominant causes of pneumonia among HIV-infected children in the absence of vaccination with any of the bacterial conjugate vaccines. In addition to the heightened burden of bacterial pneumonia, although proportionately less commonly isolated, the burden of hospitalization for common respiratory viral infections was also found to have increased, albeit less so than for bacterial pneumonia, among HIV-infected children (table 11.3).

Table 11.3 Estimated Incidence for Specific Viral-Associated Severe LRTI in HIV-1-Infected and HIV-1-Uninfected Children Age 2 to 23 Months

Virus	HIV-1-infected children (per 100,000)	HIV-1-uninfected children (per 100,000)	Relative risk, 95% CI
RSV	1,444	309	1.92, 1.29–2.83
Influenza A/B	1,268	148	8.03, 5.05–12.76
Parainfluenza 1-3	893	106	8.46, 4.95–10.47
Adenovirus	481	32	15.07, 6.62–34.33

Source: Madhi, Schoub, et al. 2000.

Further compounding the impact of the HIV epidemic on the etiology of LRTI and possibly the WHO case-management strategy for its empirical management in Sub-Saharan Africa is the dominance of other opportunistic pathogens. *Pneumocystis jiroveci,* which is an uncommon cause of LRTI in HIV-uninfected children, except perhaps those that are malnourished or who have other immuno-suppressive underlying illness (Hughes et al. 1974; Pifer et al. 1978), is commonly (10 to 45 percent of cases) identi-fied among African HIV-infected children with LRTI (Graham et al. 2000; Madhi et al. 2002). Although PCP is prevalent in various age groups according to one study in South Africa (Madhi et al. 2002), both the burden of the dis-ease and its poor outcome have consistently been found to be greatest among children less than six months of age.

A further recent observation has been the underrecog-nized importance of *Mycobacterium tuberculosis* as a cause of acute LRTI. Three separate studies from South Africa and Malawi consistently reported that *M. tuberculosis* was cul-tured from 8 percent of children with acute pneumonia (Graham et al. 2000; Madhi, Petersen, Madhi, Khoolsal, et al. 2000; Zar et al. 2001). This is even more alarming consider-ing that most of these studies were performed among children who were mainly investigated for tuberculosis by gastric washing or induced sputum samples—modalities that have a sensitivity of only 25 to 40 percent for diagnos-ing pulmonary tuberculosis. Consequently, it can be postu-lated that as many as three times more children than diagnosed by positive *M. tuberculosis* culture have acute pneumonia caused by this pathogen. Further investigation of these observations are required and, if verified, would have profound implications for the clinical algorithms used in diagnosing pulmonary tuberculosis as well as the man-agement strategies for treating LRTI in children.

THE IMPACT OF WHO MANAGEMENT STRATEGY

Following the realization that LRTI is a major contributor to childhood mortality, the WHO developed a strategy aimed at allowing primary health workers to manage LRTI speedily and effectively. The strategy, which subsequently has been incorporated into the integrated management of childhood illness (IMCI) program, is based on the premises that the majority of severe LRTI in developing countries is due to bacteria, particularly *S. pneumoniae* and *H. influenzae,* and that proper management of the disease needs to include consideration of the scarcity of health care facilities in those countries, which also coincidentally happen to be the most burdened by LRTI. A meta-analysis of this strategy has shown that it has been most effective when implemented in those countries where the infant mortality rate was greater than 100 per 1,000 live births (Sazawal and Black 2003). The meta-analysis found that the WHO LRTI case-management strategy reduced LRTI mortality by 42 percent (95 percent CI, 22–57 percent), 36 percent (95 percent CI, 20–48 per-cent), and 36 percent (95 percent CI, 20–49 percent) among neonates, infants between one and twelve months of age, and children one to four years of age, respectively (Sazawal and Black 2003). The WHO LRTI management strategy has more recently also been evaluated in a program in Malawi (Enarson and Pio 2003; Pio and Enarson 2003). The infant mortality rate in the study area prior to the intervention was 138 per 1,000, and approximately 20 percent of preg-nant women were HIV infected, resulting in approximately 4.5 percent of the birth cohort being HIV infected. Implementation of a strategy aimed at the training of dis-trict health care workers was associated with a 52 percent reduction in the LRTI mortality if the child survived beyond 24 hours of having presented at a health care facility. There was, however, only a modest nonsignificant reduction (15 percent, $P > 0.05$) in the deaths that occurred within 24 hours of attention at a health care center. Overall, the case-fatality rate for LRTI decreased from 18 percent at the time of the start of the study to 8 percent 26 months later. These reductions were observed within two years of having implemented the training of health care workers in the management of LRTI in accordance with the WHO/IMCI strategy as well as ensuring adequate access to essential drugs. The overall success of treating LRTI also improved from 55 percent at the time of the start of the program in 1999 to 82 percent 26 months later. These results, from one of the poorest nations on earth, show that standard inpa-tient case management of severe and very severe pneumonia by trained staff with a regular supply of antibiotics produced a striking impact on the number of deaths occurring after 24 hours of hospital admission, even in the adverse conditions of Malawi, where the prevalence of HIV infection is high, malnutrition is rife, the level of maternal literacy is low, and an efficient transport system from peripheral to district hospitals is lacking.

Considering the numerous challenges to expand and maintain health care provision in resource-poor countries, prevention rather than treatment of LRTI assumes even greater importance. Although some of the risk factors discussed earlier can be addressed only by a general improvement of socioeconomic conditions in these countries, a potentially more immediate measure would be vaccination. That immunization may affect the incidence of LRTI-associated mortality is probably best indicated by the success of the measles vaccine in reducing LRTI-associated deaths in Nigeria (Oyejide and Osinusi 1990). In the Nigerian study, the under-five mortality rate due to LRTI was twofold less common among children who had been immunized with measles vaccine than among children who had not received measles vaccine.

THE IMPACT OF HIB CONJUGATE VACCINES IN PREVENTING LRTI

The potential of further preventing LRTI through vaccination was shown in The Gambia during the course of evaluating the efficacy of a Hib conjugate vaccine among infants (Mulholland et al. 1997). In addition to reducing invasive Hib disease, including Hib meningitis, the vaccine was also shown to reduce the incidence of radiologically confirmed pneumonia by 21 percent (reduction of 1.3 cases per 1,000 children). The overall reduction in clinically diagnosed pneumonia was, however, more modest, with a nonsignificant reduction of 4.4 percent (95 percent CI, -5 to 12.9), although the study was not statistically powered to measure such small differences against clinically diagnosed LRTI. Interestingly, the incidence rate of clinically diagnosed LRTI requiring hospitalization in The Gambian study was only 3.6 per 1,000 children among the placebo group.

The findings from The Gambia were subsequently corroborated by an effectiveness study in Chile, where a similar reduction in radiologically (21 percent) and clinically diagnosed (5 percent) pneumonia was observed (Levine et al. 1999). The Hib conjugate vaccine was also found to prevent 2.5 cases of hospitalization for LRTI per 1,000 child-years of

observation. Although the effectiveness of the Hib conjugate vaccine against pneumonia has not been evaluated among HIV-infected children, data from South Africa suggest that the vaccine is less effective among HIV-infected than HIV-uninfected children, reducing invasive disease by 54 percent and 91 percent, respectively (Madhi et al. 2005). Consequently, it can be extrapolated that the Hib conjugate vaccine may also be less effective in preventing nonbacteremic pneumonia among HIV-infected children than HIV-uninfected children.

In The Gambia, prior to the introduction of the Hib conjugate vaccine, *H. influenzae* was identified as the second most important cause of bacterial pneumonia, with 75 percent of the isolates being of type b. The importance of *H. influenzae* is further highlighted by lung aspirate studies in children with pneumonia who did not receive antibiotics. Here, Hib accounted for an average of 27 percent (range of 14 to 45 percent) of all bacterial isolates. Indeed *H. influenzae* has been shown to be as common as *S. pneumoniae* (average of 27 percent; range of 12 to 88 percent) as a cause of pneumonia in some studies (Berman and McIntosh 1985). The incidence of bacteremic Hib pneumonia in children less than five years of age ranged between 1 and 7 per 100,000 children in developed countries, such as Finland and Israel (Dagan et al. 1998; Takala et al. 1989), whereas it was estimated to be 370 per 100,000 in developing countries if nonbacteremic cases were included (Peltola 2000). Prior to the introduction of the Hib conjugate vaccine in The Gambia, it was estimated that Hib resulted in a pneumonia-specific mortality rate of 40 per 100,000 in children zero to four years old (Greenwood 1992).

Despite Hib conjugate vaccines being available since the late 1980s, the only Sub-Saharan African country using its own resources to introduce the Hib conjugate vaccine into its routine childhood immunization program since June 1999 was, until very recently, South Africa. The vaccine has been introduced into other Sub-Saharan African countries through donor support from the Global Alliance for Vaccines and Immunisation (GAVI). GAVI has committed itself to financially supporting the introduction of the Hib conjugate vaccine into countries that have a gross domestic product of less than US$2,000 per capita for a period of five years, following which the governments of those countries would be expected to assume the responsibility of continuing to finance the use of the Hib conjugate vaccine. Whether these programs are sustainable is currently being debated. Even in an African country with relatively good resources, such as South Africa, the modest price of the vaccine (approximately US$2 per dose) has almost quadrupled the cost of vaccine procurement for the expanded program of immunization, and its continued use is under debate by policy makers. The cost of the full primary series of vaccines administered during the initial four months of life prior to the introduction of the Hib conjugate vaccine was approximately US$1.5.

THE IMPACT OF *S. PNEUMONIAE* CONJUGATE VACCINES IN PREVENTING PNEUMONIA IN CHILDREN

Despite *S. pneumoniae* having first been isolated in the 1880s and having been recognized as the leading cause of pneumonia among children, a successful vaccine aimed at preventing pneumococcal pneumonia has remained elusive until 2000 (Black et al. 2002; Klugman et al. 2003). Although Riley and colleagues (1986) showed a benefit for a pneumococcal polysaccharide vaccine in reducing childhood mortality in Papua New Guinea, other studies failed to show any benefit for the use of this vaccine, particularly among children less than 18 months of age (Broome and Breiman 1991). Following the success of the Hib conjugate vaccine, the same technology was used to produce a pneumococcal serotype-specific polysaccharide-protein conjugate vaccine. Those serotypes that were recognized as causing the majority of invasive disease among children were selected for inclusion into the vaccine. The first and currently the only licensed such vaccine is one that includes polysaccharide from seven of the pneumococcal serotypes (Prevenar), based on those serotypes that were most prevalent as a cause of invasive pneumococcal disease (IPD) among children in the United States (Zangwill et al. 1996). Inclusion of these seven serotypes was estimated to have the potential of preventing 90 percent of IPD among children in the United States (Zangwill et al. 1996). The vaccine was subsequently proved to be highly efficacious among those children and was associated with the reduction of vaccine-serotype-specific invasive disease in fully vaccinated children of 97.4 percent (95 percent CI, 82.7–99.9), with an overall reduction of invasive pneumococcal disease of 89.1 percent (95 percent CI, 73.7–95.8) (Black et al. 2000). More important, however, the vaccine was shown to reduce pneumonia associated with any chest radiograph infiltrate by 20.5 percent (95 percent CI, 4.4–34.0) and any clinically diagnosed pneumonia by 4.3 percent (95 percent CI, −3.5–11.5 percent) (Black et al. 2002). The incidence rate of pneumonia,

mainly ambulant cases, in the control group in the latter study was 55.9 per 1,000 person-years. The reduction in pneumonia confirmed by chest radiograph was striking insofar as previous epidemiological studies have shown that between 25 and 35 percent of cases of pneumonia in children are due to *S. pneumoniae* (Heiskanen-Kosma et al. 1998; Wubbel et al. 1999), indicating that the vaccine is highly efficacious even for this end point for which there was no microbiologic evaluation.

A different formulation of the vaccine that included two more serotypes than those included in Prevenar was subsequently evaluated among children in South Africa and The Gambia. These additional serotypes—serotypes 1 and 5—account for about 15 percent of IPD in Africa (Hausdorff, Siber, and Paradiso 2001; Madhi, Petersen, Madhi, Wasas, et al. 2000). In regard to the serotype-specific vaccine efficacy against IPD as well as radiologically confirmed pneumonia among HIV-uninfected children, the results from the South African study were strikingly similar to the findings in children from the United States. Among South African children, the nonavalent pneumococcal conjugate vaccine was shown to reduce culture-confirmed IPD by 83 percent and radiologically confirmed pneumonia, irrespective of microbiological diagnosis, by 20 percent (Klugman et al. 2003). Impressively, the vaccine was also shown to reduce IPD by 65 percent among HIV-infected children; however, there was no significant reduction in first-episode, radiologically confirmed pneumonia among these children (13 percent, 95 percent CI, −7–29) (Klugman et al. 2003). Further analysis of this study, however, indicated that when considering any LRTI irrespective of the chest radiograph features, the vaccine reduced LRTI by 15 percent (95 percent CI, 6–24) among HIV-infected children. This reduction in LRTI translated into a reduction of 25.7 cases of LRTI per 1,000 child-years, compared with a case reduction of 2.7 cases per 1,000 child-years in HIV-uninfected children (efficacy 17 percent; 95 percent CI, 7–26) (Madhi et al. 2005). Interestingly, the reductions in radiologically confirmed alveolar consolidation–associated LRTI were 1 and 9 per 1,000 child-years in HIV-uninfected and HIV-infected children, respectively (Madhi et al. 2005). These data suggest that the sensitivity of radiologically diagnosed pneumonia, based on WHO criteria, detected only about one-third of the cases of pneumococcal pneumonia that were prevented by vaccination. Studies that aim to define the burden of pneumonia preventable by the pneumococcal conjugate vaccine among children in other countries of Sub-Saharan Africa need to take these factors into consideration when determining the tools to be used in defining LRTI, including radiologically confirmed LRTI. Significantly, the data from the South African study included only children who required hospitalization for their episode of LRTI. Considering that only 7 to 13 percent of children with LRTI may have been hospitalized, the total burden of LRTI that may be prevented through vaccination may be much greater, especially considering that the spectrum of pathogens that cause LRTI requiring hospitalization were found to be similar to those that caused LRTI that did not require hospitalization (Selwyn 1990).

The nonavalent pneumococcal conjugate vaccine also reduced invasive pneumococcal disease (77 percent; 95 percent CI, 51–90) and radiologically confirmed pneumonia (37 percent; 95 percent CI, 25–48) in The Gambia, which is much less developed than South Africa. Impressively, in addition to a reduction in cases of pneumonia of 16 per 1,000 child-years among vaccinees in The Gambia, the nonavalent pneumococcal conjugate vaccine was also found to reduce all-cause hospitalization by 15 percent (95 percent CI, 7–21) and all-cause mortality by 16 percent (95 percent CI, 3–28) (Cutts et al. 2005). These data clearly indicate the urgency attendant on the introduction of this new vaccine into developing countries. Modification of the currently licensed product, so as to include pneumococcal serotypes that are important in Africa serotypes (1 and 5) but which are not included in the current seven-valent formulation of the vaccine, would be required to optimize the benefits of the introduction of such a vaccine into Sub-Saharan Africa.

A challenge for other Sub-Saharan Africa countries in regard to defining the potential benefit of pneumococcal conjugate vaccination would, however, include the need to define the spectrum of serotypes that cause disease among children elsewhere, as geographic variation in serotypes that cause IPD have been described even within continents (Hausdorff, Siber, and Paradiso 2001). Hence, the overall proportion of IPD and possibly pneumonia that may be prevented through vaccination may differ between geographic regions, depending on the prevalent serotypes.

Despite these positive findings, and the theoretical benefits of the pneumococcal conjugate vaccine, the greatest impending limiting factor to the introduction of the vaccine into Sub-Saharan Africa is the cost of the vaccine. Currently the vaccine is priced at $48 for the public sector in the United States. Considering the costs of the vaccine and that there are no other competing pneumococcal conjugate vaccines that are likely to be licensed any time soon, unless there is external funding support or major price tiering to assist in introducing the vaccine, it is likely to lag even beyond the 20 years that it has taken for the Hib conjugate vaccine to be introduced into Sub-Saharan Africa. Provisional data from the South African study indicate that the vaccine would be potentially cost-effective if it cost approximately US$4 per dose, based on health expenditure costs in South Africa (Ginsberg et al. unpublished data). Considering that health care expenditure in other Sub-Saharan Africa countries is much lower than in South Africa, the price at which the vaccine may be cost-effective would possibly be even lower.

OTHER POTENTIAL INTERVENTION STRATEGIES IN REDUCING THE BURDEN OF LRTI

The burden of LRTI may be reduced by as much as 45 percent in countries of Sub-Saharan Africa (Madhi, Petersen, Madhi, Wasas, et al. 2000) if effective strategies targeted at preventing HIV transmission from mother to children are implemented. Although a number of proven strategies could reduce the vertical transmission of HIV to between 2 and 13 percent, lack of infrastructure in Sub-Saharan Africa results in less than 5 percent of HIV-infected women being able to access health care to allow these interventions to be implemented (United Nations General Assembly Special Session on HIV/AIDS, unpublished data). Nevertheless, programs aimed at the prevention of the vertical transmission of HIV need to be considered a priority in reducing the overall burden of LRTI among children in Sub-Saharan Africa.

Another priority for those children who are infected with HIV is the introduction of effective strategies aimed at reducing the burden of PCP, especially considering that *P. jiroveci* has been found to be the etiological agent in as many as 15 to 45 percent of African HIV-infected children with LRTI. Although no randomized trial has evaluated the efficacy of trimethoprim-sulfamethoxazole (TMP-SMX) in preventing PCP among children, this strategy has had profound benefits when it has been implemented in developed countries as well as in such developing countries as Thailand (Chokephaibulkit et al. 2000; Simonds et al. 1995). Although recommended by the WHO and UNAIDS, data from South Africa suggest that there may be structural problems with implementing an effective TMP-SMX prophylaxis even in areas with relatively good resources, such as South Africa (Madhi et al. 2002). Of further importance regarding the widespread use of TMP-SMX is its potential to predispose to developing strains of pneumococcus that are resistant to it as well as to other classes of antibiotics (Madhi, Petersen, Madhi, Wasas, et al. 2000). Such resistance would possibly compromise the WHO management strategy in Sub-Saharan Africa, where in many areas, TMP-SMX remains the mainstay of therapy for the treatment of LRTI. It is likely that the emergence of resistant strains of pneumococcus, coupled with further dissemination of resistant strains, may render TMP-SMX obsolete in the empirical management of LRTI in Sub-Saharan Africa.

The importance of TMP-SMX in reducing morbidity and mortality in African HIV-infected children has recently been highlighted by a study in Malawi. Chintu and colleagues (2004) showed that TMP-SMX prophylaxis reduced mortality in African HIV-infected children, the majority of whom were symptomatic for AIDS, by 43 percent (hazards ratio 0.57; 95 percent CI, 0.43–0.77).

OTHER POTENTIAL WAYS TO PREVENT LRTI

Despite all the promise that the bacterial conjugate vaccines hold in preventing LRTI, it is sobering that the total burden of LRTI reduced by these vaccines is relatively small, albeit important, given the overall magnitude of the burden of LRTI in Sub-Saharan Africa. In The Gambia, the Hib conjugate vaccine prevented only 1.3 cases of hospitalization related to LRTI for every 35.1 cases (about 4 percent) that occurred per 1,000 children enrolled in the study (Mulholland et al. 1997). The nonavalent pneumococcal conjugate vaccine in The Gambia reduced the overall rate of pneumonia by 18 cases per 1,000 child-years, with an incidence rate of 249 per 1,000 child-years among the placebo group (Cutts et al. 2005). The case reduction among South African HIV-uninfected children, including only hospitalized children, was 2.7 per 1,000 child-years with the incidence in the placebo group being 15.7 cases of LRTI per 1,000 child-years (Madhi et al. 2005). These data indicate that although the most severe causes of pneumonia may have been prevented with modest to good success, there remains a large burden of LRTI that even the expensive new generation of vaccines is not able to prevent. Efforts aimed at developing vaccines against respiratory syncytial virus holds the promise that greater inroads may be made in reducing the overall LRTI morbidity even in Sub-Saharan Africa countries. Furthermore, there is a need to continue support for developing more effective vaccines against *M. tuberculosis* that are effective in preventing not only

disseminated tuberculosis but also pulmonary tuberculosis, which may be responsible for 25 percent of LRTI cases requiring hospitalization.

CONCLUSION

Although the LRTI management strategies of the WHO have the potential of reducing the burden of death from LRTI among countries where under-five mortality is greater than 100 per 1,000 live births, further advances in reducing childhood morbidity and possibly mortality depend on the effective use of bacterial conjugate vaccines in those countries that require them, but where, unjustly for the children, they are least affordable. Furthermore, the reversal of gains in reducing childhood mortality currently being experienced in Sub-Saharan Africa, largely a result of the HIV epidemic, has been associated with almost a doubling of the burden of LRTI in those countries that are heavily burdened by the epidemic. An effective approach to reducing LRTI-associated childhood mortality in Sub-Saharan Africa requires a concerted effort to prevent the vertical transmission of HIV infection, timely and effective rollout of bacterial conjugate vaccines, as well as addressing predominantly poverty-linked, predisposing factors that heighten the risk of children to develop severe and often fatal LRTI.

REFERENCES

Adegbola, R. A., A. G. Falade, B. E. Sam, M. Aidoo, I. Baldeh, D. Hazlett, H. Whittle, B. M. Greenwood, and E. K. Mulholland. 1994. "The Etiology of Pneumonia in Malnourished and Well-Nourished Gambian Children." *Pediatric Infectious Disease Journal* 13: 975–82.

Afari, E. A. 1991. "Acute Respiratory Infections in Children under Five in Two Rural Communities in Southern Ghana." *Japanese Journal of Tropical Medicine and Hygiene* 19: 275–80.

Anderson, H. R. 1978. "Respiratory Abnormalities in Papua New Guinea Children: The Effects of Locality and Domestic Wood Smoke Pollution." *International Journal of Epidemiology* 7: 63–72.

Asamoah-Odel, E., G. Asiimwe-Okiror, J. M. Garcia Calleja, and J. T. Boerma. 2003. "Recent Trends in HIV Prevalence among Pregnant Women in Sub-Saharan Africa." *AIDScience* 3 (19). http://aidscience.org/Articles/AIDScience037.asp.

Bale, J. R. 1990. "Creation of a Research Program to Determine the Etiology and Epidemiology of Acute Respiratory Tract Infection among Children in Developing Countries." *Reviews of Infectious Diseases* 12 (Suppl. 8): S861–66.

Berman, S., and K. McIntosh. 1985. "Selective Primary Health Care: Strategies for Control of Disease in the Developing World. Part 21. Acute Respiratory Infections." *Reviews of Infectious Diseases* 7: 674–91.

Black, R. E., K. H. Brown, S. Becker, and M. Yunus. 1982. "Longitudinal Studies of Infectious Diseases and Physical Growth of Children in Rural Bangladesh. I. Patterns of Morbidity." *American Journal of Epidemiology* 115: 305–14.

Black, S., H. Shinefield, B. Fireman, E. Lewis, P. Ray, J. R. Hansen, L. Elvin, et al. 2000. "Efficacy, Safety and Immunogenicity of Heptavalent Pneumococcal Conjugate Vaccine in Children." Northern California Kaiser Permanente Vaccine Study Center Group. *Pediatric Infectious Disease Journal* 19: 187–95.

Black, S. B., H. R. Shinefield, S. Ling, J. Hansen, B. Fireman, D. Spring, J. Noyes, et al. 2002. Effectiveness of Heptavalent Pneumococcal Conjugate Vaccine in Children Younger than Five Years of Age for Prevention of Pneumonia. *Pediatric Infectious Disease Journal* 21: 810–15.

Broome, C. V., and R. F. Breiman. 1991. "Pneumococcal Vaccine—Past, Present, and Future." *New England Journal of Medicine* 325: 1506–8.

Campbell, H., P. Byass, A. C. Lamont, I. M. Forgie, K. P. O'Neill, N. Lloyd-Evans, and B. M. Greenwood. 1989. "Assessment of Clinical Criteria for Identification of Severe Acute Lower Respiratory Tract Infections in Children." *Lancet* 1: 297–99.

Cherian, T., K. E. Mulholland, J. B. Carlin, H. Ostensen, R. Amin, M. de Campo, D. Greenberg, et al. 2005. "Standardised Interpretation of Paediatric Chest Radiographs for the Diagnosis of Pneumonia in Epidemiological Studies." *Bulletin of the World Health Organization* 83: 353–59.

Chintu, C., G. J. Bhat, A. S. Walker, V. Mulenga, F. Sinyinza, K. Lishimpi, L. Farrelly, et al. 2004. "Co-Trimoxazole as Prophylaxis against Opportunistic Infections in HIV-Infected Zambian Children (CHAP): A Double-Blind Randomised Placebo-Controlled Trial." *Lancet* 364: 1865–71.

Chintu, C., C. Luo, G. Bhat, H. L. DuPont, P. Mwansa-Salamu, M. Kabika, A. Zumla, et al. 1995. "Impact of the Human Immunodeficiency Virus Type-1 on Common Pediatric Illnesses in Zambia." *Journal of Tropical Pediatrics* 41: 348–53.

Chokephaibulkit, K., R. Chuachoowong, T. Chotpitayasunondh, S. Chearskul, N. Vanprapar, N. Waranawat, P. Mock, N. Shaffer, and R. J. Simonds. 2000. "Evaluating a New Strategy for Prophylaxis to Prevent *Pneumocystis carinii* Pneumonia in HIV-Exposed Infants in Thailand." Bangkok Collaborative Perinatal HIV Transmission Study Group. *AIDS* 14: 1563–69.

Cutts, F. T., S. M. Zaman, G. Enwere, S. Jaffar, O. S. Levine, J. B. Okoko, C. Oluwalana, et al. 2005. "Efficacy of Nine-Valent Pneumococcal Conjugate Vaccine Against Pneumonia and Invasive Pneumococcal Disease in The Gambia: Randomised, Double-Blind, Placebo-Controlled Trial." *Lancet* 365: 1139–36.

Dagan, R., D. Fraser, Z. Greif, N. Keller, M. Kaufstein, G. Shazberg, and M. Schlesinger. 1998. "A Nationwide Prospective Surveillance Study in Israel to Document Pediatric Invasive Infections, with an Emphasis on *Haemophilus influenzae* Type B Infections." Israeli Pediatric Bacteremia and Meningitis Group. *Pediatric Infectious Disease Journal* 17: S198–203.

Dankner, W. M., J. C. Lindsey, and M. J. Levin. 2001. "Correlates of Opportunistic Infections in Children Infected with the Human Immunodeficiency Virus Managed before Highly Active Antiretroviral Therapy." *Pediatric Infectious Disease Journal* 20: 40–48.

de Francisco, A., J. Morris, A. J. Hall, J. R. Armstrong Schellenberg, and B. M. Greenwood. 1993. "Risk Factors for Mortality from Acute Lower Respiratory Tract Infections in Young Gambian Children." *International Journal of Epidemiology* 22: 1174–82.

Demers, A.-M., P. Morency, F. Mberyo-Yaah, S. Jaffar, C. Blais, P. Somse, G. Bobossi, and J. Pepin. 2000. "Risk Factors for Mortality among Children Hospitalized Because of Acute Respiratory Infections in Bangui, Central African Republic." *Pediatric Infectious Disease Journal* 19: 424–32.

Enarson, P., and A. Pio. 2003. "Improving Pediatric Lung Health in Malawi: Lessons Learned and Next Steps." Paper presented at the American Thoracic Society (ATS) Conference, Seattle, May 16–21.

Fantahun, M. V. 1998. "Patterns of Childhood Mortality in Three Districts of North Gondar Administrative Zone. A Community Based Study Using the Verbal Autopsy Method." *Ethiopian Medical Journal* 36: 71–81.

Forgie, I. M., K. P. O'Neill, N. Lloyd-Evans, M. Leinonen, H. Campbell, H. C. Whittle, and B. M. Greenwood. 1991a. "Etiology of Acute Lower Respiratory Tract Infections in Gambian Children: I. Acute Lower Respiratory Tract Infections in Infants Presenting at the Hospital." *Pediatric Infectious Disease Journal* 10: 33–41.

———. 1991b. "Etiology of Acute Lower Respiratory Tract Infections in Gambian Children: II. Acute Lower Respiratory Tract Infection in Children Ages One to Nine Years Presenting at the Hospital." *Pediatric Infectious Disease Journal* 10: 42–47.

Foy, H. M., M. K. Cooney, A. J. Maletzky, and J. T. Grayston. 1973. "Incidence and Etiology of Pneumonia, Croup and Bronchiolitis in Preschool Children Belonging to a Prepaid Medical Care Group over a Four-Year Period." *American Journal of Epidemiology* 97: 80–92.

Garcia de Olarte, D., H. Trujillo, A. Uribe, and N. Agudelo. 1971. "Lung Puncture-Aspiration as a Bacteriologic Diagnostic Procedure in Acute Pneumonias of Infants and Children." *Clinical Pediatrics (Phila)* 10: 346–50.

George, S. A., S. S. Bai, and A. Cherian. 1996. "Blood versus Lung Aspirate Culture in Pneumonia." *Indian Pediatrics* 33: 871–72.

Graham, S. M., E. I. Mtitimila, H. S. Kamanga, A. L. Walsh, C. A. Hart, and M. E. Molyneux. 2000. "Clinical Presentation and Outcome of *Pneumocystis carinii* Pneumonia in Malawian Children." *Lancet* 355: 369–73.

Greenwood, B. 1992. "Epidemiology of Acute Lower Respiratory Tract Infections, Especially Those Due to *Haemophilus influenzae* Type B, in The Gambia, West Africa." *Journal of Infectious Diseases* 165 (Suppl. 1): S26–28.

Greenwood, B. M., A. M. Greenwood, A. K. Bradley, S. Tulloch, R. Hayes, and F. S. Oldfield. 1987. "Deaths in Infancy and Early Childhood in a Well-Vaccinated, Rural, West African Population." *Annals of Tropical Paediatrics* 7: 91–99.

Hausdorff, W. P., G. Siber, and P. R. Paradiso. 2001. "Geographical Differences in Invasive Pneumococcal Disease Rates and Serotype Frequency in Young Children." *Lancet* 357: 950–52.

Heiskanen-Kosma, T., M. Korppi, C. Jokinen, S. Kurki, L. Heiskanen, H. Juvonen, S. Kallinen, et al. 1998. "Etiology of Childhood Pneumonia: Serologic Results of a Prospective, Population-Based Study." *Pediatric Infectious Disease Journal* 17: 986–91.

Hughes, W. T., R. A. Price, F. Sisko, W. S. Havron, A. G. Kafatos, M. Schonland, and P. M. Smythe. 1974. "Protein-Calorie Malnutrition. A Host Determinant for *Pneumocystis carinii* Infection." *American Journal of Diseases of Children* 128: 44–52.

Ikeogu, M. O. 1998. "Acute Pneumonia in Zimbabwe: Bacterial Isolates by Lung Aspiration." *Archives of Disease in Childhood* 63: 1266–67.

Klugman, K. P., S. A. Madhi, R. E. Huebner, R. Kohberger, N. Mbelle, N. Pierce, and Vaccine Trialist Group. 2003. "Prevention of Pneumonia and Invasive Pneumococcal Disease by a 9-Valent Pneumococcal Conjugate Vaccine: Efficacy in Both HIV-Infected and Uninfected Children." *New England Journal of Medicine* 349: 1341–48.

Langston, C., E. R. Cooper, J. Goldfarb, K. A. Easley, S. Husak, S. Sunkle, T. J. Starc, et al. 2001. "Human Immunodeficiency Virus-Related Mortality in Infants and Children: Data from the Pediatric Pulmonary and Cardiovascular Complications of Vertically Transmitted HIV (P(2)C(2)) Study." *Pediatrics* 107: 328–38.

Leowski, J. 1986. "Mortality from Acute Respiratory Infections in Children under 5 Years of Age: Global Estimates." *World Health Statistics Quarterly* 39: 138–44.

Levine, O. S., R. Lagos, A. Munoz, J. Villaroel, A. M. Alvarez, P. Abrego, and M. M. Levine. 1999. "Defining the Burden of Pneumonia in Children Preventable by Vaccination against *Haemophilus influenzae* Type B." *Pediatric Infectious Disease Journal* 18: 1060–64.

Madhi, S. A., C. Cutland, K. Ismail, C. O'Reilly, A. Mancha, and K. P. Klugman. 2002. "Ineffectiveness of Trimethoprim-Sulfamethoxazole Prophylaxis and Importance of Concurrent Bacterial and Respiratory Viral Co-Infections among Human Immunodeficiency Virus Type-1 Infected African Children Hospitalized with *Pneumocystis carinii* Pneumonia." *Clinical Infectious Diseases* 35: 1120–26.

Madhi, S. A., C. Cutland, L. Kuwanda, and K. P. Klugman. 2005. "The Impact of a 9-Valent Pneumococcal Conjugate Vaccine on the Public Health Burden of Pneumonia in HIV Infected and Uninfected Children." *Clinical Infectious Diseases* 40: 1511–18.

Madhi, S. A., K. P. Klugman, and the Pneumococcal Vaccine Trialist Group. 2004. "A Role for *Streptococcus pneumoniae* in Virus-Associated Pneumonia." *Nature Medicine* 10: 811–13.

Madhi, S. A., H. Ludewick, Y. Abed, K. P. Klugman, and G. Boivin. 2003. "Human Metapneumovirus Associated Lower Respiratory Tract Infections among Hospitalized HIV-1 Infected and HIV-1 Uninfected African Infants." *Clinical Infectious Diseases* 37: 1705–10.

Madhi, S. A., K. Petersen, A. Madhi, M. Khoolsal, and K. P. Klugman. 2000. "Burden of Disease and Drug Resistance of Bacteria in HIV Infected Children with Severe Lower Respiratory Tract Infections." *Clinical Infectious Diseases* 31: 170–76.

Madhi, S. A., K. Petersen, A. Madhi, A. Wasas, and K. P. Klugman. 2000. "Impact of Human Immunodeficiency Virus Type-1 on the Disease Spectrum of *Streptococcus pneumoniae* in South African Children." *Pediatric Infectious Disease Journal* 19: 1141–47.

Madhi, S. A., B. Schoub, K. Simmank, N. Blackburn, and K. P. Klugman. 2000. "Increased Burden of Respiratory Virus Associated Severe Lower Respiratory Tract Infections in HIV-1 Infected Children." *Journal of Pediatrics* 137: 78–84.

Mimica, I., E. Donoso, J. E. Howard, and G. W. Ledermann. 1971. "Lung Puncture in the Etiological Diagnosis of Pneumonia. A Study of 543 Infants and Children." *American Journal of Diseases of Children* 122: 278–82.

Mofenson, L. M., R. Yogev, J. Korelitz, J. Bethel, K. Krasinski, J. Moye Jr., R. Nugent, and J. G. Rigau-Perez. 1998. "Characteristics of Acute Pneumonia in Human Immunodeficiency Virus-Infected Children and Association with Long Term Mortality Risk." National Institute of Child Health and Human Development Intravenous Immunoglobulin Clinical Trial Study Group. *Pediatric Infectious Disease Journal* 17: 872–80.

Mtango, F. D., and D. Neuvians. 1986. "Acute Respiratory Infections in Children under Five Years." Control project in Bagamoyo District, Tanzania. *Transactions of the Royal Society of Tropical Medicine and Hygiene* 80: 851–58.

Mulholland, K., S. Hilton, R. Adegbola, S. Usen, A. Oparaugo, C. Omosigho, M. Weber, et al. 1997. "Randomised Trial of *Haemophilus influenzae* Type-B Tetanus Protein Conjugate Vaccine." *Lancet* 349: 1191–97.

Murphy, T. F., F. W. Henderson, W. A. Clyde Jr., A. M. Collier, and F. W. Denny. 1981. "Pneumonia: An Eleven-Year Study in a Pediatric Practice." *American Journal of Epidemiology* 113: 12–21.

Nathoo, K. J., S. Chigonde, M. Nhembe, M. H. Ali, and P. R. Mason. 1996. "Community-Acquired Bacteremia in Human Immunodeficiency Virus-Infected Children in Harare, Zimbabwe." *Pediatric Infectious Disease Journal* 15: 1092–97.

O'Dempsey, T. J., T. F. McArdle, N. Lloyd-Evans, I. Baldeh, B. E. Laurence, O. Secka, and B. M. Greenwood. 1994. "Importance of Enteric Bacteria as a Cause of Pneumonia, Meningitis and Septicemia among Children in a Rural Community in The Gambia, West Africa." *Pediatric Infectious Disease Journal* 13: 122–28.

Oyejide, C. O., and K. Osinusi. 1990. "Acute Respiratory Tract Infections in Children in Idikan Community, Ibadan, Nigeria: Severity, Risk Factors and Frequency of Occurrence." *Reviews of Infectious Diseases* 12 (Suppl. 8): S1042–46.

Peltola, H. 2000. "Worldwide *Haemophilus influenzae* Type B Disease at the Beginning of the 21st Century: Global Analysis of the Disease Burden 25 Years after the Use of the Polysaccharide Vaccine and a Decade after the Advent of Conjugates." *Clinical Microbiology Reviews* 13: 302–17.

Pifer, L. L., W. T. Hughes, S. Stagno, and D. Woods. 1978. "*Pneumocystis carinii* Infection: Evidence for High Prevalence in Normal and Immunosuppressed Children." *Pediatrics* 61: 35–41.

Pillay, K., M. Colvin, R. Williams, and H. M. Coovadia. 2001. "Impact of HIV-1 Infection in South Africa." *Archives of Disease in Childhood* 85: 50–51.

Pio, A., and P. Enarson. 2003. "Improving Child Lung Health: The Malawi Child Lung Health Project Sponsored by the Bill and Melinda Gates Foundation." Paper presented at the American Thoracic Society (ATS) Conference, Seattle, May 16–21.

Prakash, J., D. K. Agraval, K. N. Agarval, and A. K. Kulati. 1996. "Etiologic Diagnosis of Pneumonia in Under-Five Children." *Indian Pediatrics* 33: 329–31.

Prinsloo, J. G., and A. Cicoria. 1974. "Is Lung Puncture Aspiration a Harmless Procedure?" *South African Medical Journal* 48: 597–98.

Rapkin, R. H. 1975. "Bacteriologic and Clinical Findings in Acute Pneumonia of Childhood." *Clinical Pediatrics (Phila)* 14: 130–33.

Riley, I., E. Carrad, H. Gratten, M. Gratten, K. Lovuru, P. Phillips, D. Pratt, et al. 1983. "The Status of Research on Acute Respiratory Infections in Children in Papua New Guinea." *Pediatric Research* 17: 1041–43.

Riley, I. D., D. Lehmann, M. P. Alpers, T. F. Marshall, H. Gratten, and D. Smith. 1986. "Pneumococcal Vaccine Prevents Death from Acute Lower-Respiratory-Tract Infections in Papua New Guinean Children." *Lancet* 2: 877–81.

Rudan, I., L. Tomaskovic, C. Boschi-Pinto, and H. Campbell. 2004. "Global Estimate of the Incidence of Clinical Pneumonia among Children under Five Years of Age." *Bulletin of the World Health Organization* 82: 895–903.

———. Forthcoming. "Incidence of Acute Lower Respiratory Infections (ALRI) in Children under Five Years: II Estimates for WHO Regions." *Bulletin of the World Health Organization.*

Sazawal, S., and R. E. Black. 2003. "Pneumonia Case Management Trials Group Effect of Pneumonia Case Management on Mortality in Neonates, Infants, and Preschool Children: A Meta-Analysis of Community-Based Trials." *Lancet Infectious Diseases* 3: 547–56.

Selwyn, B. J. 1990. "The Epidemiology of Acute Respiratory Tract Infection in Young Children: Comparison of Findings from Several Developing Countries." Coordinated Data Group of BOSTID Researchers. *Reviews of Infectious Diseases* 12 (Suppl. 8): S870–88.

Silverman, M., D. Stratton, A. Diallo, and L. J. Egler. 1977. "Diagnosis of Acute Bacterial Pneumonia in Nigerian Children. Value of Needle Aspiration of Lung of Countercurrent Immunoelectrophoresis." *Archives of Disease in Childhood* 52: 925–31.

Simonds, R. J., M. L. Lindegren, P. Thomas, D. Hanson, B. Caldwell, G. Scott, and M. Rogers. 1995. "Prophylaxis against *Pneumocystis carinii* Pneumonia among Children with Perinatally Acquired Human Immunodeficiency Virus Infection in the United States." Pneumocystis carinii Pneumonia Prophylaxis Evaluation Working Group. *New England Journal of Medicine* 332: 786–90.

Sofoluwe, G. O. 1968. "Smoke Pollution in Dwellings of Infants with Bronchopneumonia." *Archives of Environmental Health* 16: 670–72.

Takala, A. K., J. Eskola, H. Peltola, and P. H. Makela. 1989. "Epidemiology of Invasive *Haemophilus influenzae* Type B Disease among Children in Finland before Vaccination with *Haemophilus influenzae* Type B Conjugate Vaccine." *Pediatric Infectious Disease Journal* 8: 297–302.

UNICEF (United Nations Children's Fund). 1996. *The State of the World's Children 1996. Statistical Tables.* Geneva: UNICEF.

van den Hoogen, B. G., J. C. de Jong, J. Groen, T. Kuiken, R. de Groot, R. A. Fouchier, and A. D. Osterhaus. 2001. "A Newly Discovered Human Pneumovirus Isolated from Young Children with Respiratory Tract Disease." *Nature Medicine* 7: 719–24.

Von Schirnding, Y. E. R., D. Yach, and M. Klein. 1991 "Acute Respiratory Tract Infections as an Important Cause of Childhood Deaths in South Africa." *South African Medical Journal* 80: 79–82.

Vuori-Holopainen, E., and H. Peltola. 2001. "Reappraisal of Lung Tap: Review of an Old Method for Better Etiologic Diagnosis of Childhood Pneumonia." *Clinical Infectious Diseases* 32: 715–26.

Vuori-Holopainen, E., E. Salo, H. Saxen, K. Hedman, T. Hyypia, R. Lahdenpera, M. Leinonen, E. Tarkka, M. Vaara, and H. Peltola. 2002. "Etiological Diagnosis of Childhood Pneumonia by Use of Transthoracic Needle Aspiration and Modern Microbiological Methods." *Clinical Infectious Diseases* 34: 583–90.

Wafula, E. M., F. E. Onyango, W. M. Mirza, W. M. Macharia, I. Wamola, J. O. Ndinya-Achola, R. Agwanda, R. N. Waigwa, and J. Musia. 1990. "Epidemiology of Acute Respiratory Tract Infections among Young Children in Kenya." *Reviews of Infectious Diseases* 12 (Suppl. 8): S1035–38.

Walker, N., B. Schwartlander, and J. Bryce. 2002. "Meeting International Goals in Child Survival and HIV/AIDS." *Lancet* 360: 284–89.

Wall, R. A., P. T. Corrah, D. C. Mabey, and B. M. Greenwood. 1986. "The Etiology of Lobar Pneumonia in The Gambia." *Bulletin of the World Health Organization* 64: 553–58.

WHO (World Health Organization). 1990. *Management of the Young Child with Acute Lower Respiratory Infection.* WHO Programme for the Control of Acute Respiratory Infections. Geneva: WHO.

Williams, B. G. 2002. "Estimates of World-Wide Distribution of Child Deaths from Acute Respiratory Tract Infections." *Lancet Infectious Diseases* 2: 25–32.

Wubbel, L., L. Muniz, A. Ahmed, M. Trujillo, C. Carubelli, C. McCoig, T. Abramo, M. Leinonen, and G. H. McCracken Jr. 1999. "Etiology and Treatment of Community-Acquired Pneumonia in Ambulatory Children." *Pediatric Infectious Disease Journal* 18: 98–104.

Zangwill, K. M., C. M. Vadheim, A. M. Vannier, L. S. Hemenway, D. P. Greenberg, and J. I. Ward. 1996. "Epidemiology of Invasive Pneumococcal Disease in Southern California: Implications for the Design and Conduct of a Pneumococcal Conjugate Vaccine Efficacy Trial." *Journal of Infectious Diseases* 174: 752–59.

Zar, H. J., D. Hanslo, E. Tannenbaum, M. Klein, A. Argent, B. Eley, J. Burgess, K. Magnus, E. D. Bateman, and G. Hussey. 2001. "Aetiology and Outcome of Pneumonia in Human Immunodeficiency Virus-Infected Children Hospitalized in South Africa." *Acta Paediatrica* 90: 119–25.

Zwi, K. J., J. M. Pettifor, and N. Soderlund. 1999. "Paediatric Hospital Admissions at a South African Urban Regional Hospital: The Impact of HIV, 1992–1997." *Annals of Tropical Paediatrics* 19: 135–42.

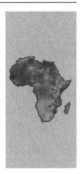

Chapter 12

Vaccine-Preventable Diseases

Mark A. Miller and John T. Sentz

Vaccines have been frequently cited as one of the most equitable low-cost, high-impact public health measures, saving millions of lives annually when programs are implemented on the national level. Over the last 40 years, the use of smallpox, measles, diphtheria, tetanus, pertussis, and poliomyelitis vaccines have eradicated smallpox and eliminated disease in those populations that have achieved and sustained programs with high implementation rates. Although there are numerous licensed vaccines that could potentially benefit the African population, only those routinely used and potential vaccines with broad application on the horizon are covered in this chapter.

HISTORY OF VACCINATION IN AFRICA

The eradication of smallpox was an outstanding display of concerted global action in a war against microbial invaders. The progress in expanding poliomyelitis and measles vaccination efforts and their elimination from many regions further demonstrates that vaccines are among the most powerful public health tools. National vaccination programs,

which grew out of the smallpox eradication initiative, have developed in many countries through the administrative, technical, and financial support of the United Nations Children's Fund (UNICEF), the World Health Organization (WHO), and many bilateral or multilateral partner agencies (figure 12.1) (WHO and UNICEF 1996). In its 1993 *World Development Report,* the World Bank classified vaccination as one of the most cost-effective public health interventions (World Bank 1993). In addition, vaccination programs have been cited as providing one of the most equitable of public health programs, providing protection to the entire population when successfully implemented.

The WHO created the Expanded Program on Immunization (EPI) in 1974 as a means to continue the great success that had been achieved earlier with the eradication of smallpox. At that time less than 5 percent of the world's children in the developing world were receiving immunizations. The six diseases chosen to be tackled under this new initiative were tuberculosis, diphtheria, tetanus, pertussis, polio, and measles. It was not until 1988 that the WHO recommended that yellow fever vaccine be added to the national immunization programs of those countries

Figure 12.1 Percentage of Target Population in Africa Vaccinated, by Vaccine Type, 1980–2002

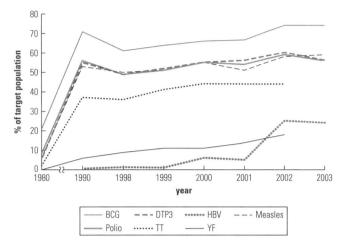

Source: WHO 2003.

Note: BCG = bacillus Calmette-Guérin; DTP3 = three doses of diphtheria, tetanus, pertussis vaccine; HBV = hepatitis B virus; TT = tetanus toxoid; and YF = yellow fever.

Table 12.1 WHO-Estimated Deaths and DALYs from Vaccine-Preventable Diseases, 2002
(thousands)

	Deaths		DALYs	
	Total	Africa[a]	Total	Africa[a]
EPI Vaccines				
Tuberculosis	1,566	348	34,736	9,266
Childhood-cluster diseases	1,124	527	41,480	18,995
Diphtheria	5	2	185	48
Tetanus	214	84	7,074	2,775
Pertussis	294	131	12,595	5,243
Poliomyelitis	1	0	151	15
Measles	611	311	21,475	10,915
EPI Plus Vaccines				
Hepatitis B				
Acute hepatitis B	103	20	2,170	582
Liver cancer	618	45	7,135	90
Cirrhosis of the liver	786	54	13,977	957
Meningitis	173	20	6,192	891
Lower respiratory infections	3,884	1,104	91,374	34,911
Otitis media	4	2	1,435	263

Source: WHO 2004.
a. WHO designated African countries.

with endemic disease (WHO and UNICEF 1996). Later, in 1992, the World Health Assembly recommended hepatitis B vaccination for all infants. Most recently the WHO has recommended that the *Haemophilus influenzae* type B (Hib) conjugate vaccines be implemented into national immunization programs unless epidemiological evidence exists of low disease burden, lack of benefit, or overwhelming obstacles to implementation (WHO 2006).

THE VACCINE-PREVENTABLE DISEASE BURDEN

The WHO-estimated disease burdens from vaccine-preventable diseases are shown for 2002 by incidence of death and disability-adjusted life years (DALYS) in table 12.1. As the WHO does not necessarily classify disease based on what may be prevented by a specific vaccine, the table includes those syndromes that may be partially mitigated by vaccines (for example, acute lower respiratory tract infection, meningitis, or conditions associated with hepatitis B infections).

As most vaccine-preventable diseases are underreported in many countries, estimates of disease burden are made by a variety of methodologies that account for the susceptible fraction of the population, as calculated from natural immunity from presumed historical infections, historical immunization coverage rates, and vaccine effectiveness. Disease burden estimates also integrate rates of infectivity, specific sequelae, and local case fatality. Life expectancies on

a national level can help to account for causes of competing mortality, allowing the assessment of health outcomes as deaths, years of life lost, or other measures (for example, DALYs). Estimates of disease burden have evolved over the years from simplistic models incorporating reported rates of disease and a reporting efficiency profile to the more complex Susceptible-Infected-Removed (SIR)–type models that can additionally account for local population-based coverage data and other deterministic data, such as socioeconomic factors and characteristics of the heterogeneity of populations throughout the region. Models are based on numerous assumptions, and their degree of accuracy is only as good as the data that support the many assumptions. Although disease burden is frequently indicated as point estimates, it is more appropriate to indicate the burden by a range of values to reflect uncertainty, sometimes by an order of magnitude or more for certain diseases.

Polio

Poliovirus is most often transmitted fecal-orally among persons living in unsanitary and crowded conditions. Acute infections are caused by any one of three serotypes of poliovirus that initially replicate in the gastrointestinal tract. Exposure to poliovirus predominantly results in asymptomatic infections. It has been estimated that 24 percent of infections result in minor illness characterized by a few days of varying symptoms, including fever, malaise, drowsiness, headache, nausea, vomiting, constipation, and sore throat (Gelfand et al. 1957). In fewer cases (4 percent), infection leads to nonparalytic polio or aseptic meningitis, which manifests as fever, vomiting, malaise, and sore throat; meningeal irritation occurs one to two days later, characterized by soreness and stiffness of the neck, back, limbs, and severe headache (Horstmann 1955). These symptoms can last up to 10 days, but recovery is usually rapid and complete. Paralytic polio, which affects less than 1 percent of those infected, is the most serious manifestation of the disease (Sabin 1951). This form of the disease presents initially as a minor fever with rapid progression to paralysis within a matter of days. Paralysis may affect the major muscles involved in respiration and therefore cause death if there is no appropriate rapid intervention.

Global efforts toward polio eradication have included vaccination campaigns and active surveillance. The annual incidence of paralytic polio was reduced from an estimated 350,000 in 1988 to about 1,000 from 2001 to 2004 (WHO 2004). Africa and South Asia are the last regions in the world where poliomyelitis is still endemic. False accusations of tainted vaccines by local leaders have led to a local resurgence of poliomyelitis cases and consequent spread to other parts of Africa (Heymann and Aylward 2004).

Two different poliomyelitis vaccines are currently used to protect against disease. Oral poliovirus vaccine (OPV) is a live attenuated vaccine containing all three serotypes of the poliovirus and induces protection as high as 95 percent in individuals who receive three doses. Additional booster doses are necessary to achieve nearly 100 percent protection. Currently the WHO recommends that OPV be given at birth, 6, 10, and 14 weeks in polio endemic or recently endemic countries (Sutter and Kew 2004). In many developed countries this vaccine is now delivered in a series of national or subnational campaigns several times a year. The majority of developing countries throughout the world rely on OPV for vaccinating their population, a combined birth cohort of 127 million people (Sutter and Kew 2004).

Because OPV is a live viral vaccine that can revert to a transmissible pathogenic virus, recipients or those in contact with them can be at increased risk of vaccine-associated paralytic poliomyelitis (VAPP) due to shedding of live virus into the environment. VAPP occurs in less than one person per 3.3 million doses administered (Sutter and Kew 2004). Viral shedding can be chronic and occur for years. Recent polio outbreaks have been blamed on continuous transmission of polioviruses derived from vaccine strains, most notably in areas with low immunization coverage rates (Kew et al. 2004). An assumption of the WHO eradication program is that countries would be able to stop vaccination after wild poliovirus ceases transmission; however, the possible threat of a resurgence because of the continued likely circulation of oral poliovirus vaccine would seriously challenge that strategy (Miller, Barrett, and Henderson 2006).

Inactivated poliovirus vaccine (IPV) is another vaccine, composed of three types of inactivated polioviruses. When IPV is administered to infants as the primary vaccine, the first two or three doses should be administered in the first six months of life, followed by a booster during the second year. It is also recommended that, when feasible, a second booster be given to children before they enter school. IPV efficacy rates have been estimated between 80 and 90 percent against paralytic polio (Plotkin and Vidor 2004). An increasing number of countries are transitioning from OPV to IPV because of the risk intolerance associated with vaccine-derived paralysis. Financial and operational barriers currently prevent many developing countries from doing the same, although costs and the ease of IPV use through combination vaccines may allow their greater use in the future.

Measles

Measles is an acute, highly infectious viral disease that is transmitted from person to person through large respiratory droplets. In the absence of vaccination, measles is estimated to infect virtually the entire population with the exception of isolated communities (Black 1976). Most children born to immune mothers are protected from the virus for the first six months of their lives from acquired maternal antibodies. More than 90 percent of infections are associated with clinical disease, which includes a range of symptoms, including fever, rhinorrhea, cough, and conjunctivitis. A rash commonly appears within three to four days after onset. Complications associated with measles include pneumonia, diarrhea, encephalitis, and blindness. The case-fatality rates in recent years have been estimated at 0.1 to 3 percent in many developing nations (Strebel, Papania, and Halsey 2004).

The number of deaths due to measles has been a subject of considerable controversy for the past several years, mostly because of the inability to specify accurately the cause of death in children afflicted with measles and other, similar conditions. Many models have been constructed that demonstrate a substantial reduction of measles deaths from the long-stated global number of 1 million deaths per year reported by the WHO prior to 1997. Large-scale urban and nationwide vaccination campaigns over the last few years have reduced measles mortality to 250,000–500,000 deaths per year, most of which still occur in Sub-Saharan Africa. Measles can coexist with several comorbid conditions that can cause death, so attribution to any one cause is somewhat arbitrary, rendering specific accounting difficult. It is likely, however, that recent implementation of mass vaccination campaigns throughout many regions, and in areas previously associated with high mortality, has dramatically reduced deaths due to measles. However, given the high transmission rate of measles virus, this reduction in mortality could only be maintained with continuous high coverage. Measles mortality can be estimated from the susceptibility profile of the population based on historical immunization coverage rates and natural immunity (Miller 2000). Transmission can be blocked if population-based immunity exceeds approximately 93 percent, limiting cases only to importations. Control in many urban parts of Africa may be difficult, given that transmission is higher in densely populated environments with low levels of hygiene (Miller 2000).

The measles vaccine is a live attenuated vaccine that can be administered by itself, combined with rubella vaccine, or with mumps and rubella vaccines. Nearly 95 percent of children vaccinated with at least one combination of the vaccine develop immunity. Most individuals who fail to develop immunity with one dose will do so upon receiving a second dose. Vaccination is believed to induce lifelong immunity. The first dose should be given on or after the first birthday. A second dose is given to children when they are about four to six years old but can be given as soon as one month after the first dose. Adverse reactions following immunization, such as fever, rash, or lowered platelet counts, have been observed in 5 to 15 percent of vaccine recipients. Many developing countries are now delivering measles vaccines in campaign style, similar to that used to deliver poliovirus vaccination.

Measles vaccination rates are sensitive indicators of functional public health systems. One to two doses of a US$0.14 vaccine could prevent a disease that practically affects 100 percent of the population with an approximate case-fatality rate of 3 to 6 percent in Sub-Saharan Africa. Given that measles vaccine is one of the most cost-effective and

Figure 12.2 Immunization Coverage with Measles-Containing Vaccines, 2003
(percent)

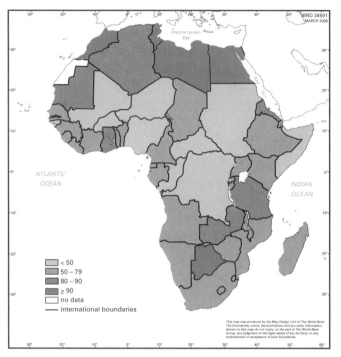

Source: WHO and UNICEF 2003.

low-cost health interventions, low coverage rates of the vaccine in the 1990s is indicative of the poor state of public health infrastructures in various Sub-Saharan Africa populations (figure 12.2).

Diphtheria-Tetanus-Pertussis

Diphtheria, tetanus, and pertussis are frequently cited together given that these three diseases are frequently controlled with a single vaccine. Each of these diseases will be covered in turn.

Diphtheria. Diphtheria is caused by toxin-producing strains of the bacterium *Corynebacterium diphtheriae*, which can be transmitted from person to person via respiratory droplets. The bacterium often affects the tonsils, pharynx, nasal mucosa, inner ear, vagina, or skin. Respiratory diphtheria presents as a sore throat often accompanying a mild fever. Death can result from severe cases in which swelling from pharyngeal and tracheal exudates obstruct the airway. Myocarditis and neuritis are two other complications associated with respiratory diphtheria. Cutaneous diphtheria presents as skin lesions and causes far fewer complications and deaths among those infected.

Estimates of the burden of diphtheria in Africa are unreliable, given the low number of diagnosed or reported cases. In The Gambia, an annual incidence rate of six cases per 1,000 persons under the age of five years was reported (Heyworth and Ropp 1973). Incidence data in Africa is limited to case series and hospital-based surveillance studies, where underreporting is likely, given that diphtheria is frequently reported as nonspecific upper respiratory infections (Rodrigues 1991).

The EPI has traditionally recommended three doses of the combined diphtheria-tetanus-pertussis (DTP) vaccine in the first year of life (in conjunction with polio vaccine). Most developed countries give subsequent booster doses in childhood and diphtheria-tetanus boosters in adulthood. There is growing concern that adolescents and adult populations are becoming more susceptible to diphtheria because repeated doses of diphtheria toxoid are needed to maintain immunity in these populations. Once a child is immunized, the immunity wanes relatively rapidly without exposure to natural *C. diphtheriae* (Galazka and Robertson 1996; Galazka, Robertson, and Oblapenko 1995; Geldermalsen and Wenning 1993). However, in Africa, the need for boosters is offset by the natural immunity provided by the presence of *C. diphtheriae* in skin ulcers as well as asymptomatic carriage in the throat, which spreads the organism throughout the population. Carrier rates in Africa have been estimated to be as high as 9.3 percent in children in the general population (Geldermalsen and Wenning 1993).

The risk of diphtheria epidemics is heightened among communities with an immunity gap in adults and a large number of susceptible children and adolescents (Galazka and Robertson 1996). As a means of controlling potential diphtheria outbreaks, immunization coverage rates should be increased among at-risk groups, cases should be promptly detected and managed, and close contacts should be recognized quickly to prevent secondary infections (Galazka, Robertson, and Oblapenko 1995). For these reasons effective vaccine and surveillance must be maintained in Sub-Saharan Africa in order to keep the prevalence of diphtheria at relatively low levels and to prevent possible epidemics. In addition, the use of booster doses should be considered, especially as immunity wanes in those populations with increasing hygiene and the consequent decrease to natural reexposure.

Pertussis. Pertussis, or whooping cough, is a highly contagious disease caused by the bacterium *Bordetella pertussis,* which is transmitted through respiratory excretions.

Pertussis is characterized as spasms (paroxysms) of coughing followed by inspiratory "whooping." The paroxysms can vary in length and severity but may become so severe, especially among infants, that respiration is compromised, resulting in hypoxia. In some cases this can cause neurological damage. Pneumonia can also be a complication of pertussis infection. In a study conducted in Canada, pneumonia occurred in 2 percent of patients younger than 30 years old and in 5 to 9 percent of older participants (De Serres et al. 2000). Severe coughing in older persons can cause serious complications, ranging from rib fractures to pneumo-thorax, inguinal hernia, and herniated lumbar disks (De Serres et al. 2000; Postels-Multani et al. 1995).

In more developed countries transmission from adults to young infants is common. Girls tend to have higher incidence rates of the disease than boys (Dragsted et al. 2004; Mahieu et al. 1978; Preziosi et al. 2002). Pertussis is highly contagious in its early stages and has a secondary attack rate in other household members as high as 90 percent (Rodrigues 1991). Reported incidence rates of pertussis in Senegal prior to any immunization campaigns were estimated to be 183 per 1,000 child-years at risk under age five years, with a 2.8 percent case-fatality rate (Preziosi 2002). Similar studies have shown incidence rates in Africa to be nearly 1,000 per 100,000 inhabitants (Galazka 1992).

Each year there are an estimated 20 million to 40 million cases of pertussis and another 200,000 to 400,000 deaths attributed to the disease, 90 percent of which occur in the developing world (WHO 1999b). The WHO believes that only 1 to 2 percent of cases are reported worldwide. Pertussis diagnosis is difficult for several reasons. Paroxysms among adults are less severe and often misdiagnosed as other respiratory illnesses. Misdiagnosis is common in areas without adequately trained personnel or technology. In a study of 3,096 patients, *B. pertussis* was found in 496 individuals; 208 (42 percent) were diagnosed by polymerase chain reaction (PCR) alone, whereas 17 (3 percent) were diagnosed by culture alone (Dragsted et al. 2004). Rapid diagnosis of pertussis using PCR techniques together with serological assays can enhance diagnosis as well as surveillance of pertussis (Fry et al. 2004). Clinical diagnosis of pertussis by a trained physician has also proved to be a reliable diagnostic tool (Granstrom, Wretlind, and Granstrom 1991) and is often characterized by a cough that lasts at least 14 days (Patriarca et al. 1988). These are important implications when considering diagnosis of pertussis in remote areas with limited laboratory resources and few trained health professionals.

The incidence rate of pertussis has declined drastically over the past half-century primarily because of the administration of the inactivated whole-cell pertussis vaccines. Due to neurological reactions associated with the whole-cell vaccines, new acellular vaccines have been developed. Either of these vaccines is usually administered with the diphtheria and tetanus toxoids (TTs). The whole-cell vaccine is cheaper than the acellular vaccine and is produced in many developing countries (WHO 1999b). A herd effect of vaccination not only protects immunized infants but decreases transmission rates to protect unvaccinated infants (Miller and Gay 1997). The introduction of pertussis vaccines through the EPI in Senegal has resulted in steady and dramatic decreases in the incidence of the disease, especially among infants under six months old (Preziosi et al. 2002).

Tetanus. Tetanus is the only EPI vaccine-preventable disease that is not communicable but acquired through environmental contamination. The bacterium *Clostridium tetani,* which can grow in dirty flesh wounds, produces a neurotoxin causing convulsions and eventual death. Neonatal tetanus (NNT), the most common form of tetanus in the developing world, is the result of contamination of the umbilical stump either by the use of nonsterile instruments after delivery or the application of animal dung to the cut cord, a custom in many cultures, especially among groups in Sub-Saharan Africa (Elmore-Meegan et al. 2001). Symptoms can appear 3 to 14 days after birth following a period of normal feeding. Infected infants will gradually lose the ability to nurse properly followed by a period of convulsions, which increase in intensity and frequency. Mortality rates of infants can range from 25 to 90 percent with care, 95 percent without (http://www.who.int/vaccines/en/neotetanus.shtml).

NNT, which causes an estimated 450,000 infant deaths, is defined as tetanus in the first month of life. Another 40,000 maternal deaths are estimated to occur from tetanus acquired during delivery (WHO 1999a). NNT remains a global problem, but the greatest burden occurs in Africa (table 12.1) (Anita-Obong, Young, and Effiong 1993; Stanfield and Galazka 1984; WHO 1999c, 2001b). Nearly 90 percent of the global burden from NNT is from 28 countries. Of these, 16 are located in Africa (Angola, Burkina Faso, Cameroon, Chad, Côte d'Ivoire, Democratic Republic of Congo, Ethiopia, Ghana, Guinea-Bissau, Liberia, Mali, Mauritania, Mozambique, Niger, Nigeria, and Senegal). Additionally, 11 of the 12 countries reporting NNT

mortality rates greater than 5 per 1,000 live births are in Africa (WHO 1999c).

The WHO estimates that approximately 3 percent of NNT cases are reported each year; this figure includes those reported from countries considered to have well-developed surveillance systems (WHO 1999b). Because death may occur within the first week of birth, it often is unreported in official mortality records and therefore is referred to as "the silent killer" (CVI 1994). Community surveys conducted in various states of Nigeria between 1990 and 1993 found that mortality rates from NNT ranged between 9 and 20 per 1,000 live births (Babaniyi and Parakoyi 1991). It was estimated in 1999 that nearly 46,000 cases of NNT occurred in Nigeria, representing 36 percent of all the NNT cases in the African region, although only 1,529 of the cases were actually reported. This problem of underreporting has serious implications for the control of the disease.

The World Health Assembly in 1989 set the goal for elimination (defined as incidence of less than 1 case per 1,000 live births) of NNT by 1995. This date was later delayed until 2005 because of operational constraints from the expanded scope of including maternal tetanus. By 1999 only 104 of the 161 developing countries in the world had eliminated neonatal tetanus. Sixteen of the 57 nations that have yet to reach this target are located in the African region (figure 12.3) (Idema et al. 2002). Included in this plan for elimination is the use of TT to protect pregnant women and the use of supplemental immunization activities, clean birthing practices, and active surveillance systems for women of childbearing age (WHO 2001b).

DTP Vaccines. Inactivated diphtheria and TTs can be combined with whole-cell or acellular pertussis vaccines, such as DTwP or DTaP, respectively, and administered as a single injection. In most of Africa, the national EPI schedule of vaccination is at 6, 10, and 14 weeks of life. Although most developed countries administer booster doses, this does not routinely occur in Africa. Pertussis vaccine efficacy is 70 to 90 percent of fully vaccinated children (Edwards and Decker 2004); however, continuous protection requires booster doses. Three doses of tetanus or diphtheria toxoids are associated with greater than 95 percent protection against disease (Cherry and Harrison 2004; Feigin, Stechenberg, and Hertel 2004; Wharton and Vitek 2004); however, periodic boosting is necessary to ensure lifelong protection. DTP vaccine has been associated with adverse effects, such as local swelling and tenderness, fever, febrile seizures, anaphylaxis, hyporesponsive episodes, and

Figure 12.3 Maternal and Neonatal Tetanus Elimination Status, 2002

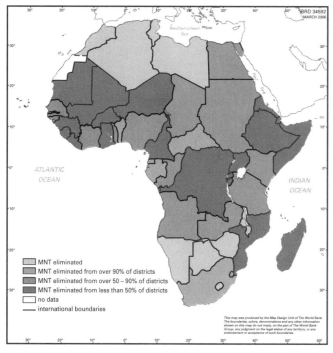

Source: WHO and UNICEF 2003.

encephalopathy (Edwards and Decker 2004). The more expensive acellular pertussis vaccines have greatly reduced these reactions.

The TT, given to immunize pregnant women to prevent neonatal and maternal tetanus, induces antibodies that can be passed from the mother to the fetus. In addition to being an effective vaccine, it is relatively cheap at about US$0.07 per dose (CVI 1994). Studies have shown that when 80 percent of women in an area have been vaccinated against tetanus with two doses, the level of seroprotection coupled with health education is adequate to eliminate tetanus (CVI 1994).

Some of the lowest coverage rates of TT are found in Africa. The EPI coverage rates among pregnant women with two doses had stagnated between 30 and 40 percent in most African nations by 1999. One of the objectives of the EPI is to increase coverage of three doses of DTP vaccine to 80 percent in all districts in the region. It is estimated that 53 percent of children under the age of one living in Sub-Saharan Africa have received three doses of the DTP vaccine (figure 12.4) (World Bank 2003).

Tuberculosis

Tuberculosis (TB) is a bacterial infection caused by *Mycobacterium tuberculosis*. Transmitted through respiratory droplets, tuberculosis is highly contagious, with studies showing a 25 to 50 percent infection rate of those in close contact with infected individuals (Smith and Starke 2004). TB presents clinically with a wide range of symptoms, depending upon the age of the individual. Infants and adolescents are most likely to have significant clinical manifestations compared with older children. Most infants will present with a nonproductive cough, shortness of breath,

Figure 12.4 Global and Regional Immunization Coverage, Three Doses DTP, 1980–2001

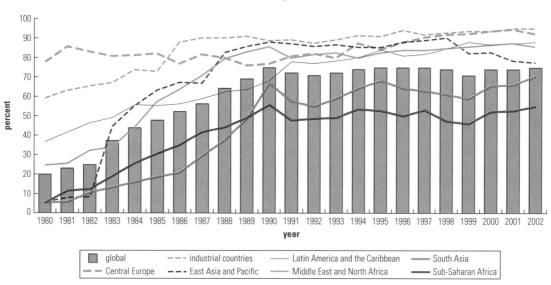

Source: WHO and UNICEF 2003.

and low grade fever. Other common symptoms include night sweats, malaise, irritability, fatigue, and weight loss. TB is often misdiagnosed as other illnesses, such as bronchitis, until it progresses to more advanced stages. TB can also present as meningitis in infants or cause a chronic infectious process almost anywhere throughout the body. The time between preclinical infection and the onset of disease can be several weeks to many decades. Adults who are able to suppress acute infections often carry the bacterium latently, which results in reactivation of the disease later in life. Accurate diagnosis of TB is a critical component for better understanding the burden of disease as well as the effectiveness of interventions. In resource-poor areas of the world in which mycobacterial cultures and radiography are not accessible, microscopy is most commonly used to identify the organism and thus diagnose the disease.

TB is blamed for nearly 2 million to 3 million deaths annually, and it is believed that another 8 million people are infected with the bacterium each year. Nearly one-third of the world's population is currently infected with TB (WHO 2001a). In much of the world the TB incidence rates continue to grow, especially in Sub-Saharan Africa, despite the widespread use of the bacille Calmette-Guérin (BCG) vaccine (Cantwell and Binkin 1996). In Africa, coinfections of human immunodeficiency virus (HIV) and TB have led to increases in the incidence rate of TB by approximately 20 percent (Smith and Starke 2004).

BCG is a live attenuated bacterial vaccine most commonly administered intradermally at birth to prevent tuberculosis. The effectiveness of the BCG vaccine against TB has been debated, with a range estimated from 0 to 80 percent (Fine 2001). Most proponents claim that it is effective against TB meningitis, but it is not commonly believed to prevent TB in adults nor its transmission. The real impact of BCG may have been confounded by many other improvements in public health that could have contributed to the decrease in disease burden associated with tuberculosis (Smith and Starke 2004).

Yellow Fever

Yellow fever is an acute viral infection transmitted by mosquito, primarily the *Aedes aegypti*. Symptoms of the infection can vary, making diagnosis difficult and leading to the underestimation of morbidity (Monath 2004). After an incubation period of three to six days, onset of symptoms—rigors, headache, nausea, joint pain, jaundice, and myalgia—is rapid. In approximately 15 to 20 percent of cases, severe disease causes multiple organ failure.

Figure 12.5 Epidemics of Yellow Fever in Africa Reported to the WHO, 1980–2003

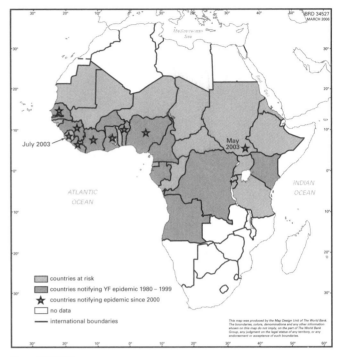

Source: WHO 2003.

Yellow fever is endemic to parts of South America as well as Sub-Saharan Africa in areas bordering jungles (figure 12.5). Between 1986 and 1995, reported incidence of yellow fever dramatically increased from previous reporting intervals, likely because of cessation of vaccinations. In Africa alone, 22,952 cases were reported, accounting for 89 percent of the total global cases during that period (Monath 2004). A case-fatality rate of 23 percent (5,357 deaths) was reported throughout Africa.

The yellow fever vaccine is a live attenuated viral vaccine recommended for anyone nine years or older living or traveling to endemic regions of South America and Africa. A single dose of the vaccine has shown to be effective for 30 to 35 years and most likely for the duration of the vaccine recipient's life (Monath 2004). Adverse effects from the vaccine have ranged from mild symptoms of headache, malaise, or low-grade fever to rare, more serious complications.

Hepatitis B

Many viral agents cause hepatitis; vaccine can counteract two of them—hepatitis A virus (HAV) and hepatitis B virus (HBV). Although a licensed vaccine against HAV is used in developed countries, it is currently not considered to be cost-effective for Africa. HBV, transmitted through blood-borne infections, sexually, or from mother to infant, can potentially cause more severe illness, including fulminant hepatitis, cirrhosis, and liver cancer. Persons infected as infants have a 70 to 90 percent chance of becoming a chronic carrier of the virus and can then either infect other persons or develop severe sequelae at a later stage in life.

National serosurveys for antibodies and antigenic markers for carrier states of HBV are available for almost all nations at various stages of resolutions due to blood-banking practices. The overall carriage rate for Sub-Saharan Africa is 12 percent. These data allow for estimations of disease burden based on a certain percentage of chronically infected persons progressing to hepatoma, fulminant hepatitis, or cirrhosis at later stages of life (Miller and McCann 2000). For Sub-Saharan Africa, this would translate into more than 500,000 deaths per year in each birth cohort at a mean age of 40 to 45 years. As life expectancy in Sub-Saharan Africa is currently declining from the HIV epidemic, actual death from hepatitis is likely to be lower.

Three doses of HBV vaccine, the first given at birth, could effectively prevent a child from becoming infected and from becoming a chronic carrier of the virus. Vaccine effectiveness is approximately 95 percent with three doses. Therefore, HBV vaccine could exert a powerful herd effect on the population by eliminating the long latency period during which persons could be infectious to others. Despite the benefits of implementing HBV into national vaccination campaigns, a minority of African nations are doing so (figure 12.6). The WHO endorses several immunization schedules so that HBV vaccine can be administered with other vaccines. The vaccine does not have any known serious effects and can be combined with other vaccines, including DTP and Hib.

As HBV is transmitted in a way similar to that of HIV, the uptake and use of this vaccine is a good proxy for the potential use of vaccines against HIV and the acquired immune deficiency syndrome (AIDS).

Haemophilus Influenzae type B

Hib is a bacterium transmitted through respiratory excretions and may be carried in the nasopharynx of about 15 percent of nonimmunized children (WHO 1998). The most common forms of invasive disease are meningitis, epiglottitis, pneumonia, arthritis, and cellulitis. Epiglottitis is characterized by swelling of the epiglottis, the tissue in the throat covering the larynx. The disease burden of Hib is highest among children between four and eighteen months, rarely occurring in infants younger than three months and after the age of six years. Hib meningitis could cause severe

Figure 12.6 African Nations Using Hepatitis B Vaccine in a National Infant Immunization Campaign, 2002

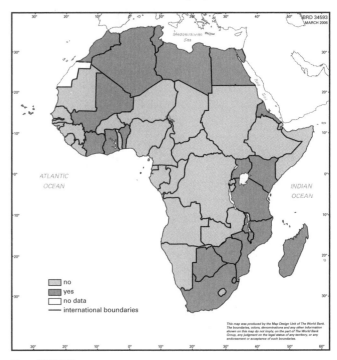

Source: WHO 2003.

mental retardation in patients who recover from the acute form of the disease.

As it is difficult to culture this organism, disease burden estimates are made through a variety of modeling studies integrating data from geographic representational populations and similar socioeconomic stratification (Miller 1998; Miller and McCann 2000). In a Hib vaccine trial in The Gambia (Mulholland et al. 1997), the vaccinated group had 21 percent fewer occurrences of severe pneumonia than the control group, indicating that up to 21 percent of cases of severe pneumonia may be due to this organism. Extrapolation to the rest of the region would indicate that this vaccine could potentially prevent 90,000 to 123,000 deaths due to bacterial pneumonia or meningitis.

Since 1988, safe and effective vaccines have been developed to prevent Hib. A conjugate vaccine can be coadministered with DTP, IPV, and HBV vaccine. A full course of vaccine confers more than 95 percent protection against invasive Hib disease and results in a herd effect (Wenger and Ward 2004). This vaccine may be given in combination with DTP. In countries that have introduced a three- to four-dose regimen, Hib disease has almost been eliminated. The relatively high cost of the Hib vaccine has hindered many low-income countries from integrating the vaccine into routine vaccine schedules. Research has been conducted to explain quantitatively the benefits of adding Hib to national immunization programs in order to assist policy makers in endemic countries. It has been estimated that from 257,000 to 317,000 deaths could be averted each year through the routine use of Hib vaccine (Miller and McCann 2000). Although Hib vaccination would be a cost-effective intervention in low-income countries, its use in Africa has been limited.

Meningococcal Disease

Neisseria meningitides is a bacterium that causes meningitis, frequently with devastating neurological sequelae (Heymann et al. 1998; Merlin et al. 1996) and a death rate often exceeding 30 percent, even with optimal treatment (Campagne et al. 1999). Infections have also resulted in limb loss. Given its acute sporadic onset and devastating impact on young healthy individuals, mostly less than 30 years of age, meningococcal disease is one of the most feared infectious diseases. Although meningococcal disease is rare in infants up to three months of age, the incidence gradually increases to a peak at about one year of age and declines thereafter.

Although there are five serogroups (A, B, C, Y, and W135), serogroup A has caused annual epidemics in the African meningitis belt, an area stretching from Senegal to Ethiopia (Greenwood 1987; Greenwood et al. 1984; Lapeyssonnie 1963). Annual incidence rates in this portion of the African continent have exceeded 1,000 cases per 100,000 population in some instances (Granoff, Feavers, and Borrow 2004). In 1996 the largest recorded meningitis outbreak occurred in Africa, resulting in more than 250,000 cases and 25,000 deaths (Tikhomirov, Santamaria, and Esteves 1997).

A polysaccharide vaccine containing polysaccharides from serotypes A, C, Y, and W135 that is approximately 85 percent effective has been licensed but has been used only in response to outbreaks triggered by a weekly incidence of 10 to 15 cases per 100,000 persons in a geographically defined region. Frequently, surveillance and logistical difficulties to timely identification of outbreaks and delivery of vaccines in these instances have had a limited impact on epidemics. The 1996 outbreak and the continuous suboptimal implementation of emergency immunization campaigns led to a reevaluation of meningococcal disease-prevention strategies in this area (Miller and Shahab 2005). Robbins and colleagues (1997) called for immediate mass immunization, followed by a routine immunization program of

four doses of polysaccharide vaccine given during the first five years of life. Others (WHO 1997) have suggested routine immunization of schoolchildren or improvement of the implementation of the current strategy of emergency response with mass immunization. To date, these vaccines are not used routinely in Sub-Saharan Africa. A conjugate meningococcal serogroup A vaccine currently being developed could routinely be administered to infants in Africa (LaForce 2004).

FUTURE VACCINES

Parallel to the successful delivery of vaccines, great advances have been made in the field of vaccine development. Since the 1985 U.S. Institute of Medicine report established priorities for vaccine development (IOM 1986), many new vaccines with the potential to dramatically reduce morbidity and mortality have been developed. Within the last 20 years new safe and effective vaccines have been developed and licensed to protect populations against HBV and Hib. Great research strides in immunology have begun to pay dividends with the more recent licensure of rotavirus vaccines against diarrhea, human papillomavirus vaccine against genital warts and possible cervical cancer, and *Streptococcus pneumoniae* (SP) vaccine against pneumonia. Although these vaccines are currently licensed, they are presently not routinely used in Africa.

VACCINATION PROGRAMS

The WHO objectives of the EPI in Africa are to strengthen the delivery of sustainable immunization services and to accelerate efforts to achieve polio eradication, measles control, neonatal tetanus elimination, and yellow fever control. Country strategic plans are prepared for the district level, with the goal of administering three doses of DTP to at least 80 percent of the target population in all districts and ensure increasing government funding for the EPI. EPI programs are strengthening health systems throughout Africa as well as implementing the use of new vaccines and technologies.

Prior to the implementation of immunization programs, vaccine-preventable diseases were highly endemic throughout Sub-Saharan Africa. During the 1990s the global immunization coverage exceeded 70 percent (figure 12.1); however, reported rates between regions and nations had great disparities. In Sub-Saharan Africa, reported immunization rates peaked in 1990 at 55 percent and remained steady throughout the decade. Immunization rates have decreased over the last 10 years in many low-income countries, particularly in Sub-Saharan Africa. For example, vaccination rates of all three doses of DTP (DTP3) in the Central African Republic decreased from 82 percent in 1990 to 29 percent in 2000. Similarly, the coverage rates with three doses of DTP vaccine dropped in the Democratic Republic of Congo from 79 percent in 1990 to 33 percent in 2000. These declines have been attributed to civil unrest and lack of political will among the national governments. As a result, millions of children have been left unvaccinated and vulnerable to disease.

The success of vaccination programs applied at the global level has had few parallels in public health. Immunizations remain one of the most cost-effective health interventions to prevent death and disability caused by infectious diseases. Despite great strides forward in vaccination development and administration throughout parts of the world, many countries, usually the poorest, struggle with vaccinating their children. This gap in immunization coverage results from many compounding problems, such as low political commitment on behalf of national and local governments, weak health service delivery systems, civil unrest, and underfunding and poor management. These problems are further compounded by relatively low levels of research and development of new vaccines to combat the predominant diseases in the developing world.

There are many possible reasons why routine vaccination has declined in Africa. Over the past decade, the budget of the WHO vaccine program has been heavily skewed toward the Poliomyelitis Eradication Initiative. Although this has led to high coverage rates against poliomyelitis virus, it likely has strained other vaccination services (Taylor, Cutts, and Taylor 1997). Additionally, throughout the 1990s, donors and the United Nations Children's Fund (UNICEF) emphasized that countries should pay for vaccine out of their own national budget rather than finance the cost through donors. The push toward self-reliance was made with good intentions, but fixed budgets within national economies may have simply moved funds from vaccine administration to vaccine purchase, with resultant declines in services.

An additional deterrent to vaccination adherence in much of the world is the threat of unsafe injections. It has been estimated that nearly 8 billion to 12 billion injections are administered in various health care settings throughout the world each year; 50 percent of these injections are believed to be unsafe and pose the risk of transmitting hepatitis, HIV, and other blood-borne pathogens (Miller and Pisani 1999). In many circumstances, especially in developing countries, disposable syringes are used multiple times, which increases the risk of disease transmission. Immunization rates drop dramatically when unsafe injection practices are publicized, whether they even are a part of vaccine campaigns.

Recognizing these factors, the WHO has recently been promoting the expansion and performance monitoring of services to local levels, with the goal of reaching routine coverage of at least 80 percent. This may rectify the maldistribution of vaccine delivery services within countries to increase the equity of benefits, especially to the populations on the margins, those likely to have the greatest disease burden.

ADOPTION OF NEW VACCINES

The traditional EPI-targeted program has been challenged by the development of new vaccines that promise to reduce the disease burden further if they can be adopted into national programs. Since the development of national vaccine programs, there has been a widening gap in the number of vaccines used in developing and developed countries (figure 12.7).

Figure 12.7 Number of Childhood Vaccines Routinely Used in Developing and Established-Market Countries

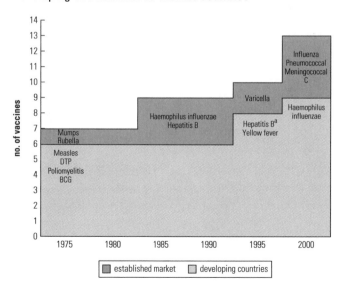

Source: WHO and UNICEF 2003.

a. Used in about 50 percent of global birth cohort.

The use of these vaccines within already existing vaccine delivery infrastructures would greatly increase the armamentarium against infectious and even cancer-causing agents. However, despite the availability of these public health tools, countries have been slow to adopt them. For example, despite the World Health Assembly's recommendation to add HBV vaccine to all member nations' vaccination programs by 1997 (WHA 1992), less than one-half the global infant birth cohort receives this vaccine. Likewise, many African countries have yet to adopt the highly efficacious Hib vaccine. Given the array of new vaccines on the horizon, and potential vaccines against HIV, malaria, and tuberculosis, what is the likelihood of their adoption, especially in those countries that have the highest mortality from those diseases?

Factors such as national infrastructure to deliver vaccines and the cost of novel vaccines relative to national income in addition to an inadequate appreciation of the disease burden have prevented the adoption of newer vaccines. The Global Alliance for Vaccines and Immunizations (GAVI) has sought to address some of these factors through the creation of vaccine purchase funds and the direct allocation of financial resources to strengthen infrastructures at the local level. It is still too early to judge the success of these tactics and sustainability in the most resource-constrained areas such as Africa. Development agencies will have limited influence on per capita gross domestic product, but they can work with manufacturers to influence the vaccine cost to the country (either by offering financial support for vaccine purchase or guaranteeing volume purchase to lower vaccine prices) and strengthen vaccination services.

VACCINATION: PROBLEMS AND BARRIERS

The barriers to vaccine adoption are presumed to be multiple. If there is poor recognition of disease burden and costs, insufficient finances, or an ineffective vaccine delivery system, the introduction of a new vaccine is unlikely. However, methodological analyses can help focus deliberations and assist countries to overcome hurdles such as these. Demonstration of a country's disease burden as well as its associated economic burden may encourage the appropriate allocation of financial resources by clarifying the value of prevention through vaccination.

Economics has frequently been sited as a barrier to the use of newer vaccines. To address this, an analysis of the health and economic implications of new vaccine introduction was conducted to help national policy makers (Miller

Table 12.2 Potential Deaths Averted by HBV, Hib, Rotavirus, and SP Vaccine Implementation

Vaccine	Estimated deaths averted (thousands)	Estimated program costs (US$ millions)
HBV	978–1,370	671
Hib	257–317	1,129
Rotavirus	149–326	1,482
SP	549–1,098	3,729

Source: Miller and McCann 2000.

and McCann 2000). Disease burden, vaccine program costs, and the potential reduction of disease from vaccination were assessed for four vaccines that have not been adopted in many countries.

Without vaccination, HBV, Hib, SP, and rotavirus contribute to more than 1 million deaths in each successive birth cohort in Africa (Miller and McCann 2000). Routine scheduled use of HBV, Hib, SP, and rotavirus vaccines could potentially prevent most of these deaths (table 12.2). Incorporation of these vaccines into routine vaccination programs was estimated to cost between US$29 and US$150 per life year saved (Miller and McCann 2000). Based on these evaluations, HBV and Hib should be considered for integration into all national immunization programs. SP and rotavirus vaccines, with the given assumptions, would also be cost-effective. Proactive analysis of the epidemiologic and economic impact of these vaccines can hasten their introduction into national vaccination schedules.

FINANCIAL IMPLICATIONS, GAVI, AND THE VACCINE FUND

GAVI is a public-private partnership devoted to the promotion and strengthening of vaccine programs in low-income countries. Through the Vaccine Fund, which is the funding arm of GAVI, financial resources are provided for eligible countries to purchase vaccines and to fund the operational costs of managing immunization campaigns. GAVI provides funding to national governments based on national income (countries with gross national income per capita below US$1,000). Approximately half of the 75 countries eligible for funding through GAVI are located in Sub-Saharan Africa. In order for an eligible country to receive funding it must demonstrate that a well-functioning national mechanism is in place to coordinate immunization activities among the various partners within the country. The immunization program must have received a comprehensive assessment by GAVI-designated technical agencies during the previous three years, a multiyear immunization plan must be complete, and finally a strategy for improving the safety of injections must be demonstrated. Currently the GAVI's Vaccine Fund is providing financial support to governments in order to improve health services; distribute safe injection materials; and acquire the HBV, Hib, and yellow fever vaccines.

In an attempt to ensure the sustainability of immunization campaigns, GAVI requires countries that receive funding to create financial sustainability plans. Financial sustainability of immunization campaigns is vital in order to reach any long-term immunization goals. These financial sustainability plans are meant to be long-term plans that can improve the countries' immunization programs and serve as a foundation to expand support from other sources, namely, their own national budgets.

Initiatives by bilateral partner and health agencies emphasize the need for nations to strengthen health system infrastructures and assume responsibility for the provision of basic services, including childhood immunizations. Concurrent with these structural changes within nations are pricing and technology changes in vaccines. The six basic EPI vaccines are currently estimated to cost approximately US$0.50 per capita. New vaccines are appreciably more costly than traditional vaccines but far less expensive than the treatment costs of the diseases they prevent. The poorer developing countries, which often have the greatest disease burden, may be inclined to reject the adoption of these vaccines without full recognition of their true value.

A determination of the value of prevented disease is not a panacea for a shortage of financial resources. However, it can support the more efficient allocation of limited resources. Indeed, many new financial resources, most notably from the World Bank and the Bill & Melinda Gates Foundation, are expanding the number of potential resources available to help finance vaccination activities. There is concurrently an expanded role for medical associations on the national, regional, and global level to highlight the value of prevention through use of some of the best tools in public health.

CONCLUSION

Traditional vaccines are among the most cost-effective interventions there are and can potentially be used to achieve several Millennium Development Goals; however, continuous vaccination must be sustainable.

In many parts of Africa, vaccine infrastructure has been suboptimal, especially for routine vaccination. Immunization campaigns versus routine services appear to be dominating given logistical and operational hurdles in Sub-Saharan Africa

In Africa, new vaccines have been slow to be adopted into national EPI programs; likely reasons have been the lack of support for routine delivery throughout the continent. Logistical and operational factors are probable barriers that require substantial continuous investments in human capital, equipment, and financing.

REFERENCES

Anita-Obong, O. E., M. U. Young, and C. E. Effiong. 1993. "Neonatal Tetanus: Prevalence before and Subsequent to Implementation of the Expanded Programme on Immunization." *Annals of Tropical Paediatrics* 13: 7–12.

Babaniyi, O., and B. Parakoyi. 1991. "Cluster Survey for Poliomyelitis and Neonatal Tetanus in Ilorin, Nigeria." *International Journal of Epidemiology* 20 (2): 515–20.

Black, F. L. 1976. "Measles." In *Viral Infections of Humans: Epidemiology and Control*, ed. A. S. Evans. New York: Plenum.

Campagne, G., A. Schuchat, S. Djibo, A. Ouseini, L. Cissé, and J. P. Chippaux. 1999. "Epidemiology of Bacterial Meningitis in Niamey, Niger, 1981–96." *Bulletin of the World Health Organization* 77: 499–508.

Cantwell, M. F., and N. J. Binkin. 1996. "Tuberculosis in Sub-Saharan Africa: A Regional Assessment of the Impact of the Human Immunodeficiency Virus and National Tuberculosis Control Program Quality." *Tubercle and Lung Disease* 77 (3): 220–25.

Cherry, J. D., and R. E. Harrison. 2004. "Tetanus." In *Textbook of Pediatric Infectious Diseases*, ed. R. D. Feigin, J. D. Cherry, G. J. Demmler, and S. L. Kaplan. Philadelphia: Elsevier.

CVI (Children's Vaccine Initiative) Forum 08. 1994. *Neonatal Tetanus: The Final Countdown*. Geneva: WHO.

De Serres, G., R. Shadmani, B. Duval, N. Boulianne, P. Dery, M. Fradet, L. Rochette, and S. Halperin. 2000. "Morbidity of Pertussis in Adolescents and Adults." *Journal of Infectious Diseases* 182: 174–79.

Dragsted, D., B. Dohn, J. Madsen, and J. Jenson. 2004. "Comparison of Culture and PCR for Detection of Bordetella Pertussis and Bordetella Parapertussis under Routine Laboratory Conditions." *Journal of Medical Microbiology* 53: 749–54.

Edwards, K. M., and M. D. Decker. 2004. "Pertussis Vaccine." In *Vaccines*, 4th ed., ed. S. A. Plotkin and W. A. Orenstein. Philadelphia: Saunders.

Elmore-Meegan, M., R. M. Conroy, S. Ole Lengeny, K. Renhault, and J. Nyangole. 2001. "Effect on Neonatal Tetanus Mortality after a Culturally-Based Health Promotion Programme." *Lancet* 358: 640–41.

Feigin, R. D., B. W. Stechenberg, and P. Hertel. 2004. "Diptheria." In *Textbook of Pediatric Infectious Diseases*, ed. R. D. Feigin, J. D. Cherry, G. J. Demmler, and S. L. Kaplan, 1305–13. Philadelphia: Elsevier.

Fine, P. E. M. 2001. "BCG Vaccines and Vaccination." In *Tuberculosis: A Comprehensive International Approach*, ed. L. B. Reichman and E. S. Hershfield. New York: Marcel Dekker.

Fry, N., O. Tzivra, T. Li, A. McNiff, N. Doshi, C. Maple, N. Crowcroft, E. Miller, R. George, and T. Harrison. 2004. "Laboratory Diagnosis of Pertussis Infections: The Role of PCR and Serology." *Journal of Medical Microbiolgy* 53: 519–25.

Galazka, A. 1992. "Control of Pertussis in the World." *World Health Statistics Quarterly* 45: 238–47.

Galazka, A., and S. Robertson. 1996. "Immunization against Diphtheria with Special Emphasis on Immunization of Adults." *Vaccine* 14 (9): 845–57.

Galazka, A., S. Robertson, and G. Oblapenko. 1995. "Resurgence of Diphtheria." *European Journal of Epidemiology* 11: 95–105.

Geldermalsen, A. A., and U. Wenning. 1993. "A Diphtheria Epidemic in Lesotho, 1989. Did Vaccination Increase the Population's Susceptibility?" *Annals of Tropical Paediatrics.* 13: 13–20.

Gelfand, H. M., D. R. LeBlanc, J. P. Fox, and D. P. Conwell. 1957. "Studies on the Development of Natural Immunity to Poliomyelitis in Louisiana. II. Description and Analysis of Episodes of Infection Observed in Study Households." *American Journal of Hygiene* 65: 367–85.

Granoff, D. M., I. M. Feavers, and R. Borrow. 2004. "Meningococcal Vaccines." In *Vaccines*, ed. S. A. Plotkin and W. A. Orenstein. Philadelphia: Saunders.

Granstrom, G., B. Wretlind, and M. Granstrom. 1991. "Diagnostic Value of Clinical and Bacteriological Findings in Pertussis." *Journal of Infection* 22: 17–26.

Greenwood, B. M. 1987. "Epidemiology of Meningitis in Tropical Africa." In *Bacterial Meningitis*, 1st ed., ed. J. D. Williams and J. Burnie, 61–91. London: Academic Press.

Greenwood, B. M., I. S. Blakebrough, A. K. Bradley, S. Wali, and H. C. Whittle. 1984. "Meningococcal Disease and Season in Sub-Saharan Africa." *Lancet* 1: 1339–42.

Heyman, S. N., Y. Ginosar, L. Niel, J. Amir, N. Marx, M. Shapiro, and S. Maayan. 1998. "Meningococcal Meningitis among Rwandan Refugees: Diagnosis, Management, and Outcome in a Field Hospital." *International Journal of Infectious Diseases* 2: 137–42.

Heymann, D. L., and R. B. Aylward. 2004. "Eradicating Polio." *New England Journal of Medicine* 351 (13): 1275–77.

Heyworth, B., and M. Ropp. 1973. "Diphtheria in The Gambia." *Journal of Tropical Medicine and Hygiene* 76 (3): 61–64.

Horstmann, D. M. 1955. "Poliomyelitis: Severity and Type of Disease in Different Age Groups." *Annals of the New York Academy of Sciences* 61: 956–67.

Idema, C. D., B. N. Harris, G. A. Ogunbanjo, and D. N. Durrheim. 2002. "Neonatal Tetanus Elimination in Mpumalanga Province, South Africa." *Tropical Medicine and International Health* 7 (7): 622–24.

IOM (Institute of Medicine). 1986. *New Vaccine Development: Diseases of Importance in Developing Countries.* Vol. 2. Washington, DC: National Academy Press.

Kew, O. M., P. F. Wright, V. I. Agol, F. Delpeyroux, H. Shimizu, N. Nathanson, and M. A. Pallansch. 2004. "Circulating Vaccine-Derived Polioviruses: Current State of Knowledge." *Bulletin of the World Health Organization* 82: 16–23.

LaForce, F. M. 2004. "Conjugate Meningococcal Vaccines for Africa." In *Vaccines: Preventing Disease and Protecting Health*, ed. C. A. de Quadros. Washington, DC: PAHO.

Lapeyssonnie, L. 1963. "La méningite cérébrospinale en Afrique [Cerebrospinal meningitis in Africa]." *Bulletin of the World Health Organization* 28 (Suppl.): 1–100.

Mahieu, J. M., A. S. Muller, A. M. Voorhoeve, and H. Dikken. 1978. "Pertussis in a Rural Area of Kenya: Epidemiology and a Preliminary Report on a Vaccine Trial." *Bulletin of the World Health Organization* 56 (5): 773–80.

Merlin, M., G. Martet, J. M. Debonne, P. Nicolas, C. Bailly, D. Yazipo, J. Bougere, A. Todesco, and R. Laroche. 1996. "Controle d'une epidemie de meningite a meningocoque en Afrique centrale [Control of an epidemic of meningococcal meningitis in Central Africa]." *Santé* 6: 87–95.

Miller, E., and N. J. Gay. 1997. "Epidemiological Determinants of Pertussis." *Developments in Biological Standardization* 89: 15–23.

Miller, M., S. Barrett, and D. A. Henderson. 2006. "Control and Eradication." In *Disease Control Priorities in Developing Countries*, 2nd ed, ed. D. T. Jamison, J. G. Breman, A. R. Measham, G. Alleyne, M. Claeson, D. B. Evans, P. Jha, A. Mills, and P. Musgrove. New York: Oxford University Press.

Miller, M. A. 1998. "An Assessment of the Value of Haemophilus Influenzae Type B Conjugate Vaccine in Asia." *Pediatric Infectious Disease Journal* 17 (Suppl. 9): S152–59.

———. 2000. "Introducing a Deterministic Model to Estimate Global Measles Disease Burden." *Journal of International Infectious Diseases* 4: 14–20.

Miller, M. A., and L. McCann. 2000. "Policy Analysis of the Use of Hepatitis B, *Haemophilus Influenzae* Type B, *Streptococcus Pneumoniae*-Conjugate and Rotavirus Vaccines in National Immunization Schedules." *Health Economics* 9: 19–35.

Miller, M. A., and E. Pisani. 1999. "The Cost of Unsafe Injections." *Bulletin of the World Health Organization* 77 (10): 808–11.

Miller, M. A., and C. K. Shahab. 2005. "Review of the Cost Effectiveness of Immunization Strategies for the Control of Meningococcal Meningitis." *Pharmacoeconomics* 23 (4): 333–43.

Monath, T. 2004. "Yellow Fever Vaccine." In *Vaccines*, ed. S. A. Plotkin and W. A. Orenstein. Philadelphia: Saunders.

Mulholland, K., S. Hilton, R. Adegbola, S. Usen, A. Oparaugo, C. Omosigho, M. Weber, et al. 1997. "Randomised Trial of *Haemophilus influenzae* Type-b Tetanus Protein Conjugate Vaccine [Corrected] for Prevention of Pneumonia and Meningitis in Gambian Infants." *Lancet* 349: 1191–97.

Patriarca, P. A., R. J. Biellik, G. Sanden, D. G. Burstyn, P. D. Mitchell, P. R. Silverman, J. P. Davis, and C. R. Manclark. 1988. "Sensitivity and Specificity of Clinical Case Definitions for Pertussis." *American Journal of Public Health* 78: 833–36.

Plotkin, S., and E. Vidor. 2004. "Poliovirus Vaccine-Inactivated." In *Vaccines*, ed. S. A. Plotkin, and W. A. Orenstein. Philadelphia: Saunders.

Postels-Multani, S., H. J. Schmitt, C. H. Wirsing von Konig, H. L. Bock, and H. Bogaerts. 1995. "Symptoms and Complications of Pertussis in Adults." *Infection* 23: 139–42.

Preziosi, M. P., A. Yam, S. G. Wassilak, L. Chabirand, A. Simaga, M. Ndiaye, M. Dia, et al. 2002. "Epidemiology of Pertussis in a West African Community before and after Introduction of a Widespread Vaccination Program." *American Journal of Epidemiology* 155 (10): 891–96.

Robbins, J., D. W. Towne, E. C. Gotschlich, and R. Schneerson. 1997. "Love's Labours Lost: Failure to Implement Mass Vaccination against Group A Meningococcal Meningitis in Sub-Saharan Africa." *Lancet* 350: 880–82.

Rodrigues, L. 1991. "EPI Target Diseases: Measles, Tetanus, Polio, Tuberculosis, Pertussis, and Diphtheria." In *Disease and Mortality in Sub-Saharan Africa*, ed. R. Feachem and D. Jamison, 173–89. New York: Oxford University Press.

Sabin, A. B. 1951. "Paralytic Consequences of Poliomyelitis Infection in Different Parts of the World and in Different Population Groups." *American Journal of Public Health* 41: 1215–30.

Smith, K. C., and J. Starke. 2004. "Baccille Calmette-Guérin Vaccine." In *Vaccines*, ed. S. A. Plotkin, and W. A. Orenstein. Philadelphia: Saunders.

Stanfield, J. P., and A. Galazka. 1984. "Neonatal Tetanus in the World Today." *Bulletin of the World Health Organization* 62: 647–49.

Strebel, P., M. Papania, and N. Halsey. 2004. "Measles Vaccine." In *Vaccines*, ed. S. A. Plotkin, and W. A. Orenstein. Philadelphia: Saunders.

Sutter, R. W., and O. M. Kew. 2004. "Poliovirus Vaccine-Live." In *Vaccines*, ed. S. A. Plotkin, and W. A. Orenstein, 651–705. Philadelphia: Saunders.

Taylor, C. E., F. Cutts, and M. E. Taylor. 1997. "Ethical Dilemmas in Current Planning for Polio Eradication." *American Journal of Public Health* 87 (6): 922–25.

Tikhomirov, E., M. Santamaria, and K. Esteves. 1997. "Meningococcal Disease: Public Health Burden and Control." *World Health Statistics Quarterly* 50: 170–77.

Wenger, J., and J. Ward. 2004. "*Haemophilus influenza* Vaccine." In *Vaccines*, ed. S. A. Plotkin and W. A. Orenstein, 229–68. Philadelphia: Saunders.

Wharton, M., and C. Vitek. 2004. "Diptheria Toxoid." In *Vaccines*, ed. S. A. Plotkin and W. A. Orenstein, 211–28. Philadelphia: Saunders.

WHA (World Health Assembly). 1992. "Immunization and Vaccine Quality." Forty-Fifth World Health Assembly, Geneva, May 4–14. Resolution WHA45.17, World Health Assembly, Geneva.

WHO (World Health Organization). 1985. "Report of the Expanded Programme on Immunization Global Advisory Group Meeting." WHO/EPI/GEN/87/1, WHO, Geneva.

———. 1997. "Minutes." WHO Informal Consultation on Operational Research on Immunization Prevention and Control Strategies for Meningococcal Disease, Annecy, France, February 18–19. WHO/EMC.97.2, WHO, Geneva.

———. 1998. "Global Programme for Vaccines Immunization." Position Paper on *Haemophilus influenzae* type B conjugate vaccines. *Weekly Epidemiological Record* 73: 64–68.

———. 1999a. *Field Manual for Neonatal Tetanus Elimination*. Geneva: WHO.

———. 1999b. "Pertussis Vaccines." *Weekly Epidemiological Record* 74: 137–44.

———. 1999c. "Progress towards the Global Elimination of Neonatal Tetanus, 1990–1998." *Weekly Epidemiological Record* 74: 73–80.

———. 2001a. *Global Tuberculosis Control: WHO Report 2001*. WHO/CDS/TB/2001.287. Geneva: WHO.

———. 2001b. *Maternal and Neonatal Tetanus Elimination: African Region*. WHO/UNICEF Five Year Regional Plan of Action, 2001–2005. Geneva: WHO.

———. 2003. *WHO Vaccine-Preventable Disease Monitoring System: 2003 Global Summary*. WHO/V&B.03.20. Geneva: WHO.

———. 2004. *The World Health Report 2004—Changing History*. Geneva: WHO.

———. 2006. "Conclusions and Recommendations from the Immunization Strategic Advisory Group." *Weekly Epidemiological Record* 81: 2–11.

WHO (World Health Organization) and UNICEF (United Nations Children's Fund). 1996. *State of the World's Vaccines and Immunization*. Geneva: WHO.

———. 2003. *State of the World's Vaccines and Immunization*. Geneva: WHO.

World Bank. 1993. *World Development Report 1993: Investing in Health*. New York: Oxford University Press.

———. 2003. *World Development Indicators*. Washington, DC: World Bank.

Chapter **13**

Tuberculosis

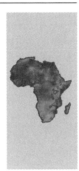

Christopher Dye, Anthony D. Harries, Dermot Maher, S. Mehran Hosseini, Wilfred Nkhoma, and Felix M. Salaniponi

About 9 million people around the world developed tuberculosis (TB) for the first time in 2004, and nearly 2 million people died with or from the disease. Globally, TB is currently responsible for more years of healthy life lost (2.5 percent of all disability-adjusted life years, or DALYs) than any other infectious disease, bar AIDS and malaria (Corbett et al. 2003; WHO 2002; WHO 2006). Only AIDS is responsible for more deaths. The full cost of the worldwide TB epidemic is rarely appreciated. The direct monetary costs of diagnosis and treatment are borne by health services and by patients and their families. Added to these are the indirect costs of lost income and production, incurred when TB patients are too sick to work and when young adults—often parents and householders—die prematurely (WHO 2000). Beyond these losses, baldly expressed in DALYs and dollars, enormous psychological and social costs are associated with TB. These extra costs are less easily quantified, but they are nonetheless real.

A decade ago the problem of TB in Africa attracted little attention, not even meriting a chapter in the first edition of *Disease and Mortality in Sub-Saharan Africa*. Part of the reason was that TB incidence was low and falling in most parts of the continent (Cauthen, Pio, and ten Dam 2002). The burden of TB in Sub-Saharan Africa is far greater today. Continuing poverty and political instability in parts of the continent has inhibited progress in implementing effective TB control measures. But the principal reason for the resurgence of TB in Africa is not the deterioration of control programs. Rather, it is the link between TB and the human immunodeficiency virus and the acquired immune deficiency syndrome (HIV/AIDS). People who are latently infected with *Mycobacterium tuberculosis*—about one-third of the inhabitants of Sub-Saharan Africa (Dye et al. 1999)—are at hugely greater risk of developing active TB if they are also immunologically weakened by a concurrent HIV infection. HIV-positive people are also more likely to develop TB when newly infected or reinfected with *M. tuberculosis*. Over the past decade, the TB caseload has increased by a factor of five or more in those countries of eastern and southern Africa that are most affected by HIV. Incidence rates in these countries are now comparable with those recorded in Europe half a century ago, before the introduction of antituberculosis drugs.

MICROBIOLOGY, TRANSMISSION, AND PATHOGENESIS

M. tuberculosis bacilli transmitted on airborne droplets cause, most importantly, a lung disease that will kill about half of all untreated patients.

Microbiology

The *M. tuberculosis* complex includes five species: *M. tuberculosis, M. bovis* (and bacillus Calmette-Guérin), *M. canetti, M. africanum,* and *M. microti.* Within the species complex, most human disease is due to *M. tuberculosis* sensu stricto. The variants within the species complex differ from the type strain biochemically and in culture. However, these differences have no known bearing on management or prognosis. The principal exception is *M. bovis,* which accounts for a small fraction of human TB cases, but which is naturally resistant to the drug pyrazinamide (which should not therefore be used in treatment).

Human disease can also be caused by species of mycobacteria other than *M. tuberculosis* (MOTT), also known as atypical mycobacteria. These organisms are widespread in nature and have been isolated from a variety of sources, including soil, dust, water, milk, animals, and birds. In humans, MOTT are low-grade pathogens and usually cause disease only in patients with preexisting lung disease or immunodeficiency. MOTT are still a rare cause of disease in Sub-Saharan Africa. The large majority of patients in Africa who are diagnosed and treated for TB, even those infected with HIV, have disease caused by *M. tuberculosis* (Nunn, Elliott, and McAdam 1994).

Mycobacteria are acid and alcohol fast, meaning that once stained by an aniline dye, such as carbolfuchsin, they resist decolorization with acid and alcohol. Mycobacteria are therefore often called "acid-fast bacilli" (AFB). In virtually all other bacteria the dye is removed by the acid-alcohol wash, and the ability of mycobacteria to retain the aniline dye despite acid and alcohol is probably due to their thick cell wall. This property allows the detection of AFB in specimens by using the simple Ziehl-Neelsen (ZN) staining technique, widely used in Sub-Saharan Africa.

Mycobacteria grow slowly, with generation times measured in hours rather than minutes. This means that the normal methods of obtaining cultures from clinical specimens are difficult because of overgrowth by other bacteria. Fortunately, the thick cell wall of mycobacteria also enables them to resist alkalis and detergents, and this property is made use of in culture techniques that use alkalis and special media to reduce contamination.

Transmission and Risk of Infection

People infected with *M. tuberculosis* carry live tubercle bacilli, but the bacilli may be present in small numbers and dormant (latent), in which case there may be no apparent disease. Disease occurs when the bacteria multiply, overcome immune defenses, and become numerous enough to cause damage to tissues.

Patients with pulmonary tuberculosis (PTB) are the most important source of infection. Infection occurs by inhaling droplet nuclei, infectious particles of respiratory secretions usually less than 5 micrometers, which contain tubercle bacilli. These are spread into the air by coughing, sneezing, talking, spitting, and singing, and they can remain suspended in the air for long periods of time. A single cough can produce 3,000 infectious droplet nuclei. Direct sunlight kills tubercle bacilli in minutes, but they can survive in dark, unventilated environments for longer periods of time. Droplet nuclei are so small that they avoid the defenses of the bronchi and penetrate into the terminal alveoli of the lungs, where multiplication and infection begins.

The risk of infection is determined by the infectiousness of the source case (that is, how many tubercle bacilli are being coughed into the air), the closeness of contact, light and humidity, and the immune status of the host (Rieder 1999). Patients with sputum smear-positive pulmonary disease (tubercle bacilli visible under the microscope when appropriate stains are used) are much more infectious than those with smear-negative sputum (Styblo 1991). Following infection, the tubercle bacilli multiply in the lungs, spread to the local lymph nodes, and then to the rest of the body. About six weeks after this primary infection, the body develops an immune response to the tubercle bacilli called delayed hypersensitivity. In the majority of cases, the immune response stops the further multiplication of the tubercle bacilli, and the only evidence of infection is a positive response to an immunological test, of which the most commonly used is the tuberculin skin test (Ewer et al. 2003; Mazurek and Villarino 2003; Von Pirquet 1909).

The proportion of any population infected depends on the rate and duration of exposure, and this varies from one group of people to another. There are, however, some common patterns. Because infection can remain dormant for many years, or because the immunological consequences of infection are long-lasting, infection rates are always observed to increase monotonically with age. Although the infection rates in boys and girls are usually indistinguishable, adult men typically show higher infection rates than adult women. Men probably suffer more from TB than women, not because they are more susceptible to disease, but because they are more exposed to infection.

Pathogenesis

The size of the infecting dose of tubercle bacilli and the immune status of the host determine the risk of progression from infection to disease. When infection progresses to disease, it is manifest as infiltrates and lesions within the lung tissue, enlarged lymph nodes within the chest, pleural effusion, or disease disseminated in other parts of the body. The immune response of the patient results in a pathological lesion, which is characteristically localized, often with extensive tissue destruction and cavitation. These cavitating lesions occur most commonly in the lungs and contain many actively dividing bacilli. Sputum from patients with these lesions is usually smear positive.

If the primary infection resolves, small numbers of tubercle bacilli can remain dormant in scarred areas of the body for many years. Postprimary TB may then occur by the process of endogenous reactivation, and it may arise in any other organ system to which the tubercle bacilli were seeded during the primary infection. Active disease can also follow from secondary or exogenous reinfection in a person who already has a latent infection.

Without HIV coinfection, the average lifetime risk of infected individuals' developing tuberculosis is 5 to 10 percent, the highest risk being within the first five years of infection (Comstock, Livesay, and Woolpert 1974; Sutherland 1976). The risk of developing TB following infection also changes with age. Infants and young children up to the age of five years who are infected with *M. tuberculosis* are at relatively high risk, particularly of severe forms (mainly miliary TB and TB meningitis), because of their immature immune systems. Children between the ages of five and fifteen years are relatively resistant to TB. The risk then rises again through adolescence, remains approximately stable during adulthood, but increases again in the elderly.

Other factors that enhance the risk of developing TB following infection include undernutrition, toxins (tobacco, alcohol, corticosteroids, immunosuppressive drugs), and other diseases (diabetes mellitus, silicosis, leukemia, measles, and whooping cough in children), but none is as important as HIV (Crofton, Horne, and Miller 1999; Rieder 1999).

CLINICAL MANIFESTATIONS AND DIAGNOSIS

Clinical diagnoses of tuberculosis distinguish between pulmonary and extrapulmonary disease, the former being of much greater importance epidemiologically.

Pulmonary Tuberculosis

Patients with pulmonary TB present with a chronic productive cough, fever, and weight loss. Cough occurs in a variety of circumstances, notably in acute upper and lower respiratory infections. However, these acute infections often resolve within three weeks. Therefore a patient with a cough longer than three weeks, which persists after a course of antibiotics, should be investigated for PTB.

The diagnosis of PTB in most hospitals in African countries is based on sputum smear microscopy and chest radiography. Most countries have a reference laboratory where *M. tuberculosis* can be cultured from clinical specimens, such as sputum. Because *M. tuberculosis* is a slow-growing organism taking two to three months to become visible on culture medium, cultures are not usually helpful in making an individual diagnosis. Mycobacterial cultures are commonly used for monitoring drug-sensitivity patterns in patients with recurrent TB and for monitoring the community prevalence of drug-resistant TB.

Taking sputum specimens (three per suspect) for smear microscopy of AFB is a cheap and simple way to screen for PTB. However, sputum smears may be negative in pulmonary TB patients for three reasons. First, the patient has genuine smear-negative pulmonary tuberculosis, that is, expectorating small numbers of AFB. AFB can be detected on microscopy only if there are 10,000 organisms or more per milliliter of sputum. Second, the clinical diagnosis of TB is incorrect and the patient has another condition, such as left ventricular failure, asthma, bacterial pneumonia, *Pneumocystis carinii* pneumonia, or pulmonary Kaposi's sarcoma. Third, the result is a false negative resulting from technical inadequacies (poor sputum sample, faulty smear preparation, inadequate time spent examining the smear) or administrative failures (incorrect labeling of specimens).

If sputum smear examination shows no AFB, patients suspected of having PTB should be referred for chest radiography. Classical patterns of TB with upper lobe disease, bilateral disease, and cavitations are more common in HIV-negative patients and in HIV-positive patients who have relatively well preserved immune function. However, no chest radiographic pattern is absolutely diagnostic of TB (Hargreaves et al. 2001).

Extrapulmonary TB

The common signs or forms of extrapulmonary TB (EPTB) are pleural effusion, lymphadenopathy, pericardial effusion, miliary disease, and meningitis. Patients usually present with constitutional symptoms and local features related to the site of disease. EPTB is found in a higher proportion of female TB patients than male patients. If patients cough for longer than three weeks, sputum smear examination and chest radiography are often carried out, because patients may have coexisting pulmonary disease. Definitive diagnosis of EPTB depends on having diagnostic tools, such as radiographs, ultrasound scans, procedures to obtain and analyze fluid samples, and procedures for tissue biopsies and histological analysis. This degree of diagnostic sophistication is often unavailable in district hospitals in Africa. For example, in one study in Tanzania only 18 percent of patients diagnosed with EPTB had laboratory confirmation of the diagnosis (Richter et al. 1991).

Childhood TB

Children are most commonly infected with *M. tuberculosis* as a result of transmission from an adult (often a family member) with smear-positive disease. Most children remain asymptomatic, and a positive tuberculin test may be the only evidence of infection. For those who do progress to disease, PTB is the most common manifestation in both HIV-infected and HIV-uninfected children, although extrapulmonary disease is more frequent in those who are HIV positive. The patterns of EPTB in children and the diagnostic problems encountered are similar to those described for adults, although meningitis makes up a higher proportion of EPTB cases in young children.

The diagnosis of childhood PTB has always been difficult because children rarely produce sputum for smear examination. Diagnosis therefore usually requires a combination of clinical features, history of contact with a sputum-positive case, growth faltering, chest X-ray, and tuberculin skin test. Chest X-ray findings on their own are nonspecific, as are clinical features, but the most important symptoms are weight loss and poor appetite. Gastric aspiration, induced sputum, and nasopharyngeal aspiration show promise as alternative diagnostic techniques but are not practical under routine clinical conditions in Africa.

Given the problems with diagnosis and the low frequency of routine childhood screening, the real burden of childhood TB in Sub-Saharan Africa is not known. One nationwide study in Malawi found that 12 percent of all registered TB cases were children less than 15 years of age (Harries, Hargreaves, Graham et al. 2001). Such investigations are a useful starting point for much-needed, population-based studies of the burden of TB in children.

Consequences of HIV Coinfection

Untreated HIV infection causes a progressive decline in the number of CD4$^+$ T lymphocytes and progressive dysfunction of those lymphocytes that survive. CD4$^+$ cells play a major role in the body's defense against tubercle bacilli, and it is therefore not surprising that HIV infection is the most powerful known risk factor for progression to active disease in those with a latent *M. tuberculosis* infection. In HIV-positive people infected with *M. tuberculosis* the annual risk of developing active disease is 5 to 15 percent, with a lifetime risk of 50 percent or higher (Lienhardt and Rodrigues 1997; Raviglione et al. 1997; Rieder et al. 1989). HIV-infected people are also more susceptible to new tuberculous infections (Di Perri et al. 1989) and to reinfection, and they progress more frequently and more quickly to overt disease (Sonnenberg et al. 2001). After the end of a primary episode, HIV increases the likelihood that TB will recur (Fitzgerald, Desvarieux et al. 2000), either by reactivation (true relapse) or reinfection (Daley 1993).

People who are coinfected with *M. tuberculosis* and HIV can develop TB across a wide spectrum of immunodeficiency (Ackah et al. 1995; Mukadi et al. 1993), but the risk of developing active disease increases as the CD4$^+$ cell count declines (figure 13.1). HIV-positive patients with moderate to severe immunosuppression show atypical forms of TB, which complicates radiographic diagnosis. Some HIV-infected TB patients have normal chest radiographs and negative sputum smears, and the diagnosis may therefore be missed unless there are pronounced clinical signs or symptoms. Among children, the highest rates of HIV infection are observed in those age one to four years, and the accurate diagnosis of TB has become especially difficult in this age group (Graham, Coulter, and Gilks 2001). In children and adults who are infected with *M. tuberculosis* and who are also HIV positive, immunosuppression frequently leads to negative tuberculin skin tests.

The presentation of HIV-related EPTB is generally no different from that of HIV-negative EPTB, although there are sometimes complications. The enlargement of TB

Figure 13.1 Relative Incidence of TB in HIV-Infected Individuals as a Function of CD4$^+$ Cell Count

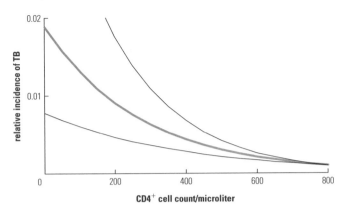

Source: Williams and Dye 2003.

Note: TB incidence is nominally set to 100 per 100,000 people at 800 CD4$^+$ per microliter. The middle line is the best estimate, and the outer lines, 95 percent confidence limits (CL), were obtained from a combined analysis of data from three separate studies.

lymph nodes in HIV-positive patients can occasionally be rapid and resemble an acute abscess. It is possible that a diagnosis of miliary or disseminated TB is regularly missed. Diagnosis is often more difficult in patients who are severely immunosuppressed. For example, disseminated TB was diagnosed only after death in 44 percent of patients with HIV wasting syndrome in Côte d'Ivoire; TB was not recognized during life (Lucas et al. 1994).

EPIDEMIOLOGY

About one-third of the population of Sub-Saharan Africa is infected with *M. tuberculosis* (Dye et al. 1999). In the year 2000, an estimated 17 million people in Sub-Saharan Africa were infected with both *M. tuberculosis* and HIV—70 percent of all people co-infected worldwide (Corbett et al. 2003). As more people have become infected and coinfected with HIV, especially in eastern and southern Africa, the incidence of TB has been driven upward, as reflected in estimates derived from population-based surveys and from routine TB surveillance data (figures 13.2 and 13.3) (WHO 2002, 2006). In 2004, the incidence rate of TB in the WHO African region was growing at approximately 3 percent per year (table 13.1), and at 4 percent per year in eastern and southern Africa (the areas most affected by HIV), faster than on any other continent, and considerably faster than the 1 percent per year global increase (WHO 2006). In several African countries, including those with well-organized control programs (Harries et al. 1996; Kenyon et al. 1999), annual TB case-notification rates have risen more than fivefold since the mid-1980s, reaching more than 400 cases per 100,000 people (WHO 2006). HIV infection is the most important single predictor of TB incidence across the African continent (figure 13.4). Despite the emphasis placed

Figure 13.2 Estimated Incidence Rates of New TB Cases and Percentages of TB Patients Infected with HIV, by Country, 2004

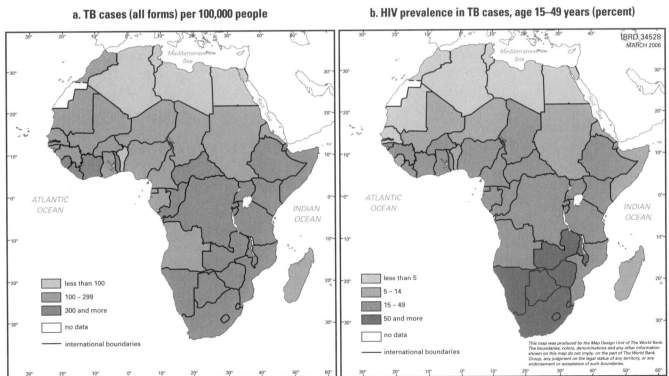

Source: Data from WHO 2006.

Figure 13.3 Trends in TB (All Forms) Case Notifications in the WHO African Region Contrasted with Trends in Other Parts of the World

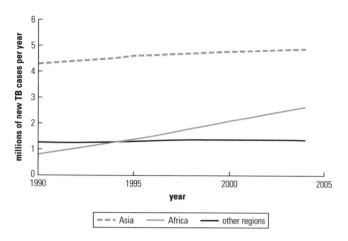

Source: Data from WHO 2006.

Note: Asia includes the WHO Southeast Asia and Western Pacific regions.

Figure 13.4 Estimated TB Incidence in Relation to Estimated HIV Prevalence in Adults Age 15 to 49 for 42 Countries in the WHO African Region
(per 100,000 people)

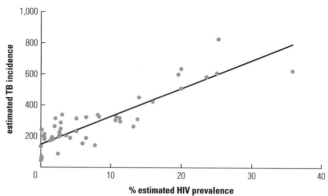

Source: Corbett et al. 2003.

Table 13.1 The Contribution of Sub-Saharan Africa to the Global TB Epidemic

	Estimated New Cases of TB				HIV-related TB			Deaths				
	Population (millions)	New cases of TB (thousands)	Incidence rate (per 100,000 per year)	Increase in incidence rate 2003–2004 (% per year)	HIV prevalence in new adult cases (%)	No. of adult TB cases attributable to HIV (thousands)	Adult TB cases attributable of HIV (%)	Deaths from TB (thousands)	Deaths from TB (per 100,000)	Deaths from TB in HIV-infected adults (thousands)	TB deaths attributable to HIV (%)	HIV/AIDS deaths attributable to TB, 2003 (%)
WHO African Region	722	2,573	356	3	33	600	28	587	81	206	32	11
Rest of the world	5,665	6,345	112	−1	3	141	3	1,106	20	43	4	8
Global	6,387	8,918	140	1	13	741	12	1,693	27	248	14	11

Source: WHO estimates for 2004, updated from Corbett et al. 2003.

on finding smear-positive cases under DOTS and the new WHO Stop TB Strategy (Raviglione and Uplekar, forthcoming), the proportion of cases reported to be smear-positive has fallen in recent years in several African countries with high rates of HIV. Although there are uncertainties about diagnosis, these data conform with the expectation that there will be more smear-negative TB where there is more HIV. Because HIV infection rates are higher in women than men, more TB cases are also being reported among women, especially those between the ages of 15 and 24 years. TB case reports are typically male-biased (WHO 2006), but in several African countries with high rates of HIV infection, the majority of notified TB cases are now women.

The increase in HIV prevalence has also been accompanied by a rise in the TB case-fatality rate, and hence the TB death rate in the general population. One recent estimate put the fraction of AIDS deaths due to TB at 12 percent in the WHO African region in 2000 (Corbett et al. 2003), although this fraction could be higher. In an autopsy study in Abidjan, Côte d'Ivoire, TB was found to be the cause of death of 54 percent of patients with HIV infection or AIDS (Lucas et al. 1993). Malawi has reported high early death rates of HIV-infected TB patients during the first one to two months of treatment (Harries, Hargreaves, Gausi et al. 2001). Whether this reflects late presentation and consequently severe TB disease or severe HIV-related illness,

Figure 13.5 Prevalence of HIV in TB Cases (All Forms) in Relation to HIV Prevalence in Adults Age 15 to 49

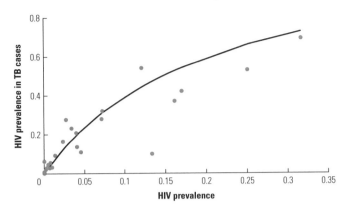

Source: Corbett et al. 2003.

Note: Each point represents a different African population in which HIV prevalence was measured both in TB patients and in the adult population. The fitted line estimates the incidence-rate ratio to be 5.8 (95 percent CL, 5.2–6.5), that is, the ratio of TB incidence rates in HIV-infected and HIV-uninfected populations.

such as bacteremia or cryptococcal meningitis, is not known. The precise cause of death in patients with HIV-related TB has been difficult to determine because there have been so few autopsy studies.

Although the ratio of TB incidence rates in HIV-infected and HIV-uninfected individuals is expected to vary during the course of the HIV epidemic (as the average level of immunocompetence declines), recent studies have shown that this incidence-rate ratio takes an average value of about six (figure 13.5) (WHO 2002). Knowing both the incidence-rate ratio and the HIV infection rate in the general population, we can calculate the proportion of people newly diagnosed with TB who are infected with HIV. Estimates vary widely between countries, from less than 1 percent on some African islands (for example, Comoros, Mauritius) to over 50 percent in some countries, including Botswana, Malawi, South Africa, Zambia, and Zimbabwe. Overall, about one-third (34 percent) of all adults who had TB in Sub-Saharan Africa were infected with HIV in 2004.

Resistance to Antituberculosis Drugs

Drug resistance, and eventually multidrug resistance (MDR-TB; that is, resistance to at least isoniazid and rifampicin), is expected to occur whenever patients fail a course of anti-TB chemotherapy. An assessment of the number and distribution of drug-resistant TB cases is important for planning TB control, because the treatment of resistant cases is more costly and more complex if second-line drugs are used, and failures and deaths are more frequent.

Surveys coordinated by the WHO and the International Union against TB and Lung Disease (IUATLD) between 1996 and 2002 yielded data on anti-TB drug resistance among new and previously treated cases from sites in 10 countries in Sub-Saharan Africa (Espinal et al. 2001; WHO 2004a). This limited number of surveys suggests that MDR-TB is not a widespread problem in the region. Low resistance rates (MDR-TB prevalence typically less than 3 percent among patients suffering a first episode of TB) could be explained by the recent introduction of rifampicin in Africa, by the use of rifampicin-free treatment regimens in the continuation phase (during months three to eight), by the growing use of directly observed treatment as recommended under the directly observed treatment, short course (DOTS) strategy, and by the use of fixed-dose combination tablets in a few countries (Espinal et al. 2001).

Implementation of the DOTS Strategy for Tuberculosis Control

Population Coverage, Case Detection, and Treatment Outcome. The key components of the WHO Stop TB Strategy are listed in box 13.1. The new strategy builds on the foundations laid by DOTS, and the main aim is still to prevent illness, transmission, and death by curing active TB cases (Raviglione and Uplekar, forthcoming; WHO 2006). With respect to the implementation of DOTS, the primary goals of national TB programs are to detect 70 percent of new smear-positive cases arising each year and to successfully treat 85 percent of these. The target year was set by WHO to be 2005, but the achievements made by 2005 will not be fully known until the end of 2006. With the correct application of antituberculosis drugs (short-course chemotherapy), it is possible to cure over 90 percent of new smear-positive TB patients who are neither resistant to first-line drugs nor infected with HIV. Before the spread of HIV, countries that met these two targets could expect to see a decline in TB incidence rates of 5 to 10 percent per year or more (Dye et al. 1998).

By the end of 2004, the core DOTS strategy was available in principle to 84 percent of people living in the WHO African region (WHO 2006). The estimated case detection rate by DOTS programs was 48 percent, somewhat below the global average of 53 percent, and not increasing as quickly as the global average (figure 13.6). However, much uncertainty surrounds this assessment of case detection. First, for countries that have estimates of the true TB incidence rate based on population surveys, these are typically

Box 13.1 The WHO Stop TB Strategy

Vision: A world free of TB

Goal: To dramatically reduce the global burden of TB by 2015 in line with the Millennium Development Goals and the Stop TB Partnership targets

Objectives:

- Achieve universal access to high-quality diagnosis and patient-centered treatment
- Reduce the human suffering and socioeconomic burden associated with TB
- Protect poor and vulnerable populations from TB, TB/HIV, and multidrug-resistant TB
- Support development of new tools and enable their timely and effective use

Targets: • MDG 6, Target 8: Halt and begin to reverse the incidence of TB by 2015

- Targets linked to the MDGs and endorsed by the Stop TB Partnership:
  - By 2005: detect at least 70% of new sputum smear-positive TB cases and cure at least 85% of these cases
  - By 2015: reduce TB prevalence and deaths rates by 50% relative to 1990
  - By 2050: eliminate TB as a public health problem (1 case per million population)

Components of the strategy and implementation approaches

1. **Pursue high-quality DOTS expansion and enhancement**
   a. Political commitment with increased and sustained financing
   b. Case detection through quality-assured bacteriology
   c. Standardized treatment with supervision and patient support
   d. An effective drug supply and management system
   e. Monitoring and evaluation system, and impact measurement

2. **Address TB/HIV, MDR-TB, and other challenges**
   - Implement collaborative TB/HIV activities
   - Prevent and control multidrug-resistant TB
   - Address prisoners, refugees, and other high-risk groups, and special situations

3. **Contribute to health system strengthening**
   - Actively participate in efforts to improve systemwide policy, human resources, financing, management, service delivery, and information systems
   - Share innovations that strengthen systems, including the Practical Approach to Lung Health (PAL)
   - Adapt innovations from other fields

4. **Engage all care providers**
   - Public–Public and Public–Private Mix (PPM) approaches
   - International Standards for Tuberculosis Care (ISTC)

5. **Empower people with TB, and communities**
   - Advocacy, communication, and social mobilization
   - Community participation in TB care
   - Patients' Charter for Tuberculosis Care

6. **Enable and promote research**
   - Programme-based operational research
   - Research to develop new diagnostics, drugs, and vaccines

Source: Raviglione and Uplekar 2006.

Figure 13.6 Progress toward the Target of 70 Percent Case Detection in the WHO African Region, Compared with the Average Progress Worldwide
(percent)

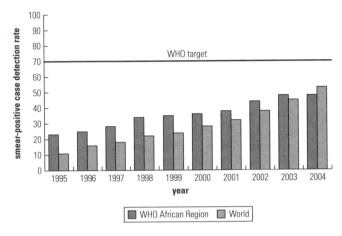

Source: Data from WHO 2006.

tuberculin surveys of the prevalence (and hence, risk) of infection carried out before the emergence of HIV (Cauthen, Pio, and ten Dam 2002). Few countries have surveyed the prevalence of infection during the last decade, the exceptions being Kenya (Odhiambo et al. 1999) and Tanzania (Tanzanian Tuberculin Survey Collaboration 2001). There are no recent national surveys in Africa of the prevalence of active TB. For the many African countries that have no survey data at all, the estimate of case detection is little more than an expert guess, based on what is known (mostly qualitatively) about the method of surveillance. Second, the apparent upward trend in case detection could be explained partly by improved case finding and partly by the real rise in incidence due to HIV. In sum, the data describing incidence rates and their trends, and, hence, case-detection rates, are poor for most African countries.

The outcome of treatment in the African region is somewhat clearer. The treatment success rate for more than 480,000 smear-positive patients enrolled under DOTS in 2003 was 72 percent (WHO 2006). Treatment success under DOTS in Africa was low in part because the death rate was 7 percent, higher than in any other region of the world. More important was the large proportion of patients for whom the outcome of treatment was not known: 20 percent of patients defaulted from treatment, were transferred to other treatment centers without follow-up, or were simply not evaluated. It is highly likely that death was the outcome for some patients recorded as defaulters or transfers. Although the high reported death rates might be attributable

to HIV coinfection in some countries, the failure to record treatment outcomes is evidently a problem of program management. It would be extremely useful to have comprehensive and reliable data on TB deaths and their trends in African populations, but no country in Sub-Saharan Africa, except South Africa, has a national system for recording and reporting deaths by cause.

Treatment of TB Patients Infected with HIV. HIV-positive TB patients suffer significant HIV-related morbidity during the course of TB treatment. Adverse reactions to anti-TB drugs are more frequent and lead to treatment interruptions and fatalities (Raviglione et al. 1997). Several studies in Africa have reported an increase in recurrent TB in HIV-positive patients (Korenromp et al. 2003), and national programs with good registration systems routinely record high rates of recurrent disease.

HIV-positive TB patients have a much higher mortality rate during and after anti-TB treatment than HIV-negative patients (Mukadi, Maher, and Harries 2001). This may change with wider use of antiretroviral (ARV) therapy, but clinical studies have shown that, without ARV therapy, 20 to 30 percent of HIV-positive and smear-positive PTB patients die before the end of treatment, and about 25 percent of those who survive die during the following 12 months. The immune status of a patient is an important predictor of death: lower CD4$^+$ cell counts at the time of diagnosis in HIV-positive and smear-positive patients are associated with higher mortality rates (Graham, Coulter, and Gilks 2001). HIV-positive patients who present with smear-negative PTB have higher case-fatality rates during treatment than those who present with smear-positive PTB, probably because they are typically more immunosuppressed.

HIV-infected patients given drug regimens with no rifampicin have higher case-fatality rates, and higher relapse rates, than those given regimens with rifampicin (Korenromp et al. 2003). Rifampicin-containing regimens improve survival, possibly because they act more strongly against *M. tuberculosis* and, through the broad spectrum antibiotic activity of rifampicin, they may prevent other bacterial infections.

Notwithstanding the problems of implementation, DOTS has made a bigger contribution to the management of TB in Africa than any other strategy (for example, bacillus Calmette-Guérin [BCG] vaccination). DOTS has been enlarged as the new Stop TB Strategy, in part to confront the complexities that HIV adds to TB epidemiology (Raviglione and Uplekar, forthcoming; box 13.1).

The Stop TB Strategy must be implemented in Africa by improving the population coverage of DOTS and by adding other key elements, including intensified TB case finding, TB preventive treatment, HIV testing and ARV therapy for TB patients, and various interventions against HIV (and therefore indirectly against TB) (De Cock and Chaisson 1999; Maher, Floyd, and Raviglione 2002). The Global Plan to Stop TB 2006–2015 (Stop TB Partnership and WHO 2006) is a blueprint for the implementation of the Stop TB Strategy in all regions of the world, including Africa. Implementation of this wider strategy should complement efforts to improve the basic tools for TB control, such as a more efficacious vaccine (http://www.aeras.org; Young and Dye forthcoming), more accurate diagnostic tests (http://www.finddiagnostics.org.), and better drugs for prevention and treatment (http://www.tballiance.org).

Intensified TB Case Finding. DOTS has traditionally relied on passive case detection. It is possible that more cases could be found by searching more actively among certain population groups, although the evidence that active case finding can yield more cases at acceptable cost remains weak. Groups that might be targeted in Africa for improved case finding include people with respiratory symptoms attending general hospitals (outpatients and inpatients); health service providers and health care workers in the public, private, and nongovernmental organization (NGO) sectors (Harries, Maher, and Nunn 1997); people attending centers for HIV testing and voluntary counseling (Aisu et al. 1995); prisoners (Coninx et al. 2000); and household contacts of those with infectious TB, including patients and contacts known to be HIV positive (Nunn et al. 1994). The screening of child contacts, often neglected, can be an important benefit to individual children, although, because children with TB are usually not infective to others, it will not decrease transmission (Topley, Maher, and Nyong'onya Mbewe 1996).

TB Preventive Treatment. Individuals at high risk of developing TB can benefit from preventive treatment, usually six months of isoniazid. Isoniazid preventive treatment (IPT) is recommended for children who are household contacts of an infectious case of TB and who, after screening, are found not to have active TB themselves (Harries and Maher 2004). Up to 15 percent of tuberculin-positive, HIV-positive adults will develop TB each year (WHO 1999), and IPT can reduce the short-term risk of TB in this group by about 60 percent, although there is little improvement in survival (Quigley et al. 2001). IPT may also be valuable for HIV-infected individuals even without tuberculin testing.

IPT probably protects HIV-positive people from active TB by reducing the risk of progression from recent and latent infection. Where the transmission rate of *M. tuberculosis* is relatively high, repeated exposure to infection probably accounts for the limited duration of benefit of up to 2.5 years (Quigley et al. 2001) following completion of a six-month course of IPT. Not surprisingly, the duration of protection depends on the duration of preventive treatment (Fitzgerald, Morse et al. 2000).

Although cheap, IPT is at present used mostly for the protection of individuals, rather than to prevent transmission. This is because children rarely develop infectious TB, and because it is hard to administer IPT to healthy adults on a large scale. Because IPT requires consumption of the drug daily for at least six months, a process that is difficult for health services and patients alike, many people who could benefit from treatment drop out before completion. The proportion of HIV-infected people who do complete a course of IPT is typically small. For IPT to be effective in preventing a large number of TB cases associated with HIV, it will be necessary to find ways of minimizing the dropout rate and to expand the provision of voluntary counseling services for HIV-positive patients (Hawken and Muhindi 1999).

IPT can also prevent TB from recurring in patients who have already suffered one episode. Studies by Perriens and colleagues (1995) in the Democratic Republic of Congo (formerly Zaire) and by Fitzgerald, Desvarieux, and colleagues (2000) in Haiti showed a higher rate of recurrent TB in HIV-infected individuals than in non-HIV-infected individuals treated with a six-month regimen containing rifampicin throughout (the regimen used in the study in the Democratic Republic of Congo had a four-drug initial phase and that in Haiti had a three-drug initial phase). In both studies, posttreatment prophylaxis (isoniazid and rifampicin in the study in the Democratic Republic of Congo and isoniazid in the study in Haiti) decreased the number of TB recurrences in HIV-positive patients but did not prolong survival. Based on these successes, further studies are needed before posttreatment prophylaxis can be used more widely; they must confirm the benefits, establish optimum regimens (drugs and duration), and assess operational feasibility.

BCG Immunization. Most of the 75 percent of infants in Africa who were vaccinated with BCG in 2003 (WHO 2004b) will be protected against disseminated and severe TB (for example, meningeal and miliary TB) for the first few years of their lives (WHO 1995). The efficacy of BCG against severe forms of TB in children is 70 to 80 percent, but it takes about 3,400 inoculations to prevent one case of meningitis and 9,300 inoculations to prevent one case of miliary TB (Bourdin Trunz, Fine, and Dye forthcoming). However, most people who are vaccinated as children in Africa will not be protected against pulmonary TB as adults, because the vaccine is unlikely to protect for longer than 15 years and, in many populations, has low efficacy against adult pulmonary disease. Even though BCG is not expected to have any significant impact in reducing transmission and incidence, the WHO recommends vaccination for all neonates in Africa, except those with symptoms of HIV disease or AIDS (WHO 1996).

Interventions against HIV. In pilot projects, controlled trials, and national programs in less-developed countries, all of the following interventions have been shown to be effective in preventing HIV infection: increased condom use, treatment of sexually transmitted infections, reduction in the number of sexual partners, safe injections, and drugs to prevent mother-to-child transmission of HIV (Merson, Dayton, and O'Reilly 2000). If HIV control programs can encourage the use of, or provide greater access to, these interventions, we can expect concomitant reductions in the burden of HIV-related TB. However, in a comparative modeling analysis of DOTS and various other strategies to control TB and HIV-related TB, incidence and death rates were far more sensitive to improvements in TB case detection and cure than to the introduction of TB preventive therapy and ARV therapy, even when rates of HIV infection are high (figure 13.7) (Currie et al. 2003).

Although ARV therapy can prevent TB by preserving or restoring immunity, early therapy plus high levels of coverage and compliance will be needed to avert a significant fraction of TB cases (figure 13.8). The reason is that TB emerges as an AIDS-related illness at a median CD4$^+$ cell count of about 250 per micrometer (Williams and Dye 2003). Beginning ARV therapy at 200 per microliter in the absence of an AIDS-related illness (WHO 2003) means that a high proportion of HIV-infected people that are destined to develop TB will progress to active disease before they are offered ARV therapy. Nonetheless, ARV therapy could greatly extend the lives of HIV-infected TB patients, and the

Figure 13.7 Expected Reductions in the Number of TB Cases in Kenya over 10 Years

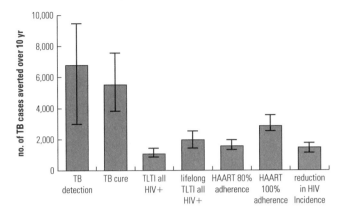

Source: Currie et al. 2003.

Note: TLTI = treatment of latent TB infection; HAART = highly active antiretroviral therapy. Reductions (±95 percent CL) based on increase in coverage of each intervention by 1 percent over present values (i.e., 50 percent case detection, 70 percent cure, zero otherwise) and on stabilization of HIV prevalence at the estimated value of 14 percent among adults age 15 to 49.

Figure 13.8 Proportional Reduction in the Incidence of TB over 20 Years among HIV-Positives as a Function of Effective Coverage and the CD4$^+$ Count per Microliter at Which People Start ARV Therapy

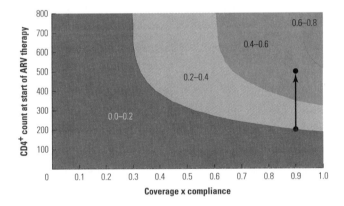

Source: Adapted from Williams and Dye 2003.

Note: Shaded areas of the graph show proportional reductions in lifetime risk of TB. ARV therapy is assumed to reduce the incidence of TB to the level immediately after seroconversion. Even with 90 percent effective coverage, we can expect no more than a 20 percent reduction in incidence if patients begin therapy at 200 CD4$^+$ cells per microliter (lower point, at base of arrow). Beginning at 500 CD4$^+$ cells per microliter would prevent 40 to 60 percent of TB cases (upper point, at tip of arrow).

diagnosis of TB could provide an important entry point for the treatment of HIV/AIDS.

Besides efficacy, we must also consider affordability and value for money. DOTS was known to be a relatively low-cost and cost-effective strategy to improve health before the emergence of HIV/AIDS (Murray et al. 1991). Among the diversity of interventions available under the Stop TB Strategy, the detection and treatment of active TB cases is still the most cost-effective approach to TB control in Africa (Currie et al. 2005).

Cotrimoxazole Prophylaxis. Prophylaxis against common intercurrent infections (for example, bacterial causes of pneumonia and diarrhea and their complications) is another way to decrease the morbidity and mortality rates of HIV-infected TB patients. Two studies in Côte d'Ivoire have shown a beneficial effect of cotrimoxazole. One found that the drug reduced deaths of HIV-infected TB patients by 48 percent; the other showed a significant reduction in morbidity, but not mortality (Anglaret et al. 1999; Wiktor et al. 1999). As a result, cotrimoxazole prophylaxis has been provisionally recommended for HIV-infected individuals in Africa as part of the minimum package of care (UNAIDS 2001). In Malawi, voluntary counseling and HIV testing for TB patients, with treatment including cotrimoxazole, reduced case-fatality rates by almost 20 percent compared with a control group (Zachariah et al. 2003). Further studies in other sites are necessary to confirm and evaluate the benefits and the duration of effectiveness, and the feasibility of using cotrimoxazole under routine conditions.

CONCLUSION

Before HIV infection and AIDS emerged and spread in Africa, TB incidence rates were typically under 100 per 100,000 persons per year and falling. HIV has turned a slow decline into a rapid resurgence, especially in eastern and southern Africa. However, the worst HIV epidemics are now almost certainly decelerating, and even turning downward in some countries (UNAIDS and WHO 2005). Because the interval between HIV infection and the onset of TB is four to six years, we can expect TB incidence rates to continue increasing for some years in some African countries. But we are now, at least, in a position to evaluate the maximum size of the TB problem created by HIV in Africa. Beyond peak TB incidence rates, the future of TB in Africa will remain unpredictable as long as the direction of HIV epidemics is also unknown. Will the significant reduction in HIV infection documented in Uganda (Parkhurst 2002) be replicated across eastern and southern Africa? Or can we expect HIV infection rates in other countries to stabilize at close to peak levels?

As the spread of HIV infection and AIDS adds to the complexity of health care, studies that can identify the limiting factors in TB control will have great value. The national TB program managers of some African countries have attempted to identify the main constraints to improving their program's performance (WHO 2006), but the list in box 13.2 needs to be refined, quantified, and customized for different countries. More money is needed for TB control, as set out in the Global Plan to Stop TB 2006–2015 (Stop TB Partnership and WHO 2006) but money is not the only essential commodity. The mechanisms to identify other necessary materials and processes will include better analyses of the abundant surveillance data that have already been collected by national TB programs. Good operational research, which need not be costly or complex, will also suggest ways to improve the performance of the programs. For example, following investigations in several African countries, it is now clear that community-based care can give, under a wide range of circumstances, satisfactory treatment results at lower cost (Floyd et al. 2003; Moalosi et al. 2003; Nganda et al. 2003; Okello et al. 2003; Sinanovic 2003). Pragmatic field studies must continue to explore better ways of using the current tools for TB control as new vaccines, drugs, and diagnostics begin to emerge from laboratories.

Whatever the impact of HIV on TB in the next few years, African countries will continue to need vigorous TB control programs that fully implement the new Stop TB Strategy, founded on DOTS. Even with high rates of HIV infection, DOTS implementation is relatively cheap and cost-effective.

Other methods for the prevention and treatment of HIV and AIDS will be needed too, but they should be introduced in ways that will be complementary to DOTS. Tuberculosis and HIV control programs now clearly have mutual concerns: the prevention of HIV infection and the treatment of AIDS should be components of TB control, and TB care and prevention should be priorities in the management of HIV/AIDS. Until recently, TB programs and HIV/AIDS programs have pursued separate courses. They can no longer afford to do so.

REFERENCES

Ackah, A. N., D. Coulibaly, H. Digbeu, K. Diallo, K. M. Vetter, I. M. Coulibaly, A. E. Greenberg, and K. M. De Cock. 1995. "Response to Treatment, Mortality, and CD4 Lymphocyte Counts in HIV-Infected Persons with Tuberculosis in Abidjan, Cote d'Ivoire." *Lancet* 345: 607–10.

Aisu, T., M. C. Raviglione, E. van Praag, P. Eriki, J. P. Narain, L. Barugahare, G. Tembo, D. McFarland, and F. A. Engwau. 1995. "Preventive Chemotherapy for HIV-Associated Tuberculosis in Uganda: An Operational Assessment at a Voluntary Counselling and Testing Centre." *AIDS* 9: 267–73.

Anglaret, X., G. Chene, A. Attia, S. Toure, S. Lafont, P. Combe, K. Manlan, T. N'Dri-Yoman, and R. Salamon. 1999. "Early Chemoprophylaxis with Trimethoprim-Sulphamethoxole for HIV-1-Infected Adults in Abidjan, Côte d'Ivoire: A Randomized Trial." *Lancet* 353: 1463–68.

Bourdin Trunz, B., P. E. M. Fine, and C. Dye. Forthcoming. "Global Impact of BCG Vaccination on Childhood Tuberculous Meningitis and Miliary Tuberculosis." *Lancet*.

Cauthen, G. M., A. Pio, and H. G. ten Dam. 2002. "Annual Risk of Tuberculous Infection. 1988." *Bulletin of the World Health Organization* 80: 503–11.

Comstock, G. W., V. T. Livesay, and S. F. Woolpert. 1974. "The Prognosis of a Positive Tuberculin Reaction in Childhood and Adolescence." *American Journal of Epidemiology* 99: 131–38.

Coninx, R., D. Maher, H. Reyes, and M. Grzemska. 2000. "Tuberculosis in Prisons in Countries with High Prevalence." *British Medical Journal* 320: 440–42.

Corbett, E. L., C. J. Watt, N. Walker, D. Maher, B. G. Williams, M. C. Raviglione, and C. Dye. 2003. "The Growing Burden of Tuberculosis: Global Trends and Interactions with the HIV Epidemic." *Archives of Internal Medicine* 163: 1009–21.

Crofton, J., N. Horne, and F. Miller. 1999. *Clinical Tuberculosis*, 2nd ed. London: Macmillan Education.

Currie, C. S., K. Floyd, B. G. Williams, and C. Dye. 2005. "Cost, Affordability and Cost-effectiveness of Strategies to Control Tuberculosis in Countries with High HIV Prevalence." *BMC Public Health* 5: 130.

Currie, C. S. M., B. G. Williams, R. C. Cheng, and C. Dye. 2003. "Tuberculosis Epidemics Driven by HIV: Is Prevention Better Than Cure?" *AIDS* 17: 2501–8.

Daley, C. L. 1993. "Tuberculosis Recurrence in Africa: True Relapse or Re-infection?" *Lancet* 342: 756–57.

De Cock, K. M., and R. E. Chaisson. 1999. "Will DOTS Do It? A Reappraisal of Tuberculosis Control in Countries with High Rates of HIV Infection." *International Journal of Tuberculosis and Lung Disease* 3: 457–65.

Di Perri, G., M. Cruciani, M. C. Danzi, R. Luzzati, G. De Checchi, M. Malena, S. Pizzighella, et al. 1989. "Nosocomial Epidemic of Active Tuberculosis in HIV Infected Patients." *Lancet* 2: 1502–4.

Dye, C., G. P. Garnett, K. Sleeman, and B. G. Williams. 1998. "Prospects for Worldwide Tuberculosis Control under the WHO DOTS Strategy. Directly Observed Short-Course Therapy." *Lancet* 352: 1886–91.

Dye, C., S. Scheele, P. Dolin, V. Pathania, and M. C. Raviglione. 1999. "Global Burden of Tuberculosis: Estimated Incidence, Prevalence and Mortality by Country." *Journal of the American Medical Association* 282: 677–86.

Espinal, M. A., A. Laszlo, L. Simonsen, F. Boulahbal, S. J. Kim, A. Reniero, S. Hoffner, et al. 2001. "Global Trends in Resistance to Anti-TB Drugs." *New England Journal of Medicine* 344: 1294–1303.

Ewer, K., J. Deeks, L. Alvarez, G. Bryant, S. Waller, P. Andersen, P. Monk, and A. Lalvani. 2003. "Comparison of T-Cell-Based Assay with Tuberculin Skin Test for Diagnosis of Mycobacterium Tuberculosis Infection in a School Tuberculosis Outbreak." *Lancet* 361: 1168–73.

Fitzgerald, D. W., M. Desvarieux, P. Severe, P. Joseph, W. D. Johnson Jr., and J. W. Pape. 2000. "Effect of Post-Treatment Isoniazid on Prevention of Recurrent Tuberculosis in HIV-1-Infected Individuals: A Randomised Trial." *Lancet* 356: 1470–74.

Fitzgerald, D. W., M. M. Morse, J. W. Pape, and W. D. Johnson Jr. 2000. "Active Tuberculosis in Individuals Infected with Human Immunodeficiency Virus after Isoniazid Prophylaxis." *Clinical Infectious Diseases* 31: 1495–97.

Floyd, K., J. Skeva, T. Nyirenda, F. Gausi, and F. Salaniponi. 2003. "Cost and Cost-Effectiveness of Increased Community and Primary Care Facility Involvement in Tuberculosis Care in Lilongwe District, Malawi." *International Journal of Tuberculosis and Lung Disease* 7 (9 Suppl. 1): S29–37.

Graham, S. M., J. B. S. Coulter, and C. F. Gilks. 2001. "Pulmonary Disease in HIV-Infected African Children." *International Journal of Tuberculosis and Lung Disease* 5: 12–23.

Hargreaves, N. J., O. Kadzakumanja, S. Phiri, C. H. Lee, X. Tang, F. M. Salaniponi, A. D. Harries, and S. B. Squire. 2001. "What Causes Smear-Negative Pulmonary Tuberculosis in Malawi, an Area of High HIV Seroprevalence?" *International Journal of Tuberculosis and Lung Disease* 5: 1–10.

Harries, A. D., N. J. Hargreaves, F. Gausi, J. H. Kwanjana, and F. M. Salaniponi. 2001. "High Early Death Rate in Tuberculosis Patients in Malawi." *International Journal of Tuberculosis and Lung Disease* 5: 1000–05.

Harries, A. D., N. J. Hargreaves, S. M. Graham, C. Mwansambo, P. Kazembe, R. L. Broadhead, D. Maher, and F. M. Salaniponi. 2001. "Childhood Tuberculosis in Malawi: Nationwide Case-Finding and Treatment Outcomes." *International Journal of Tuberculosis and Lung Disease* 6: 424–31.

Harries, A. D., and D. Maher. 2004. *TB/HIV: A Clinical Manual*. 2nd ed. WHO/HTM/TB/2004.329. Geneva: WHO.

Harries, A. D., D. Maher, and P. Nunn. 1997. "Practical and Affordable Measures for the Protection of Health Care Workers from Tuberculosis in Low-Income Countries." *Bulletin of the World Health Organization* 75: 477–89.

Harries, A. D., L. Nyong'Onya Mbewe, F. M. Salaniponi, D. S. Nyangulu, J. Veen, T. Ringdal, and P. Nunn. 1996. "Tuberculosis Programme Changes and Treatment Outcomes in Patients with Smear-Positive Pulmonary Tuberculosis in Blantyre, Malawi." *Lancet* 347: 807–9.

Hawken, M., and D. W. Muhindi. 1999. "Tuberculosis Preventive Therapy in HIV-Infected Persons: Feasibility Issues in Developing Countries." *International Journal of Tuberculosis and Lung Disease* 3: 646–50.

Kenyon, T. A., M. J. Mwasekaga, R. Huebner, D. Rumisha, N. Binkin, and E. Maganu. 1999. "Low Levels of Drug-Resistance Amidst Rapidly

Increasing Tuberculosis and Human Immunodeficiency Virus Co-Epidemics in Botswana." *International Journal of Tuberculosis and Lung Disease* 3: 4–11.

Korenromp, E. L., F. Scano, B. G. Williams, C. Dye, and P. Nunn. 2003. "Effects of Human Immunodeficiency Virus Infection on Recurrence of Tuberculosis after Rifampicin-Based Treatment: An Analytical Review." *Clinical Infectious Diseases* 37: 101–12.

Lienhardt, C., and L. C. Rodrigues. 1997. "Estimation of the Impact of the Human Immunodeficiency Virus Infection on Tuberculosis: Tuberculosis Risks Revisited?" *International Journal of Tuberculosis and Lung Disease* 1: 196–204.

Lucas, S. B., K. M. De Cock, A. Hounnou, C. Peacock, M. Diomande, M. Honde, A. Beaumel, L. Kestens, and A. Kadio. 1994. "The Contribution of Tuberculosis to Slim Disease in Africa." *British Medical Journal* 308: 1531–33.

Lucas, S. B., A. Hounnou, C. Peacock, A. Beaumel, G. Djomand, J. M. N'Gbichi, K. Yeboue, et al. 1993. "The Mortality and Pathology of HIV Infection in a West African City." *AIDS* 7: 1569–79.

Maher, D., K. Floyd, and M. Raviglione. 2002. "Strategic Framework to Decrease the Burden of TB/HIV." WHO/CDS/TB/2002.296, WHO, Geneva.

Mazurek, G. H., and M. E. Villarino. 2003. "Guidelines for Using the QuantiFERON-TB Test for Diagnosing Latent Mycobacterium Tuberculosis Infection." *Morbidity and Mortality Weekly Report* 52 (RR-2): 15–18.

Merson, M. H., J. M. Dayton, and K. O'Reilly. 2000. "Effectiveness of HIV Prevention Interventions in Developing Countries." *AIDS* 14 (Suppl. 2), S68–84.

Moalosi, G., K. Floyd, J. Phatshwane, T. Moeti, N. Binkin, and T. Kenyon. 2003. "Cost-Effectiveness of Home-Based Care versus Hospital Care for Chronically Ill Tuberculosis Patients, Francistown, Botswana." *International Journal of Tuberculosis and Lung Disease* 7 (9 Suppl. 1): S80–85.

Mukadi, Y. D., D. Maher, and A. Harries. 2001. "Tuberculosis Case Fatality Rates in High HIV Prevalence Populations in Sub-Saharan Africa." *AIDS* 15: 143–52.

Mukadi, Y., J. H. Perriens, M. E. St. Louis, C. Brown, J. Prignot, J. C. Willame, F. Pouthier, et al. 1993. "Spectrum of Immunodeficiency in HIV-1-Infected Patients with Pulmonary Tuberculosis in Zaire." *Lancet* 342: 143–46.

Murray, C. J., E. DeJonghe, H. J. Chum, D. S. Nyangulu, A. Salomao, and K. Styblo. 1991. "Cost Effectiveness of Chemotherapy for Pulmonary Tuberculosis in Three Sub-Saharan African Countries." *Lancet* 338: 1305–8.

Nganda, B., J. Wang'ombe, K. Floyd, and J. Kangangi. 2003. "Cost and Cost-Effectiveness of Increased Community and Primary Care Facility Involvement in Tuberculosis Care in Machakos District, Kenya." *International Journal of Tuberculosis and Lung Disease* 7 (9 Suppl. 1): S14–20.

Nunn, P., A. M. Elliott, and K. P. W. J. McAdam. 1994. "Impact of Human Immunodeficiency Virus on Tuberculosis in Developing Countries." *Thorax* 49: 511–18.

Nunn, P., M. Mungai, J. Nyamwaya, C. Gicheha, R. J. Brindle, D. T. Dunn, W. Githui, J. O. Were, and K. P. McAdam. 1994. "The Effect of Human Immunodeficiency Virus Type 1 on the Infectiousness of Tuberculosis." *Tubercle and Lung Disease* 75: 25–32.

Odhiambo, J. A., M. W. Borgdorff, F. M. Kiambih, D. K. Kibuga, D. O. Kwamanga, L. Ng'ang'a, R. Agwanda, et al. 1999. "Tuberculosis and the HIV Epidemic: Increasing Annual Risk of Tuberculous Infection in Kenya, 1986–1996." *American Journal of Public Health* 89: 1078–82.

Okello, D., K. Floyd, F. Adatu, R. Odeke, and G. Gargioni. 2003. "Cost and Cost-Effectiveness of Community-Based Care for Tuberculosis Patients in Rural Uganda." *International Journal of Tuberculosis and Lung Disease* 7 (9 Suppl. 1): S72–79.

Parkhurst, J. O. 2002. "The Ugandan Success Story? Evidence and Claims of HIV-1 Prevention." *Lancet* 360: 78–80.

Perriens, J. H., M. E. St Louis, Y. B. Mukadi, C. Brown, J. Prignot, F. Pouthier, F. Portaels, et al. 1995. "Pulmonary Tuberculosis in HIV-Infected Patients in Zaire. A Controlled Trial of Treatment for Either 6 or 12 Months." *New England Journal of Medicine* 332: 779–84.

Quigley, M. A., A. Mwinga, M. Hosp, I. Lisse, D. Fuchs, J. D. H. Porter, and P. Godfrey-Faussett. 2001. "Long Term Effect of Preventive Therapy for Tuberculosis in a Cohort of HIV-Infected Zambian Patients." *AIDS* 15: 215–22.

Raviglione, M. C., A. D. Harries, R. Msiska, D. Wilkinson, and P. Nunn. 1997. "Tuberculosis and HIV: Current Status in Africa." *AIDS* 11 (Suppl. B): S115–23.

Raviglione, M. C., and M. W. Uplekar. Forthcoming. "The New Stop TB Strategy of WHO." *Lancet.*

Richter, C., B. Ndosi, A. S. Mwammy, and R. K. Mbwambo. 1991. "Extrapulmonary Tuberculosis—a Simple Diagnosis?" *Tropical and Geographical Medicine* 43: 375–78.

Rieder, H. L. 1999. *Tuberculosis Epidemiology.* 1st ed. Paris: IUATLD.

Rieder, H. L., G. M. Cauthen, G. W. Comstock, and D. E. Snider. 1989. "Epidemiology of Tuberculosis in the United States." *Epidemiologic Reviews* 11: 79–98.

Sinanovic, E., K. Floyd, L. Dudley, V. Azevedo, R. Grant, and D. Maher. 2003. "Cost and Cost-Effectiveness of Community-Based Care for Tuberculosis in Cape Town, South Africa." *International Journal of Tuberculosis and Lung Disease* 7 (9 Suppl. 1): S56–62.

Sonnenberg, P., J. Murray, J. R. Glynn, S. Shearer, B. Kambashi, and P. Godfrey-Faussett. 2001. "HIV-1 and Recurrence, Relapse, and Reinfection of Tuberculosis after Cure: A Cohort Study in South African Mineworkers." *Lancet* 358: 1687–93.

Stop TB Partnership and WHO (World Health Organization). 2006. *The Global Plan to Stop TB, 2006–2015.* WHO/HTM/STB/2006.35. Geneva: WHO.

Styblo, K. 1991. *Epidemiology of Tuberculosis. Selected Papers.* Vol. 24. The Hague: Royal Netherlands Tuberculosis Association KNCV.

Sutherland, I. 1976. "Recent Studies in the Epidemiology of Tuberculosis, Based on the Risk of Being Infected with Tubercle Bacilli." *Advances in Tuberculosis Research* 19: 1–63.

Tanzania Tuberculin Survey Collaboration. 2001. "Tuberculosis Control in the Era of the HIV Epidemic: Risk of Tuberculosis Infection in Tanzania, 1983–98." *International Journal of Tuberculosis and Lung Disease* 5: 103–12.

Topley, J., D. Maher, and L. Nyong'onya Mbewe. 1996. "Transmission of Tuberculosis to Contacts of Sputum Positive Adults in Malawi." *Archives of Disease in Childhood* 74: 140–43.

UNAIDS (Joint United Nations Programme on HIV/AIDS). 2001. "Provisional Recommendations on the Use of Cotrimoxazole as Part of a Minimum Package of Care in Adults and Children Living with HIV/AIDS in Africa."

UNAIDS (Joint United Nations Programme on HIV/AIDS) and WHO (World Health Organization). 2005. *AIDS Epidemic Update, December 2005.* UNAIDS/05.19E. Geneva: UNAIDS and WHO.

Von Pirquet, C. 1909. "Frequency of Tuberculosis in Childhood." *Journal of the American Medical Association* 52: 675–78.

WHO (World Health Organization). 1995. "Global Tuberculosis Programme and Global Programme on Vaccines." Statement on BCG Revaccination for the Prevention of Tuberculosis. *Weekly Epidemiological Record* 70: 229–36.

———. 1996. *Immunisation Policy.* Global Programme on Vaccines. Geneva: WHO.

———. 1999. "Preventive Therapy against Tuberculosis in People Living with HIV." *Weekly Epidemiological Record* 74: 385–98.

———. 2000. *The Economic Impacts of Tuberculosis.* Stop TB Initiative 2000 Series. WHO/CDS/STB/2000.5. Geneva: WHO.

———. 2002. *The World Health Report—Reducing Risks, Promoting Healthy Life.* Geneva: WHO.

———. 2003. "Scaling Up Anti-Retroviral Therapy in Resource-Limited Settings: Treatment Guidelines for a Public Health Approach." WHO, Geneva.

———. 2004a. *Anti-Tuberculosis Drug Resistance in the World. Report Number 3.* WHO/HTM/TB/2004.343. Geneva: WHO.

———. 2004b. "WHO Vaccine-Preventable Disease Monitoring System. 2004 Global Summary." WHO/IVB/2004, WHO, Geneva.

———. 2006. *Global Tuberculosis Control: Surveillance, Planning and Financing.* WHO/HTM/TB/2006.362. Geneva: WHO.

Wiktor, S. Z., M. Sassan-Morokro, A. D. Grant, L. Abouya, J. M. Karon, C. Maurice, G. Djomand, et al. 1999. "Efficacy of Trimethoprim-Sulphamethoxazole Prophylaxis to Decrease Morbidity and Mortality in HIV-1-Infected Patients with Tuberculosis in Abidjan, Côte d'Ivoire: A Randomised Controlled Study." *Lancet* 353: 1469–75.

Williams, B. G., and C. Dye. 2003. "Antiretroviral Drugs for Tuberculosis Control in the Era of HIV/AIDS." *Science* 301: 1535–37.

Young, D. B., and C. Dye. Forthcoming. "The Development and Impact of Tuberculosis Vaccines." *Cell.*

Zachariah, R., M-P. Spielmann, C. Chinji, P. Gomani, V. Arendt, N. J. Hargreaves, F. M. L. Salaniponi, and A. D. Harries. 2003. "Voluntary Counselling, HIV Testing and Adjunctive Cotrimoxazole Reduces Mortality in Tuberculosis Patients in Thyolo, Malawi." *AIDS* 17: 1053–61.

Chapter 14

Malaria

Robert W. Snow and Judy A. Omumbo

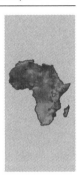

Plasmodium falciparum is the most common of the four human malaria parasites across much of Sub-Saharan Africa. (The other three parasites are *P. vivax*, *P. malariae*, and *P. ovale.*) The distribution of *P. vivax* is concentrated in the Horn of Africa, covering Djibouti, Eritrea, Ethiopia, Somalia, and Sudan. *P. falciparum* accounts for almost all the malaria mortality in Sub-Saharan Africa, and it is often stated that the continent bears over 90 percent of the global *P. falciparum* burden. Recent bioinformatics analysis of changes in human ecology suggest that about 6,000 years ago, *P. falciparum* populations expanded rapidly in Africa and spread worldwide, coincident with human population growth and subsequent diasporas facilitated by the dawn of agriculture (Joy et al. 2003). This parasite has exacted a heavy mortality toll on Africa's population, evidenced by the selection for several human survival mechanisms, such as the genetic polymorphisms associated with red cell structure and function (Hill 1992).

Malaria infection is common in Sub-Saharan Africa, but death directly attributed to the parasite is comparatively rare, largely because of acquired functional immunity. Unlike the human immunodeficiency virus (HIV) and the acquired immune deficiency syndrome (AIDS) or tuberculosis, infection with the malaria parasite is almost always universal in a population, and the presence of the pathogen is not a sufficient marker of disease. Individuals who die from malaria represent the public health costs of developing immunity at a population level. These deaths are concentrated among those with poorly developed immunity, and, generally, young children bear the brunt of the mortality burden. Individuals born into areas of stable *P. falciparum* transmission frequently acquire and clear infections without becoming ill, but most will, at some stage in their lives, develop an overt clinical response to infection, often manifested as fever. These clinical events may lead to severe complications, which may resolve naturally, require medical intervention, or result in death. Figure 14.1 shows a typical age-structured series of risks of infection, mild clinical disease, severe disease, and death due to *P. falciparum* for a population living on the Kenyan coast (Snow and Gilles 2002). Many individuals naturally acquire functional immune responses to severe disease and death early in life; immunity to the milder consequences of infection occurs later in childhood, but the ability to sterilize blood-stage infection probably does not occur until adulthood.

Figure 14.1 Malarial Risks in Children Age 0 to 14 Years in a Stable Endemic Area of the Kenyan Coast

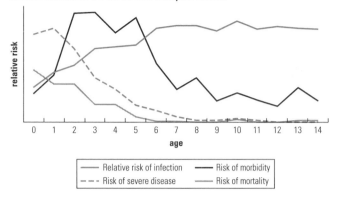

Source: Snow and Gilles 2002.

Note: Scale of y axis has arbitrarily been fitted to demonstrate relative change in risk by age.

The relation between the frequency of parasite exposure and disease outcome is complex. The speed with which a population acquires functional immunity to the severe consequences of *P. falciparum* infection depends on the frequency of parasite exposure from birth as measured by the intensity of parasite transmission in a given locality (see Snow and Marsh 2002). The shape of the severe disease and mortality curves shown in figure 14.1 may therefore be shifted to the right for areas where parasite transmission is of low, stable intensity and to the left for areas where transmission is of high, stable intensity. Where infection is rare the risk of mortality is likely to be directly related to the risk of infection, because acquired functional immunity is

unlikely to affect health outcomes. Understanding this relationship is important for defining the age-specific mortality burdens in Sub-Saharan Africa, an area able to support infection rates ranging from one infection every three years to hundreds of new infections per year (Hay et al. 2000).

In addition to the morbidity and mortality directly attributed to *P. falciparum*, other consequential and indirect effects are linked to each step of the infection and disease process. Chronic, subclinical infections cause anemia or may encourage undernutrition, which in turn may increase susceptibility to severe clinical outcomes of subsequent malarial or other pathogenetic infection. During pregnancy, asymptomatic infection of the placenta significantly reduces birthweights and infant survival rates. Patients who survive severe disease may be left with debilitating sequelae, such as spasticity or epilepsy. Subtler consequences include behavioral disturbances or cognitive impairment (Holding and Snow 2001; Holding and Wekulo 2004). These combined effects are summarized in figure 14.2. In the absence of measures aimed at reducing the risk of infection, the risks shown in figure 14.2 largely depend on extrinsic factors, such as those that determine the speed with which a population develops acquired immunity and the access to effective case management, and on intrinsic factors, such as host genetics.

This chapter describes the determinants and distribution of *P. falciparum* infection risk in Sub-Saharan Africa and

Figure 14.2 Public Health Effects of *Plasmodium falciparum* Malaria

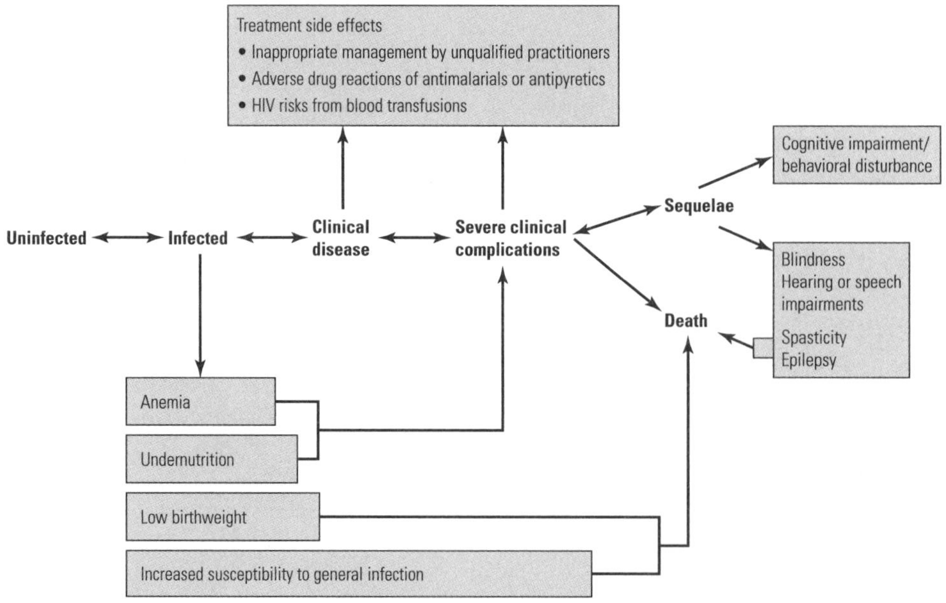

Source: Snow and Gilles 2002.

uses populations at risk to estimate mortality from malaria. It also considers the evidence for consequential and indirect mortality and describes *P. falciparum* as a risk factor for rather than a cause of pediatric mortality. The chapter concludes with a description of the relationship between poverty and malaria and recent trends in malaria mortality in Sub-Saharan Africa to provide some context for current international efforts to halve the malaria burden by the year 2010 (Nabarro and Taylor 1998).

PLASMODIUM FALCIPARUM DISTRIBUTION IN AFRICA

Climate, local ecology, and active control affect the ability of malaria parasites and their anopheline mosquito vectors to coexist long enough to enable transmission. The frequency of transmission, or endemicity, depends on the density and infectivity of anopheline vectors. These features depend on a range of climatic, physical, and population characteristics, for example, rainfall, location of human settlements near or at rivers or other mosquito larval breeding sites, and the density of human populations in a village. The most significant determinant of the intensity of parasite transmission is climate.

Climate Determinants of *P. falciparum* Transmission in Africa

The development of both the vector and parasite is temperature dependent. The optimum temperature range for parasite development in the female *Anopheles* (sporogony) is between 25°C and 30°C, and development ceases below 16°C. Intermittent low temperatures delay sporogony, and the period immediately after the infective bite by the mosquito on an infected human host is the most sensitive to drops in temperature. Above 35°C sporogony slows down considerably. Extremely high temperatures are associated with the development of smaller and less fecund adult mosquitoes. Thermal death of mosquitoes occurs at 40°C to 42°C. Altitude and temperature are strongly correlated: with every 100-meter increase in altitude, the temperature drops by 0.5°C. Overall, the use of altitude as a marker of endemicity or disease risk is vague, yet there is a tendency within the literature to refer to *highland malaria* in East Africa and the Horn of Africa.

Numerous studies have demonstrated the association between *Anopheles gambiae sensus lato* (the most important vector of *P. falciparum* in Africa) abundance and rainfall. Without surface water the female *Anopheles* cannot lay eggs.

Rainfall is also related to humidity and saturation deficit, both affecting mosquito survival (adult vector longevity increases with humidities over 60 percent).

Mapping Malaria Risks

Using the climatic determinants of transmission identified above, the Mapping Malaria in Africa Project (http://www.mara.co.za) developed a series of risk maps for stable *P. falciparum* transmission across the continent (Craig, Snow, and le Sueur 1999). In brief, the project used long-term mean monthly temperature and rainfall data to define the limits of distribution of stable endemic malaria across Africa. Temperature and rainfall profiles in sample areas, where malaria endemicity was known, were translated into a model of "climate suitability." The temperature limits were related to the requirements for the extrinsic parasite development cycle. The model made the following assumptions: (a) the optimal temperature range was 18°C to 22°C; (b) optimal rainfall values were greater than or equal to 80 millimeters; (c) conditions of rainfall and temperature had to coincide on a month-to-month basis for at least five consecutive months (three months for the northern fringes of Sub-Saharan Africa); and finally, (d) a frost factor (mean monthly minimum temperature of less than 5°C for any one month) was used to eliminate transmission at any point. The model provided fuzzy climate suitability (FCS) values, ranging from zero (unsuitable, hence malaria absent) to one (very suitable, malaria endemic).

During earlier attempts to describe the malaria burden in Sub-Saharan Africa the climate suitability maps for *P. falciparum* transmission were combined with interpolated maps of population distribution (Deichmann 1996; Snow et al. 1999). The population data were initially constructed using population totals from the last available censuses for administrative units (communities, towns, or districts). These data were then converted into a regular raster grid of population totals, and auxiliary information was used to distribute the population within the administrative unit across its raster grid cells. The process heuristically incorporated information on where people tend to live: in or close to towns and cities, close to transportation infrastructure, around protected areas, near water bodies, and not at very high elevations. Using the Geographical Information System (GIS)–based information on the location and size of towns and cities, roads, railroads, navigable rivers, and uninhabitable areas, population density was weighted, a high value implying a high density and a low or zero value implying low or no population. These weights were then used to proportionately distribute population to grid cells. The digital map extracted population distributions according to each cell in a regular raster grid with a resolution of 5 kilometers at the equator. It was then combined with the maps of malaria risk to provide simple population totals of those exposed to stable, unstable, or no malaria risk.

The *P. falciparum* risk-to-population distribution for Africa has subsequently been refined through use of an improved link between mortality data and transmission intensity (Snow et al. 2003). New criteria were adopted following an improved understanding of the variations in disease outcomes and risks congruent with variations in stable *P. falciparum* transmission. The relation between the exact number of new infections a population is exposed to each year (annual entomological inoculation rates, or EIR) and parasite prevalence is nonlinear, but quartiles of the prevalence of infection have been shown to approximate logarithmic increases in the EIR (Beier, Killeen, and Githure 1999). This principle has been used previously to categorize pediatric malaria and all-cause mortality according to parasite prevalence estimates from childhood cross-sectional surveys (Snow, Korenromp, and Gouws 2004; Snow and Marsh, 2002). When infection prevalence quartiles (less than 25 percent, 25 to 49 percent, 50 to 74 percent, and 75 percent and greater) are used, mortality indicators saturate at the highest two classes of endemicity and rise sharply from the x–y intercept within the first class. Analysis of 217 independent parasitological surveys among children in Kenya suggests that most areas (81 percent) with a FCS value of less than 0.75 are represented by communities supporting parasite prevalence rates of less than 25 percent (Omumbo et al. 2004). It seems appropriate, therefore, to distribute the population of Sub-Saharan Africa into areas of no risk, unstable transmission risk, low stable risk, and moderate to high stable endemic risk.

The fuzzy membership model developed by Craig, Snow, and le Sueur (1999) was used to delineate four ecologically distinct areas of Africa (figure 14.3). First, there are areas with no human settlement, or FCS values of zero (class 1). Some countries have minimal and only very localized risks of malaria transmission, with over 90 percent of their population residing in class 1 areas, the western Sahara region (Algeria, the Arab Republic of Egypt, Lesotho, Libya, Morocco, and Tunisia). It is assumed that these countries have a negligible malaria burden; thus, they are excluded from the Sub-Saharan Africa malaria burden estimations. Second, areas with marginal risks of malaria transmission

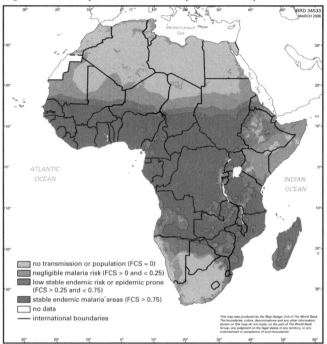

Figure 14.3 Fuzzy Climate Suitability Membership for Malaria

Source: Modified from Craig, Snow, and le Sueur 1999.

Note: Areas of no transmission or population: class1, FCS = 0; areas of negligible malaria risk: class 2, FCS > 0 and < 0.25; areas of low, stable endemic risk or epidemic prone: class 3, FCS ≥ 0.25 and < 0.75; and stable endemic malaria areas: class 4, FCS ≥ 0.75.

are represented by a FCS greater than zero but less than 0.25 (class 2). Parasite prevalence rates are likely to be extremely low or zero; however, these populations often border areas of higher infection risk and may be subject to aberrations in climate that lead to localized transmission. Third, in some areas populations are exposed to a FCS value between 0.25 and 0.75 (class 3). Communities living in these areas are likely to support cross-sectional parasite prevalence estimates in childhood of less than 25 percent, and transmission is likely to be acutely seasonal with a tendency toward epidemics. In practice it would be hard to distinguish between classes 2 and 3 in many areas of Sub-Saharan Africa outside of southern Africa, and therefore they are grouped together here. Finally, some areas of the continent have stable endemic malaria transmission (FCS greater than or equal to 0.75), which may still vary seasonally, but support parasite prevalence rates greater than or equal to 25 percent (class 4). In southern Africa (Botswana, Namibia, South Africa, Swaziland, and Zimbabwe) a different approach was taken, because classes 2 and 3 represent the historical extents of transmission and do not reflect contemporary distributions of risk (M. Craig, personal communication). Class 4 areas are the only areas where malaria still poses a risk, and its extent and transmission potential are determined by

Table 14.1 Populations at Risk During 2000
(thousands)

Region	Age 0–4 years	Age 5–14 years	Age 15+ years	Total
North Africa (exclusion)	17,020	33,663	95,038	145,721
Southern Africa (classes 1–3: no malaria risk)	4,190	10,682	29,195	44,067
Rest of Africa (class 1: no malaria risk)	7,366	11,680	23,033	42,079
Southern Africa (class 4: stable malaria risk)	2,049	3,709	8,687	14,445
Rest of Africa (classes 2, 3: epidemic to low stable risk; FCS < 0.75; parasite prevalence < 25%)	22,018	34,668	69,126	125,812
Rest of Africa (class 4: stable endemic risk; FCS ≥ 0.75; parasite prevalence ≥ 25%)	73,351	115,261	228,105	416,717

Source: Compiled by authors.

Note: The medium variant assumptions of changing fertility, mortality, and migration on population growth were selected for the year 2000. The database also provided the estimated proportion of the population age less than 5 years, 5–14 years, and 15 years or older and the crude birth rate (CBR). The CBR was used to estimate the approximate number of live births in 2000.

The residents of Comoros, Réunion, and the Seychelles are assumed to be at negligible malaria risk and during the burden estimations formed part of the excluded Sub-Saharan Africa populations. Conversely it seems reasonable to assume that the islands of Cape Verde and São Tomé and Principe are subject to stable transmission; however, they have proved difficult to characterize at effective resolutions using the GIS malaria risk models, and their small contribution to populations at risk (less than 0.5 million people) have not been included.

aggressive vector control. The combined malaria-risk and population models were used to estimate populations resident in each malaria-risk class by using country-level data available from the World Population Prospects Population Database (United Nations Population Division 2001). The summed extractions for the continent are shown in table 14.1.

The current distribution maps of *P. falciparum* depend entirely on the biotic effects of climate on transmission. They fail to capture the more localized yet marked effects, such as urbanization and localized control. The *Anopheles gambiae* complex is less prolific in urban areas because there are fewer appropriate breeding sites. People living in urban areas are on average 10 times less likely to receive an infective bite than their rural counterparts (Hay et al. 2000; Robert et al. 2003; Trape et al. 1992). In 2000, 38 percent of Africa's population were urban dwellers (United Nations Population Division 2001). The current estimations of populations at risk under different endemicity conditions (table 14.1) will overrepresent those in the higher-risk classes. New satellite imagery makes it possible to map the extent of land use, land cover, and urbanization, a refinement important for subsequent iterations of the disease burden models for Sub-Saharan Africa (Hay et al. 2005).

Several aggressive, and highly successful, vector control programs in Africa have had significant effects upon transmission (Bradley 1991; Le Sueur, Sharp, and Appleton 1993). More recently, such countries as South Africa and Mozambique have successfully reduced or eliminated transmission in areas that are currently classified as prone to

transmission (Barnes and Folb 2003; LSDI 2001). It will never be possible to account for all local vector control activities on a continent-wide map, but it is important to recognize that because current estimations of disease burden will be overestimated.

Other important factors that determine localized transmission intensity are currently not captured in the climate-driven models shown in figure 14.3. These include widespread use of insecticide-treated bednets, leading to a decrease in local parasite transmission in only a few areas of Sub-Saharan Africa; drug resistance, leading to increased parasite transmission carriage; population displacement due to conflict or resettlement, altering transmission characteristics of newly settled areas; man-made ecological changes, such as deforestation; and agricultural practices, such as rice-field cultivation, that change the breeding site availability for local mosquito vector populations. More detailed models of malaria risk in Mali and Kenya have included some of these factors on more recent maps (Kleinschmidt et al. 2001; Snow et al. 1998). However, at present these more complex models are not available at a continental scale.

Finally, because population estimates in the United Nations Population Division's figures are based on estimations incorporating assumptions about fertility and mortality in a country, these totals may differ from the total populations in each administrative unit reported by the country. More refined microcensus data or models of population projections below the national level are required for future mapping of disease burdens.

DIRECT MALARIA MORTALITY

Malaria is often difficult to diagnose on a purely clinical basis. Fever is common to almost every infectious disease, and the severe pathology caused by *P. falciparum*, such as acidosis, anemia, and altered consciousness, are also complications of other infections. When a person is ill, demonstrating the presence of malaria infection increases the likelihood that symptoms are directly due to the infection, but the high prevalence of asymptomatic infections makes it difficult to exclude other diagnoses. Our earlier understanding of the pathophysiology of malaria derived from clinical descriptions among adults in Southeast Asia and only recently have the mechanisms of death been more precisely defined for pediatric African populations (Marsh et al. 1995; Warrell 2002). Several detailed clinical studies in African hospital settings have described the principal, sometimes overlapping, routes to a fatal outcome. These include cerebral involvement from sequestered infection in the vasculature of the brain, metabolic disturbances, respiratory distress, and severe anemia. For epidemiological purposes it is convenient to define two major syndromes, cerebral malaria (CM) and severe malarial anemia (SMA). CM is a condition in which patients present in coma with several underlying causes, ranging from a primarily neurological condition to a systemic metabolic disturbance (Marsh and Snow 1999; Newton and Krishna 1998). Severe anemia is a pathology of life-threatening malaria with a complex etiology combining rapid hemolysis during acute infection or a slow insidious process compounded by antimalarial drug resistance. SMA is a life-threatening condition in young children and often warrants blood transfusion.

Measuring Malaria-Specific Mortality

Africa presents an epidemiological challenge, because although it has high mortality rates, existing vital registration systems are not reliable or comprehensive. Most deaths occur outside the formal health service, and national government systems of civil registration in Sub-Saharan Africa are incomplete. Epidemiologists interested in defining malaria-specific mortality have established demographic surveillance systems (DSS) of large populations (between 20,000 and 100,000 people) to prospectively monitor population migration, births, and deaths (INDEPTH Network 2002; Smith and Morrow 1996).

The attribution of causes of death during DSS surveys is often performed through a verbal autopsy (VA) interview with bereaved relatives about symptoms and signs associated with the terminal illness. The VA details are either reviewed by a panel of clinicians or subjected to diagnostic algorithms. The sensitivity and specificity of VA diagnosis for malaria as a cause of death have been estimated in seven hospital-based validation studies in Africa. There is considerable variation in both the specificity (77 to 100 percent) and the sensitivity (45 to 75 percent) (Korenromp et al. 2003). The sensitivity of verbal autopsies for malaria will depend on the intensity of malaria transmission: in high-transmission areas, severe malaria is more likely to present as SMA than as CM (Snow et al. 1997a). SMA in a young child is often difficult to distinguish from acute respiratory infections (ARI), although CM among older children is less ambiguous. Similarly, the sensitivity and specificity of verbal autopsies for malaria will vary with the local spectrum of other diseases. ARI, acute gastroenteritis, and meningitis all share common clinical features with malaria, including cough, difficulties in breathing, diarrhea, or cerebral dysfunction. Despite these limitations, the VA-diagnosed risks of malaria mortality represent our only source of contemporary information on the direct, fatal consequences of infection in areas with stable transmission in Africa.

The data presented in this chapter derive largely from the Burden of Malaria in Africa (BOMA) project, supported by the Wellcome Trust, United Kingdom, and the Bill & Melinda Gates Foundation. The BOMA project began in 1998 and has completed a comprehensive search for published and unpublished empirical measures of malaria morbidity, disability, and death. The data include historical accounts of mortality from colonial administration records and detailed descriptions of recent DSS surveys. Details of the search methods and applications of the data are presented elsewhere (Snow, Korenromp, and Gouws 2004; Snow and Marsh 2002; Snow, Trape, and Marsh 2001). The estimates of malaria-specific mortality in childhood outside of southern Africa use only mortality reports based on a VA within a DSS framework after 1989. This time restriction was made because of recent temporal changes in pediatric risks of mortality from malaria in Sub-Saharan Africa (see "Trends in Malaria Mortality" section). Where DSS and VA methods were used during community or household randomized intervention trials, only control communities were included. In order to structure risks according to transmission classes shown in table 14.1, DSS surveys of malaria-specific mortality were also limited only to those in which there was a congruent estimation of malaria transmission intensity.

Adult malaria-specific mortality data from DSS sites are rare, and VA methods have not been well developed nor widely validated for the description of malaria deaths in this group. At Kilifi, Kenya, in the absence of obvious signs of respiratory disease an algorithm was used based on detailed exclusion criteria (for example, well-defined deaths or hospital-diagnosed conditions) involving an acute febrile event (R. W. Snow, unpublished data). In Tanzania a similar approach was used (Y. Hemed, personal communication). Both approaches are likely to overestimate the number of adult deaths from malaria in endemic areas. Owing to the paucity of empirical data in this age group, these two contemporary estimates have been included with other sources of historical data on adult malaria mortality from detailed, preindependence civil registration systems when causes of death were investigated by medical personnel from circumscribed, censused populations. It seems reasonable to assume that under stable transmission conditions adult mortality from malaria is unlikely to have changed much over time, as deaths would normally occur in individuals who, for some ill-defined reasons, failed to acquire functional immunity in childhood or lost their functional immune response. The intention has been to attempt, where possible, to fill an important data gap using imperfect data, and therefore the risks reported must be interpreted with caution.

Civil and vital registration systems in southern Africa are more comprehensive than those in other parts of Sub-Saharan Africa. Data from southern Africa, however, also underreport events and must be viewed as minimum estimates. Data have been extracted from reports provided during subregional malaria control program meetings and malaria deaths (reported only for all age groups combined) and expressed per projected population estimates for administrative areas of known malaria risk (figure 14.3). Data were available for the three areas of KwaZulu-Natal Province in South Africa, seven areas of Botswana, four areas of Namibia, and eight areas of Zimbabwe.

The spatial coordinates of the study location were used to identify a time and location-specific estimate of infection prevalence for the geographical areas covered by the mortality data. Data were identified primarily through the MARA/ARMA database (http://www.MARA/ARMA.or.za) or correspondence with authors of original data on the disease burden. The estimates of malaria risk have been used to provide empirical ecological categorization for each data point in accordance with the cartography of risk described in figure 14.3 and table 14.1. Median and interquartile ranges (IQR) have been used to describe the risk data per malaria risk class (table 14.2), and the estimated numbers of deaths directly attributed to *P. falciparum* in 2000 are shown in table 14.3 according to populations at various continental risk classes shown in table 14.1.

Table 14.2 Median and Interquartile Ranges of Malaria-Specific Mortality Estimates per 1,000 People per Year

Region	Age 0–4 years	Age 5–14 years	Age 15+ years	Bibliographic sources
Southern Africa (malaria risk areas; class 4)	0.13 [0.08–0.21] (study sites 22)			Diseko 1994; Kamwi 1998; Piotti 1997; South African Medical Research Council 1998, unpublished data
Rest of Africa (low, stable epidemic risk; classes 2, 3; FCS < 0.75; parasite prevalence < 25%)	2.62 (287/109,412 PYO) (study sites 3)	0.94 (158/167,598 PYO) (study sites 2)	0.71 (265/372,777 PYO) (study sites 2)	Charlwood et al. 2001; Government of Tanzania 1997
Rest of Africa (stable endemic risk; class 4; FCS ≥ 0.75; parasite prevalence ≥ 25%)	9.33 [7.38–14.57] (study sites 12)	1.58 [0.66–2.77] (study sites 10)	0.6 [0.37–0.94] (study sites 15)	Delacollette and Barutwanayo 1993; Ghana VAST 1993; Jaffar et al. 1997; Snow, Mung'ala et al. 1994; Trape et al. 1998; Barnish et al. 1993; Premji et al. 1997; Government of Tanzania 1997; Salum et al. 1994; D'Allesandro et al. 1995; Pasha et al. 2003; Government of Colony of Gold Coast 1912–48; Colbourne and Edington 1956; Government of the Colony and Protectorate of Kenya 1935; Government of Colony and Protectorate of Nigeria 1934–35; Bruce-Chwatt 1952; Government of Colony and Protectorate of Sierra Leone 1913–17

Source: Compiled by authors. For low, stable endemic risks for "rest of Africa," G. D. Shanks and R. W. Snow provided unpublished data in Kenya; additional information from the Ghana VAST project were provided by the late Nicola Dollimare and Gilly Maude; unpublished VA data reconstructed by R. W. Snow to provide estimates of malaria-specific mortality in the study described by Snow, Mung'ala et al. 1994; additional information provided by Brian Greenwood for the Barnish et al. 1993 study.

Note: First numbers in each entry represent the median; numbers in square brackets represent the IQR; PYO = person-years of observation. For southern Africa, the figures in the first column include all age groups.

Table 14.3 Estimated Numbers of Malaria-Specific Deaths and Interquartile Ranges during 2000

Region	Age 0–4 years	Age 5–14 years	Age 15+ years	Total
Southern Africa (malaria risk areas; class 4)				1,878
Rest of Africa (low, stable epidemic risk; classes 2 & 3; FCS < 0.75; parasite prevalence < 25%)	57,688	32,588	49,079	139,355
Rest of Africa (stable endemic risk; class 4; FCS ≥ 0.75; parasite prevalence ≥ 25%)	684,364 [541,330–1,068,723]	182,113 [76,072–319,274]	136,863 [84,399–214,419]	1,003,340 [701,801–1,602,416]

Source: Compiled by authors.

Note: The total for southern Africa includes all age groups. Numbers in square brackets represent the IQR.

Empirical Estimates of Malaria-Specific Mortality by Age

Twelve independent estimates of malaria mortality among children under five years living under conditions of stable transmission were used from DSS sites in Burundi, The Gambia, Ghana, Kenya, Senegal, Sierra Leone, and Tanzania. The median malaria-specific mortality rate among these communities was 9.33 per 1,000 children per year and represented 28.2 percent of all mortality among children under five. Under similar transmission conditions the median malaria-specific mortality among older children, age 5 to 14 years, was 1.58 per 1,000 per year (from 10 study sites), representing 52.2 percent of all deaths in this age group. Among adult populations surveyed as part of colonial administration civil registration systems or recent DSS sites in stable endemic areas, the median malaria mortality rates were 0.6 per 1,000 per year (15 reports), or 6 percent of all deaths among populations age 15 years or older.

There are few DSS or colonial administration civil registration data from low, stable endemic or epidemic conditions (parasite rate less than 25 percent; classes 2 and 3) outside southern Africa. Approximations to the DSS from the populations of a tea estate in the highlands of Kenya (Shanks and Snow, unpublished data) and a settled refugee camp in Sudan (Charlwood et al. 2001) provided data on malaria-specific mortality rates among censused childhood populations at low risk of malaria infection. In addition, the one true DSS site at Hai district in Tanzania provided a VA estimate of malaria mortality (Government of Tanzania 1997). All three studies covered periods after 1990. Only the Kenyan and Tanzanian studies provided information on older children and adults. Rather than being used to provide a median estimate from the limited data, the combined person-years of observation (PYO) and malaria deaths have been used to define direct risks of death from malaria under these transmission conditions. For children under five years the overall mortality rate was 2.62 per 1,000 per year (three studies); for children age 5 to 14 years the

mortality rate was 0.94 per 1,000 per year (two studies); and for adults age 15 years and over the rate was 0.71 per 1,000 per year (two studies).

An ongoing rural DSS site at Agincourt, South Africa (Kahn et al. 1999), located at the fringes of malaria risk (Brink 1958), also provided additional data. A malaria-specific mortality rate of 0.065 per 1,000 per year (2 out of 216 deaths) was measured among children under five years between 1992 and 1995. Of the 785 deaths recorded in the population older than five years of age, only one was attributed to malaria. This single estimate is an inadequate representation of the malaria mortality across southern Africa. The civil registration data in malaria-risk districts of southern Africa suggest that the median estimate of malaria-specific mortality among the entire population in these areas was 0.13 per 1,000 per year. Although these estimates represent minimal approximations of the true mortality burden, they fall within the ranges of mortality described for the single DSS site (Kahn et al. 1999) and those sites described in the more detailed analysis of malaria mortality data from civil registers in two districts of KwaZulu-Natal Province between 1996 and 1999: 0.02 to 0.52 per 1,000 people per year (Tsoka, Sharp, and Kleinschmidt 2002).

Overall malaria-specific mortality in children is approximately 3.5 times higher in areas of stable endemic transmission than in areas of low intensity, stable, or epidemic-prone malaria in Sub-Saharan Africa, excluding southern Africa. Mortality declines rapidly with increasing age, and this is especially striking under conditions of stable endemic transmission. The mortality rates for all ages from *P. falciparum* in southern Africa are considerably lower than those described for the rest of Africa, reflecting a low risk of infection combined with effective control. Even with the use of all the tools described earlier in this chapter, approximately 1.14 million people might have died in Sub-Saharan Africa as a direct consequence of infection with *P. falciparum* in 2000.

CONSEQUENTIAL MORTALITY

The consequences of disease that are related to the clinical event include the consequences of clinical management, such as the immediate effects of adverse drug reactions or the longer-term effects of HIV-acquired infection through blood transfusion. Nonintervention-related consequences of clinical events also include the short- and long-term residual impairments resulting from cerebral malaria.

Adverse Drug Reactions to Commonly Used Antimalarial Drugs

Drugs used to manage malarial fevers have adverse effects. We can assume that most of the severe adverse drug-related events are described as direct mortality during DSS VA studies, as they are likely to occur close to the febrile event. They are mentioned here, however, to emphasize that fevers are common in Africa and the use of antimalarial drugs is prolific. Adverse drug reactions (ADR) are likely to increase with the greater use of new, more complex drug combinations and agents, although the increase of ADR will probably never surpass the alternative of using ineffective drugs. There have been too few epidemiological studies of the human toxicity of many antimalarial drugs among African populations repeatedly exposed to these compounds. Most data derive from an examination of chemoprophylactic drug use among nonimmune travelers (Philips-Howard and Bjorkman 1990; Philips-Howard and West 1990). The majority of adverse reactions due to sulfonamides and 4-aminoquinolines are idiosyncratic. Severe adverse reactions to the commonly available antimalarial drugs in Africa, when used as recommended, include severe cutaneous reactions (Stevens-Johnson and Lyell's disease syndromes), aplastic anemia, severe neutropenia, thrombocytopenia, keratopathy, agranulocytosis, and hepatic failure (Reynolds 1993). It has been estimated that 2,350 deaths were probably caused by treatment rather than the disease itself in a single year among the children outside of southern Africa (Snow et al. 2003).

Anemia, Transfusion, and HIV

Severe anemia is a common feature of children hospitalized with complicated malaria. Transfusion is a common pediatric practice in Africa and adherence to guidelines for transfusion are often poor (English et al. 2004; Lackritz et al. 1992). Greenberg and colleagues (1988) examined the HIV and malaria status of 167 admissions of children to an emergency ward at the Mama Yemo Hospital in Kinshasa, the Democratic Republic of the Congo. The authors propose an unadjusted odds ratio for acquired HIV infection of 3.5 for malaria patients between 1 month and 12 years of age transfused once, 21.5 for those transfused twice, and 43.0 for those transfused three times during a single admission. In a study of transfusion practices in 1994 at six government hospitals in Kenya, Moore and colleagues (2001) calculated a 2 percent risk of transmission of HIV antibody positive blood from screened donations through blood transfusion to HIV-negative patients. This study did not include the risk from pre-seroconversion donations, nor did it allow for the sensitivity of test kits or the use of unscreened blood. The probability that an HIV antibody negative unit of blood is HIV infected has been estimated to be between 0.5 and 1.1 percent (Savarit et al. 1992). The probability of seroconversion following HIV-contaminated blood is assumed to be 96 percent (Colebunders et al. 1991). From estimates of hospitalized patients with severe malaria anemia, transfusion rates, and relative risks of seroconversion from HIV-infected blood donation, it has been estimated that between 5,000 and 8,000 children might become infected with HIV each year as a consequence of poor management of their malaria in the hospital (Snow et al. 2003).

Neurological Disability Associated with Severe Malaria

The case-fatality rate of cerebral malaria in most hospital settings is high, often over 30 percent (Newton and Krishna 1998). Prolonged coma and seizures are associated with neurological impairment in survivors. The immediate and prolonged sequelae associated with CM among African children includes hemiparesis, quadriparesis or severe deficit, hearing and visual impairments, speech and language and nonverbal construction difficulties, behavioral problems, and epilepsy (Mung'ala-Odera, Snow, and Newton 2004). These impairments are estimated to occur in about 4,000 children each year in Sub-Saharan Africa.

Those with severe deficits have a higher mortality risk soon after the disease event. For less dramatic impairments, such as epilepsy, increased mortality rates have been described (Coleman, Loppy, and Walraven 2002; Jillek-All and Rwiza 1992; Snow, Mung'ala, et al. 1994). In Western countries, the risk of premature mortality could be as high as two to three times that described in age-comparable groups without epilepsy (Cockerell et al. 1994; Hauser, Annegers, and Elveback 1980; Zielinski 1974), but in Africa the risk could be as high as nine times (Coleman, Loppy, and Walraven 2002). This is likely to be caused by poorly managed epilepsy resulting in status epilepticus or accidents, such as drowning or burns.

INDIRECT MORTALITY

Indirect consequences of *P. falciparum* infection include anemia (unless anemia is linked to acute high-density parasitemia as a direct cause), low birthweight, growth retardation, or undernutrition. In addition, malaria infection can increase the severity of other comorbid infectious diseases through immune suppression or enhanced invasive capacities across physical barriers to infection (for example, blood and tissue). Previous approaches to the global burden of disease have assumed that each death must be attributed to a single cause and can be fitted into the fixed disease-mix matrix of all causes (Murray and Lopez 1997).

During randomized controlled intervention trials aimed at reducing the incidence of infection (but not 100 percent protective), the all-cause mortality of children is often reduced more than would be attributed by VA diagnosis of malaria. For example, in Kilifi the proportion of deaths of children under five years attributed to malaria by VA was 34 percent (R. W. Snow, unpublished data). During a randomized controlled trial of insecticide-treated bednets in the same area, the incidence of malaria infection was reduced by 50 percent (Snow et al. 1996), which was sufficient to reduce all-cause mortality by 33 percent (Nevill et al. 1996). More dramatically, in The Gambia, insecticide-treated bednets reduced all-cause mortality by over 60 percent, and yet the VA-diagnosed contribution of malaria to all-cause mortality among control populations was only 16 percent (Alonso et al. 1993). This has led some to speculate that malaria infection is a contributor to broad causes of mortality beyond the direct fatal consequences of infection (Molineaux 1997).

Attempts have been made to distinguish between factors that affect the direct outcomes of malaria infection and the effects of malaria infection on the outcome of other health burdens. This is particularly important when the interaction between malaria and HIV or undernutrition is considered. Especially important is the role malaria infection plays as a risk for the extended, indirect consequences of infection on the public health burden posed by *P. falciparum*. A recent model relates infection prevalence to all-cause pediatric mortality outcomes in Sub-Saharan Africa (Snow,

Korenromp, and Gouws 2004). The model regards *P. falciparum* infection as a risk factor for all-cause mortality rather than attempting to directly estimate malaria's contribution to all-cause mortality (one cause, one death).

Malaria during Pregnancy

Despite a poor understanding of the precise mechanisms of pathology (Menendez 1995), the morbid outcomes of malaria infection during pregnancy have been well described (Brabin 1983; Guyatt and Snow 2001a, 2001b; Steketee, Wirima, Hightower et al. 1996; Steketee et al. 2001). In endemic settings in Africa, pregnant women experience relatively little malaria-specific morbidity (for example, fever) but do have increased risk of infection and higher density parasitemia leading to anemia and placental sequestration of the parasite. These effects operate across a broader range of endemicities used to describe morbid and fatal risks among nonpregnant populations (that is, areas covered by classes 3 and 4 shown in figure 14.1). Maternal anemia has been shown to be an important contributor to maternal mortality with a relative risk for mortality of 1.35 for moderate anemia and 3.51 for severe anemia (Brabin, Hakimi, and Pelletier 2001). Brabin and colleagues further estimate that malaria contributes to maternal anemia and that 9 percent of anemia-associated maternal mortality can be attributed to malaria in Sub-Saharan Africa; this figure predicts approximately 5,300 maternal deaths annually from malaria anemia in areas of Sub-Saharan Africa outside of southern Africa classified as classes 3 and 4.

Prematurity and low birthweight (less than 2,500 grams) are associated with maternal malaria, including the contribution from both malaria-associated maternal anemia and placental infection. The contribution of malaria during pregnancy to low birthweight and subsequent mortality in the first year of life has been estimated to range from 3 to 8 percent of infant mortality (Greenwood et al. 1992; Steketee, Wirima, Hightower et al. 1996; Steketee et al. 2001). If this range had been applied to the expected numbers of live births in 2000 among populations in low endemic, epidemic prone, and endemic malaria areas of Sub-Saharan Africa outside of southern Africa, there may have been between 71,000 and 190,000 infant deaths indirectly attributable to malaria in pregnancy.

In very low endemic settings or areas where malaria is epidemic prone and in southern Africa, malaria in nonimmune pregnant women can be devastating and lead to maternal death and abortion. For example, in urban

Mozambique, 15.5 percent of all maternal deaths in one hospital over a five-year period were attributed directly to malaria (Granja et al. 1998). In an epidemic-prone setting of Ethiopia, maternal malaria carried an approximately eight-fold increased risk of abortion (R. Newman, unpublished data). Similarly, in a low-endemicity setting in Southeast Asia even single malaria infections were associated with increased risk of low birthweight (Luxemburger et al. 2001).

Malaria and Anemia

Anemia among African children is a hematological state determined by combinations of nutritional deficiencies (iron, folic acid, other micronutrients, and protein-calorie malnutrition), iron loss through helminth infection, red cell destruction, red cell production decreased by infectious diseases, and the genetic constitution of red cell hemoglobin (Menendez, Fleming, and Alonso 2000; Nussenblatt and Semba 2002). Malaria has long been recognized as a major contributor to anemia in children, reducing hemoglobin concentrations through several mechanisms. The primary mechanism increases rates of destruction and removal of red blood cells and decreases the rate of erythrocyte production in the bone marrow. Other mechanisms are associated with acute clinical states (for example, hemolysis or cytokine disturbances), whereas chronic or repeated infections are more likely to involve dyserythropoiesis (Menendez, Fleming and Alonso 2000). Data from randomized controlled trials of malaria-specific interventions to reduce the incidence of new infections through insecticide-treated bednets or the prevalence of blood-stage infections through chemoprophylaxis or intermittent presumptive treatment suggest a halving of anemia risks through intervention (Korenromp et al. 2004). This substantial reduction in the risks of anemia demonstrates the importance of *P. falciparum* in maintaining the poor hematological health of children. This finding, however, cannot be extrapolated to subsequent morbid or fatal consequences, because few detailed prospective studies focus on describing the effects of reduced hemoglobin concentrations on health outcomes.

Malaria and Undernutrition

It has been postulated that nutritional status is related to the threats posed by infection and disease and to the role of infectious disease in perpetuating undernutrition (Pelletier, Frongillo, and Habicht 1993; Pelletier et al. 1995). Most studies have generally focused on severe malnutrition and specific nutrient deficiency, and only a few have examined the role of malaria. One striking feature of the global distribution of anthropometric markers of undernutrition is its congruence with the distribution of endemic malaria. Although *P. falciparum* malaria and malnutrition are both highly prevalent in Sub-Saharan Africa, the existence of a synergistic interaction has not been well established. Evidence from intervention trials aimed at reducing the frequency of new infections suggests that malaria infection might have some indirect effects upon the generalized nutritional status of African children. A study in Nigeria on the use of chemoprophylaxis in the treatment of malaria in children showed a reduction in the incidence of infection and clinical attacks that was accompanied by a reduction in the incidence of malnutrition (Bradley-Moore et al. 1985). Improved growth among young children has more recently been demonstrated in The Gambia and Kenya in studies comparing those protected by insecticide-treated bednets with those left unprotected (D'Allessando et al. 1995; Snow et al. 1997b; Ter Kuile et al. 2003). Despite the biological plausibility of synergism between infection and growth, the precise relationship between undernutrition and severe malaria continues to be difficult to quantify empirically within disease burden frameworks.

Malaria and HIV Interactions

In Sub-Saharan Africa the HIV epidemic has been superimposed on the long-standing malaria pandemic. The wide geographical overlap and the concurrent high prevalence of both HIV and malaria mean that even modest interactions could substantially affect public health among populations exposed to both (Chandromohan and Greenwood 1998). Studies during the 1990s observed that malaria infection was more common and of higher parasite density in HIV-positive than in HIV-negative pregnant women in a range of malaria endemic settings, and in women of all gravidity, and that those who have had multiple pregnancies were most affected (Parise et al. 1998; Shulman 1999; Steketee, Wirima, Bloland et al. 1996; van Eijk, Ayisi, and ter Kuile 2001, p. 405; van Eijk et al. 2001; Verhoeff et al. 1999). Additionally, two longitudinal cohort studies in Uganda and Kenya and one hospital-based case-control study in Uganda have demonstrated that HIV-infection approximately doubles the risk of malaria parasitemia and clinical malaria in nonpregnant adults, and that increasing HIV-immunosuppression is associated with higher-density parasitemias (Francesconi et al. 2001; French et al. 2001; Whitworth et al. 2000). Thus, some evidence shows that HIV infection increases the incidence and severity of clinical malaria in adults.

In order to define the indirect consequences of *P. falciparum* it is important to know whether the high intensity of exposure to malaria infections increases the rate of progression of HIV disease in Africa. In a recent study in Malawi, HIV blood viral levels were found to be seven times higher in HIV-infected adults with acute uncomplicated malaria than in HIV-infected blood donors without malaria (Hoffman et al. 1999). As with other acute infections, the increased viral burden was reversed by effective malaria therapy (Hoffman et al. 1999). These findings are consistent with in vitro laboratory studies in which HIV-1 replication was increased 10-fold to 100-fold in peripheral blood mononuclear cells exposed to soluble malaria antigens or malaria pigment (Xiao et al. 1998).

The evidence on the potentiation of malaria by HIV or HIV by malaria is currently insufficient to quantify the specific HIV-malaria interaction risks for inclusion in malaria burden estimates.

The Combined Indirect Effects of Malaria on All-Cause Mortality

The effects of malaria infection on low birthweight seem conclusive; the overall role of malaria infection on anemia is clear, but its extrapolation to indirect mortality is difficult; the effects of infection on undernutrition and HIV is at present less conclusive and impossible to enumerate. It seems reasonable to assume that these additional consequential or indirect risks contribute to all-cause mortality beyond that described from estimates of the causes of death directly attributed to malaria.

To examine these conclusions and assumptions further, data on all-cause mortality of children under five from DSS studies undertaken across a broad range of malaria transmission settings in Sub-Saharan Africa were analyzed against the prevalence of *P. falciparum* infection at each site. Weighted least-squares regression was used to model the contiguous relationships between all-cause mortality and parasite prevalence rates, allowing for the square of parasite prevalence (for possible saturation of parasite prevalence), timing, location, and the sampling precision of each study (Snow, Korenromp, and Gouws 2004). The unadjusted median all-cause child mortality rate for low prevalence areas of childhood infection (less than 25 percent) was 10.9 per year per 1,000 children under five (IQR 7.8–17.6). This rose dramatically to 39.1 per year per 1,000 children (IQR 32.8–52.2) among populations exposed to childhood parasite prevalence risks greater than

or equal to 25 percent. In the regression model, mortality increased significantly with parasite prevalence, but this effect leveled off at higher prevalence rates. The model suggested that, in rural DSS sites throughout Sub-Saharan Africa, all-cause mortality increases by more than twofold (25–30 deaths per 1,000 children under five years old) over the prevalences of malaria infection covered by the DSS sites, and parasite prevalence explained 64 percent of the variation between sites in all-cause under-five mortality. By contrast, the direct estimation of malaria-specific mortality presented earlier for children living under stable endemic conditions was only 28.2 percent.

These comparisons of direct versus indirect contributions of malaria infection to child survival must be viewed with some caution. Ecological analyses are constrained by multiple confounders, notably, influences of socioeconomic status, access to and effectiveness of health services, prevalence of HIV, exposure to other parasitic diseases, nutrition, and the genetic makeup of the population. Still, such an approach to estimating malaria's contribution to child mortality in Sub-Saharan Africa suggests that the influence of *P. falciparum* infection is greater than that described by the direct, single-cause attribution of childhood deaths. The effects of malaria during pregnancy on low birthweight and to a lesser extent the nutritional and hematological influences of malaria infection may explain the difference between direct and indirect estimates.

MALARIA AND POVERTY

Recent global, cross-country regression analysis of malaria risk and gross domestic product have found the disease to be a significant influence on long-term economic growth. As much as half the gross domestic product is lost in highly endemic areas over 25 years as a direct result of malaria (Gallup and Sachs 2001; McCarthy and Wu 2000). Although persuasive to international donors, such a macroeconomic analysis fails to identify the mechanisms of these economic losses (Malaney, Speilman, and Sachs 2004). It seems reasonable to assume that national levels of economic loss are a composite of economic burdens at the household level. Shepard and colleagues (1991) estimated the household cost of malaria in Burkina Faso, Chad, the Republic of Congo, and Rwanda. The authors concluded that a case of malaria in Africa cost US\$9.84 in 1987, of which US\$1.83 was direct and US\$8.01 was accrued indirectly as a result of forgone income associated with malaria morbidity and mortality. The total estimated cost of US\$0.8 billion represents 0.6 percent of the gross domestic product of the economies in Sub-Saharan Africa. Thus, microeconomic analyses of household economic burden posed by malaria are only a fraction of macroeconomic analyses of national economic loss. Malaney, Speilman, and Sachs (2004) suggest that this difference might arise either because of inadequate methodologies or because the macroeconomic national burden encompasses household financial costs and ill-defined financial "externalities," such as trade, tourism, and investment.

Whether malaria drives household or national poverty requires better definition. However, the converse is irrefutable: poor people are less able to prevent infection or afford effective disease management. In Africa, malaria is largely a disease of the rural populations, and often these communities are home to some of the poorest of the poor in Africa. There is increasing evidence that strategies promoted to prevent infection, such as insecticide-treated bednets, are not reaching the poor when cost-retrieval is part of the strategy. The recent Kenyan Demographic and Health Survey showed that less than 7 percent of children described as living in households at the lowest wealth index quartile sleep under an insecticide-treated bednet compared with 35 percent of children in the top wealth quartile households (http://www.measuredhs.org/). Similar findings have been reported for Uganda (Mugisha and Arinatwe 2003). In Tanzania, poor children were less likely to receive antimalarials when febrile than children from wealthier families (Schellenberg et al. 2003). A household survey in Malawi focused on low-income households whose mean annual income was US$115 and where the costs of malaria prevention and treatment represented about 20 percent of annual income (Ettling et al. 1994).

TRENDS IN MALARIA MORTALITY

One of the earlier applications of the BOMA project was to examine long-term changes in the estimates of malaria mortality in Sub-Saharan Africa (Snow, Trape, and Marsh 2001). A comparison of preindependence malaria-specific and all-cause childhood mortality data derived from circumscribed colonial medical records and civil registration with early DSS data before 1990 and contemporary DSS data post-1990 is shown in figure 14.4. The period 1960–89 was characterized by a median malaria-specific mortality of 7.8 per 1,000 children under five per year, a decline of 18 percent from the estimates recorded before 1960 (9.5 per 1,000 children under five per year). However, the 11 studies of childhood malaria-specific mortality during the 1990s provided

Figure 14.4 Malaria-Specific and All-Cause Mortality Estimates per Year for Children under Five
(per 1,000)

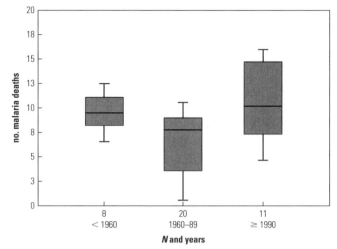

a. Malaria-Specific Mortality

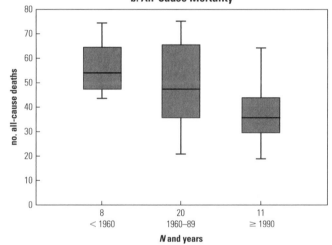

b. All-Cause Mortality

Source: Snow, Trape, and Marsh 2001.

Note: Central horizontal lines = median quartile range; box width and T = median and upper/lower limits of mortality estimates, respectively. Single outlier is more than three times the box width.

a median estimate of 10.2 per 1,000 children under five per year, similar to that described in the preindependence surveillance data (figure 14.4a). In contrast, the annualized risks of all-cause mortality recorded at the same sites demonstrate a continued decline over the three time periods (figure 14.4b), and overall childhood mortality during the early 1990s was 34 percent lower than the median estimates of all-cause mortality recorded during the preindependence surveys. The net result has been a rise in the proportion of all deaths attributed to malaria: 18 percent before 1960, 12 percent between 1960 and 1989, rising to 30 percent during the 1990s.

The BOMA data were reanalyzed to define more precisely the recent trends in malaria-specific mortality estimates from DSS sites among children under five years, allowing for variation in the VA performance, malaria endemicity, and region (Korenromp et al. 2003). In West African DSS sites, malaria mortality was on average 7.8 per 1,000 child-years throughout the 1980s and 1990s without a significant change over time. Although conclusive evidence of temporal increases in malaria-specific mortality was observed within a series of DSS sites in Senegal (Trape et al. 1998). In East and southern African DSS sites the estimated malaria mortality increased from 6.5 per 1,000 child-years between 1982 and 1990 to 11.9 per 1,000 child-years between 1990 and 1998. Nonmalaria mortality, in contrast, decreased over time in both regions. Figure 14.5 summarizes the combined Sub-Saharan Africa data for 1982–98, allowing for parameters of region, parasite prevalence, and VA performance.

There are several possible explanations for the observed trends in malaria mortality in Sub-Saharan Africa over the last 20 years, such as declining household wealth linked to a changing health sector based on cost retrieval and the general deterioration in the quality of clinical care. Although access to and quality of health care is undoubtedly suboptimal in many areas, this has not had a similar impact on nonmalaria childhood mortality. Global warming has been debated as a general cause of expanding malaria risk and thereby increasing malaria-specific mortality in several parts of Africa. However, this seems an unlikely explanation for the areas included in figures 14.4a and 14.5, as long-term data for areas likely to be affected by changes in ambient temperature do not support a trend in favor of increased malaria transmission (Hay et al. 2002). For many years chloroquine provided a cheap, effective, and easily available treatment. The past 20 years have seen a precipitous decline in the efficacy of chloroquine across Africa (EANMAT 2003; Talisuna, Bloland, and D'Alessandro 2004), and this represents the most likely factor contributing to the change in malaria-specific childhood mortality. Such an explanation would also be entirely consistent with observations of increased hospitalization and morbidity in other parts of Africa (Asindi et al. 1993; Greenberg et al. 1989; Shanks et al. 2000) and the sharp rises in malaria morbidity associated with declining first-line therapy in KwaZulu-Natal Province of South Africa and its reversal following the introduction of effective artemisinin-based combination therapies (Barnes and Folb 2003).

CONCLUSION

During 2000 approximately 1.14 million people may have died as a direct result of infection with *P. falciparum*. Eighty-eight percent of these deaths would have occurred in areas of stable endemic malaria and the majority of these would have been among young children. The empirical evidence for indirect or consequential mortality may explain an additional 10 percent of mortality directly attributed to malaria infection. This would be consistent with observations made during randomized controlled trials that suggest that reducing the risks of infection in a community has an impact beyond what might readily be described by verbal autopsy as direct malaria mortality. Recent ecological analyses of all-cause pediatric mortality suggest that the difference between direct and indirect attribution of malaria as cause of death might be substantially higher than 10 percent.

The Roll Back Malaria movement proposes to halve malaria mortality by the year 2010 (http://www.rbm.int). This goal has been set even though existing, affordable therapeutics are rapidly failing, health service provision is breaking down, there are no immediate prospects of widespread vaccination, and poverty continues to afflict most endemic countries. There are strong reasons to believe that over the past 15 years malaria-specific mortality has risen and now accounts for an increasing proportion of overall childhood mortality. The starting point for new efforts to "roll back malaria" is not a level playing field but a mortality burden that has returned to levels described before Africa gained independence.

Figure 14.5 Malaria-Specific, Nonmalaria, and All-Cause Mortality Rates among Children under Five
(per 1,000 per year from 28 DSS sites)

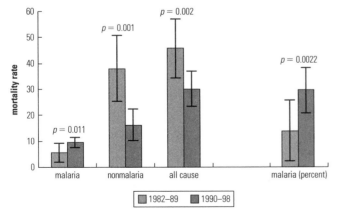

Source: Adapted from Korenromp et al. 2003.

Note: Data analyzed by least-squares linear regression to allow for interactions of determinants of VA-adjusted mortality, the square of parasite prevalence, and region.

One million deaths due to malaria each year in Africa resonate with earlier claims of a similar figure proposed as far back as the 1950s (Bruce-Chwatt 1952; Greenwood 1990; Schwartlander 1997; Sturchler 1989). These estimations are hard to comprehend without a methodological framework or empirical evidence to support them. How much further forward are we in estimating malaria's contribution to the mortality burden in Sub-Saharan Africa? The estimates provided in this chapter continue to be driven by informed approximations, in part because of the paucity of reliable and accurate data, but also due to the inherent difficulties of unique diagnosis. The estimates, however, have been made from empirical epidemiological measures of mortality risks, structured according to age and malaria transmission. The method is similar to one previously used to define the malaria burden in Sub-Saharan Africa (Snow et al. 1999) but takes into account new data, refined endemicity classifications, broader health consequences, and the temporal effects associated with changing antimalarial drug sensitivity. This data-driven method allows for a more transparent review of the evidence.

Such reviews of available evidence reveal as much about what we do know as about what we do not know. Many aspects of the malaria burden in Sub-Saharan Africa require further empirical investigation or modeling. In the continued absence of wide-area, reliable coverage of cause-specific mortality data there is a need for increased research to help in an understanding of the spatial determinants of risk. The assumption that urban versus rural, East versus West African, or poor versus affluent populations experience similar risks of poor health outcomes from malaria infection is clearly an oversimplification of complex interactions. The precise cartography of risk requires improved population distribution maps. This is now being addressed at a global scale through a new initiative, the Malaria Atlas Project, funded by the Wellcome Trust, United Kingdom (http://www.map.ox.ac.uk). The emphasis within the literature on measuring childhood risks of disease and death from malaria would seem justified from the current understanding of immunity, but there is comparative ignorance about the true public health consequences of malaria among older children and adults. The impact of infection and disease on undernutrition, anemia, and HIV remain at best speculative and require further investigation before these composite risks can be defined. The most significant challenge facing the malaria epidemiologist today is to describe malaria health outcomes in Africa and how these risks change from birth through adulthood according to the dependent factors of infection, immunity, and control.

NOTE

This review was made possible because of a large contribution over the years from malaria epidemiology colleagues, notably Marlies Craig, Uwe Deichmann, Simon Hay, Eline Korenromp, Claire Mackintosh, Kevin Marsh, Charles Newton, Dennis Shanks, Rick Steketee, and Jean-François Trape. The Burden of Malaria in Africa Project is principally supported by the Wellcome Trust, United Kingdom (project number 058992), with additional support from the Bill & Melinda Gates Foundation (project number 17408); the Disease Control Priorities Project, World Bank; and the Kenyan Medical Research Institute. Robert W. Snow is supported by the Wellcome Trust, United Kingdom, as a senior research fellow.

REFERENCES

Alonso, P. L., S. W. Lindsay, J. R. M. Armstrong-Schellenberg, K. Keita, P. Gomez, F. C. Shenton, A. G. Hill, et al. 1993. "A Malaria Control Trial Using Insecticide-Treated Bed Nets and Targeted Chemoprophylaxis in a Rural Area of The Gambia, West Africa." *Transactions of the Royal Society of Tropical Medicine and Hygiene* 87 (Suppl. 2): 37–44.

Asindi, A. A., E. E. Ekanem, E. O. Ibia, and M. A. Nwangwa.1993. "Upsurge of Malaria-Related Convulsions in a Paediatric Emergency Room in Nigeria. Consequence of Emergence of Chloroquine-Resistant *Plasmodium falciparum*." *Tropical and Geographic Medicine* 45: 110–13.

Barnes, K., and P. Folb. 2003. "The Role of Artemisinin-Based Combination Therapy in Malaria Management." In *Reducing Malaria's Burden: Evidence of Effectiveness for Decision Makers*, ed. C. Murphy, K. Ringheim, S. Woldehanna, and J. Volmink, 25–31. Washington, DC: Global Health Council.

Barnish, G., G. H. Maude, M. J. Bockarie, T. A. Eggelte, and B. M. Greenwood. 1993. "The Epidemiology of Malaria in Southern Sierra Leone." *Parasitologia* 35: 1–4.

Beier, J. C., G. F. Killeen, and J. I. Githure. 1999. "Entomologic Inoculation Rates and *Plasmodium falciparum* Malaria Prevalence in Africa." *American Journal of Tropical Medicine and Hygiene* 61: 109–13.

Brabin, B. J. 1983. "An Analysis of Malaria in Pregnancy in Africa." *Bulletin of the World Health Organization* 61: 1005–16.

Brabin, B. J., M. Hakimi, and D. Pelletier. 2001. "An Analysis of Anemia and Pregnancy-Related Maternal Mortality." *Journal of Nutrition* 131 (Suppl.): 604S–615S.

Bradley, D. J. 1991. "Morbidity and Mortality at Pare-Taveta, Kenya and Tanzania, 1954–66: The Effects of a Period of Malaria Control." In *Disease and Mortality in Sub-Saharan Africa,* ed. R. G. Feachem and D. T. Jamison, 248–63. New York: Oxford University Press.

Bradley-Moore, A. M., B. M. Greenwood, A. K. Bradley, B. R. Kirkwood, and H. M. Gilles. 1985. "Malaria Prophylaxis with Chloroquine in Young Nigerian Children. III. Its Effect on Nutrition." *Annals of Tropical Medicine and Parasitology* 79: 575–84.

Brink, C. J. H. 1958. "Malaria Control in the Northern Transvaal." *South African Medical Journal* 32: 800–08.

Bruce-Chwatt, L. J. 1952. "Malaria in African Infants and Children in Southern Nigeria." *Annals of Tropical Medicine and Parasitology* 46: 173–200.

Chandramohan, D., and B. M. Greenwood. 1998. "Is There an Interaction between Human Immunodeficiency Virus and *Plasmodium falciparum*?" *International Journal of Epidemiology* 27: 296–301.

Charlwood, J. D., M. Qassim, E. I. Elnsur, M. Donnelly, V. Petrarca, P. F. Billingsley, J. Pinto, and T. Smith. 2001. "The Impact of Indoor Residual Spraying with Malathion on Malaria in Refugee Camps in Eastern Sudan." *Acta Tropica* 80: 1–8.

Cockerell, O. C., A. L. Johnson, J. W. Sander, Y. M. Hart, D. M. Goodridge, and S. D. Shorvon. 1994. "Mortality from Epilepsy: Results from a Prospective Population-Based Study." *Lancet* 344: 918–21.

Colbourne, M. J., and G. M. Edington. 1954. "Mortality from Malaria in Accra." *Journal of Tropical Medicine and Hygiene* 57: 203–10.

Colebunders, R., R. Ryder, H. Francis, W. Nekwei, Y. Bahwe, I. Lebughe, M. Ndilu, G. Vercauteren, K. Nseka, and J. Perriens. 1991. "Seroconversion Rate, Mortality and Clinical Manifestations Associated with the Receipt of a Human Immunodeficiency Virus-Infected Transfusion in Kinshasa, Zaire." *Journal of Infectious Diseases* 164: 450–56.

Coleman, R., L. Loppy, and G. Walraven. 2002. "The Treatment Gap and Primary Health Care for People with Epilepsy in Rural Gambia." *Bulletin of the World Health Organization* 80: 378–83.

Craig, M. H., R. W. Snow, and D. le Sueur. 1999. "A Climate-Based Distribution Model of Malaria Transmission in Sub-Saharan Africa." *Parasitology Today* 15: 105–11.

D'Alessandro, U., B. O. Olaleye, W. McGuire, P. Langerock, S. Bennett, M. K. Aikins, M. C. Thompson, M. K. Cham, B. A. Cham, and B. M. Greenwood. 1995. "Mortality and Morbidity from Malaria in Gambian Children after the Introduction of an Impregnated Bed Net Programme." *Lancet* 345: 479–83.

Deichmann, U. 1996. African Population Database. Digital database and documentation. National Center for Geographic Information and Analysis, Santa Barbara, CA. http://grid2.cr.usgs.gov/globalpop/africa/.

Delacollette, C., and M. Barutwanayo. 1993. "Mortalité et morbidité aux jeunes ages dans une région a paludisme hyperendemique stable, commune de Nyanza Lac, Imbo Sud, Burundi." *Bulletin de la Société de Pathologie Exotique* 86: 1–7.

Diseko, R. 1994. "Malaria in Botswana." Minutes of Annual Malaria Conference, St. Lucia, South Africa, October.

EANMAT (East African Network for Monitoring Antimalarial Therapy). 2003. "The Efficacy of Antimalarial Monotherapies Sulphadoxine-Pyrimethamine and Amodiaquine in East Africa: Implications for Sub-Regional Policy." *Tropical Medicine and International Health* 8: 860–67.

English, M., F. Esamai, A. Wasunna, F. Were, A. Wamae, R. W. Snow, and N. Peshu. 2004. "In-Patient Paediatric Care at the First Referral Level in Kenya." *Lancet* 363: 1948–53.

Ettling, M., D. A. McFarland, L. J. Schultz, and L. Chitsulo. 1994. "Economic Impact of Malaria in Malawian Households." *Tropical Medicine and Parasitology* 45: 74–79.

Francesconi, P., M. Fabiani, M. G. Dente, M. Lukwiya, R. Okwey, J. Ouma, R. Ochakachon, F. Cian, and S. Declich. 2001. "HIV, Malaria Parasites, and Acute Febrile Episodes in Ugandan Adults: A Case-Control Study." *AIDS* 15: 2445–50.

French, N., J. Nakiyingi, E. Lugada, C. Watera, J. A. Whitworth, and C. F. Gilks. 2001. "Increasing Rates of Malarial Fever with Deteriorating Immune Status in HIV-1-Infected Ugandan Adults." *AIDS* 15: 899–906.

Gallup, J., and J. Sachs. 2001. "The Economic Burden of Malaria." *American Journal of Tropical Medicine and Hygiene* 64S: 85–96.

Ghana VAST (Vitamin A Supplementation Treatment) Study Team. 1993. "Vitamin A Supplementation in Northern Ghana: Effects on Clinic Attendance, Hospital Admissions and Child Mortality." *Lancet* 342: 7–12.

Government of Colony of Gold Coast. 1912–48. *Annual Reports of the Medical Department for the Years Ending 31st December 1912–1916.* London: Waterlow & Sons.

Government of the Colony and Protectorate of Kenya. 1935. *Medical Department Annual Report, Including the Medical Research Laboratory Annual Report for 1933.* Nairobi, Kenya: Government Printers.

Government of Colony and Protectorate of Nigeria. 1934–35. *Annual Reports of the Medical and Health Department for the Years 1932 and 1933.* Lagos, Nigeria: Government Printers.

Government of Colony and Protectorate of Sierra Leone. 1913–17. *Annual Reports of the Medical Department for the Years ending 31st December 1912–1916.* London: Waterlow & Sons.

Government of Tanzania. 1997. *Policy Implications of Adult Morbidity and Mortality: End of Phase 1 Report.* Dar es Salaam, Tanzania: Ministry of Health.

Granja, A. C., F. Machungo, A. Gomes, S. Bergstrom, and B. Brabin. 1998. "Malaria-Related Maternal Mortality in Urban Mozambique." *Annals of Tropical Medicine and Parasitology* 92: 257–63.

Greenberg, A. E., P. Nguyen-Dinh, J. M. Mann, N. Kabote, R. L. Colebunders, H. Francis, T. C. Quinn, et al. 1988. "The Association between Malaria, Blood Transfusions, and HIV Seropositivity in a Pediatric Population in Kinshasa, Zaire." *Journal of the American Medical Association* 259: 545–49.

Greenberg, A. E., M. Ntumbanzondo, N. Ntula, L. Mawa, J. Howell, and F. Davachi. 1989. "Hospital-Based Surveillance of Malaria-Related Pediatric Morbidity and Mortality in Kinshasa, Zaire." *Bulletin of the World Health Organization* 67: 189–96.

Greenwood, A. M., J. R. M. Armstrong, P. Byass, R. W. Snow, and B. M. Greenwood. 1992. "Malaria Chemoprophylaxis, Birth Weight and Child Survival." *Transactions of the Royal Society of Tropical Medicine and Hygiene* 86: 483–85.

Greenwood, B. M. 1990. "Populations at Risk." *Parasitology Today* 6: 188.

Guyatt, H. L., and R. W. Snow. 2001a. "Malaria in Pregnancy as an Indirect Cause of Infant Mortality in Sub-Saharan Africa." *Transactions of the Royal Society of Tropical Medicine and Hygiene* 95: 569–76.

———. 2001b. "The Epidemiology and Burden of *Plasmodium falciparum*–Related Anemia among Pregnant Women in Sub-Saharan Africa." *American Journal of Tropical Medicine and Hygiene* 64: 36–44.

Hauser, W. A., J. F. Annegers, and L. R. Elveback. 1980. "Mortality in Patients with Epilepsy." *Epilepsia* 21: 399–412.

Hay, S. I., J. Cox, D. J. Rogers, S. E. Randolph, D. I. Stern, D. G. Shanks, M. F. Myers, and R. W. Snow. 2002. "Climate Change and the Resurgence of Malaria in the East African Highlands." *Nature* 415: 905–9.

Hay, S. I., C. A. Guerra, A. J. Tatem, P. M. Atkinson, and R. W. Snow. 2005. "Urbanization, Malaria Transmission and Disease Burden in Africa." *Nature Microbiology Review* 3: 81–90.

Hay, S. I., D. J. Rogers, J. F. Toomer, and R. W. Snow. 2000. "Annual *Plasmodium falciparum* Entomological Inoculation Rates (EIR) across Africa: Literature Survey, Internet Access and Review." *Transactions of the Royal Society of Tropical Medicine and Hygiene* 94: 113–27.

Hill, A. V. S. 1992. "Malaria Resistance Genes: A Natural Selection." *Transactions of the Royal Society of Tropical Medicine and Hygiene* 86: 225–26.

Hoffman, I. F., C. S. Jere, T. E. Taylor, P. Munthali, J. R. Dyer, J. J. Wirima, S. J. Rogerson, et al. 1999. "The Effect of *Plasmodium falciparum* Malaria on HIV-1 RNA Blood Plasma Concentration." *AIDS* 13: 487–94.

Holding, P. A., and R. W. Snow. 2001. "The Impact of *Plasmodium falciparum* Malaria on Performance and Learning: A Review of the Evidence." *American Journal of Tropical Medicine and Hygiene* 64 (Suppl. 1): 68–75.

Holding, P. A., P. K. K. Wekulo. 2004. "Child Development: What Should We Be Measuring and How Can We Measure It?" *American Journal of Tropical Medicine and Hygiene* 71 (Suppl. 2): 71–79.

INDEPTH Network 2002. *Population and Health in Developing Countries.* Vol. 1: *Population, Health and Survival at INDEPTH Sites.* Ottawa: International Development Research Centre.

Jaffar, S., A. Leach, A. M. Greenwood, A. Jepson, O. Muller, M. O. C. Ota, K. Bojang, S. Obaro, and B. M. Greenwood. 1997. "Changes in the Pattern of Infant and Childhood Mortality in Upper River Division, The Gambia, from 1989 to 1993." *Tropical Medicine and International Health* 2: 28–37.

Jillek-All, L., and H. T. Rwiza. 1992. "Prognosis of Epilepsy in a Rural African Community: A 30-Year Follow-up of 164 Patients in an Outpatient Clinic in Rural Tanzania. *Epilepsia* 33: 645–50.

Joy, D. A., X. R. Feng, J. B. Mu, T. Furuya, K. Chotivanich, A. U. Krettli, M. Ho, et al. 2003. "Early Origin and Recent Expansion of *Plasmodium falciparum.*" *Science* 300: 318–21.

Kahn, K., S. M. Tollman, M. Garenne, and J. S. S. Gear. 1999. "Who Dies from What? Determining Cause of Death in South Africa's Rural North-East." *Tropical Medicine and International Health* 4: 433–41.

Kamwi, M. 1998. "Report on Malaria Situation." Ministry of Health and Social Services Epidemiology Section, Government of Namibia.

Kleinschmidt, I., J. A. Omumbo, O. Briet, N. van de Giesen, N. Sogoba, N. K. Mensah, P. Windermeijer, M. Moussa, and T. Teuscher. 2001. "An Empirical Malaria Distribution Map for West Africa." *Tropical Medicine and International Health* 6: 779–86.

Korenromp, E. L., J. R. M. Armstrong-Schellenberg, B. G. Williams, B. Nahlen, and R. W. Snow. 2004. "Impact of Malaria Control on Childhood Anemia in Africa—A Quantitative Review." *Tropical Medicine and International Health* 9: 1050–65.

Korenromp, E. L., B. G. Williams, E. Gouws, C. Dye, and R. W. Snow. 2003. "Measuring Trends in Childhood Malaria Mortality in Africa: A New Assessment of Progress toward Targets Based on Verbal Autopsy." *Lancet Infectious Diseases* 3: 349–58.

Lackritz, E. M., C. C. Campbell, T. K. Ruebush II, A. W. Hightower, W. Wakube, R. W. Steketee, and J. B. O. Were. 1992. "Effect of Blood Transfusion on Survival among Children in a Kenyan Hospital." *Lancet* 340: 524–28.

Le Sueur, D., B. L. Sharp, and C. C. Appleton. 1993. "Historical Perspective of the Malaria Problem in Natal with Emphasis on the Period 1928–1932." *South African Journal of Science* 89: 232–39.

LSDI (Lubombo Special Development Initiative). 2001. "Annual Report, 2001." LSDI Malaria Control. Medical Research Council Report, Durban, South Africa.

Luxemburger, C., R. McGready, A. Kham, L. Morison, T. Cho, T. Congsuphajaisiddhi, N. J. White, and F. Nosten. 2001. "Effects of Malaria during Pregnancy on Infant Mortality in an Area of Low Malaria Transmission." *American Journal of Epidemiology* 154: 459–65.

Malaney, P., A. Speilman, and J. Sachs. 2004. "The Malaria Gap." *American Journal of Tropical Medicine and Hygiene* 71 (Suppl. 2): 141–6.

Marsh, K., D. Forster, C. Waruiru, I. Mwangi, M. Winstanley, V. Marsh, C. Newton, et al. 1995. "Life-Threatening Malaria in African Children: Clinical Spectrum and Simplified Prognostic Criteria." *New England Journal of Medicine* 332: 1399–404.

Marsh, K., and R. W. Snow. 1999. "Malaria Transmission and Morbidity." *Parassitologia* (Rome) 41: 241–46.

McCarthy, D. H. W., and Y. Wu. 2000. *Malaria and Growth.* Policy Research Working Paper 2303, World Bank, Washington, DC.

Menendez, C. 1995. "Malaria during Pregnancy: A Priority Area of Malaria Research and Control." *Parasitology Today* 11: 178–83.

Menendez, C., A. F. Fleming, and P. L. Alonso. 2000. "Malaria-Related Anaemia." *Parasitology Today* 16: 469–76.

Molineaux, L. 1997. "Malaria and Mortality: Some Epidemiological Considerations." *Annals of Tropical Medicine and Parasitology* 91: 811–25.

Moore, A., G. Herrera, J. Nyamongo, E. Lackritz, B. Nahlen, A. Oloo, G. Opondo, R. Muga, and R. Janssen. 2001. "Estimated Risk of HIV Transmission by Blood Transfusion in Kenya." *Lancet* 358: 657–60.

Mugisha, F., and J. Arinatwe. 2003. "Sleeping Arrangements and Mosquito Net Use among Under Fives: Results from the Uganda Demographic and Health Survey." *Malaria Journal* 2: 40–50.

Mung'ala-Odera, V., R. W. Snow, and C. R. J. C. Newton. 2004. "The Burden of the Neuro-Cognitive Impairment Associated with *Plasmodium Falciparum* Malaria in Sub-Saharan Africa." *American Journal of Tropical Medicine and Hygiene* 71 (Suppl. 2): 55–63.

Murray, C. J. L., and A. D. Lopez. 1997. "Mortality by Cause for Eight Regions of the World: Global Burden of Disease Study." *Lancet* 349: 1269–76.

Nabarro, D. N., and E. Taylor. 1998. "The 'Roll Back Malaria' Campaign." *Science* 280: 2067–68.

Nevill, C. G., E. S. Some, V. O. Mung'ala, W. Mutemi, L. New, K. Marsh, C. Lengeler, and R. W. Snow. 1996. "Insecticide-Treated Bednets Reduce Mortality and Severe Morbidity from Malaria among Children on the Kenyan Coast." *Tropical Medicine and International Health* 1: 139–46.

Newton, C. R. J. C. and S. Krishna. 1998. "Severe Falciparum Malaria in Children: Current Understanding of Pathophysiology and Supportive Treatment." *Pharmacology and Therapeutics* 79: 1–53.

Nussenblatt, V., and R. D. Semba. 2002. "Micronutrient Malnutrition and the Pathogenesis of Malarial Anemia." *Acta Tropica* 82: 321–37.

Omumbo, J. A., C. A. Guerra, S. I. Hay, and R. W. Snow. 2004. "The Relationship between the Parasite Ratio in Childhood and Climate Estimates of Malaria Transmission in Kenya." *Malaria Journal* 3: 1–8.

Parise, M. E., J. G. Ayisi, B. L. Nahlen, L. J. Schultz, J. M. Roberts, A. Misore, R. Muga, A. J. Oloo, and R. W. Steketee. 1998. "Efficacy of Sulfadoxine-Pyrimethamine for Prevention of Placental Malaria in an Area of Kenya with a High Prevalence of Malaria and Human Immunodeficiency Virus Infection." *American Journal of Tropical Medicine and Hygiene* 59: 813–22.

Pasha, O., J. D. Rosso, M. Mukaka, and D. Marsh. 2003. "The Effect of Providing Fansidar (sulfadoxine-pyrimethamine) in Schools on Mortality in School-Age Children in Malawi." *Lancet* 361: 577–8.

Pelletier, D. L., E. A. Frongillo, and J. P. Habicht. 1993. "Epidemiologic Evidence for a Potentiating Effect of Malnutrition on Child Mortality." *American Journal of Public Health* 83: 1130–33.

Pelletier, D. L., E. A. Frongillo, D. G. Schroeder, and J. P. Habicht. 1995. "The Effects of Malnutrition on Child Mortality in Developing Countries." *Bulletin of the World Health Organization* 73: 443–48.

Philips-Howard, P., and A. B. Bjorkman. 1990. "Ascertainment of Risk of Serious Adverse Reactions Associated with Chemoprophylactic Antimalarial Drugs." *Bulletin of World Health Organization* 68: 493–504.

Philips-Howard, P., and L. J. West. 1990. "Serious Adverse Drug Reactions to Pyrimethamine-Sulphadoxine, Pyrimethamine-Dapsone and to Amodiaquine in Britain." *Journal of the Royal Society of Medicine* 83: 82–85.

Piotti, A. 1997. "Memo on Collection of Malaria Clinical Case Incidence Rates, December 1995 to April 1996 and December 1996 to April 1997." Report, Ministry for Health, Zimbabwe, July 4.

Premji, Z., P. Ndayanga, C. Shiff, J. Minjas, P. Lubega, and J. MacLeod. 1997. "Community Based Studies on Childhood Mortality in a Malaria Holoendemic Area on the Tanzanian Coast." *Acta Tropica* 63: 101–9.

Reynolds, J. E. F., ed. 1993. *Martindale: The Extra Pharmacopoeia.* 13th ed. London: Pharmaceutical Press.

Robert, V., K. MacIntyre, S. Keating, J. F. Trape, J. B. Duchemin, M. Wilson, and J. C. Beier. 2003. "Malaria Transmission in Urban Sub-Saharan Africa." *American Journal of Tropical Medicine and Hygiene* 68: 169–76.

Salum, F. M., T. J. Wilkes, K. Kivumbi, and C. F. Curtis. 1994. "Mortality of Under Fives in a Rural Area of Holoendemic Malaria Transmission." *Acta Tropica* 58: 29–34.

Savarit, D., K. M. De Cock, R. Schutz, S. Konate, E. Lackritz, and A. Bondurand. 1992. "Risk of HIV Infection from Transfusion with Blood Negative for HIV Antibody in a West African City." *British Medical Journal* 305: 498–501.

Schellenberg, J. R. M. A., C. G. Victora, A. Mushi, D. De Savigny, D. Schellenberg, H. Mshinda, and J. Bryce. 2003. "Inequities among the Very Poor: Health Care Children in Rural Southern Tanzania." *Lancet* 361: 561–66.

Schwartlander, B. 1997. "Global Burden of Disease." *Lancet* 350: 141–42.

Shanks, G. D., K. Biomondo, S. I. Hay, and R. W. Snow. 2000. "Changing Patterns of Clinical Malaria Since 1965 among a Tea Estate Population Located in the Kenyan Highlands." *Transactions of the Royal Society of Tropical Medicine and Hygiene* 94: 253–55.

Shepard, D. S., M. B. Ettling, U. Brinkmann, and R. Sauerborn. 1991. "The Economic Cost of Malaria in Africa." *Tropical Medicine and Parasitology* 42: 199–203.

Shulman, C. E. 1999. "Malaria in Pregnancy: Its Relevance to Safe-Motherhood Programmes." *Annals of Tropical Medicine and Parasitology* 93 (Suppl. 1): S59–66.

Smith, P. G., and R. H. Morrow. 1996. *Field Trials of Health Interventions in Developing Countries: A Toolbox.* 2nd ed. London: Macmillan Education.

Snow, R. W., M. H. Craig, U. Deichmann, and K. Marsh. 1999. "Estimating Mortality, Morbidity and Disability Due to Malaria among Africa's Non-Pregnant Population." *Bulletin of the World Health Organization* 77: 624–40.

Snow, R. W., M. H. Craig, C. R. J. C. Newton, and R. W. Steketee. 2003. "The Public Health Burden of *Plasmodium falciparum* Malaria in Africa: Deriving the Numbers." Disease Control Priorities Project Working Paper 11, Fogarty International Center, National Institutes of Health, Bethseda, Md. http://www.fic.nih.gov/dcpp.

Snow, R. W., and H. M. Gilles. 2002. "The Epidemiology of Malaria." In *Bruce-Chwatt's Essential Malariology,* 4th ed., ed. D. A. Warrell and H. M. Gilles, 85–106. London: Arnold Publishers.

Snow, R. W., E. Gouws, J. Omumbo, B. Rapuoda, M. H. Craig, F. C. Tanser, D. le Sueur, and J. Ouma. 1998. "Models to Predict the Intensity of *Plasmodium falciparum* Transmission: Applications to the Burden of Disease in Kenya." *Transactions of the Royal Society of Tropical Medicine and Hygiene* 92: 601–6.

Snow, R. W., E. L. Korenromp, and E. Gouws. 2004. "Pediatric Mortality in Africa: *Plasmodium Falciparum* Malaria as a Cause or a Risk?" *American Journal of Tropical Medicine and Hygiene* 71 (Suppl. 2): 16–24.

Snow, R. W., and K. Marsh. 2002. "The Consequences of Reducing *Plasmodium falciparum* Transmission in Africa." *Advances in Parasitology* 52: 235–64.

Snow, R. W., C. S. Molyneux, P. A. Warn, J. Omumbo, C. G. Nevill, S. Gupta, and K. Marsh. 1996. "Infant Parasite Rates and Immunoglobulin M Seroprevalence as a Measure of Exposure to *Plasmodium falciparum* during a Randomized Controlled Trial of Insecticide-Treated Bed Nets on the Kenyan Coast." *American Journal of Tropical Medicine and Hygiene* 55: 144–49.

Snow, R. W., V. O. Mung'ala, D. Forster, and K. Marsh. 1994. "The Role of the District Hospital in Child Survival at the Kenyan Coast." *African Journal of Health Sciences* 1: 71–75.

Snow, R. W., J. A. Omumbo, B. Lowe, S. M. Molyneux, J. O. Obiero, A. Palmer, M. W. Weber, et al. 1997a. "Relation between Severe Malaria Morbidity in Children and Level of *Plasmodium falciparum* Transmission in Africa." *Lancet* 349: 1650–54.

———. 1997b. "The Effects of Malaria Control on Nutritional Status in Infancy." *Acta Tropica* 65: 1–10.

Snow, R. W., J. F. Trape, and K. Marsh. 2001. "The Past, Present and Future of Childhood Malaria Mortality in Africa." *Trends in Parasitology* 17: 593–97.

Snow, R. W., R. E. M. Williams, J. E. Rogers, V. O. Mung'ala, and N. Peshu. 1994. "The Prevalence of Epilepsy among a Rural Kenyan Population: Its Association with Premature Mortality." *Tropical and Geographical Medicine* 46: 175–79.

Steketee, R. W., B. L. Nahlen, M. E. Parise, and C. Menendez. 2001. "The Burden of Malaria in Pregnancy in Malaria-Endemic Areas." *American Journal of Tropical Medicine and Hygiene* 64 (Suppl.): 28–35.

Steketee, R. W., J. J. Wirima, P. B. Bloland, B. Chilima, J. H. Mermin, L. Chitsulo, and J. G. Breman. 1996. "Impairment of a Pregnant Woman's Acquired Ability to Limit *Plasmodium falciparum* by Infection with Human Immunodeficiency Virus Type-1." *American Journal of Tropical Medicine and Hygiene* 55 (Suppl.): 42–49.

Steketee, R. W., J. J. Wirima, A. W. Hightower, L. Slutsker, D. L. Heymann, and J. G. Breman. 1996. "The Effect of Malaria and Malaria Prevention in Pregnancy on Offspring Birthweight, Prematurity, and Intrauterine Growth Retardation in Rural Malawi." *American Journal of Tropical Medicine and Hygiene* 55 (Suppl.): 33–41.

Sturchler, D. 1989. "How Much Malaria is There World-Wide?" *Parasitology Today* 5: 39–40.

Talisuna, A. O., P. Bloland, and U. D'Alessandro. 2004. "History, Dynamics and Public Health Importance of Malaria Parasite Resistance." *Clinical Microbiology Reviews* 17: 235–54.

Ter Kuile, F. O., D. J. Terlouw, S. K. Kariuki, P. A. Phillips-Howard, L. B. Mirel, W. A. Hawley, J. F. Friedman, et al. 2003. "Impact of Permethrin-Treated Bednets on Malaria, Anemia and Growth in Infants in an Area of Intense Perennial Malaria Transmission in Western Kenya." *American Journal of Tropical Medicine and Hygiene* 68 (Suppl. 4): 68–77.

Trape, J. F., E. Lefebvre-Zante, F. Legros, G. Ndiaye, H. Bouganali, P. Druille, and G. Salem. 1992. "Vector Density Gradients and the Epidemiology of Urban Malaria in Dakar, Senegal." *American Journal of Tropical Medicine and Hygiene* 47: 181–89.

Trape, J. F., G. Pison, M. P. Preziosi, C. Enel, A. Desgrees du Lou, V. Del Aunay, B. Samb, E. Lagarde, J. F. Molez, and F. Simondon. 1998. "Impact of Chloroquine Resistance on Malaria Mortality." *Comptes Rendus de l'Académie des Sciences Paris, Série III* 321: 689–97.

Tsoka, J. M., B. L. Sharp, and I. Kleinschmidt. 2002. "Malaria Mortality in a High Risk Area of South Africa." Paper presented at the Third MIM Pan-African Malaria Conference: "Global Advances in Malaria Research: Evidence-Based Decision Making for Malaria Control Policy," Arusha, Tanzania, November.

United Nations Population Division. 2001. *World Population Prospects: The 2000 Revision* and *World Urbanization Prospects: The 2001 Revision.* http://esa.un.org/unpp.

van Eijk, A. M., J. G. Ayisi, and F. O. ter Kuile. 2001. "Human Immunodeficiency Virus Increases the Risk of Malaria in Women of All Gravidities in Kisumu, Kenya." Abstract 405 in *Proceedings of 50th Annual Meeting of the American Society of Tropical Medicine and Hygiene,* Atlanta, Ga.

van Eijk, A. M., J. G. Ayisi, F. O. ter Kuile, A. Misore, J. A. Otieno, M. S. Kolczak, P. A. Kager, R. W. Steketee, and B. L. Nahlen. 2001. "Human Immunodeficiency Virus Seropositivity and Malaria as Risk Factors for Third-Trimester Anemia in Asymptomatic Pregnant Women in Western Kenya." *American Journal of Tropical Medicine and Hygiene* 65: 623–30.

Verhoeff, F. H., B. J. Brabin, C. A. Hart, L. Chimsuku, P. Kazembe, and R. L. Broadhead. 1999. "Increased Prevalence of Malaria in HIV-Infected Pregnant Women and Its Implications for Malaria Control." *Tropical Medicine and International Health* 4: 5–12.

Warrell, D. A. 2002. "Clinical Features of Malaria." In *Bruce-Chwatt's Essential Malariology*, 4th ed., ed. D. A. Warrell and H. M. Gilles, 191–205. London: Arnold Publishers.

Whitworth, J., D. Morgan, M. Quigley, A. Smith, B. Mayanja, H. Eotu, N. Omoding, M. Okongo, S. Malamba, and A. Ojwiya. 2000. "Effect of HIV-1 and Increasing Immunosuppression on Malaria Parasitaemia and Clinical Episodes in Adults in Rural Uganda: A Cohort Study." *Lancet* 356: 1051–56.

Xiao, L., S. M. Owen, D. L. Rudolph, R. B. Lal, and A. A. Lal. 1998. "*Plasmodium falciparum* Antigen-Induced Human Immunodeficiency Virus Type 1 Replication Is Mediated through Induction of Tumor Necrosis Factor-Alpha." *Journal of Infectious Diseases* 177: 437–45.

Zielinski, J. J. 1974. "Epilepsy and Mortality Rate and Cause of Death." *Epilepsia* 15: 191–201.

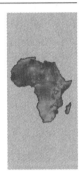

Chapter **15**

Onchocerciasis

Uche Amazigo, Mounkaila Noma, Jesse Bump, Bruce Benton,
Bernhard Liese, Laurent Yaméogo, Honorat Zouré,
and Azodoga Seketeli

Onchocerciasis, commonly called river blindness, is a parasitic disease particularly prevalent in Africa, where more than 99 percent of all cases occur. In total, 30 countries are infested, ranging from Senegal across to Ethiopia in the north and as far south as Angola and Malawi.

TRANSMISSION

Onchocerciasis is caused by worms, *Onchocerca volvulus*. The adult worms measure nearly a meter long and live in coiled mating pairs in nodules under the skin. Reproducing adult females spawn about 2,000 immature worms every day. These tiny juvenile worms migrate throughout the skin and eyes, causing the various symptoms of the disease. Although they are damaging, these immature worms cannot mature to adulthood without being transmitted by a blackfly of the genus *Simulium*. This fly breeds in rapidly flowing streams and rivers, and thus the name "river blindness." The most important vector is *Simulium damnosum sensus lato*, which has a wide range throughout Africa and the Middle East. In East Africa, *S. neavei* also transmits onchocerciasis.

There are many vectors in the Western hemisphere, but *S. ochraceum*, *S. metallicum*, *S. oyapockense*, *S. guianense*, and *S. exiguum* are among the most important. In the island of Bioko, the vector is *S. yahense*, Bioko form.

Blackflies serve as the intermediate host of the parasite. Flies ingest immature worms when they bite infected people. As the worms live in the fly, they mature sexually over the course of a week. Then, should the fly bite a person, the maturing worm will grow to adulthood inside the human body. Upon finding mating partners, the adults become encapsulated and produce more immature worms, completing the full transmission cycle.

THE DISEASE BURDEN

The most severe consequences of onchocerciasis is blindness, which may affect one-third of the adult population of the most highly affected communities. The prevention of blindness was the main clinical reason for initiating the Onchocerciasis Control Programme (OCP) in West Africa in 1974 (Benton et al. 2002). Onchocerciasis causes several symptoms, including unrelenting itching, physical scars from constant scratching, de-pigmentation and thickening of the skin, impaired vision, and complete blindness.

Important pioneering studies in the last decade, sponsored by the United Nations Development Programme (UNDP), the World Bank, and the World Health Organization (WHO) Special Programme for Research and Training in Tropical Diseases (TDR), have shown that onchocercal skin disease (OSD) is associated with a greater degree of morbidity than was hitherto appreciated. These studies demonstrated that severe OSD causes suffering to millions of people, particularly to those in the forest zone, where the blinding form of the disease is less prevalent (Amazigo 1993; WHO 1995b). OSD not only causes psychosocial problems, ostracism, and stigma (Brieger et al. 1998b; Okello, Ovuga, and Ogwal Okeng 1995; Ovuga et al. 1995) but also has a demonstrably negative socioeconomic impact on the productivity of farmers, breastfeeding, and school attendance (Amazigo 1994; Benton 1998; Kim et al. 1997; Oladepo et al. 1997; Vlassoff et al. 2000).

The relative contributions of both ocular and dermal symptoms to the burden of onchocercal disease and their socioeconomic consequences are substantial (Kale 1998). The unbearable itching and blindness that accompany the disease hinder the ability of individuals to contribute to their own well-being, and they undermine the emotional and economic health of the household and the community. Consequently, onchocerciasis, which predominantly affects poor people in remote areas, can be directly linked to poverty.

THE SOCIOECONOMIC TOLL

In the 1970s, when investigations of onchocerciasis in the endemic villages and districts of West Africa began, scientists made astonishing and disturbing discoveries. More than 60 percent of the savanna population carried the parasite; 10 percent of the adult population and half of the males over 40 years of age were blind, 30 percent of the people were visually impaired, and early signs of onchocerciasis were common among children (WHO 1973, 1987, 1995a).

Scientists revealed the huge socioeconomic consequences of the high infection rates they had found. As village blindness reached epidemic proportions, it left too few able-bodied people to tend fields. Food shortages and economic collapse forced residents to abandon homelands in fertile river valleys. Moving to hardscrabble highlands and forested areas

offered some protection from further infection, but then farmers struggled with poor soil and water shortages on overcrowded lands. Onchocerciasis often ultimately sent a prosperous community into poverty. Armed with this new knowledge about the economic impact, and with many fertile lands and water sources off-limits because of endemic onchocerciasis, development agencies made the disease a priority.

RAPID EPIDEMIOLOGICAL MAPPING OF ONCHOCERCIASIS

Continued research has led to the development of Rapid Epidemiological Mapping of Onchocerciasis (REMO), a tool that provides data on the distribution and prevalence of the disease. REMO is a simple, noninvasive, and practicable process that is easy to apply over a wide range of bioecological zones, with no sociocultural or religious restrictions. This tool was vital to rapid mapping and accelerating the scaling-up process of identifying endemic villages for mass treatment with ivermectin in control areas. Integration of REMO data into the Geographical Information System (GIS) allowed delineation of zones of different levels of endemicity, which is an important step in the planning process for onchocerciasis control. Zones, and communities in these zones, are included or excluded from the community-directed treatment with ivermectin (CDTI), depending on whether their levels of onchocercal endemicity reach the threshold set by the control program. Prevalence rates of infection in the OCP areas prior to control activities were high in all the countries.

POPULATION AT RISK AND POPULATION INFECTED

In 1995 it was estimated that 18 million persons were infected, of whom 270,000 were blind and about 500,000 persons severely visually impaired (WHO 1995a). However, the large-scale REMO that was undertaken by the African Programme for Onchocerciasis Control (APOC), covering the 19 remaining endemic countries in Africa, provides recent and more accurate estimates. From the REMO results it was estimated in 2004 that about 87 million persons were at high risk of contracting onchocerciasis in APOC countries. This figure is higher than the number at risk (about 58 million persons) reported two years earlier by Noma and colleagues (2002), when countrywide mapping of the disease had not been carried out in Angola and Burundi and had been implemented (only partially) in very few areas in the Democratic Republic of Congo and Sudan.

The results of REMO, also used to determine the number of infected persons in the APOC countries, showed that the mean infection rate was 38.2 percent, or approximately 37 million people. This represents almost three times the number estimated (13.7 million people) at the planning phase of the APOC program, when only partial data were available for few countries.

ONCHOCERCIASIS CONTROL PROGRAMS

In 1970, funded by the UNDP, a team of WHO scientists and consultants began to lay the technical groundwork for a major regional initiative to defeat river blindness. By 1972 the international development community mobilized funds to aid in the control of the disease. In 1974 the affected countries and four agencies (the World Bank, the WHO, the Food and Agriculture Organization [FAO], and the UNDP) launched an unprecedented partnership. The "river blindness partnership" has had two distinct phases: the OCP between 1974 and 2002 and APOC between 1996 and 2010. The OCP had a dual mandate: to eliminate river blindness as a public heath problem and as an obstacle to socioeconomic development. The APOC mandate in East Africa and central Africa does not express the same socioeconomic development needs as did the OCP mandate in West Africa. This is because the strain of parasite prevalent outside the savanna belt is less likely to cause blindness. Instead, it exacts its toll in greater skin disease. The stigma and disability from these dermatologic effects are difficult to quantify, and humanitarian reasons alone were more than sufficient to justify the expense of control.

Partnership of the Control Programs

The onchocerciasis control programs in Sub-Saharan Africa—the OCP and, in particular, APOC—developed a unique partnership structure. More than 80 partners are involved in this rich coalition, including 26 donors; 30 African countries; a major pharmaceutical firm, Merck & Co.; and 12 major nongovernmental development organizations (NGDOs) over 120,000 local communities within the OCP and APOC ambit of operations. This broad coalition is complex to maintain but has created synergies that have yielded enormous advantages, including rapid expansion of ivermectin distribution to remote communities. The partners have ably demonstrated how to deliver medicines to reach those who need them most, the poorest. With lessons from the OCP, the partners of APOC are making efforts to mentor national or local nongovernmental organizations (NGOs) in different countries to play major roles in sustaining ivermectin distribution by supporting the health system, especially after the withdrawal of external support.

Vector Control

Onchocerciasis control is complicated by the long life of the adult worms, which remain fertile throughout most of their 10- to 15-year lifespan. The immature worms live in the skin for about two years, but their numbers are continually refreshed as long as adults are alive in the body. This means that even with instant and complete transmission control, the disease would not die out naturally for 15 years; hence, control attempts must last at least the life span of the adult worm. The control program in West Africa, the OCP, initially attacked the disease by killing the larvae of the flies that transmit the worms. It depended on killing these larvae over a long enough time that the adult worms would all die out. Then, when fly control stopped, biting flies would no longer ingest any parasites, and the transmission cycle would be broken. The key to this approach lies in reducing the fly population sufficiently to stop transmission and then sustaining the effort for two decades or more.

The principal strategy of the OCP from its inception was vector control. Covering Burkina Faso and six neighboring countries, the control began in 1974 in West Africa as a large regional project. Vector control, treating the breeding sites of disease-transmitting flies with larvicides, was the only available approach.

Prior control attempts dating back to the 1950s had shown that the disease is transmitted on a regional scale. The first projects were small, and the savanna was consistently reinfested. Accordingly, the OCP was established as a large program to cover entire endemic zones. Even this ambitious start was not sufficient; in 1986 the program doubled in size and was expanded to cover 11 countries in all.

Since blackflies migrate across international borders, the affected governments and international experts were convinced that only a regional program could control river blindness. Thus, the OCP targeted seven West African countries (Benin, Burkina Faso, Côte d'Ivoire, Ghana, Mali, Niger, and Togo; figure 15.1). With the collaboration and

Figure 15.1 Prevalence of Onchocerciasis Infection in 1974 and Gradual Expansion, 1977–92

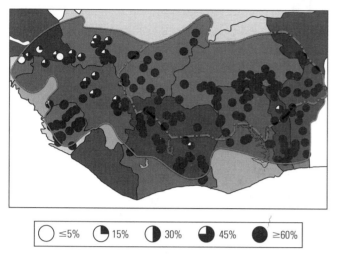

| ○ ≤5% | ◔ 15% | ◑ 30% | ◕ 45% | ● ≥60% |

Source: Onchocerciasis Coordination Unit, World Bank.

Note: The dotted green line indicates the original seven-country control area. The solid green line encloses 11 countries and shows the extensions made during program implementation.

political commitment of these nations, control operations were planned. As the primary method of control, aircraft would spray environmentally safe larvicides around fast-flowing rivers—the breeding grounds of the intermediate host of the disease, the blackfly.

Initially, operations covered 660,000 square kilometers in seven countries, an area believed to be large enough to contain the blackfly vector (WHO 1995a). However, in 1975, after three initial months of successful operations, many migrant blackflies from untreated watercourses reappeared, threatening to reintroduce the disease into the program area. Scientists found that the flies were coming from up to 600 kilometers away from the area being treated (Le Berre et al. 1990; WHO 1995a). In response, the program extended operations to another four West African countries (Guinea, Guinea-Bissau, Senegal, and Sierra Leone; figure 15.1). The program area increased geographic coverage from 780,000 square kilometers to 1.3 million square kilometers, enabling the campaign to increase the number of people protected from 10 million to 30 million.

Ivermectin Treatment and Approaches to Disease Control

The advent of ivermectin (Mectizan) and its donation by Merck & Co. in 1987, for as long as needed, provided a second string to OCP's control operations. The first extensive field studies on the suitability of the drug for use on a mass scale were conducted by the OCP (Awadzi et al. 1985).

The favorable results of these studies led to the OCP's adopting mass distribution of Mectizan as an adjunct to vector control. In 1990 the program began full-scale distribution in extension areas—to the south and west of the original core area in West Africa—using mobile teams in jeeps plus local health staff support.

In this first step toward scaling up, OCP-paid local health professionals called communities to a central location for dosing. In more than 30 river basins, therapeutic coverage averaged about 65 percent in 1987, improving to more than 70 percent by 1995. However, it was expensive to use trained health staff at the local level. In light of high, recurring costs, the program considered various cost-recovery schemes to no avail. The answer to the high cost of mobile teams arrived indirectly. Invariably, when drugs were distributed, some villagers were away, either hunting, working, or traveling. In response, the program authorized the mobile teams to leave doses upon departure for absent community members, once it became clear that ivermectin's safety profile allowed unsupervised dosing. In the second step toward scaling up, national health services combined with local health staff to distribute the drug, forming a community-based distribution approach.

In some areas the OCP used ivermectin alone (Awadzi et al. 1985; Dadzie et al. 1990, 1991; Remme et al. 1989, 1990; Whitworth et al. 1991,1992) and effectively so. Ivermectin is effective against only the juvenile parasites, killing 95 percent with one dose. Even when a patient takes ivermectin, the adult worms continue to live, churning out offspring. However, because the juvenile parasites cause the disease, ivermectin relieves the symptoms and allows the body to begin healing itself. Treatment with ivermectin is required only once per year but must be taken for as long as any adults are still alive, up to 15 years. By killing almost all the immature worms, ivermectin also dramatically lowers the chance of parasite ingestion by biting flies.

The application of the two strategies by the OCP has led to the virtual elimination of onchocerciasis as a public health problem and as an obstacle to socioeconomic development in 10 of the 11 countries in which the program was carried out (figure 15.2), leading to the recognition of OCP as one of the most successful programs in the history of development assistance (Kim and Benton 1995). Figure 15.3 shows the other health interventions implemented using the CDTI network in APOC countries in 2004. By the end of the OCP, the program had covered 11 countries, protecting 40 million persons at risk and 1.3 million square kilometers of land. By the end of APOC in 2010, the program's two

Figure 15.2 Prevalence of Onchocerciasis Infection in 2002

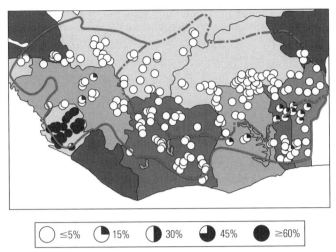

○ ≤5% ◔ 15% ◑ 30% ◕ 45% ● ≥60%

Source: Onchocerciasis Coordination Unit, World Bank.

Note: The dotted green line indicates the original seven-country control area. The solid green line encloses 11 countries. The map shows the larger area covered in 2002, and the much lower rate of infection obtained after 28 years of OCP, from 1974 to 2002.

Figure 15.3 Scaling Up with Additional Interventions

A community-directed network offers a key entry point for many health interventions in the most remote, rural communities. Phase II reaches the poorest of the poor in areas where National Health Services are weak or nonexistent.

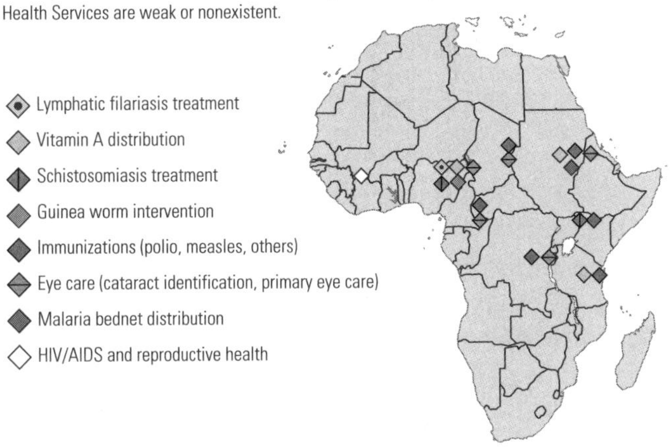

◈ Lymphatic filariasis treatment

◇ Vitamin A distribution

◧ Schistosomiasis treatment

◆ Guinea worm intervention

◆ Immunizations (polio, measles, others)

◆ Eye care (cataract identification, primary eye care)

◆ Malaria bednet distribution

◇ HIV/AIDS and reproductive health

Source: Onchocerciasis Coordination Unit, World Bank.

phases will have protected an estimated 150 million people in 30 countries.

The initial efforts at mass distribution of ivermectin outside OCP were made by NGDOs. The first of the NGDO-facilitated ivermectin distribution programs in Africa was established in Nigeria in 1989 (Duke and Dadzie 1993). Many of the pioneering NGDOs were already well known through their activities in prevention of blindness and were already with the WHO Prevention of Blindness Programme.

The NGDOs soon recognized the need to coordinate their separate and independent efforts if they were to achieve their common goal. Therefore, in 1992 they came together to form the NGDO Coordination Group for Ivermectin Distribution. By 1995 the group needed considerably more resources than they could generate on their own for a significant expansion in the scope of their activities. Furthermore, the various NGDOs and programs used mobile teams and the clinic-based and community-based treatment with ivermectin in the distribution of the drug. These methods were proved inappropriate or not cost-effective for large-scale sustainable distribution of the drug for several years. In 1995 the Task Force on Onchocerciasis Operational Research of the UNDP, World Bank, and WHO Special Program for Research and Training in Tropical Diseases, in collaboration with the OCP, addressed the problem in a multicountry research study (WHO 1995b).

The study concluded that community-directed treatment with ivermectin (CDTI) was feasible and effective in a wide range of geographical and cultural settings in Africa, and likely to be replicable in other endemic communities in Africa. It recommended that this approach become a principal method for onchocerciasis control in Africa. (WHO 1996). The scaling up to community-directed treatment was a major turning point for the onchocerciasis control programs.

Two successful regional programs, APOC and the Onchocerciasis Elimination Program for the Americas (OEPA), were introduced to distribute ivermectin (Remme 1995; Richards et al. 2001). APOC was launched in 1995 to cover 19 countries in the remainder of infested Africa. In 1997 the program adopted the CDTI as its principal strategy for ivermectin distribution. In 2001, 42 million tablets of ivermectin donated by Merck & Co. were used in the 28 countries in Sub-Saharan Africa for onchocerciasis control. Ivermectin is distributed by community workers, trained and supported by the external partners.

In 1996 APOC had approved four CDTI projects, and by the end of 2003 the Programme totaled 107 projects to be implemented (table 15.1), of which 97 were CDTI projects. Sixty-two projects delivered more than 32 million treatments in 2003 alone (table 15.1). By 2010 the total treatments are expected to reach 90 million people. The distribution network is also being tested to deliver other health interventions. This enticing possibility opens the door to further scaling up to help control other diseases and presents the opportunity to deliver other basic health interventions in the river-blindness areas, all of which are remote, rural, and poor. Most are not reached by other programs, and some are not reached by the national governments themselves.

Table 15.1 Scaling up APOC, 1996–2003

	1996	1997	1998	1999	2000	2001	2002	2003	Total
Projects approved (including CDTI, Vector Elimination, and National Onchocerciasis Task Forces HQ support)	4	25	16	12	6	6	11	27	107
Annual treatments	n.a.	1.5	14.1	16.9	20.4	24.6	29.0	32.2	138.7
Geographic coverage (percent)[a]	n.a.	36.6	39.5	42.3	73.0	69.8	75.3	84.8	n.a.
Therapeutic coverage (percent)[b]	n.a.	52.7	54.2	57.8	58.6	54.8	58.2	68.1	n.a.

Source: APOC.
Note: n.a. = not applicable.
a. Geographic coverage is the percentage of communities treated per total communities at high risk.
b. Therapeutic coverage is the percentage of people covered per total population at high risk.

In 2003, through community-directed treatment, APOC countries achieved ivermectin therapeutic coverage of 68.1 percent on average in the targeted communities. It augmented these distribution efforts with a strong commitment to increasing capacity.

The introduction of ivermectin presented challenges and opportunities that became a catalyst for scaling up on all levels. It transformed onchocerciasis control from a technologically driven categorical health initiative to a community-directed process of treatment and empowerment of communities. This grassroots approach contributed, as shown in table 15.1, to high coverage of the population and empowered communities to take charge of their own health. It also planted the seeds for sustainability—absolutely vital for a disease that must be treated for at least 15 years to interrupt transmission. Systematic assessments of 48 CDTI projects in 10 countries (Cameroon, Chad, the Democratic Republic of Congo, Ethiopia, Malawi, Nigeria, the Republic of Congo, Sudan, Tanzania, and Uganda) at four levels—namely, the central level (the state, regional, and provincial levels of the different health systems in Sub-Saharan Africa), the district and local government authorities level, the subdistrict and frontline health facility level, and the community level—were undertaken between 2002 and 2004. These sustainability assessments were carried out with outside technical assistance. A total of 304 district and local government authorities and 468 communities were evaluated. The performance of health care service providers and community workers was assessed using quality-of-implementation indicators designed for the multicountry evaluation of CDTI. The results of these in-depth evaluations show that 35 (73 percent) of the 48 projects are making satisfactory progress toward sustainability, and 13 (27 percent) are not.

Benefits of the Onchocerciasis Control Programs

The 20 percent economic rate of return of OCP from the inception of phase 1 in 1975 to 2002 compares well with other development projects, including those outside the health sector (Kim and Benton 1995). In the study by Kim and Benton (1995) the benefits taken into account were an increase in the labor force due to prevention of blindness (25 percent of benefits) and increased land use (75 percent of benefits).

By 2010 the total budget for the OCP and APOC will amount to approximately US$735 million in donor financing; these funds were allocated primarily to larviciding and entomological evaluation. Other costs were for administration, including extensive meetings aimed at ensuring transparency within the wide-ranging partnership; ivermectin delivery; training; and research and development. The cost of protection from OCP operations per person per year was well under US$1. The target cost per treatment is about US$0.15 for APOC.

Normally, a 10 percent rate of return for World Bank projects in the "productive sector" (excluding social projects, such as education and health) is considered a success. By 2010, the economic rate of return for APOC is expected to reach 18 percent. Moreover, every U.S. dollar invested in APOC activities is expected to add 27 labor-productive days between 1996 and 2017.

CONCLUSION

Over the last 30 years a large international partnership has successfully attacked onchocerciasis. This partnership has defeated the disease in 10 of the 11 countries in West Africa and is making progress in the remaining endemic countries in central Africa and East Africa. The program, spanning 30 countries across Sub-Saharan Africa, encompasses more than 107 projects to create a comprehensive approach to eliminating the disease as a public health problem. The onchocerciasis control programs have yielded the following results:

- 1989–90—60,000 people treated in 11 countries
- 1994—2 million people treated
- 2002 (end of phase 1)—40 million people protected in 11 countries; 600,000 cases of blindness prevented; 18 million children spared the risk of onchocerciasis
- 2003—33 million people treated in 69,641 communities in the APOC countries; more than 162,000 community distributors and 18,000 health workers trained or retrained
- 2010—a projected 102 million people and about 100,000 communities protected in 16 countries and a projected 150 million people protected in 30 countries.

Prior to 2002, when the OCP closed, 25 million hectares of relatively fertile land in the river valleys were freed for resettlement and for agriculture; the socioeconomic impact of OCP is considered to be enormous. More than 40 million people in the 11 countries were considered free from infection and eye lesions. Sixteen million children born after 1974, when OCP activities began, are free of onchocerciasis; more than 1.5 million people originally infected are no longer so; and more than 200,000 cases of blindness have been prevented.

The second phase of the studies to determine the impact of APOC are under way, but the program is considered to be highly cost-effective. The cost per disability-adjusted life year of APOC operations is US$6.50. A study is also being conducted to demonstrate the feasibility and cost-benefit of onchocerciasis elimination with ivermectin.

The community-directed distribution network can get primary health care to the poorest of the poor through simple, once- or twice-a-year interventions by nonmedical staff. In some areas, additional activities have been carefully tested and planned; in other areas, communities themselves took spontaneous action. Effective interventions exist, but they do not reach the people who need them most—the poor. Prior to the launching of APOC, not enough was known about what works to reach the poor, that is, what systems can ensure that poor and very remote populations have access to the benefits of health services, to available drugs, regardless of their locations.

Participating countries, donors, and the partnership's governing board have all endorsed the integration of community-directed treatment into existing health systems through other health interventions. Some countries, such as Uganda, have begun reorganizing their rural health services to use the community-based network as a national strategy. Some communities within the 30 African countries, along with NGDOs, such as Helen Keller International and The Carter Center, have begun distributing bednets to prevent malaria, and medications, including vitamin A, to prevent malnutrition, pediatric blindness, and death; Praziquantel to control schistosomiasis; and ivermectin and albendazole to control the transmission of lymphatic filariasis.

REFERENCES

Amazigo, U. 1993. "Onchocerciasis and Women's Reproductive Health: Indigenous and Biomedical Concepts." *Tropical Doctor* 23 (4): 149–51.

———. 1994. "Detrimental Effects of Onchocerciasis on Marriage Age and Breastfeeding." *Tropical and Geographical Medicine* 46: 322–25.

Awadzi, K., K. Y. Dadzie, H. Shulz-Key, D. R. Haddock, H. M. Gilles, and M. A. Aziz. 1985. "The Chemotherapy of Onchocerciasis X. An Assessment of Four Single Dose Treatment Regimes of MK-933 (Ivermectin) in Human Onchocerciasis." *Annals of Tropical Medicine and Parasitology* 79 (1): 63–78.

Benton, B. 1998. "Economic Impact of Onchocerciasis Control through the African Programme for Onchocerciasis Control: An Overview." *Annals of Tropical Medicine and Parasitology* 92: S33–39.

Benton, B., J. Bump, A. Seketeli, and B. Liese. 2002. "Partnership and Promise: Evolution of the African River-Blindness Campaigns." *Annals of Tropical Medicine and Parasitology* 96 (Supplement 1–March): 5–14.

Brieger, W. R., A. K. Awedoba, C. I. Eneanya, M. Hagan, D. Okello, K. F. Ogbuagu, O. O. Osanga, and E. B. L. Ovuga. 1998a. "The Effect of Ivermectin on Onchocercal Skin Disease and Severe Itching: Results of a Multi-Centre Trial." *Tropical Medicine and International Health* 3: 951–61.

Brieger, William R., Frederick O. Oshiname, and Oladele O. Ososanya. 1998b. "Stigma Associated with Onchocercal Skin Disease among Those Affected Near the Ofiki and Oyan Rivers in Western Nigeria." *Social Science and Medicine* 47 (7): 841–852.

Dadzie, K. Y., J. Remme, E. S. Alley, and G. de Sole. 1990. "Changes in Ocular Onchocerciasis Four and Twelve Months after Community-Based Treatment with Ivermectin in a Holoendemic Onchocerciasis Focus." *Transactions of the Royal Society of Tropical Medicine and Hygiene* 84: 103–8.

Dadzie, K. Y., J. Remme, G. de Sole, B. Boatin, E. S. Alley, O. Ba, and E. M. Samba. 1991. "Onchocerciasis Control by Large-Scale Ivermectin Treatment. *Lancet* 337: 1358–59.

Duke, B. O. L., and K. Y. Dadzie. 1993. *Procedural Manual for Ivermectin Distribution Programmes.* Geneva: World Health Organization.

Kale, O. O. 1998. "Onchocerciasis: The Burden of Disease." *Annals of Tropical Medicine and Parasitology* 92 (Suppl. 1): S101–15.

Kim, A., and B. Benton. 1995. "Cost–Benefit Analysis of the Onchocerciasis Control Program (OCP)." Technical Paper 282, World Bank, Washington, DC.

Kim, A., A. Tandon, A. Hailu, H. Birrie, N. Berhe, A. Aga, G. Mengistu, et al. 1997. "Health and Labour Productivity: The Economic Impact of Onchocercal Skin Disease (OSD)." Policy Research Working Paper 1836, World Bank, Washington, DC.

Le Berre, R., J. F. Walsh, B. Philippon, P. Poudiougo, J. E. Henderickx, P. Guillet, A. Seketeli, D. Quillevere, J. Grunewald, and R. A. Cheke. 1990. "The WHO Onchocerciasis Control Programme: Retrospect and Prospects." *Philosophical Transactions of the Royal Society of London. Series B Biological Sciences* 328 (1251): 721–27.

Noma, M., B. E. Nwoke, I. Nutall, P. A. Tambala, P. Enyong, A. Namsenmo, J. Remme, U. V. Amazigo, O. O. Kale, and A. Seketeli. 2002. "Rapid Epidemiological Mapping of Onchocerciasis (REMO): Its Application by the African Programme for Onchocerciasis Control (APOC)." *Annals of Tropical Medicine and Parasitology* 96 (Suppl. 1): S29–39.

Okello, D. O., E. B. Ovuga, and J. W. Ogwal Okeng. 1995. "Dermatological Problems of Onchocerciasis in Nebbi District, Uganda." *East African Medical Journal* 72: 295–98.

Oladepo, O., W. R. Brieger, S. Otusanya, O. O. Kale, S. Offiong, and M. Titiloye. 1997. "Farm Land Size and Onchocerciasis, Status of Peasant Farmers In South–Western Nigeria." *Tropical Medicine and International Health* 2: 334–40.

Ovuga, E. B., D. O. Okelo, J. W. Ogwal Okeng, N. Orwortho, and F. O. Opoka. 1995. "Social and Psychological Aspects of Onchocercal Skin Disease in Nebbi District of Uganda." *East African Medical Journal* 72: 449–53.

Remme, J. H. F. 1995. "The African Programme for Onchocerciasis Control: Preparing to Launch." *Parasitology Today* 11: 403–06.

Remme, J., R. H. Baker, G. de Sole, K. Y. Dadzie, J. F. Walsh, M. A. Adams, E. S. Alley, and H. S. Avissey. 1989. "A Community Trial of Ivermectin in the Onchocerciasis Focus of Asubende, Ghana. I. Effect on the microfilarial reservoir and the transmission of *Onchocerca volvulus*." *Tropical Medicine and Parasitology* 40 (3): 367–74.

Remme, J., G. de Sole, K. Y. Dadzie, E. S. Alley, R. H. A. Baker, J. D. F. Habbema, A. P. Plaisier, G. J. van Oortmarssen, and E. M. Samba. 1990.

"Large Scale Ivermectin Distribution and Its Epidemiological Consequences." *Acta Leidensia* 59: 177–91.

Richards Jr., F. O., B. Boatin, M. Sauerbrey, and A. Seketeli. 2001. "Control of Onchocerciasis Today: Status and Challenges." *Trends in Parasitology* 17 (12): 558–63.

Vlassoff, C., M. Weiss, E. B. Ovuga, C. Eneanya, P. T. Nwel, S. S. Babalola, A. K. Awedoba, B. Theophilus, P. Cofie, and P. Shatabi. 2000. "Gender and the Stigma of Onchocercal Skin Disease in Africa." *Social Science and Medicine* 50: 1353–54.

Whitworth, J. A. G., C. E. Gilbert, D. M. Mabey, G. H. Maude, D. Morgan, and D. W. Taylor. 1991. "Effects of Repeated Doses of Ivermectin on Ocular Onchocerciasis: Community-Based Trial in Sierra Leone." *Lancet* 338: 1100–03.

Whitworth, J. A., D. Morgan, G. H. Maude, A. J. Luty, and D. W. Taylor. 1992. "A Community Trial of Ivermectin for Onchocerciasis in Sierra Leone: Clinical and Parasitological Responses to Four Doses Given at Six-Monthly Intervals." *Transactions of the Royal Society of Tropical Medicine and Hygiene* 86 (3): 277–80.

WHO (World Health Organization). 1973. *PAG Mission: Controle de l'Onchocercose dans la Région du Bassin de la Volta: Rapport de la Mission d'Assistance Preparatoire aux Gouvernements de Côte d'Ivoire, Dahomey, Ghana, Haute-Volta, Mali, Niger, Togo.* Geneva: WHO.

———. 1987. *WHO Expert Committee on Onchocerciasis, Third Report.* Technical Report Series 752. Geneva: WHO.

———. 1995a. "Onchocerciasis and Its Control. Report of a WHO Expert Committee on Onchocerciasis Control." *World Health Organization Technical Report Series* 852: 1–104.

———. 1995b. *The Pan-African Study Group on Onchocercal Skin Disease. Report of a Multi-country Study.* Document TDR/AFR/RP/95.1. Geneva: WHO.

———. 1996. *Report of a Multi-country Study on Community Directed Treatment with Ivermectin.* Document TDR/AFR/RP/96.1. Geneva: WHO.

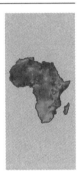

Chapter **16**

Maternal Mortality

Khama O. Rogo, John Oucho, and Philip Mwalali

At the close of the last century, Sub-Saharan Africa still had high maternal morbidity and mortality rates, with the goals of safe motherhood eluding many governments. The Programme of Action of the International Conference on Population and Development of 1994 and the Fourth World Conference on Women of 1995 were created in an attempt to tackle these issues and drew unprecedented attention to reproductive health and rights as well as to gender equity and equality. The scourge of the human immunodeficiency virus and acquired immune deficiency syndrome (HIV/AIDS) has ravaged the region's population and has left in its wake untold destruction in the demographic, economic, and social spheres (UN 2003). Demographic events of the last decade are a sharp contrast to those in the 1980s, when decreasing infant, child, and adult mortality rates and maternal mortality ratios (MMRs) were leading to steadily increasing life expectancy and improved health status for women in the region.

Data sets assembled since the 1990s are the basis for the analysis of maternal mortality in Sub-Saharan Africa in this chapter. Beginning with an examination of measurement approaches and data sources of maternal mortality, the chapter continues with a description of the levels and trends in maternal mortality in the decade 1990–2000. The causes and correlates of maternal mortality, as well as priority interventions, are examined. The last section of the chapter points to what Sub-Saharan African countries could do to meet the maternal health component of the Millennium Development Goals.

MEASUREMENT AND DATA SOURCES

Measuring maternal mortality remains one of the more difficult issues in maternal health, and yet an accurate picture of the scope of the problem is important to implement approaches to improve maternal health care.

Definitions

The World Health Organization's (WHO's) 10th revision of the *International Statistical Classification of Diseases and Related Health Problems* (ICD-10) defines *maternal mortality* as "the death of a woman while pregnant or within 42 days of termination of pregnancy irrespective of the duration and the site of the pregnancy, from any cause related to or aggravated by the pregnancy or its management but not from accidental or incidental causes" (WHO 1992). Furthermore, the ICD-10 introduced a new category, namely, *late maternal death,* that is defined as "the death of a woman from direct or indirect obstetric causes more than 42 days but less than one year after termination of pregnancy." The ICD-10 defined *direct obstetric deaths* as "maternal deaths resulting from obstetric complications of the pregnant state (pregnancy, labor, and the puerperium), from interventions, omissions, incorrect treatment, or from a chain of events resulting from any of the above." *Indirect obstetric deaths,* by contrast, are "those resulting from previous existing disease or disease that developed during pregnancy and which was not due to obstetric causes, but was aggravated by physiologic effects of pregnancy." Because accidental deaths are excluded from the definition of maternal deaths, the ICD-10 introduced the term *pregnancy-related death,* defined as "the death of a woman while pregnant or within 42 days of termination of pregnancy, irrespective of the cause of death" (WHO 1992).

Maternal mortality is associated with neonatal mortality, but a lack of data, especially for Sub-Saharan Africa, constrains conclusive findings. A review of the literature suggests that a relationship exists between maternal mortality and perinatal mortality, including stillbirths and early neonatal deaths, and that interventions that save the lives of mothers are also effective in reducing neonatal mortality (Bang, Bang, and Reddy 2005; Darmstadt et al. 2005; Jacobson 1991; Kwast 1996; Lompo et al. 1993; Onuh and Aisien 2004).

Measures of Maternal Mortality

Three measures of maternal mortality are commonly used. First, the *maternal mortality ratio* is expressed as the number of maternal deaths during a given time period per 100,000 live births during the same period:

$$\text{MMR} = \frac{\text{No. of maternal deaths}}{\text{No. of live births}} \times 100,000 \qquad (16.1)$$

The MMR represents a measure of the risk of death once a woman has become pregnant. As a ratio, it is not a true risk, as it involves two different populations, pregnant women and live newborns. The ratio can be influenced by the prevalence of stillbirths as well as the prevalence of induced abortions.

Second, the *maternal mortality rate* is the number of maternal deaths in a given period per 100,000 women of reproductive age during the same period:

$$\text{Maternal mortality rate} =$$
$$\frac{\text{No. of maternal deaths}}{\text{No. of women age 15–49}} \times 100,000 \qquad (16.2)$$

The maternal mortality rate is a cause-specific mortality rate for women of reproductive age in the presence of other causes of death.

Third, the *lifetime risk of maternal death* is the risk a woman has of dying during her reproductive years, given current rates of fertility and the risk of maternal mortality. Given the length of the reproductive period (about 35 years), the lifetime risk is calculated as $[1 - (1 - \text{maternal mortality rate})^{35}]$ (AbouZahr and Wardlaw 2003).

Data Sources

Estimation of maternal mortality indicators is difficult and subject to error because the data on which the estimates are based are frequently inaccurate. In the estimates produced jointly by the WHO, the United Nations Children's Fund (UNICEF), and the United Nations Population Fund (UNFPA) (AbouZahr and Wardlaw 2003), countries are classified into one of the following four categories:

1. countries with complete civil registration and good cause-of-death attribution
2. those with complete or nearly complete civil registration of the number of births and deaths but with poor cause-of-death attribution
3. those without a reliable system of civil registration, where maternal deaths, like other vital events, go unrecorded
4. those with estimates of maternal mortality based on household surveys, using direct or indirect sisterhood methods.

Most Sub-Saharan African countries fall into the last two categories. This implies that estimates of maternal mortality in Sub-Saharan Africa are derived from the methods mentioned in category 4 above. When estimating maternal mortality for these countries, the WHO, UNICEF, and the UNFPA use an approach that includes adjusting country data to account for underreporting and misclassification and a statistical model to generate estimates. Maternal deaths are generally identified by medical certification when vital registration exists; in household surveys, censuses, and

Reproductive Age Mortality Studies (RAMOS), a time of death definition is used, making these "pregnancy-related deaths" rather than "maternal deaths." Several sources of data on which estimates of maternal mortality rely are described briefly below.

Vital Registration. This source is generally used in developed countries, where maternal mortality is estimated from deaths registered by cause of death. It permits calculation of period-specific maternal mortality ratios in which the numerator is registered maternal deaths and the denominator is the registered live births (see equation 16.1). Where the degree of underreporting of maternal deaths is almost similar to that of live births, the resulting maternal mortality ratio will give a reasonable population-based estimate. In Sub-Saharan Africa, vital registration is lacking in all countries, with the exception of Mauritius. In the rest of Sub-Saharan Africa, vital registration-based maternal mortality estimates are inadequate because of the failure to register vital events, as well as the misclassification of causes of death, due to the absence of medical personnel and for social, religious, and emotional reasons (Graham 1991). In view of these shortcomings, the vital registration system is ruled out as a reliable source of measuring maternal mortality in the region.

Population-Based Data. In the absence of complete vital registration, the main sources of population-based data are censuses and surveys, which use one of the following approaches to estimate maternal mortality: RAMOS, sisterhood method, sibling-history method, and household deaths methods. The key characteristics of each of them in the context of Sub-Saharan Africa follow.

Decennial census counts can generate both national and subnational data with questions on deaths in the household in a defined reference period (one or two years before the census), followed by detailed questions that permit identification of maternal deaths according to time of death relative to pregnancy. Estimates of maternal mortality derived from censuses in this way are believed to be fairly accurate (Stanton et al. 2001). A problem is that censuses of Sub-Saharan African countries ask questions that are often not useful for identification of maternal deaths, which, in addition, are often not fully reported.

A RAMOS study seeks to identify all deaths of females of reproductive age in a defined population by investigating all relevant sources of information, namely, household interviews, hospital and health center records, vital registration,

or word of mouth. Generally, a team of physicians studies the information collected by the study team to determine maternal mortality (Stanton, Abderrahim, and Hill 1997).

Investigation of maternal mortality by the sisterhood method, an indirect approach, entails asking respondents about ever-married sisters: how many have died, and how many died while they were pregnant or during childbirth or six weeks following the end of the pregnancy (Stanton, Abderrahim, and Hill 2000). This method has been used frequently in population-based approaches, such as household surveys. Originated by W. J. Graham and W. Brass (Graham 1991) in a field trial in The Gambia in 1987, it is a simple and low-cost technique with considerable appeal in maternal mortality studies. The method provides a retrospective rather than a current estimate, averaging experience over a lengthy time period, 35 years, with a midpoint of about 12 years before the survey. The estimates have wide confidence intervals, making short-term monitoring of maternal mortality trends difficult (AbouZahr and Wardlaw 2003).

The direct sibling-history method has been employed by the Demographic and Health Surveys (DHSs), and permits the calculation of a maternal mortality ratio for a more recent period of time; results are typically calculated for a reference period of seven years before the survey, with a point estimate some three to four years before the survey (AbouZahr and Wardlaw 2003). The data requirements for this method are more demanding than for the indirect approach because respondents are asked three sets of questions. First, they are asked how many children the mother has given birth to and how many of the children were born before the respondent. The second set of questions asks about the siblings' sex, age, and survival, or how many years ago she or he died and age at death. Finally, three questions are asked about dead sisters to determine maternal mortality: whether she was pregnant when she died, whether she died during childbirth, and whether she died within two months after the end of pregnancy or childbirth (Stanton, Abderrahim, and Hill 2000).

The final method entails undertaking a survey of households to ascertain maternal deaths. Unlike the sibling-history method, in which a sibling reports on the deaths of female siblings, the direct household method involves reporting by household heads or any other persons volunteering such information. When household information is screened, maternal and nonmaternal deaths can be distinguished. Although useful in direct estimation of maternal mortality, this type of household survey is expensive and often too complex to implement in many countries because it requires large sample sizes. An alternative approach is provided by demographic surveillance systems (DSSs) that exist in selected districts in a few Sub-Saharan African countries, notably the Navrongo DSS in Ghana and the Nouna DSS in Burkina Faso (http://www.indepth-network.org/dss_site_profiles/dss_sites.htm). DSSs continually collect births and deaths in households in the populations in the sites. Unfortunately, the DSSs generally cover small areas, typically a district in a country, so that the maternal mortality estimates based on them do not permit generalization; they can be treated as estimates based on case studies.

Health Services Data. Hospitals generally collect data on causes of deaths, including maternal deaths. But lower-level facilities, such as clinics, dispensaries, or health posts, are sometimes omitted in inquiries about maternal mortality. As a result, health services data in Sub-Saharan Africa are often incomplete and misclassified, especially because deaths related to ectopic pregnancy and abortion are recorded in female wards rather than maternity wards. In addition, deaths outside health facilities are generally excluded from the health services data. In Sub-Saharan Africa, where 58 percent of deliveries take place outside of health facilities, maternal mortality using health services data is underestimated (WHO 2005).

LEVELS AND TRENDS IN MATERNAL MORTALITY

Estimates of maternal mortality based on survey data and models have been compiled at the WHO for 1990, 1995, and 2000. Table 16.1 presents estimates of MMR and the total deaths relating to maternal mortality in the years 1990, 1995, and 2000, but trends should be interpreted with caution, as the estimates are based on different models. Among regions, Sub-Saharan Africa had the highest MMR over the period 1990–2000. The wide margins of error (not shown in table 16.1) of the MMR estimates, and the methodological approaches employed in the three years, limit analysis of trends over the period (AbouZahr and Wardlaw 2003).

Table 16.2 shows maternal mortality measures (number of maternal deaths, MMR, and lifetime risk of maternal death) in Sub-Saharan Africa over the period 1990–2000. MMRs of 1,000 or more per 100,000 live births were recorded in 16 of the Sub-Saharan Africa countries in 1990; that level of MMR was recorded in 21 countries in 1995, and 17 countries in 2000 (table 16.2). Many of the countries with civil war or unstable governments—including Angola, Burundi, Central African Republic (since 1995), Chad, Eritrea, Ethiopia, Mozambique (except for 1995), Niger, Nigeria, Rwanda, Sierra Leone, and Somalia—fell into that category in the 1990s. Kenya and Tanzania, although not

Table 16.1 Maternal Mortality Measures, 1990, 1995, and 2000

Region	MMR (per 100,000 live births)			Maternal deaths (thousands)		
	1990	1995	2000	1990	1995	2000
World total	430	400	400	585	515	529
Developed regions	27	21	20	4	2.8	2.5
Europe	36	28	28	3.2	2.2	1.7
Developing regions	480	440	440	582	512	527
Africa	870	1,000	830	235	273	251
North Africa	340	200	130	16	7.2	4.6
Sub-Saharan África	823[a]	1,100	920	219[a]	265	247
Asia	390	280	330	323	217	253
East Asia	95	55	55	24	13	11
South-central Asia	560	410	520	227	158	207
Southeast Asia	440	300	210	56	35	25
Western Asia	320	230	190	16	11	9.8
Latin America and the Caribbean	190	190	190	23	22	22
Oceania	680	260	240	1.4	0.6	0.5

Sources: AbouZahr and Wardlaw 2001, 2003; WHO and UNICEF 1996.
Note: The estimates are based on models, which were specified differently for each of the years. The data are therefore not strictly comparable, and trends should be interpreted with caution.
a. Average for Sub-Saharan Africa subregions: eastern, middle, southern, and western.

Table 16.2 Maternal Mortality Measures in Sub-Saharan Africa, by Country, 1990–2000

Country	No. of maternal deaths			MMR (per 1,000 births)			Lifetime risk of maternal death (1 in the numbers below)		
	1990	1995	2000	1990	1995	2000	1990	1995	2000
1. Angola	7,200	7,100	11,000	1,500	1,300	1,700	8	9	7
2. Benin	2,300	2,000	2,200	990	880	850	12	15	17
3. Botswana	120	250	50	250	480	100	65	38	200
4. Burkina Faso	4,000	6,700	5,400	930	1,400	1,000	14	7	12
5. Burundi	3,400	5,100	2,800	1,300	1,900	1,000	9	21	12
6. Cameroon	2,600	3,800	4,000	550	720	730	26	21	23
7. Cape Verde	..	20	20	..	190	150	..	120	160
8. Central African Republic	850	1,500	1,600	700	1,200	1,100	21	14	15
9. Chad	3,700	4,500	4,200	1,500	1,500	1,100	9	9	11
10. Comoros	260	130	130	950	570	480	12	29	33
11. Congo, Democratic Republic of	16,000	20,000	24,000	870	940	990	14	13	13
12. Congo, Republic of	890	1,300	690	890	1,100	510	15	12	26
13. Côte d'Ivoire	4,900	6,000	3,900	810	1,200	690	14	13	25
14. Djibouti	110	120	180	570	520	730	24	29	19
15. Equatorial Guinea	130	240	180	820	1,400	880	17	10	16
16. Eritrea	1,900	1,600	930	1,400	1,100	630	10	12	24
17. Ethiopia	33,000	46,000	24,000	1,400	1,800	850	9	7	14
18. Gabon	210	250	200	500	620	420	32	25	37
19. Gambia, The	460	500	270	1,100	1,100	540	13	14	31
20. Ghana	4,800	4,000	3,500	740	590	540	18	26	35
21. Guinea	4,700	3,600	2,700	1,600	1,200	740	7	12	18
22. Guinea-Bissau	380	420	590	910	910	1,100	16	15	13
23. Kenya	7,000	13,000	11,000	650	1,300	1,000	20	13	19
24. Lesotho	420	370	380	610	530	550	26	32	32
25. Liberia	690	1,100	1,200	560	1,000	760	22	12	16
26. Madagascar	2,800	3,400	3,800	490	580	550	27	25	26
27. Malawi	2,700	2,800	9,300	560	580	1,800	20	21	7
28. Mali	5,700	3,000	6,800	1,200	630	1,200	10	19	10
29. Mauritania	750	850	1,200	930	870	1,000	16	17	14
30. Mauritius	25	10	5	120	45	24	300	880	1,700
31. Mozambique	9,800	7,400	7,900	1,500	980	1,000	9	13	14
32. Namibia	190	210	190	370	370	300	42	44	54
33. Niger	5,100	4,300	9,700	1,200	920	1,600	9	13	7
34. Nigeria	44,000	45,000	37,000	1,000	1,100	800	13	14	18
35. Reunion	..	5	5	..	39	41	..	930	970
36. Rwanda	400	6,300	4,200	1,300	2,300	1,400	9	6	10
37. Senegal	3,900	4,100	2,500	1,200	1,200	690	11	12	22
38. Sierra Leone	3,600	4,200	4,500	1,800	2,100	2,000	7	6	6
39. Somalia	7,000	7,100	5,100	1,600	1,600	1,100	7	7	10
40. South Africa	2,700	3,600	2,600	230	340	230	85	70	120
41. Swaziland	160	130	120	560	370	320	29	45	49
42. Tanzania	8,700	13,000	21,000	770	1,100	1,500	18	14	10
43. Togo	1,000	1,700	1,000	640	980	570	20	13	26
44. Uganda	11,000	10,000	10,000	1,200	1,100	880	10	11	13
45. Zambia	3,500	3,100	3,300	940	870	750	14	17	19
46. Zimbabwe	2,300	2,200	5,000	570	610	1,100	28	33	16

Sources: AbouZahr, Wardlaw, and Hill 2001; WHO and UNICEF 1996.

Note: .. = negligible. Countries for which data are not available for two of the three years are excluded. The estimates are based on models, which were specified differently for each of the years; the data are therefore not strictly comparable, and trends should be interpreted with caution.

having suffered a conflict, are notable for maintaining maternal mortality ratios above 1,000 maternal deaths per 100,000 live births since 1995. Mauritius and Reunion in the Indian Ocean, and Cape Verde in the Atlantic Ocean, and the landlocked country of Botswana have low maternal mortality ratios, atypical of Sub-Saharan Africa.

CAUSES AND CORRELATES OF MATERNAL MORTALITY

Understanding the causes and correlates of maternal mortality is crucial in confronting the challenge of unyielding high rates in Sub-Saharan Africa. Abraham Lilienfeld, a prominent epidemiologist, very appropriately remarked, "the better we know about the root cause of a problem, the better we are in a position to address the problem," and in his book, *Foundations of Epidemiology,* cites Benjamin Disraeli's statement, "The more extensive a man's knowledge of what has been done, the greater will be his power of knowing what to do" (Lilienfeld 1980). Despite the 1978 Alma Ata Declaration and the 1987 Safe Motherhood Initiative, the reduction of maternal mortality has been minimal worldwide. The slow improvement in the MMR in the developing world is due not only to the trend in Sub-Saharan Africa but also to stagnating declines in the regions of Latin America and the Caribbean and South Central Asia. In other regions, notably North Africa and Southeast Asia, the MMR is estimated to have declined substantially during the 1990s. Such divergent trends call for a closer examination of the factors correlated with the MMR.

Different interactive factors contribute to maternal morbidity and mortality. The range is wide and includes the behavior of families and communities, social status, education, income, nutritional status, age, parity, and availability of health services. It is important to note that non–health sector activities, such as education, water and sanitation, roads and communication, agriculture, and internal security, also influence maternal outcome. In Sub-Saharan Africa, some of the highest MMRs have been recorded in countries that are in conflict or have large refugee populations, such as Angola and Sierra Leone.

Causes of Maternal Deaths

About 60 percent of the maternal deaths occur during childbirth and the immediate postpartum period, with 50 percent of these deaths occurring within the first 24 hours of delivery. In a recent study in Eritrea, 16 percent of maternal deaths occurred during pregnancy, 48 percent during childbirth, and 36 percent postpartum (Ghebrehiwot 2004). These findings imply that the causes of the deaths in this critical period are either the result of labor or worsened by labor and delivery.

As noted earlier, the causes of maternal mortality have traditionally been classified as direct and indirect, although the distinction is not always easy to discern (both were grouped under pathogenic causes in the previous edition of this book). Pathogenic causes are purely medical and therefore best determined by health professionals. Most of the information on pathogenic causes is derived from hospital studies; thus, data from health institutions will continue to be an important source of information for direct and indirect causes of maternal deaths. Implicit is the need to educate health professionals on the ICD and provide updates whenever the ICD definition changes. As an example, the 10th revision of ICD has introduced a much broader definition of maternal death and has expanded on the categorization of the causes (WHO 1992). This will make analysis of trends increasingly more difficult because past data will need to be adjusted to accommodate the new definition in order to make them comparable with more recent data.

Availability and accuracy of data sources influence the study of causes and correlates. For instance, data from hospitals or health institutions are limited in that medically certified deaths at these institutions involve only a small and selective fraction of total deaths. This limitation is greatest in Sub-Saharan Africa, where a large proportion of deliveries take place at home (WHO 2005).

The main direct causes of maternal deaths, accounting for up to 80 percent of cases in Africa, are obstetric hemorrhage, puerperal sepsis, pregnancy-induced hypertension (including eclampsia), obstructed labor and ruptured uterus, and complications of unsafe abortion (see figure 16.1). Three causes—hemorrhage, sepsis, and eclampsia—account for a vast majority of deaths, considering that even some cases of abortion or obstructed labor eventually succumb to either bleeding or sepsis.

Indirect causes account for 20 to 25 percent of maternal deaths and are attributable to illnesses aggravated by pregnancy (WHO 2005). They include anemia; malaria; HIV/AIDS; diseases of the heart, lung, liver, or kidneys; and ectopic pregnancies. Physical violence and accidents are not included in this group.

As documented by several DHS surveys, many African women enter pregnancy in a state of nutritional deficit and therefore are unprepared to cope with the extra physiological

Figure 16.1 Major Causes of Maternal Mortality in Sub-Saharan Africa

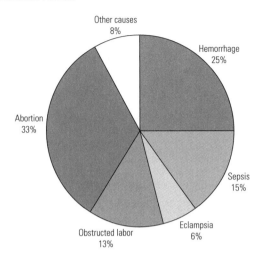

Source: WHO 1992.

demands of pregnancy. In Eritrea, for example, 37.3 percent of women have a low body mass index, which is an indicator of chronic energy deficiency (Eritrea National Statistics and Evaluation Office and ORC Macro 2002). The nutritional deficit, macro- or micronutrient, predisposes these women to anemia in pregnancy, among other problems. Anemia is highly prevalent in Africa, with up to three-fifths of pregnant women in Africa having some degree of anemia, and about one-third classified as having severe anemia (Isah et al. 1985; Massawe et al. 1996; Massawe et al. 1999; Van den Broek and Letsky 2000). Anemia may cause death on its own or predispose a woman to severe postpartum hemorrhage leading to death (Harrison 1997).

The growing HIV/AIDS pandemic is also having a severe impact on women's health. It is estimated that there were 5 million new HIV infections in 2003, of which 40 percent were among women and 20 percent among children (United Nations 2003). In eastern and southern Africa, between 20 and 30 percent of pregnant women are infected with HIV, and available evidence indicates that HIV/AIDS currently accounts for at least 18 percent of maternal deaths. Death in this case results from opportunistic infections, puerperal sepsis, meningitis, tuberculosis, pneumonia, postabortion sepsis, encephalitis, and probably malaria (Mbaruku 2005; Pattinson et al. 2005).

Unsafe abortion deserves special mention in Africa, the only region where complications of abortion are the most common cause of maternal mortality. Globally, unsafe abortion accounts for about 13 percent of maternal deaths compared with 30 to 50 percent in Sub-Saharan Africa (AGI 1999; Henshaw, Singh, and Haas 1999). Of the estimated

46 million induced abortions globally every year, about 20 million are considered unsafe. It is estimated that 95 percent of unsafe abortions occur in the developing world (Henshaw, Singh, and Haas 1999). The WHO (1998) estimated that there were about 5 million induced abortions in Africa annually, whereas Rogo (1993), using the results of several DHS surveys, estimated that there were 1.5 million induced abortions, most of which were unsafe. The tragedy of abortion-related mortality in Africa is that most of the victims are teenagers.

The unsafe abortion conundrum in Africa begins with unprotected sex among teenagers who are ill-informed about their sexuality; an unwanted or ill-timed pregnancy follows. Living in countries where induced abortions are legally restricted, the young victims resort to back street abortionists or quacks. Crude methods used in the pregnancy termination, delay in seeking medical attention when and if there is a problem, and the poor quality of postabortion care lead to a significant proportion of the victims sustaining serious injuries with life-threatening complications, resulting in either death or disability. For survivors the psychological impact is immense and lifelong (Rogo 2004). Postabortal sepsis is worse in HIV/AIDS-infected women (Mbaruku 2005).

Determinants of Maternal Mortality and Morbidity

Available evidence indicates that there are several factors that predispose a woman to greater risk of maternal death. The common biomedical approach to the determinants of maternal morbidity and mortality usually divides them into distal and proximal factors.

The seminal work by McCarthy and Maine (1992) is credited with the conceptual model of analyzing determinants of maternal mortality that could be applied to research as well as programs. The concept grouped the determinants as:

- distant, or socioeconomic, factors;
- intermediate factors (health behavior and status, access to services, and unknown factors);
- outcomes (pregnancy, morbidity, and mortality).

The McCarthy and Maine concept has since been modified, most notably by UNICEF (1999), to facilitate strategic programming for maternal health. From the pediatric perspective, the Mosley and Chen (1984) framework for the study of child survival in developing countries has also found, with various modifications, utility in the analysis of determinants of maternal morbidity and mortality. The original model proposed three levels of determinants of child mortality (socioeconomic determinants, proximate and biological determinants, and outcomes expressed in terms of growth and death), but subsequent modifications have expanded the levels to five: household characteristics (behavioral), intermediate variables (behavioral and biological), risk factors (biological), malnutrition-infection syndrome, and demographic outcome (van Norren and van Viannen 1986). The Poverty Reduction Strategy approach developed by the World Bank and sector-wide approaches to the health sector have generated new interest for incorporating government policies and actions, within or outside the health sector, that focus on health outcomes. Edwards (2001), by expanding on previous models, introduced the macroeconomic evaluation of non–health sector policies that influence health.

These developments are relevant to maternal health and can be applied to generating a more comprehensive understanding of determinants and correlates of maternal health in Africa. The following modified framework is proposed as appropriate for discussing the correlates of maternal mortality in Africa:

- household and community characteristics (behavior, cultural-religious values, and income poverty)
- biological-demographic variables and risk factors
- malnutrition-infection syndrome (including protein-energy malnutrition [PEM], micronutrient deficiencies, anemia, malaria, and HIV/AIDS)
- health systems
- national policies and related investments (health and nonhealth).

Household and Community Characteristics. Pregnancy outcome and maternal survival have strong correlations with household behavior and decision making. Enlightened communities value their mothers and seek prompt attention at the earliest indication of problems. Low status of women in the household and society as a whole, as exemplified by inequality in education, employment, property ownership, participation, and decision making, is another important correlate (Wall 1998). Gender-based violence is common in situations in which the status of women is low and legal protection inadequate, and in turn it is correlated with high rates of maternal mortality.

Harmful traditional practices and religious beliefs also adversely affect maternal health. They vary from one ethnic group to another and cover a wide range of activities and practices; from the sexual or genitally linked ones, such as female genital cutting, to feeding and nutritional practices. In addition, a plethora of harmful beliefs and practices around pregnancy and childbirth affect health-seeking behavior during pregnancy and parturition. The disproportionately low use of health facilities for delivery care is testimony to the strength of these beliefs (Ghebrehiwot 2004).

Household poverty, allocation of resources, and the control of those resources also influence maternal mortality. Delivery of infants is not free of charge in many African countries. Indeed, it was never without cost in traditional societies either. Even in countries where delivery is declared to be free in public facilities, the cost of accessing care, both direct and indirect, can be prohibitive, quality notwithstanding. The relationship to poverty is bi-directional; complications of pregnancy were cited as one of the most common causes of household poverty (Borghi et al. 2003; Claeson et al. 2001).

Biological-Demographic Variables and Risk Factors. Standard biological variables, such as age, height, and parity, apply to maternal mortality in Africa as elsewhere. In many countries of Sub-Saharan Africa, at least 50 percent or more of women will have started childbearing by age 19. Adolescents comprise about 20 percent of maternal deaths, most of which are due to complications of unsafe abortion. Early marriage and childbearing are associated with high parity and therefore higher risk of maternal death (Ghebrehiwot 2004). Various indicators of maternal status during pregnancy and childbirth may also be predictors of maternal outcome, including edema, hypertension, and history of previous complications (Garenne et al. 1997). Sociodemographic factors are correlates of maternal mortality. Marital status, first pregnancy, and level of education are commonly cited (Garenne et al. 1997).

Malnutrition-Infection Syndrome. Malaria remains a major killer of women in pregnancy and a leading indirect cause of maternal mortality. There are effective interventions, such as intermittent preventive treatment and insecticide-treated bednets that are affordable but often not available where they are most needed. The changing complexities of malaria chemotherapy and the rising cost of newer, more effective combinations pose new challenges, including safety in pregnancy (Heymann et al. 1990; Shulman et al. 1999).

HIV/AIDS and its effect on maternal outcomes in Africa is grossly underreported. HIV is not regarded as a primary cause of death unless AIDS is diagnosed. A study in South Africa reported a 25 percent increase in seropositivity, from 50 to 75 percent between 1997–99 and 2000, in maternal deaths due to non–pregnancy-related sepsis in Pretoria (Pattinson and Moodley 2002). HIV infection in pregnancy is also associated with anemia and severe malaria infections (Antelman et al. 2000).

As previously mentioned, both PEM and micronutrient deficiencies are prevalent in African women. Pregnancy aggravates the situation and increases vulnerability to any concurrent condition or opportunistic infection. Paul (1993), in analyzing maternal mortality in Africa from 1980 to 1987 found a strong correlation with calorie supply as a percentage of requirements. Maternal anemia, however mild, also increases several-fold the risk of life-threatening postpartum hemorrhage.

Health Systems. Poorly financed and unaccountable health systems, including weak referral systems, are a key determinant of maternal outcome. Another determinant is poor access to quality maternal health care services because of geographical terrain and poor roads. Maternal health care services are deemed to be of poor quality if, for example, they lack skilled health providers, the providers have negative attitudes, treatment guidelines and protocols are inappropriate, and they lack essential drugs, equipment, and supplies. A low health personnel-to-population ratio is a chronic issue in Sub-Saharan Africa. For instance, the health personnel-to-population ratio in Sub-Saharan Africa is reported as 1:23,540, ranging from 1:750 in South Africa to 1:72,000 in Rwanda. For nurses, the Sub-Saharan African health personnel-to-population ratio is 1:3,460, ranging from 1:600 in Zambia to 1:5,470 in Tanzania (Howson, Harrison, and Law 1996).

Given that skilled birth attendants working within a supportive health system are the most important factor in keeping women healthy and safe in pregnancy, inadequate numbers and distribution of human resources are a major underlying cause of maternal mortality in Sub-Saharan Africa. Although the use of skilled attendants at delivery increased significantly in the developing world as a whole, from 41 percent in 1990 to 57 percent in 2003, the greatest improvements were in Southeast Asia and North Africa and the least in Sub-Saharan Africa (http://unstats.un.org/unsd/mi/goals_2005/goal_5.pdf). A recent WHO report indicates an average of 42 percent in the Africa Region,

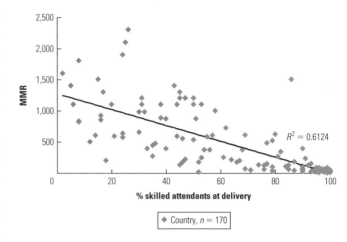

Figure 16.2 Relation between Skilled Attendant at Delivery and MMR for All Countries, 1995

Source: Safe Motherhood Initiative and Maternal Mortality in 1995. Estimates developed by WHO, UNICEF, and UNFPA 2001.

implying no change from the 1990 global average (WHO 2005).

Although there is no specific comparative rate, in its global estimates on births attended by skilled personnel the WHO (2005) reported 46.2 percent for Africa with the lowest rates in East Africa (32.5 percent) and West Africa (39.7 percent) (http://www.who.int/reproductive-health/global_monitoring/skilled_attendant.html).

Figure 16.2 shows that the higher the proportion of deliveries with a skilled attendant in a country, the lower the country's MMR. Furthermore, most of the Sub-Saharan Africa countries (not labeled) are above the regression line. Lack of or poorly functioning health management information systems with an effective feedback loop as well as weak supervision are further challenges influencing the quality of maternal services and MMRs.

National Policies and Investments. For any program or strategy on maternal health and safe motherhood to succeed, it must have the support of the highest level of national authority. Such support facilitates the allocation of adequate financial and human resources; improves the infrastructure and communications; and puts in place effective and implementable standards, policies, and protocols. Most countries in Sub-Saharan Africa have not addressed policy issues, even where the policies have been shown to have significant influence on maternal mortality. Romania provides the best example for the developing world of the impact of changes in policy. Figure 16.3 clearly demonstrates the trends of maternal mortality that occurred with the change in the country's abortion law in 1966 and 1989

Figure 16.3 Effects of the Introduction in Romania of an Anti-Abortion Law in 1966 and Legalization of Abortion in 1989

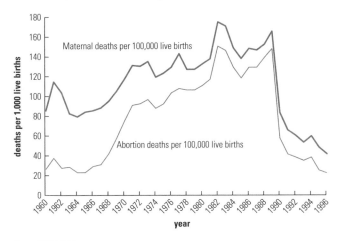

Source: WHO 1998.

REDUCING MATERNAL MORTALITY: PRIORITY INTERVENTIONS AND LESSONS

Many lessons have been learned on what works in maternal health. These have led to the identification of key interventions for the reduction of maternal morbidity and mortality in the developing world.

Priority Interventions

The past two decades have witnessed significant shifts in thinking about effective interventions for improving maternal outcomes in poor countries, from the Maternal and Child Health program to the Safe Motherhood Initiative, with its "Pillars," and the Making Pregnancy Safer program (Starrs 1998; http://w3.whosea.org/pregnancy/chap1f.htm). More recently, the case for identifying and investing in the most effective interventions for safe motherhood has dominated the debates (AbouZahr, Wardlaw, and Hill 2001). There is evidence of effective clinical interventions that save lives, but less is known about the best strategies for accelerating reduction of maternal mortality in developing countries, especially in Africa and South Asia (De Brouwere and Van Lerberghe 2002; Donnay 2002; Koblinski, Campbell, and Heichelheim 1999; Liljestrand 2000). The findings of the World Bank's analysis for the decline in maternal mortality in Malaysia and Sri Lanka in the past 50 to 60 years and the magnitude of health system expenditures on maternal health are relevant to Africa (World Bank 2003).

Malaysia and Sri Lanka have succeeded in reducing maternal mortality to levels comparable to those in industrial countries in the last few decades. Expanded female literacy in Sri Lanka and strong economic performance by Malaysia helped promote these gains. The World Bank analysis confirmed that maternal mortality can be halved in developing countries every 7 to 10 years and is affordable, regardless of income level and economic growth rate; steady, modest investment in poverty reduction and in maternal health services to improve access to and quality of emergency obstetric care are required.

Removal of financial barriers to maternal care was an important step in both countries, as was increased access to skilled birth attendance and emergency obstetric care. Recording and reporting of maternal deaths was a prerequisite to addressing the challenges of reducing maternal mortality in both countries. Other important lessons were that governments can afford to provide the critical elements of maternal care free of charge to clients and that different

(http://www.who.int/docstore/world-health-day/en/pages1998/whd98_10.html). In the 1950s and early 1960s, the law provided for access to abortion and was associated with relatively low mortality ratios. The restrictions on abortion that followed was associated with significant increase in the MMR in the 1980s. Immediately after the December 1989 revolution that overthrew President Nicolae Ceauşescu, restrictions on contraceptives were removed and abortion legalized. Subsequently, with the precipitous drop in abortion-related mortality, the MMR dropped.

Changing the abortion policy reduced maternal mortality by more than half in less than 10 years. Therefore, by changing the underlying policy-related causes, Sub-Saharan African countries have the potential of achieving reductions in maternal mortality. In most Sub-Saharan African countries, despite many international pronouncements, high-level support for maternal health and measures to reduce maternal mortality and unsafe abortion is weak or nonexistent.

Inadequate financing and sustainability of the health sector in general and of reproductive health in particular, are other barriers. In most African countries, health expenditures have not increased substantially while major problems in allocation efficiency and inequities exist (World Bank 2005). With various competing priorities for a dwindling financial resource base, the health sector needs to do a better job in reclaiming its rightful share. Moreover, given the inadequate investment, the number of health personnel trained is often small, and once trained, many open private clinics or emigrate to developed countries to earn a better living.

tactics are needed at different stages of the development of health systems. The transition from high to low MMR passes through several phases characterized by the following:

- high MMR: low levels of skilled attendance and emergency obstetric care (EmOC)
- declining MMR: medium levels of skilled attendance and EmOC
- low MMR: high levels of skilled attendance and EmOC.

Except for South Africa and Botswana, most of Sub-Saharan Africa falls in the first category, "high MMR—low levels of skilled attendance and EmOC." This status calls for establishing a solid foundation for effective maternity care, increasing access to care, and ensuring appropriate use of available services through community mobilization and improved quality. Elements of the foundation to support effective maternal care in Malaysia and Sri Lanka included professionalization of midwifery, civil registration of births, compilation of data on maternal deaths, and replication of local success. These elements do not always need additional resources but require focused leadership and effective management.

Improving Emergency Obstetric Care: The Three Levels of Delay

It is clear from the foregoing that accelerating the decline of maternal mortality in Sub-Saharan Africa and realization of the Millennium Development Goals will require the provision of a synergistic package of health and social services that reaches everyone, especially deprived populations.

The framework model of three delays has been applied to analyze the constraints, opportunities, and systems required at different levels of a safe motherhood program (box 16.1). This framework serves as a useful planning tool for the actions required at every level of health care while emphasizing the need to link these levels through transport and communication, supervision, and community outreaches. Thus, community awareness and trust and better access to and quality of emergency transport reinforce each other to improve maternal outcome. In an integrated essential health care package, this network enhances provision of other services, such as family planning and immunization, while promoting emphasis on skilled attendance.

The model is advocated by the Regional Prevention of Maternal Mortality Network (PMMN 1995) and is rapidly gaining ground in Africa. Using a modified "Four Levels of

---

Box 16.1 Model of Three Levels of Delay

Level 1 delay: decision making at community level—examines decision-making process on pregnancy and childbirth at household and community level, including birth preparedness

Level 2 delay: accessibility, transport, and communication—examines options for communication and transport from community to a health facility

Level 3 delay: availability of appropriate care, including quality—examines perceived and actual quality of care provided to the client on arrival at the facility

Source: Thaddeus and Maine 1994.

Delay" approach to analyze maternal mortality in Eritrea, Ghebrehiwot (2004) attributed the causes of death to the following processes:

- Delay One: failure or delay in recognition of danger signs—33 percent of maternal deaths
- Delay Two: delay in deciding to seek care—40 percent of the cases
- Delay Three: delay in reaching appropriate care—19 percent of cases
- Delay Four: delay in receiving appropriate care—52 percent of cases.

This simple framework appears ideal for Sub-Saharan Africa. It works well and supports local partners in finding tailor-made solutions to challenges posed in each specific setting and making service more responsive to local community needs. It can also be used to improve data collection and use at the local level.

The first level involves a primary health care bottoms-up approach with active community involvement (men and women) and focused comprehensive development programs wherein reproductive health and safe motherhood are appropriately integrated into the district health system. The second level entails expanding access to quality services, including functional linkages between communities and health facilities in regard to transport and communication. This leads to the final level, where appropriate quality of services is provided to clients on arrival at the health facility.

A Tanzania case study (Urassa et al. 1997) depicts a typical finding from most maternal mortality reviews in Africa. A large proportion of women die because of delayed decision making at home, lack of transport, and inappropriate care if they make it alive to a health facility. This confirms the observation that reduction of high maternal mortality demands a strong focus on each level of delay through creation of an effective system providing EmOC. Links between the different levels of the health care system, from community through the basic health center (basic EmOC) to the referral hospital (comprehensive EmOC) are critical.

CONCLUSION

Countries in Sub-Saharan Africa face the challenge of identifying the base MMR to be reduced by the prescribed proportion in view of the conflicting MMR statistics from country-based studies and global estimates. Because of the difficulties in assessing MMR, different methodologies have been used. The use of different approaches complicates the comparison and study of trends and causes of maternal mortality, owing to variations in coverage, reference dates, and data presentation.

Two Millennium Development Goals are of direct relevance to maternal and newborn health: goal 4, to reduce child mortality, and goal 5, to improve maternal health. The latter goal is aimed at reducing the 1990 MMRs by 75 percent by 2015. The probability of reaching this goal in most Sub-Saharan Africa countries is highly questionable given that most countries have shown little or no change in their MMRs and in a few countries they have even increased (World Bank 2004). Evidence from Sri Lanka and Malaysia shows that maternal mortality reduction can be accelerated through joint government and community action. For Sub-Saharan Africa, this calls for the establishment of a solid foundation for effective maternity care and increasing access and use of services. Monitoring of maternal care services and audits of maternal deaths are crucial to this effort.

Further exploration into maternal mortality, especially the underlying factors in Sub-Saharan Africa, is necessary, as are improved data collection systems, credibility in dissemination of data, and realistic estimates where information is deficient. Without good sources of data, Sub-Saharan Africa will continue to rely on model estimates, which could be misleading and de-motivating. For instance, the WHO, UNICEF, and UNFPA estimates, the best and most quoted, vary significantly from those obtained from country-based studies (AbouZahr and Wardlaw 2003). In some countries,

the estimates are double those reported from country-based studies, and underreporting was presented as the main factor. For instance, WHO, UNFPA, and UNICEF estimates reflect Kenya's MMR of 1,300 maternal deaths per 100,000 live births against the 590 maternal deaths per 100,000 live births reported by the DHS (AbouZahr and Wardlaw 2003). Also, the WHO, UNFPA, and UNICEF estimate for Tanzania was 1,500 maternal deaths per 100,000 live births, compared with the DHS estimate of 529 maternal deaths per 100,000 live births (AbouZahr and Wardlaw 2003). These discrepancies are enormous and have significant implications in regard to the Millennium Development Goals.

Increasing interest in the "near-miss population" provides an opportunity to explore the underlying causes and correlates of maternal morbidity and mortality. *Near-miss population* is defined as individuals who present to the health facilities with life-threatening conditions or develop life-threatening complications while under management (Filippi et al. 2000; Kaye et al. 2003; Mantel et al. 1998). This is a special category of survivors, whose stories provide unique insights and valuable information on maternal mortality. In the absence of accurate and detailed information on maternal deaths in Sub-Saharan Africa, increased use of studies on the near-miss population could provide useful lessons. Such studies could provide information on the sequence of events leading to complications and describe critical life-saving interventions. Comparative studies between the near misses and deaths occurring in the same institution or communities could further clarify the factors contributing to or averting deaths.

REFERENCES

AbouZahr, C., and T. Wardlaw. 2001. "Maternal Mortality at End of a Decade: Signs of Progress." *Bulletin of the World Health Organization* 79: 32–34.

———. 2003. "Maternal Mortality in 2000: Estimates Developed by WHO/UNICEF/UNFPA." WHO, Geneva.

AbouZahr, C., T. Wardlaw, and K. Hill. 2001. "Maternal Mortality in 1995: Estimates Developed by WHO, UNICEF, UNFPA." WHO/RHR/01.9, WHO, Geneva.

AGI (Alan Guttmacher Institute). 1999. *Sharing Responsibility; Women, Society and Abortion Worldwide.* New York: AGI.

Antelman, G., G. I. Msamanga, D. Spiegelman, E. J. N. Urassa, R. Nahr, D. J. Hunter, and W. W. Fawzi. 2000. "Nutritional Factors and Infectious Disease Contribute to Anemia among Pregnant Women with HIV in Tanzania." *Journal of Nutrition* 130: 1950–57.

Bang, A. T., R. A. Bang, and H. M. Reddy. 2005. "Home-Based Neonatal Care: Summary and Applications of the Field Trial in Rural Gadchiroli, India 1993–2003." *Journal of Perinatology* 25: S108–122.

Borghi, J., K. Hanson, C. Adjei Acquah, G. Ekanmian, V. Filippi, C. Ronsmans, R. Brugha, E. Browne, and E. Alihonou. 2003. "Costs of

Near-Miss Obstetric Complications for Women and Their Families in Benin and Ghana." *Health Policy and Planning* 18 (4): 383–92.

Claeson, M., C. C. Griffin, T. A. Johnston, M. McLachlan, A. L. B. Soucat, A. Wagstaff, and A. S. Yazbeck. 2001. *Poverty Reduction and the Health Sector.* Washington, DC: World Bank.

Darmstadt, G. L., Z. A. Bhutta, S. Cousens, T. Adam, N. Walker, L. de Bernis, and the Lancet Neonatal Survival Steering Team. 2005. "Evidence-Based, Cost-Effective Interventions : How Many Newborn Babies Can We Save?" *Lancet* 365: 977–88.

De Brouwere, V., and W. Van Lerberghe. 2002. "Safe Motherhood Strategies: A Review of the Evidence." *Studies in Health Services Organization and Policy* 17: 415–48.

Donnay, F. 2002. "Maternal Survival in Developing Countries. What Can Be Done in the Next Decade?" *International Journal of Gynecology and Obstetrics* 70: 89–97.

Edwards, R. T. 2001. "Paradigms and Research Programs: Is It Time to Move from Health Care Economics to Health Economics?" *Health Economics* 19: 635–49.

Eritrea National Statistics and Evaluation Office and ORC Macro. 2003. *Eritrea Demographic and Health Survey 2002.* Calverton, MD: Eritrea National Statistics and Evaluation Office and ORC Macro.

Filippi, V., C. Ronsmans, T. Gandaho, W. Graham, E. Alihonow, and P. Santos. 2000. "Women's Reports of Severe (Near-miss) Obstetric Complications in Benin." *Studies in Family Planning* 31 (4): 309–24.

Garenne, M., K. Mbaye, M. D. Bah, and P. Correa. 1997. "Risk Factors for Maternal Mortality: A Case-Control Study in Dakar Hospitals (Senegal)." *African Journal of Reproductive Health* 1 (1): 14–24.

Ghebrehiwot, M. 2004. "Measurement of Maternal Mortality in Eritrea." PhD diss., Johns Hopkins Bloomberg School of Public Health, Baltimore.

Graham, W. J. 1991. "Maternal Mortality: Levels, Trends and Data Deficiencies." In *Disease and Health in Sub-Saharan Africa,* ed. R. G. Feachem and D. R. Jamison, 101–16. New York: Oxford University Press.

Harrison, K. 1997. "Maternal Mortality in Nigeria: The Real Issues." *African Journal of Reproductive Health* 1 (1): 7–13.

Henshaw, S. K., S. Singh, and T. Haas. 1999. "The Incidence of Abortion Worldwide." *International Family Planning Perspective* 25: S30–38.

Heymann, D. L., R. W. Steketee, J. J. Wirima, D. A. McFarland, C. O. Khoromana, and C. C. Campbell. 1990. "Antenatal Chloroquine Prophylaxis in Malawi: Chloroquine Resistance, Compliance, Protective Efficacy and Cost." *Transactions of the Royal Society of Tropical Medicine and Hygiene* 84: 496–98.

Howson, C. P., P. F. Harrison, and M. Law. 1996. *In Her Lifetime: Female Morbidity and Mortality in Sub-Saharan Africa.* Washington, DC: National Academy Press.

Isah, H. S., A. F. Fleming, I. A. O. Ujah, and C. G. Ekwempu. 1985. "Anemia and Iron Status of Pregnant and Non-Pregnant Women in the Guinea Savanna of Nigeria." *Annals of Tropical Medicine and Parasitology* 79 (5): 485–93.

Jacobson, J. L. 1991. "Zimbabwe Birth Force." *World Watch* 4 (4): 5–6.

Kaye, D., F. Mirembe, F. Aziga, and B. Namulema. 2003. "Maternal Mortality and Associated Near-Misses among Emergency Intrapartum Obstetric Referrals in Mulago Hospital, Kampala, Uganda." *East African Medical Journal* 80 (3): 144–49.

Koblinski, M. A., O. Campbell, and J. Heichelheim. 1999. "Organizing Delivery Care: What Works for Safe Motherhood?" *Bulletin of the World Health Organization* 77 (5): 399–406.

Kwast, B. E. 1996. "Reduction of Maternal and Perinatal Mortality in Rural and Peri-Urban Settings: What Works." Review. *European Journal of Obstetrics, Gynecology, and Reproductive Biology* 69 (1): 47–53.

Lilienfeld, A. 1980. *Foundations of Epidemiology.* 2nd ed. New York: Oxford University Press.

Liljestrand, J. 2000. "Strategies to Reduce Maternal Mortality Worldwide." *Current Opinion in Obstetrics and Gynecology* 12 (6): 513–17.

Lompo, K., Y. J. Hutin, G. Traore, F. Tall, J. B. Guiard-Schmid, G. Yameogo, and B. Fabre-teste. 1993. "Morbidity and Mortality Related to Obstetrical Referral Patients to the Hospital of Bobo-Dioulasso, Burkina Faso." *Annales de la Societe Belge de Medecine Tropicale* 73 (2): 153–63.

Mantel, G. D., E. Buchmann, H. Rees, and R. C. Pattinson. 1998. "Severe Acute Maternal Morbidity: A Pilot Study of a Definition for a Near-Miss." *British Journal of Obstetrics and Gynaecology* 105 (9): 985–90.

Massawe, S. N., E. Urassa, G. Lindmark, B. Moller, and L. Nystrom. 1996. "Anemia in Pregnancy: A Major Health Problem with Implications for Maternal Health Care." *African Journal of Health Sciences* 3: 126–32.

Massawe, S. N., E. N. Urassa, M. Mmari, G. Ronquist, G. Lindmark, and L. Nystrom. 1999. "The Complexity of Pregnancy Anemia in Dar es Salaam." *Gynecologic and Obstetric Investigation* 47: 76–82.

Mbaruku, G. 2005. "Enhancing Survival of Mothers and Their Newborns in Tanzania." PhD diss., Karolinska Institute, Stockholm.

McCarthy, J., and D. Maine. 1992. "A Framework for Analyzing the Determinants of Maternal Mortality." *Studies in Family Planning* 23: 23–33.

Mosley, W. H., and L. C. Chen. 1984. "An Analytical Framework for the Study of Child Survival in Developing Countries." *Population and Development Review* 10: S24–45.

Onuh, S. O., and A. O. Aisien. 2004. "Maternal and Fetal Outcome in Eclamptic Patients in Benin City, Nigeria." *Journal of Obstetrics and Gynecology* 24 (7): 765–68.

Pattinson, R. C., and J. Moodley. 2002. *Saving Mothers.* Second Report on Confidential Enquiries into Maternal Deaths in Pretoria, South Africa, 1999–2001. Department of Health, South Africa.

Pattinson, R. C., H. Vandecruys, A. P. Macdonald, and G. D. Mantel. 2005. "Why Do Women Die during Childbirth?" *Science in Africa,* April 11.

Paul, B. K. 1993. "Maternal Mortality in Africa: 1980–87." *Social Science and Medicine* 37 (6): 745–52.

PMMN (Prevention of Maternal Mortality Network). 1995. "Situation Analyses of Emergency Obstetric Care: Examples from Eleven Operations Research Projects in West Africa." *Social Science and Medicine* 40 (5): 657–67.

Rogo, K. 1993. "Induced Abortion in Sub-Saharan Africa." *East African Medical Journal* 70 (6): 386.

———. 2004. "Improving Technologies to Reduce Abortion-Related Morbidity and Mortality." *International Journal of Gynecology and Obstetrics* 85: 552–61.

Shulman, C. E., E. K. Dorman, F. Cutts, K. Kawuondo, J. Bulmer, and K. Marsh. 1999. "Intermittent Sulphadoxine-Pyrimethamine to Prevent Severe Anemia Secondary to Malaria in Pregnancy: Randomized Placebo Controlled Trial." *Lancet* 353: 632–36.

Stanton, C., N. Abderrahim, and K. Hill. 1997. *DHS Maternal Mortality Indicators: An Assessment of Data Quality and Implications for Data Use.* DHS Analytical Reports 4. Calverton, MD: Macro International.

———. 2000. "An Assessment of DHS Maternal Mortality Indicators." *Studies in Family Planning* 31: 111–23.

Stanton, C., J. Hobcraft, K. Hill, N. Kodjogbe, and W. T. Mapeta. 2001. "Every Death Counts: Measurement of Maternal Mortality Via Census." *Bulletin of the World Health Organization* 79 (7): 657–64.

Starrs, A. 1998. *The Safe Motherhood Action Agenda: Priorities for the Next Decade.* New York: Family Care International.

Thaddeus, S., and D. Maine. 1994. "Too Far to Walk: Maternal Mortality in Context." *Social Science and Medicine* 38 (8): 1091–110.

UNICEF (United Nations Children's Fund). 1999. *Programming for Safe Motherhood: Guidelines for Maternal and Neonatal Survival.* New York: UNICEF.

United Nations. 2003. "Workshop in HIV/AIDS and Adult Mortality in Developing Countries." UN/POP/2003/3, United Nations, New York.

Urassa, E., S. Massawe, G. Lindmark, and L. Nystrom. 1997. "Operational Factors Affecting Maternal Mortality in Tanzania." *Health Policy Plan* 12 (1): 50–57.

Van den Broek, N. R., and E. A. Letsky. 2000. "Etiology of Anemia in Pregnancy in South Malawi." *American Journal of Clinical Nutrition* 72: 247S–56S.

Van Norren, B., and H. A. W. van Viannen. 1986. *The Malnutrition Infection Syndrome and Its Demographic Outcome in Developing Countries.* Publication 4. The Hague: Programming Committee for Demographic Research.

Wall, L. L. 1998. "Dead Mothers and Injured Wives: The Social Context of Maternal Morbidity and Mortality among the Hausa of Northern Nigeria." *Studies in Family Planning* 29: 341–59.

WHO (World Health Organization). 1992. *International Statistical Classification of Diseases and Related Health Problems.* 10th rev. ed. Geneva: World Health Organization.

———. 1998. "Unsafe Abortion: Global and Regional Estimates of Incidence of and Mortality Due to Unsafe Abortion with a Listing of Available Country Data." WHO/RHT/MSM/97.16, WHO, Geneva.

———. 2005. *Reducing Maternal Deaths: The Challenge of the New Millennium in the African Region.* Brazzaville: WHO.

WHO and UNICEF. 1996. *Revised 1990 Estimates of Maternal Mortality: A New Approach by WHO and UNICEF.* Geneva: WHO.

World Bank. 2003. *Investing in Maternal Health: Learning from Malaysia and Sri Lanka.* Washington, DC: World Bank.

———. 2004. *Making Services Work for Poor People.* World Development Report. Washington, DC: World Bank.

———. 2005. *Improving Health, Nutrition, and Population Outcomes in Sub-Saharan Africa: The Role of the World Bank.* Washington, DC: World Bank.

Chapter 17

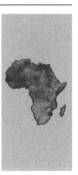

HIV/AIDS

Souleymane Mboup, Rosemary Musonda, Fred Mhalu, and Max Essex

The acquired immune deficiency syndrome (AIDS) was first recognized as a disease in the early 1980s. Within about five years it became clear that a new epidemic of unprecedented proportions was spreading throughout Sub-Saharan Africa. Destruction of the immune system, the main characteristic of the disease, caused patients to die from a range of opportunistic infections. As the opportunistic infections that occurred reflected the prevalence of given pathogens in the afflicted population, tuberculosis was one of the most common outcomes in Africa. Soon after the recognition of AIDS, a new group of retroviruses, subsequently designated the human immunodeficiency virus (HIV), was identified as the probable cause (Barre-Sinoussi et al. 1983; Gallo et al. 1984; Kitchen et al. 1984; Popovic et al. 1984). Some people were reluctant to accept the evidence that HIV was the cause of AIDS, both in the West and in Africa (Duesberg 1988). Many political leaders also chose to ignore or deny the importance of the expanding epidemic until after widespread transmission of HIV had already occurred.

DEVELOPMENT OF THE AIDS PANDEMIC

In retrospect, it is clear that several characteristics of HIV/AIDS resulted in a serious underestimation of the importance of the epidemic by both individuals and societies. One feature of HIV/AIDS that is highly unusual for an infectious disease is its consistently long incubation period combined with a high rate of disease development. Most organisms cause clinical signs or symptoms in only a fraction of those they infect. When infection occurs, as in diseases such as measles or smallpox, the induction period is short. HIV/AIDS is unique in that it regularly causes lethal disease after a prolonged induction period that lasts several years. As a result, the vast majority of HIV-infected people are clinically asymptomatic and do not know they are infected unless they undergo serologic testing. Because HIV-infected asymptomatic people can transmit the virus to others, the epidemic accelerates robustly. In some settings, a significant fraction of the population becomes infected before disease and death have provided the most evident lesson of the need for vigilance.

HIV/AIDS is also difficult to control because it is a sexually transmitted disease. In most societies both leaders and citizens are reluctant to discuss sex. Although condoms are efficient in preventing infection, they are often not an available option, for example, when couples wish to have children. The image of AIDS as a sexually transmitted disease also contributes to the stigmatization of infected people, which in turn may cause many to avoid testing to determine their status.

The variability in clinical outcomes also contributed to the difficulty in controlling the spread of HIV, particularly during the early stages of the epidemic. Tuberculosis, Kaposi's sarcoma, and chronic diarrhea can all occur in the absence of HIV infection. In the absence of testing for HIV, it is still possible for AIDS patients with such outcomes, and their families, to deny the infection and perhaps avoid some of the associated discrimination and stigma. As a societal problem, AIDS is also devastating because it usually attacks young adults during their most productive years of employment and parenting. Because both parents are often infected, AIDS epidemics ordinarily leave large numbers of orphans behind.

RATES OF HIV/AIDS IN AFRICA

In its most recent projections, the Joint United Nations Programme on HIV/AIDS (UNAIDS) has estimated that about 40 million people are currently infected with HIV, of whom about 25.8 million, or 64 percent of the total, are in Sub-Saharan Africa (UNAIDS and WHO 2005). The estimates are that 4.9 million people became infected during 2005, of whom 3.2 million, or 65 percent, were in Sub-Saharan Africa. During the same year, 77 percent of an estimated global burden of 3.1 million AIDS deaths were projected for Sub-Saharan Africa. During recent years, the use of antiretroviral (ARV) drugs in the United States and other developed countries has dramatically reduced AIDS death rates, but until now, only a small proportion of AIDS patients in Sub-Saharan Africa have received treatment (see figure 17.1).

Several factors account for the low fraction of AIDS patients receiving ARV treatment. One of the largest is the cost of the drugs. Until recently, all the major ARV drugs were prohibitively expensive in developing countries. This situation is now changing, but ARV drugs and medical care are still out of reach for the majority of AIDS patients in Africa. The global burden of AIDS is disproportionate in

Figure 17.1 Disease Burden and Treatment of AIDS in Relation to Global Population and Economy

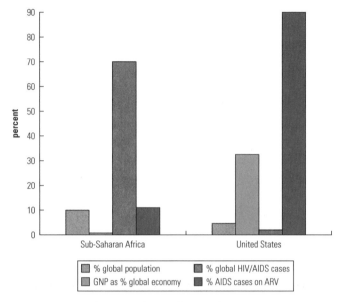

Source: CIA 2006; UNAIDS 2004; UNAIDS and WHO 2005; WHO 2005.

Figure 17.2 Global Burden of HIV-1 Infection

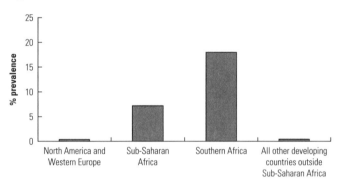

Source: UNAIDS 2004.

countries whose gross national productivity represents a small fraction of the global economy (see figure 17.1).

Wide variation in HIV prevalence rates also occurs within Africa (Essex and Mboup 2002). However, overall adult rates of HIV in Sub-Saharan Africa are about 7.2 percent, much higher than in other regions of the world, including other regions with large populations living in developing countries (see figure 17.2). Rates of HIV are low in North Africa, although countries that span the Sahara, such as Sudan, have higher rates than those countries on the northern coast.

Within Sub-Saharan Africa, the AIDS epidemic was noticed first in central Africa (Clumeck et al. 1983). Soon after, the epidemic was observed in East Africa, and subsequently in West Africa (Essex and Mboup 2002). The epidemic seemed to occur last in southern Africa, although rates there are now the highest in Africa and in the world. Six countries of southern Africa have adult prevalence rates of 20 percent or higher, and the mean prevalence rate for all of southern Africa is about 18 percent.

The mean adult prevalence rate in Sub-Saharan Africa is 7.2 percent, whereas the mean rates in Asia are 0.4 percent (see table 17.1). Haiti, with a prevalence rate of 5.6 percent, has the highest outside of Africa, and Cambodia, with 2.6 percent, has the highest in Asia (UNAIDS 2004). Brazil, one of the few countries outside of the West that began ARV treatment at an early stage, has an estimated adult prevalence rate of 0.7 percent.

Table 17.1 HIV-1 Prevalence in Representative Regions and Countries

Regions and countries	Prevalence (%)	Dominant subtype
East Africa	*6.7*	*A (50%)*
Tanzania	8.8	Various
Uganda	4.1	A (60%)
North Africa	*0.3*	*B (> 95%)*
Egypt, Rep. of	< 0.1	B (> 95%)
Morocco	0.1	B (> 95%)
Southern Africa	*18.0*	*C (> 95%)*
Botswana	37.3	C (> 95%)
Mozambique	12.2	C (> 95%)
South Africa	21.5	C (> 95%)
West Africa	*4.4*	*CRF 02 (70%)*
Côte d'Ivoire	7.0	CRF 02 (80%)
Nigeria	5.4	CRF 02 (70%)
Senegal	0.8	CRF 02 (60%)
Asia	*0.4*	*Various*
Cambodia	2.6	CRF 01 (> 90%)
China	0.1	CRF 07,08 (80%)
India	0.9	C (80%)
Thailand	1.5	CRF 01 (> 90%)
Caribbean	*1.6*	*B (90%)*
Haiti	5.6	B (90%)
Latin America	*0.6*	*B (90%)*
Brazil	0.7	B (80%)
North America	*0.6*	*B (> 90%)*
United States	0.6	B (> 90%)
Western Europe	*0.3*	*B (> 90%)*
Italy	0.5	B (70%)

Source: Country-specific prevalence data from UNAIDS 2004. Regional prevalence data from UNAIDS and WHO 2005 or adapted from UNAIDS 2004. Dominant subtype information from Essex and Mboup 2002.

Note: CRF = circulating recombinant form.

The overall burden that HIV/AIDS has placed on Sub-Saharan Africa is unprecedented. It is now the most common cause of death in the region (WHO 1999). It has been estimated that by the year 2010 life expectancy at birth could be decreased by at least 15 years in most of the region and by 30 years or more in five countries (Stanecki and Walker 2002). Population growth rates would fall and infant mortality rates would increase. It has been estimated that mortality rates for children under five could experience a fivefold increase in Botswana and Zimbabwe (Stanecki and Walker 2002). All these projections, however, assume that ARV drugs are not being used to save lives in the region. This is an assumption that, fortunately, is no longer valid.

RETROVIRUSES

Prior to the AIDS epidemic and the discovery of HIV, retroviruses were known to exist and were associated with certain leukemias of animals and people. Such "oncoretroviruses" were characterized by an ability to replicate without killing the cells they infect. Lentiretroviruses, which include the HIVs, usually replicate at higher levels and kill the cells they infect. All retroviruses use reverse transcription of the virion RNA to replicate, and they produce a proviral DNA form that can remain latent in host cell chromosomes. All retroviruses also generate a high rate of mutations when transcribing the RNA, but the error rate is highest for those viruses that replicate to high levels, such as HIV.

The high mutation rate facilitates a rapid rate of evolutionary change for HIVs. Another feature of the viruses that promotes rapid variation is the diploid nature of the viral RNA. With two complete copies of the genome packaged in each virus particle, recombinational events are also frequent, allowing progeny viruses to pick up large segments of somewhat different genetic information in a short period of time.

An extremely important aspect of the rate of evolutionary variation for HIVs is the selection pressure exerted by the host. This aspect is vividly illustrated by the rapid emergence of drug-resistant variations of HIV. Resistance occurs rapidly in a single individual, particularly when only one drug is used. The same type of competition occurs during host-mediated immunoselection pressure, in which viral variants emerge to avoid control by epitope-specific host immune responses. The process is repeated frequently and cyclically; the dominant clone of the virus elicits a new immune response, becomes controlled, and a new mutational variant takes over as the next dominant viral clone.

Many of the mutations and recombinational events result in the emergence of genomes that are incapable of replication. This occurs because viruses, to be viable, must fold their proteins in specific ways and retain reactive sites that signal key events. All HIVs, for example, must retain the ability to bind to the CD4 receptors and chemokine coreceptors, such as CCR5 and CXCR4, on T lymphocytes and macrophages. This in turn forces a certain level of convergent evolution.

As progressive cycles of HIV mutant clones begin to exhaust the immune control capacity of the host, the number of dying lymphocytes exceeds the capacity for cell replacement and the number of CD4 lymphocytes rapidly falls. As plasma viral load reaches levels of 50,000 copies per milliliter and above, and the number of CD4 lymphocytes drops to 300 per cubic millimeter and below, the ability of the body to resist opportunistic infections is largely lost, and clinical AIDS develops.

REGIONAL VARIATION

Soon after HIV-1 was identified, other lentiretroviruses were identified in primates. These included a wide range of simian immunodeficiency viruses (SIVs) and a second category of HIVs in people in West Africa, designated HIV-2s (Barin et al. 1985). The SIVs naturally infected large fractions of populations of various species of African monkeys, apparently without causing disease (Kanki, Homma, et al. 1985). The SIVs did, however, cause clinical AIDS when artificially injected into Asian macaques (Daniel et al. 1985; Kanki, McLane, et al. 1985).

Some of the SIVs were virtually indistinguishable from HIV-2s at the genetic level, although SIVs and HIV-2s were usually 50 to 60 percent different from HIV-1s. HIV-2s also cause an AIDS-like disease in people, but with considerably less efficiency than HIV-1s (Marlink et al. 1994). HIV-2s were much less transmissible, both by sexual contact and by mother-to-infant transmission (Kanki, Sankale, and Mboup 2002). Presumably because of this dramatic reduction in transmission efficiency, HIV-2 has been largely limited to West Africa, and it has not caused any of the large epidemics typical of HIV-1.

Many different categories of HIV-1s have been identified, with at least six of them linked to major epidemics. The different categories of HIV-1s are usually designated clades, or subtypes, and viruses of one subtype differ from those of another subtype by an average of 20 to 30 percent in genetic sequence. Two of the six common categories of HIV-1s were found to be circulating recombinant forms (CRFs) (McCutchan 2000).

The first major category of HIV-1 to be identified and categorized was subtype HIV-1B, which is responsible for the epidemics in the Americas and Western Europe. These epidemics have been characterized by patterns that reflect primary transmission via homosexual contact and injection drug use. HIV-1B has also been found in other sites, such as India, South Africa, and Thailand. Even in these sites, HIV-1B infections have not been associated with heterosexual epidemics, although heterosexual epidemics due to other HIV subtypes have occurred concurrently in the same sites (Hudgens et al. 2002; Janssens, Buve, and Nkengasong 1997).

The most common HIV in the world and in Africa is HIV-1 subtype C (HIV-1C). HIV-1C accounts for as many infections as all other HIVs combined, both in the world and in Africa (Essex 1999). It is responsible for the massive epidemic in southern Africa, and all the countries in Africa that have the highest rates of HIV have HIV-1C epidemics. Along with an epidemic expansion that plateaued at the highest levels, the HIV-1C epidemic in southern Africa expanded faster than other HIV epidemics, although it started later (Essex and Mboup 2002).

The next most important HIV virus in Africa, and in the world, is CRF 02, a recombinant form that originated from an HIV-1A and an HIV-1G. This virus accounts for about 25 percent of the world's infections (Essex and Mboup 2002). It is largely responsible for the epidemics in West Africa and central Africa. Although mean prevalence rates in these regions are only 5 percent and 6 percent, respectively, they represent some sites with large populations, such as Nigeria. East Africa has had epidemics of HIV-1A and HIV-1D, often coexisting in the same populations (Rayfield et al. 1998). A few countries, such as Tanzania in the east and Cameroon in the west, have a wide variety of viruses present in the same site (Fonjungo et al. 2000; Renjifo et al. 1999). In Tanzania, for example, an earlier epidemic of HIV-1A and HIV-1D fused with the northward expansion of the HIV-1C epidemic. This apparently resulted in the generation of a large number of recombinant viruses (Renjifo et al. 1999). A schematic distribution of the major subtypes and CRFs in Africa is illustrated in figure 17.3.

Phenotypic distinctions between the HIV-1 subtypes and CRFs are much less apparent than the differences between

Figure 17.3 Distribution of Major HIV-1 Subtypes and Circulating Recombinant Forms in Africa

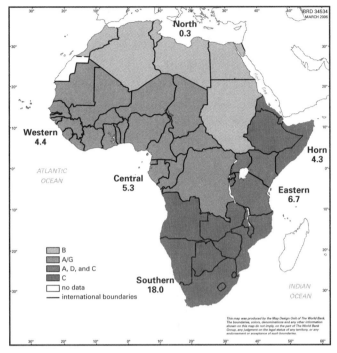

North 0.3
Western 4.4
Horn 4.3
Central 5.3
Eastern 6.7
Southern 18.0

B
A/G
A, D, and C
C
no data
international boundaries

ATLANTIC OCEAN
INDIAN OCEAN

IBRD 34534
MARCH 2006

This map was produced by the Map Design Unit of The World Bank. The boundaries, colors, denominations and any other information shown on this map do not imply, on the part of The World Bank Group, any judgment on the legal status of any territory, or any endorsement or acceptance of such boundaries.

Source: Essex and Mboup 2002; UNAIDS 2004; UNAIDS and WHO 2005.

HIV-1s and HIV-2s. HIV-1C genomes ordinarily have three NFκB enhancer sequences, whereas other subtypes have only two, and in the case of HIV-2s, only one (Montano et al. 1997). This is almost certainly associated with the higher transcriptional activation rates seen for HIV-1Cs (Montano et al. 2000). It is also a possible explanation for the higher rates of genomic variation (Novitsky et al. 1999) and the higher viral loads reported for HIV-1Cs (Neilson et al. 1999). The efficient spread of HIV-1C is also compatible with this subtype's preference for the CCR5 coreceptor (Ping et al. 1999; Tscherning et al. 1998). HIV-1Ds and HIV-1Bs, for example, are much more likely to use the CXCR4 coreceptor than the HIV-1Cs (Tscherning et al. 1998), and neither HIV-1B nor HIV-1D has spread to cause large epidemics in Africa.

Coinfection of individuals with two different HIVs— different subtypes; different types, such as HIV-1 and HIV-2; or different variants within a subtype—can occur. These events appear to occur less often than might be expected (Travers et al. 1995), perhaps because of some level of cross-protection due to activation of chemokines, receptor competition, or specific immunity. When the same cells are coinfected, the opportunity for generation of infectious recombinants is substantial.

PROGRESSION OF INFECTION

After initial exposure to HIV occurs, several weeks go by before the virus can be detected in blood. At least in the case of HIV-1B infections in homosexual men, an acute, influenza-like illness then occurs in the majority of the infected. This is characterized by high levels of virus replication reflected in the blood as viremia. Whether the same flu-like illness occurs at the same rate in heterosexual infections of other HIV-1 subtypes is unclear.

During the stage of acute viremia large numbers of T lymphocytes become infected in lymph nodes (Pantaleo et al. 1993), and patients are highly infectious to other potential contacts (Quinn and Chaisson 2003). The acute viremia then falls precipitously, presumably because of an effective immune response, albeit a response that later becomes largely ineffective as mutant variants emerge. The magnitude of the acute viremia and the depth of the subsequent resolution, sometimes called the set point, probably determine the subsequent rate of disease progression. For a minority of those infected, a rapid and well-controlled set point apparently results in the development of clinical AIDS only after a very prolonged period of time. Such individuals are sometimes called "long-term nonprogressors."

The length of time before disease development may also be related to other factors, such as the infected individual's genetic background (Winkler and O'Brien 2002), nutritional state, and parasite burden of coinfecting microorganisms. Antigenic stimulation of infected cells causes DNA synthesis, which in turn causes activation and replication of latent HIV. The tissue damage caused by other infections also stimulates the release of inflammatory cytokines, which also causes transcriptional activation of HIV (Montano et al. 2000). With all these variables, however, clinical AIDS rarely occurs before 4 to 5 years after infection, and almost always occurs within 10 to 12 years after infection. In the absence of therapy, death usually occurs within 1 to 3 years after the onset of clinical AIDS.

PREVENTION

Methods of preventing HIV infection can be divided into those that are currently available, such as education, and those that are not yet available but are being pursued through research, such as vaccines.

HIV transmission through blood transfusion, although an important issue at the early stages of the pandemic, now occurs only rarely. The serology tests used to determine if blood is contaminated are highly sensitive and specific, although an infectious unit of blood can occasionally be missed if the donor was infected within the two to three weeks before donation, before antibodies had time to develop. The use of contaminated needles or injection equipment is sometimes an important method of transmission in defined populations, but it is not nearly as important as sexual transmission, at least in Africa.

Voluntary testing and counseling programs are extremely important to reduce sexual transmission. A major limitation in most countries is the reluctance of most people to get tested and thus learn their status. Such reluctance may be particularly evident where infected individuals have few or no opportunities for treatment with ARV. In such situations concerns about stigma and death from the infection may provide disincentives for the individual to learn his or her status.

Condoms are highly effective when used properly. Abstinence provides a guarantee against sexual infection. But neither abstinence nor condoms allow couples to have children.

The use of ARVs for chemoprophylaxis is effective in preventing transmission of HIV from infected mothers to their infants. In the absence of intervention, 25 to 45 percent of infants born to HIV-positive mothers become infected. The infection occurs in utero, during the process of birth, and through breastfeeding. The use of ARVs, such as zidovudine (AZT), was shown to reduce neonatal transmission by as much as 67 percent in nonbreastfeeding populations if given at least six to eight weeks before birth (Connor et al. 1994). Even when given only at the time of labor, nevirapine (NVP) apparently reduced intrapartum transmissions by as much as 50 percent (Guay et al. 1999). The use of drug combinations early in gestation can presumably reduce in utero and intrapartum transmission to only a few percent.

Avoidance of breastfeeding can obviously eliminate postnatal infections by this route. However, in many cultures recommendations for formula feeding are not well received, in part because of the stigma associated with bottle feeding of the infant. The effectiveness of chemoprophylaxis to the infant or the mother, or both, while breastfeeding is being evaluated.

ARV drugs can also be used to block transmission of HIV by accidental needlestick infections, such as those that might occur among medical personnel treating AIDS patients (Bouvet, Laporte, and Tarantola 2002). The same three-drug combinations, such as AZT, lamivudine (3TC), and NVP,

that are used for treatment of AIDS, are highly effective if given within hours after the presumed exposure. The same interventions can be used for victims of sexual violence.

VACCINES AND MICROBICIDES

Effective vaccines that exist against other viral diseases are based on the injection of either killed virus, purified viral surface proteins, or live attenuated virus. All three types are commonly used in people. The Salk polio vaccine is killed virus, the vaccine used against hepatitis B is a purified viral surface protein, and the Sabin oral polio vaccine is a live attenuated virus. The killed virus and viral protein approaches can function only by inducing virus-neutralizing antibodies. The live attenuated types of vaccine often induce both neutralizing antibodies and cytolytic T cell immunity.

The use of live attenuated HIV as a vaccine was largely dismissed, even at the earliest stages, because of safety concerns. Killed HIV was similarly dismissed for safety concerns and because it was assumed that subunit surface proteins would work as well as killed virus without the same safety concerns, as was true of the hepatitis B vaccine. As a result, almost all the initial experimental vaccines were based on the use of HIV proteins gp120 or gp160 that protrude from the outer surface of the virus.

As HIVs grown in cultured cell lines provided the highest titers for subsequent purification, the first vaccines were made from T-cell-line adapted gp120/160 proteins. It was soon recognized that the neutralizing antibodies these vaccines induced were ineffective against naturally occurring HIVs. Subsequently it was also recognized that monomeric gp120/160 proteins induced antibodies that would work only against the exact strain selected. The profound sequence variation seen among HIVs created a situation in which matching the vaccine gp120 to the field challenge strain was not possible.

The next wave of HIV vaccine research was based primarily on the development of cytolytic T cell (CTL) vaccines. Most were based on the use of nonvirulent viruses, such as vaccinia, the vaccine used for smallpox, or adenoviruses. Genes, or parts of genes, of HIV that were suspected of being able to induce CTL responses were inserted in the "vaccine vector viruses" through gene splicing. HIV antigens or "CTL epitopes" must be delivered in this way, because for immunity to be effective, recognition of the immunogen must be in conjunction with cell processing to match the HIV antigens to the histocompatibility antigens of the recipient.

Several CTL vaccines have now been evaluated in people for safety and immunogenicity. In general, they appear to be quite safe, but they do not appear to be sufficiently stimulating to elicit strong immune responses that are likely to be protective. Developing CTL vaccines using other viruses as vectors is an entirely new area of vaccine science. If these methods can be mastered, they could probably also be extrapolated for use in combating many other diseases.

A major part of the rationale for CTL vaccines was the assumption that they would be more broadly cross-reactive than gp120 vaccines. Viral core proteins are usually more genetically conserved than viral surface proteins, thus reducing antigenic variation and reducing opportunities for immune selection in the vaccinee to evade effectiveness. Even for CTL vaccines, however, it seems prudent to use the relevant HIV-1 subtype or regional strain to increase the likelihood of protection.

To maximize the chances that a vaccine may work, most researchers endorse the use of vaccines or vaccine combinations that might induce both neutralizing antibodies and CTL responses. This is ordinarily done using a "prime-boost" strategy of several inoculations, in which the first (prime) would allow the induction of CTL responses, and the boost would encourage both CTL and antibody responses.

Recently, research to design gp120 antigens that would induce cross-reactive neutralizing antibodies has also begun a new generation of vaccine approaches (Fouts et al. 2000). The concept is based on the stabilization of a conformational state of the HIV-1 gp120 at the time it interacts with the CD4 receptor or the CCR5 receptor or both. This and other approaches serve to illustrate that HIV vaccine research is alive and well in providing new designs, but is also unlikely to yield a final product of high efficacy in less than 5 to 10 years. Thus, the prevention of further spread of HIV within the next decade must be centered on other measures.

THERAPY

The first phase of therapy using ARV drugs was AZT. Initially it was the only drug, and when used alone it often gave AIDS patients another six months or so in partial remission. Soon, other related drugs, nucleoside analogue reverse transcriptase inhibitors (NRTIs) such as lamivudine (3TC), didanosine (DDI), and stavudine (D4T), were also available. One of these drugs used with AZT clearly worked better than using just one drug alone. However, their use posed two significant problems. One was drug toxicities,

which ranged from gastrointestinal problems and anemias to peripheral neuropathies. The other was the rapid generation of drug-resistant variants of HIV, which soon grew just as well in the patient as before the drugs were first used. Using two drugs at once lowered HIV viremia even better than using one drug and delayed the time to development of drug resistance. However, even with two NRTIs, drug resistance often developed within a year, and resistance to one of the NRTIs often prompted resistance to other NRTIs of the same class.

The next class of drugs available was the nonnucleoside reverse transcriptase inhibitors (NNRTIs), such as nevirapine (NVP) and efavirenz (EFV). These drugs were even easier for the virus to mutate around to cause drug resistance, and this happened within weeks when one of these drugs was given alone, as "monotherapy." However, when given with two or more other drugs, they could often be given for long periods of time.

The third major class of drugs, the protease inhibitors, work on an entirely different gene of HIV, so they provided an additional, separate mechanism to keep down virus replication. However, unlike the NRTIs and the NNRTIs, which could often be made "off patent" or as "generics," the protease inhibitors are still expensive and generally not available in developing countries.

The standard drug regimen for most developing countries is now a three-drug combination that includes two NRTIs, especially AZT and 3TC, and one NNRTI, such as NVP. In most cases this regimen works well, unless resistance to any of the drugs is already present. This happens, for example, if women have recently been treated with AZT or NVP alone, as part of a chemoprevention strategy to block infection of their infant. The use of NVP alone during labor, for example, can cause resistance to the whole NNRTI class of drugs in 20 percent or more of mothers, even when only one dose is given (Eshleman et al. 2001).

In the West, combination three-drug therapy usually begins earlier than the current recommendations projected for the developing world. In the United States, for example, drug therapy would usually be recommended by the time the patient fell below 350 CD4+ cells per cubic millimeter or a viral load of less than 25,000 RNA per milliliter. In Africa a consensus is building that the most logical time to initiate therapy is when CD4+ cells fall below 200, or when the patient has experienced an AIDS-defining illness. By this time, most patients have viral loads in excess of 50,000 RNA per milliliter. In early studies, disease-free one-year survival rates for patients given a three-drug combination with initiation below 200 CD4$^+$ cells per cubic millimeter seem to be quite good (Djomand et al. 2003). Rigorous adherence to taking the drugs is essential to increase the time to development of drug-resistant variants. Many newer drugs and drug combinations reduce the difficulty of dosing because they are taken only once per day and have fewer gastrointestinal side effects.

Studies using several combinations of three drugs to treat AIDS patients have now been conducted in several African countries (Coetzee et al. 2004; Djomand et al. 2003; Laurent et al. 2002; Weidle et al. 2002; Wester et al. 2005). The results indicate a high degree of success. Despite the initiation of therapy at low levels of immune competence (for example, 10–200 CD4$^+$ cells per cubic millimeter), responses have been good (Coetzee et al. 2004; Laurent et al. 2002; Weidle et al. 2002; Wester et al. 2005). These include survival rates of 85 percent or higher, and escalation of CD4 cell counts of 150 CD4$^+$ cells per cubic millimeter or more by a year after drug initiation. Even patients who began drug therapy at cell counts below 50 CD4$^+$ cells per cubic millimeter, most of whom would probably die within a year if left untreated, had surprisingly positive responses.

The positive responses occurred in part because most patients showed a strong commitment to adhere to the prescribed regimen of drugs. Although different viral subtypes may show different profiles of drug mutations (Quan et al. 2003; Turner et al. 2004), high levels of adherence reduced rates of clinical failure due to drug resistance (Coetzee et al. 2004; Laurent et al. 2002; Wester et al. 2005). It is too early to know whether HIV drug resistance will become a major problem in Africa. However, the widespread use of just one or two drugs in perinatal chemoprophylaxis clearly results in high levels of genotypic resistance in mothers who may soon need the same drugs for their own therapy. Whether such drug-resistant variants will be transmitted by sexual contact remains to be determined.

The cost of a basic three-drug regimen, such as AZT, 3TC, and NVP, is now as low as about US$1 per day. Although this is far below the original cost for the same drugs, it is still above a level that is possible for many in the poorest countries. The actual cost of treatment, including costs of health care personnel, infrastructure, and laboratory diagnosis and monitoring, is generally substantially higher than the cost of the drugs alone. Initiation on ARV therapy should be possible in many sites in Africa, but costs will also increase as patients become resistant to any of those drugs used in the "first-line" regimen. Switching to different regimens may require the use of protease inhibitors or other

drugs that cost more, as do monitoring costs and the involvement of personnel with more specialized skills. The use of CD4 counts alone may be adequate for initiation, for example, but viral load tests and drug resistance tests may be necessary if drug failure occurs. The latter tests are more expensive, but they may be needed to validate the efficacy of second- or third-line drug regimens.

CONCLUSION

The epidemic of HIV/AIDS is unprecedented, having expanded from a new disease to the leading cause of death in Sub-Saharan Africa in just over two decades. Despite some clear examples of success, such as Senegal for prevention, and Uganda for control, major new measures are needed to avoid further devastation. The epidemic in Africa is uneven, with the greatest burden in southern Africa, where populations are already experiencing major reductions in life expectancy and a reversal of progress in the management of national economies.

About two-thirds of the world's HIV infections are in Sub-Saharan Africa in just 10 percent of the world's population. Because HIV/AIDS in the Americas and Europe is uncommon in women and rare in children, Africa holds more than 90 percent of the world's burden on such issues as child mortality and the care of orphans.

At present, prevention strategies are largely limited to education for changes in sexual practices and the use of condoms. Vaccines and microbicides represent an extremely important area of research, but useful products are not likely to be available in less than 5 to 10 years. ARV drug treatment programs have begun in Africa but are as yet very modest in impact. Operational research to maximize the benefits of ARV use will be important to address treatment efficacy and drug resistance, the impact on health manpower resources, and cost-effectiveness. The full devastation of AIDS in Africa has yet to be fully appreciated. Still, an increase in awareness and willingness to act should give cause for optimism.

REFERENCES

Barin, F., S. Mboup, F. Denis, P. Kanki, J. S. Allan, T. H. Lee, and M. Essex. 1985. "Serological Evidence for Virus Related to Simian T-Lymphotropic Retrovirus III in Residents of West Africa." *Lancet* 2: 1387–89.

Barre-Sinoussi, F., J. C. Chermann, F. Rey, M. T. Nugeyre, S. Chamaret, J. Gruest, C. Dauguet, et al. 1983. "Isolation of a T-Lymphotropic

Retrovirus from a Patient at Risk for Acquired Immune Deficiency Syndrome (AIDS)." *Science* 220: 868–71.

Bouvet, E., A. Laporte, and A. Tarantola. 2002. "Postexposure Prophylaxis for Occupational Exposure and Sexual Assault." In *AIDS in Africa*, ed. M. Essex, S. Mboup, P. Kanki, R. Marlink, and S. Tlou, 571–83. New York: Kluwer Academic/Plenum Publishers.

CIA (Central Intelligence Agency). 2006. *The World Factbook.* http://www. cia.gov/cia/publications/factbook/ (accessed January 13, 2006).

Clumeck, N., F. Mascart-Lemone, J. de Maubeuge, D. Brenez, and L. Marcelis. 1983. "Acquired Immune Deficiency Syndrome in Black Africans." *Lancet* 1: 642.

Coetzee, D., K. Hildebrand, A. Boulle, G. Maartens, F. Louis,, V. Labatala, H. Reuter, N. Ntwana, and E. Goemaere. 2004. "Outcomes after Two Years of Providing Antiretroviral Treatment in Khayelitsha, South Africa." *AIDS* 18: 887–95.

Connor, E. M., R. S. Sperling, R. Gelber, P. Kiselev, G. Scott, M. J. O'Sullivan, R. VanDyke, et al. 1994. "Reduction of Maternal-Infant Transmission of Human Immunodeficiency Virus Type 1 with Zidovudine Treatment." Pediatric AIDS Clinical Trials Group Protocol 076 Study Group. *New England Journal of Medicine* 331: 1173–80.

Daniel, M. D., N. L. Letvin, N. W. King, M. Kannagi, P. K. Sehgal, R. D. Hunt, P. J. Kanki, M. Essex, and R. C. Desrosiers. 1985. "Isolation of T-Cell Tropic HTLV-III-Like Retrovirus from Macaques." *Science* 228: 1201–4.

Djomand, G., T. Roels, T. Ellerbrock, D. Hanson, F. Diomande, B. Monga, C. Maurice, et al. 2003. "Virologic and Immunologic Outcomes and Programmatic Challenges of an Antiretroviral Treatment Pilot Project in Abidjan, Côte d'Ivoire." *AIDS* 17: S5–S15.

Duesberg, P. 1988. "HIV Is Not the Cause of AIDS." *Science* 241: 514-17.

Eshleman, S. H., M. Mracna, L. A. Guay, M. Deseyve, S. Cunningham, M. Mirochnick, P. Musoke, et al. 2001. "Selection and Fading of Resistance Mutations in Women and Infants Receiving Nevirapine to Prevent HIV-1 Vertical Transmission (HIVNET 012)." *AIDS* 15: 1951–57.

Essex, M. 1999. "Human Immunodeficiency Viruses in the Developing World." *Advances in Virus Research* 53: 71–88.

Essex, M., and S. Mboup. 2002. "Regional Variations in the African Epidemics." In *AIDS in Africa*, ed. M. Essex, S. Mboup, P. Kanki, R. Marlink, and S. Tlou, 631–40. New York: Kluwer Academic/Plenum Publishers.

Fonjungo, P. N., E. N. Mpoudi, J. N. Torimiro, G. A. Alemnji, L. T. Eno, J. N. Nkengasong, F. Gao, et al. 2000. "Presence of Diverse Human Immunodeficiency Virus Type 1 Viral Variants in Cameroon." *AIDS Research and Human Retroviruses* 16: 1319–24.

Fouts, T. R., R. Tuskan, K. Godfrey, M. Reitz, D. Hone, G. K. Lewis, and A. L. DeVico. 2000. "Expression and Characterization of a Single-Chain Polypeptide Analogue of the Human Immunodeficiency Virus Type 1 Gp120-CD4 Receptor Complex." *Journal of Virology* 74, 11427–36.

Gallo, R. C., S. Z. Salahuddin, M. Popovic, G. M. Shearer, M. Kaplan, B. F. Haynes, T. J. Palker, et al. 1984. "Frequent Detection and Isolation of Cytopathic Retroviruses (HTLV-III) from Patients with AIDS and at Risk for AIDS." *Science* 224: 500–03.

Guay, L. A., P. Musoke, T. Fleming, D. Bagenda, M. Allen, C. Nakabiito, J. Sherman, et al. 1999. "Intrapartum and Neonatal Single-Dose Nevirapine Compared with Zidovudine for Prevention of Mother-to-Child Transmission of HIV-1 in Kampala, Uganda: HIVNET 012 Randomised Trial." *Lancet* 354: 795–802.

Hudgens, M. G., I. M. Longini Jr., S. Vanichseni, D. J. Hu, D. Kitayaporn, P. A. Mock, M. E. Halloran, G. A. Satten, K. Choopanya, and T. D. Mastro. 2002. "Subtype-Specific Transmission Probabilities for Human Immunodeficiency Virus Type 1 among Injecting Drug Users in Bangkok, Thailand." *American Journal of Epidemiology* 155: 159–68.

Janssens, W., A. Buve, and J. N. Nkengasong. 1997. "The Puzzle of HIV-1 Subtypes in Africa." *AIDS* 11: 705–12.

Kanki, P., J. L. Sankale, and S. Mboup. 2002. "Biology of Human Immunodeficiency Virus Type 2." In *AIDS in Africa*, ed. M. Essex, S. Mboup, P. Kanki, R. Marlink, and S. Tlou, 74–103. New York: Kluwer Academic/Plenum Publishers.

Kanki, P. J., T. Homma, T. H. Lee, N. W. King Jr., R. D. Hunt, and M. Essex. 1985. "Antibodies to Human T-Cell Leukemia Virus-Membrane Antigens in Macaques with Malignant Lymphoma." *Haematology and Blood Transfusion* 29: 345–49.

Kanki, P. J., M. F. McLane, N. W. King Jr., N. L. Letvin, R. D. Hunt, P. Sehgal, M. D. Daniel, R. C. Desrosiers, and M. Essex. 1985. "Serologic Identification and Characterization of a Macaque T-Lymphotropic Retrovirus Closely Related to HTLV-III." *Science* 228: 1199–1201.

Kitchen, L. W., F. Barin, J. L. Sullivan, M. F. McLane, D. B. Brettler, P. H. Levine, and M. Essex. 1984. "Aetiology of AIDS—Antibodies to Human T-Cell Leukaemia Virus (type III) in Haemophiliacs." *Nature* 312: 367–69.

Laurent, C., N. Diakhaté, N. F. N. Gueye, M. A. Touré, P. S. Sow, M. A. Faye, M. Gueye, et al. 2002. "The Senegalese Government's Highly Active Antiretroviral Therapy Initiative: An 18-Month Follow-Up Study." *AIDS* 16: 1363–70.

Marlink, R., P. Kanki, I. Thior, K. Travers, G. Eisen, T. Siby, I. Traore, C. C. Hsieh, M. C. Dia, and E. H. Gueye. 1994. "Reduced Rate of Disease Development after HIV-2 Infection as Compared to HIV-1." *Science* 265: 1587–90.

McCutchan, F. E. 2000. "Understanding the Genetic Diversity of HIV-1." *AIDS* 14 (Suppl. 3): S31–44.

Montano, M. A., C. P. Nixon, T. Ndung'u, H. Bussmann, V. A. Novitsky, D. Dickman, and M. Essex. 2000. "Elevated Tumor Necrosis Factor-Alpha Activation of Human Immunodeficiency Virus Type 1 Subtype C in Southern Africa Is Associated with an NF-Kappab Enhancer Gain-of-Function." *Journal of Infectious Diseases* 181: 76–81.

Montano, M. A., V. Novitsky, J. Blackard, N. Cho, D. Katzenstein, and M. Essex. 1997. "Divergent Transcriptional Regulation among Expanding Human Immunodeficiency Virus Type 1 Subtypes." *Journal of Virology* 71: 8657–65.

Neilson, J. R., G. C. John, J. K. Carr, P. Lewis, J. K. Kreiss, S. Jackson, R. W. Nduati, et al. 1999. "Subtypes of Human Immunodeficiency Virus Type 1 and Disease Stage among Women in Nairobi, Kenya." *Journal of Virology* 73: 4393–4403.

Novitsky, V., M. Montano, M. McLane, B. Renjifo, F. Vannberg, B. Foley, T. Ndung'u, et al. 1999. "Molecular Cloning and Phylogenetic Analysis of Human Immunodeficiency Virus Type 1 Subtype C: A Set of 23 Full-Length Clones from Botswana." *Journal of Virology* 73: 4427–32.

Pantaleo, G., C. Graziosi, J. F. Demarest, L. Butini, M. Montroni, C. H. Fox, J. M. Orenstein, D. P. Kotler, and A. S. Fauci. 1993. "HIV Infection Is Active and Progressive in Lymphoid Tissue during the Clinically Latent Stage of Disease." *Nature* 362: 355–58.

Ping, L., J. Nelson, I. Hoffman, J. Schock, S. Lamers, M. Goodman, P. Vernazza, et al. 1999. "Characterization of V3 Sequence Heterogeneity in Subtype C Human Immunodeficiency Virus Type 1 Isolates from Malawi: Underrepresentation of X4 Variants." *Journal of Virology* 73: 6271–81.

Popovic, M., M. G. Sarngadharan, E. Read, and R. C. Gallo. 1984. "Detection, Isolation, and Continuous Production of Cytopathic Retroviruses (HTLV-III) from Patients with AIDS and Pre-AIDS." *Science* 224: 497–500.

Quan, Y., B. Brenner, R. Marlink, M. Essex, T. Kurimura, and M. Wainberg. 2003. "Drug Resistance Profiles of Recombinant Reverse Transcriptases from HIV-1 Subtypes A/E, B, and C." *AIDS Research and Human Retroviruses* 19: 743–53.

Quinn, T. C., and R. E. Chaisson. 2003. "International Epidemiology of Human Immunodeficiency Virus." In *Infectious Diseases*, ed. S. L. Gorback, J. G. Bartlett, and N. R. Blacklow, 970–86. Philadelphia: Lippincott Williams & Wilkins.

Rayfield, M. A., R. G. Downing, J. Baggs, D. J. Hu, D. Pieniazek, C. C. Luo, B. Biryahwaho, R. A. Otten, S. D. Sempala, and T. J. Dondero. 1998. "A Molecular Epidemiologic Survey of HIV in Uganda." HIV Variant Working Group. *AIDS* 12: 521–27.

Renjifo, B., P. Gilbert, B. Chaplin, F. Vannberg, D. Mwakagile, G. Msamanga, D. Hunter, W. Fawzi, and M. Essex. 1999. "Emerging Recombinant Human Immunodeficiency Viruses: Uneven Representation of the Envelope V3 Region." *AIDS* 13: 1613–21.

Stanecki, K. A., and N. Walker. 2002. "Current Estimates and Projections for the Epidemic." In *AIDS in Africa*, ed. M. Essex, S. Mboup, P. Kanki, R. Marlink, and S. Tlou, 281–96. New York: Kluwer Academic/Plenum Publishers.

Travers, K., S. Mboup, R. Marlink, A. Gueye-Ndiaye, T. Siby, I. Thior, Traore, et al. 1995. "Natural Protection against HIV-1 Infection Provided by HIV-2." *Science* 268: 1612–15.

Tscherning, C., A. Alaeus, R. Fredriksson, A. Bjorndal, H. Deng, D. R. Littman, E. M. Fenyo, and J. Albert. 1998. "Differences in Chemokine Coreceptor Usage between Genetic Subtypes of HIV-1." *Virology* 241: 181–88.

Turner, D., B. Brenner, D. Moisi, M. Detorio, R. Cesaire, T. Kurimura, H. Mori, M. Essex, S. Maayan, and M. A. Wainberg. 2004. "Nucleotide and Amino Acid Polymorphisms at Drug Resistance Sites in Non-B-Subtype Variants of Human Immunodeficiency Virus Type 1." *Antimicrobial Agents and Chemotherapy* 48: 2993–98.

UNAIDS (Joint United Nations Programme on HIV/AIDS). 2004. *Report on the Global HIV/AIDS Epidemic*. Geneva: UNAIDS and WHO.

UNAIDS and WHO (World Health Organization). 2005. *AIDS Epidemic Update: December 2005*. Geneva: UNAIDS and WHO.

Weidle, P. J., S. Malamba, R. Mwebaze, C. Sozi, G. Rukundo, R. Downing, D. Hanson, et al. 2002. "Assessment of a Pilot Antiretroviral Drug Therapy Programme in Uganda: Patients' Response, Survival, and Drug Resistance." *Lancet* 360: 34–40.

Wester, C. W., S. Kim, H. Bussmann, A. Avalos, N. Ndwapi, T. F. Peter, T. Gaolathe, et al. 2005. "Initial Response to Highly Active Antiretroviral Therapy in HIV-1C Infected Adults in a Public Sector Treatment Program in Botswana." *Journal of Acquired Immune Deficiency Syndrome* 40: 336–43.

WHO (World Health Organization). 1999. *The World Health Report 1999—Making a Difference*. Geneva: WHO.

———. 2005. *Progress on Global Access to HIV Antiretroviral Therapy : An Update on "3 by 5"*. Geneva: World Health Organization.

Winkler, C., and S. O'Brien. 2002. "Effect of Genetic Variation on HIV Transmission and Progression to AIDS." In *AIDS in Africa*, ed. M. Essex, S. Mboup, P. Kanki, R. Marlink, and S. Tlou. 52–73. New York: Kluwer Academic/Plenum Publishers.

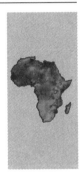

Chapter 18

Lifestyle and Related Risk Factors for Chronic Diseases

Krisela Steyn and Albertino Damasceno

Chronic diseases, often referred to as noncommunicable diseases (NCDs), usually emerge in middle age after long exposure to an unhealthy lifestyle involving tobacco use, a lack of regular physical activity, and consumption of diets rich in highly saturated fats, sugars, and salt, typified by "fast foods." This lifestyle results in higher levels of risk factors, such as hypertension, dyslipidemia, diabetes, and obesity that act independently and synergistically. The risk factors are frequently undiagnosed or inadequately managed in health services designed to treat acute conditions.

Chronic conditions are frequently incorrectly considered to have limited impact on the burden of disease in Sub-Saharan Africa, because of the known high relevance of the infectious diseases. Nevertheless, these diseases occur in younger age groups more commonly in Sub-Saharan Africa than in the developed countries and are at least as common in the poor sector of society as in the more affluent.

The current burden of chronic diseases reflects the cumulative effects of unhealthy lifestyles and the resulting risk factors over the life span of people. Some of these influences are present from before a child is born.

ANTENATAL INFLUENCES ON THE EMERGENCE OF RISK FACTORS FOR CHRONIC DISEASES

The fetal origins of adult chronic diseases play a particularly important role in Sub-Saharan Africa countries. The adequacy of the mother's nutrition before and during pregnancy is the first key component in determining the infant's birthweight. The latter in its own right is associated with the emergence of chronic disease risk factors in these children (Barker 1993, 1994). In The Gambia, an inverse relationship was found between the weight gain of women in the last trimester of pregnancy and the blood pressure of their children at age eight years (Margetts et al. 1991).

Another critical factor during pregnancy is cigarette smoking, which results in high rates of low birthweight (LBW) babies and other complications in pregnancy. This association has been reported in some Sub-Saharan Africa countries (Odendaal, Van Schie, and De Jeu 2001; K. Steyn, unpublished data). Fortunately, smoking tobacco products during pregnancy or the reproductive years is not a common phenomenon in African women, particularly if they still live according to their traditional lifestyles. However, surveys of women who progressively adopt Western lifestyles show that smoking during pregnancy or during the reproductive years is becoming far more common (Steyn et al. 1994; Steyn et al. 1997).

LBW is common in Sub-Saharan Africa countries. For example, Kinabo, Kissawke, and Msuya (1997) reviewed the birth records of 40,595 full-term live singleton infants and found a 15.4 percent prevalence of birthweight below 2,500 grams. In a five-year randomized control trial of maternal supplementation in a rural primary health care setting in The Gambia, 15.9 percent of LBW babies were born in the control group. The intervention group received high-energy groundnut biscuits for about the last 20 weeks of their pregnancy, and that significantly reduced the LBW rate to 10.7 percent. These data highlight the need to ensure adequate nutrition for women in Sub-Saharan Africa during pregnancy (Ceesay et al. 1997).

Levitt, Steyn, De Wet, and colleagues (1999) showed that LBW predicted systolic blood pressure level at age five years in the children in Soweto, South Africa. The data show that children who had a LBW and had gained the most weight during the five years since birth had the highest systolic blood pressure. Those children who were of normal weight at birth and maintained a normal weight had the lowest systolic blood pressure (Levitt, Steyn, De Wet, et al. 1999). A glucose tolerance test done on these children when they were seven years old showed that LBW in conjunction with rapid childhood weight gain, especially if there was a large gain of subcutaneous fat, produced poor glucose tolerance (Crowther et al. 1998).

A study by Longo-Mbenza and colleagues (1999) in Kinshasa, Democratic Republic of Congo, of 2,409 schoolchildren age 5 to 16 years also showed a significant inverse relationship between LBW (less than 2,500 grams) and blood pressure, as well as heart rate. In Cape Town, South Africa, Levitt, Steyn, Lambert, and colleagues (1999) found the same relationship in adults age 20 years who had LBW. These young adults also had impaired glucose tolerance, as well as increased plasma cortisol and cortisol axis activation, compared with young adults who had a birthweight of 2,500 grams or more (Levitt et al. 2000; Longo-Mbenza et al. 1999).

The association between poor intrauterine growth because of inadequate nutrition and smoking tobacco during pregnancy, resulting in LBW and increased NCD risk in children in Sub-Saharan Africa, could possibly increase in the twenty-first century. At the beginning of this century most of the Sub-Saharan Africa countries were in the grip of serious food shortages as well as unopposed promotion of tobacco products targeting women and youth. This situation led to more starvation and more smoking during pregnancy and thus to the birth of more LBW babies in these countries.

TOBACCO USE

As tobacco-control activities in the developed world have increased, the tobacco industry has shifted its marketing to middle- and low-income countries. Not only do these countries have fewer formal tobacco-control activities in place, but they also have a much larger population, which can provide future consumers of tobacco products. In Sub-Saharan Africa countries, most people are young and have relatively low levels of education. They rarely receive the necessary health education to allow them to critically evaluate the material provided by the tobacco industry promotions.

The following five countries participated in the global Youth Tobacco Survey: Ghana, Malawi, Nigeria, South Africa, and Zimbabwe (Global Youth Tobacco Survey Collaborative Group 2002). The data from the five Sub-Saharan Africa countries are shown in table 18.1. Although a significant number of youths age 13 to 15 smoked cigarettes, many more used other tobacco products. Relatively few of the youth smoked at home. These data also raise concern about the pattern and impact of tobacco marketing in Sub-Saharan Africa. Overall, more than 10 percent of the youth had been offered free cigarettes by the tobacco industry, and about 40 percent of them thought boys who smoked had more friends. Despite the traditional taboos against smoking by women, about 20 percent thought that those girls who smoked had more friends than those who didn't.

More than 60 percent of the youth had seen antismoking media messages, and between one-third and two-thirds had been taught the dangers of smoking at school. Of the youth who smoked, 74 percent and 54 percent in South Africa and Zimbabwe, respectively, had tried to quit in the previous year (Global Youth Tobacco Survey Collaborative Group 2002).

The impact of tobacco marketing on five-year-olds has been shown in children living in Johannesburg and Soweto in the Birth-to-Ten study (Levitt, Steyn, De Wet, et al. 1999). This birth cohort comprised children who were born in 1990, and by the time they were five years old the new political dispensation had been established and the country had a new South African flag. When these children were shown pictures of well-known logos of cigarettes available in South Africa along with that of the new flag and the logos of other well-known South African brands, over 90 percent of the

Table 18.1 Exposure to Tobacco Products of Participants, Age 13–15 Years, in the Global Youth Tobacco Survey, 1999–2001

Students		Site						
	Ghana	Blantyre, Malawi	Lilongwe, Malawi	Cross River State, Nigeria	South Africa	Harare, Zimbabwe	Maricaland, Zimbabwe
Number	1,088	783	1,083	914	2,579	621	700
Currently smoking cigarettes	4.2 (1.7)	2.4 (2.2)	6.1 (1.9)	7.0 (3.0)	17.6 (2.5)	10.7 (3.4)	10.0 (3.7)
Currently using other tobacco products[a]	14.5 (3.4)	14.7 (2.8)	12.9 (2.1)	14.0 (3.2)	11.8 (3.4)	9.5 (3.4)	13.2 (4.5)
Current smokers who usually smoke at home	24.4 (14.0)	n.a.	30.4 (12.2)	22.2 (15.3)	18.8 (4.2)	25.2 (12.2)	26.0 (10.7)
Exposed to smoke from others in their home	22.2 (3.8)	19.0 (4.5)	16.0 (2.3)	34.3 (5.1)	43.6 (4.6)	36.2 (5.0)	35.0 (6.0)
Think boys who smoke have more friends	41.1 (5.0)	41.6 (4.9)	48.8 (5.2)	42.5 (4.6)	48.1 (6.2)	43.1 (5.8)	43.8 (3.7)
Think girls who smoke have more friends	30.1 (5.2)	21.1 (4.2)	20.3 (3.4)	26.9 (4.0)	30.7 (4.0)	23.3 (3.9)	18.6 (2.8)
Think smoking should be banned from public places	58.2 (8.8)	90.1 (3.0)	85.1 (6.8)	60.2 (4.6)	53.4 (9.1)	43.2 (11.1)	31.6 (8.1)
Think ETS is harmful to themselves	41.6 (9.7)	83.1 (3.6)	81.8 (6.1)	35.4 (5.9)	57.3 (7.5)	45.3 (6.2)	31.0 (6.3)
Reported having seen ads for cigarettes on billboards	52.7 (3.5)	57.7 (9.2)	55.8 (3.5)	59.6 (5.7)	76.4 (4.6)	76.6 (5.3)	64.6 (5.1)
Reported having seen ads for cigarettes in newspapers or magazines	48.7 (5.3)	72.6 (6.8)	64.0 (3.4)	51.7 (3.6)	80.7 (3.9)	74.7 (4.9)	66.7 (4.0)
Reported having seen ads for cigarettes at sporting and other events	53.4 (6.3)	57.1 (4.1)	55.1 (3.8)	56.7 (5.2)	78.3 (5.3)	73.1 (5.8)	62.2 (6.2)
Reported having been offered free cigarettes by tobacco company	11.0 (2.1)	13.3 (2.5)	14.4 (2.5)	13.7 (2.9)	15.2 (4.4)	8.7 (3.7)	14.5 (3.4)
Reported having seen anti-smoking media messages	69.0 (4.8)	83.6 (2.7)	85.7 (2.5)	65.9 (4.2)	79.8 (2.8)	80.7 (3.6)	69.7 (6.1)
Reported having been taught the dangers of smoking in class	57.7 (7.0)	68.7 (5.2)	68.9 (2.5)	42.1 (4.8)	38.7 (4.8)	34.1 (5.9)	51.6 (5.7)
Reported having discussed reasons why people their age smoke in class at school	32.1 (5.0)	44.5 (8.3)	50.7 (4.1)	28.7 (3.0)	29.4 (4.3)	26.7 (5.7)	34.9 (5.5)

Source: Global Youth Tobacco Survey Collaborative Group 2002.
Note: Numbers in parentheses = confidence interval, percent; n.a. = not applicable (fewer than 35 participants answered this question); ETS = environmental tobacco smoke.
a. Currently smoking cigarettes or used other tobacco products on at least 1 of the previous 30 days.

children identified the new flag. This showed clearly that this new South African symbol had been internalized by the age of five years. Therefore, it was of great concern when it was found that between 51 and 76 percent of these children could identify the logos of popular cigarette brands. The highest level of recognition was for the cigarette brand of the company that sponsored the soccer tournament in the previous year. Seven percent of these five-year-old children had experimented with cigarettes at least once (Thea de Wet, unpublished data).

Only 23 of the Sub-Saharan Africa countries had any data on cigarette-use prevalence rates available in 2000, and only a few had data on rates based on adequate national surveys (Corrao et al. 2000). These data are shown in table 18.2.

Generally, men smoke much more than women do. With the exception of women in Guinea, Kenya, and Namibia, only 20 percent or fewer of the women smoke. However, these figures probably underestimate tobacco use, as cigarettes are not the only form of tobacco used in Sub-Saharan Africa. A substantial number of people use hand-rolled cigarettes or smoke a pipe, and the use of smokeless tobacco is common in women. In South Africa, Steyn and colleagues (2002) found that 12.6 percent of black women used snuff, a higher rate than the 5.3 percent of black women who

Table 18.2 Prevalence of Adults Who Smoke Cigarettes, by Country

Country	Age in years	Year of survey	Total (%)	Men (%)	Women (%)
Benin	≥10	1988	37	—	—
Botswana	≥15	1998	21	—	—
Cameroon	Adult	1994	37.5	—	—
Chad	≥15	1994	—	24.1	—
Congo, Dem. Rep. of	≥15	1998	—	23.6	5.5
Côte d'Ivoire	≥15	1977	—	42.3	1.8
Ethiopia	Adult	1995	15.8	—	—
Ghana	≥16	1980	—	28.4	3.5
Guinea	11–72	1998	—	59.5	43.8
Kenya	≥20	1995	—	66.8	31.9
Lesotho	≥15	1992	—	38.5	1
Malawi	Adult	—	—	20	9
Namibia	Adult	1994	—	65	35
Nigeria	≥15	1998	—	15.4	1.7
Senegal	12–100	1998	—	32	4.6
Sierra Leone	≥15	1998	18.5	—	—
South Africa	≥15	1998	—	42	11
Swaziland	Adult	1994	—	24.7	2.1
Tanzania	Adult	—	—	49.5	12.4
Uganda	Adult	1995	—	52	17
Zambia	Adult	1996	—	35	10
Zimbabwe	≥15	1993	—	34.4	1.2

Source: Corrao et al. 2000.
Note: — = data not available.

smoke regularly. Black women in Cape Town believe that snuff has medicinal value as well as that of pain relief (Marks, Steyn, and Ratheb 2001).

It is traditionally taboo for black women of Sub-Saharan Africa to smoke during their reproductive years. Marks, Steyn, and Ratheb (2001) found that Xhosa women in Cape Town manifested this attitude, as 72 percent of the women participating in the survey thought it disgraceful, shameful, and taboo for them to smoke. The women who smoked did so in private settings or in secret. Almost all women who smoked said they did not smoke in front of their elders or parents.

In their promotion of tobacco products in Sub-Saharan Africa, tobacco companies target women and youth with images of "attractive, successful, upwardly mobile black women." They have thus overwhelmed many of the traditional taboos. This was revealed by Marks, Steyn, and Ratheb (2001), who found in their Cape Town study that 5 percent of nonsmoking black women were found to be

pro-smoking in orientation and on the verge of smoking, whereas another 53 percent were found to have only a shallow commitment to not smoking.

It has been reported from South Africa that black women start to smoke at a later age than do women elsewhere in the world (Steyn et al. 2002). The implication is that intervention programs in Sub-Saharan Africa should be targeting women in their reproductive years to prevent the onset of smoking and for smoking cessation programs.

Commercially manufactured cigarettes in Sub-Saharan Africa are characteristically sold singly. It has been estimated that in Nigeria up to 80 percent of cigarettes are sold in singles. Either people cannot afford to buy packs of 20 or they sometimes supplement other forms of tobacco use with manufactured cigarettes (Saloojee 2000).

Saloojee (2000) suggests that Sub-Saharan Africa has the lowest tobacco consumption rates and tobacco-related mortality in the world but that the current trend of tobacco consumption implies that it is only a matter of time before it succumbs to the same pattern of tobacco-related diseases as the rest of the world. Projections suggest that the tobacco epidemic can peak in Sub-Saharan Africa in the middle of this century. Saloojee emphasizes that it is extraordinary to be able to predict an epidemic so far in the future and have the knowledge to prevent it. Price increases are the single most important factor in reducing smoking rates in a country. The price elasticity, defined as the degree to which tobacco consumption decreases with increasing price, is higher in developing countries than in richer countries. Significant price increases for cigarettes and other tobacco products, therefore, would be a major step toward improved tobacco control for Sub-Saharan Africa (Saloojee 1995). Although smuggling may account for up to 50 percent of consumption in some settings and may limit the impact of price increases, economic policies have been effective in limiting tobacco consumption.

NUTRITION IN TRANSITION

A diet high in fat, particularly saturated fat, low in carbohydrates, fruit, and vegetables, along with a high salt intake leads to the emergence of chronic risk factors. Traditional diets in Sub-Saharan Africa, which are low in fat and high in unrefined carbohydrates, protect people against chronic diseases. The nutrition transition refers to large shifts in the composition and structure of diets (Popkin 2001a). The dietary changes of the nutrition transition involve large increases in the consumption of fat (especially saturated fat) and sugar, marked increases in animal products, and a decline in unrefined cereal and, thus, in fiber intakes (Popkin 2001a, 2001b).

Nutrition patterns in Sub-Saharan Africa countries are influenced by many factors, including individual preference; culture, traditions, and beliefs; and price. However, availability and accessibility are the principal factors that shape dietary patterns (N. P. Steyn, WHO, personal communication). In the Sub-Saharan context, war and internal strife, drought and poor agricultural practices, and rapid urbanization are particularly influential. In addition, multinational food companies market their products aggressively in the region. For example in West Africa, consumption has changed from that of locally produced coarse grains, such as millet and sorghum, to imported wheat and rice (Teklu 1996).

In the black population of Cape Town, it was found that a larger proportion of life spent in the city was associated with an increased consumption of fat and a decrease in carbohydrates (figure 18.1). This is reflected in an increased use of dairy produce, meat, fat, and nonbasic food items and a decreased intake of cereals (Bourne, Lambert, and Steyn 2002).

An examination of food balance sheets, based on the amount of food sold in South Africa indicates that per capita available fat consumption increased by 27 percent between 1993 and 1999 (figure 18.2). This increase was accompanied by a decrease in carbohydrate consumption.

An enigma in the proposed relationship of a diet high in cholesterol and fat, but with little fruit and vegetables, and raised blood cholesterol levels was reported for the pastoral

Figure 18.2 Macronutrient Intakes in South Africans, per Capita, 1993 and 1999

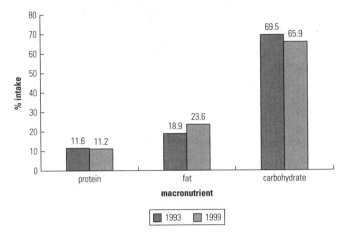

Source: Steyn, Senekal et al. 2000; data extrapolated from food balance sheets.

Masai in Tanzania. Although their traditional diet was high in cholesterol and fat from whole milk, blood, and meat, and included little green vegetables or fruit, they maintained low serum cholesterol levels (Gibney and Burstyn 1980). It was suggested that this unexpected relationship could be explained by the cholesterol-lowering effect of the high levels of fermented milk consumed by the Masai and the substantial amounts of saponins and phenolic compound in the plant dietary additives used by them (Johns et al. 1999; St-Onge, Farnworth, and Jones 2000). Unfortunately, these protective dietary practices have declined and new dietary changes have been observed in the pastoral Masai; consequently there has been a significant increase in their serum total cholesterol levels (McCormick and Elmore-Meegan 1992). Not even the physically active Masai of Sub-Saharan Africa could escape the impact of the nutrition transition.

AEROBIC EXERCISE

Adequate physical activity has been shown to have many health-promoting properties and has a direct, independent role in reducing cardiovascular disease mortality (Haskell, Leon, and Caspersen 1992; McBride et al. 1992). Traditionally, it has been thought that a high level of physical exercise could in part explain the low levels of chronic diseases found in Sub-Saharan Africa countries. However, the amounts of physical exercise have been decreasing as a result of the high degree of urbanization that has been occurring across the continent. In urban settings, public transport replaces the

Figure 18.1 Fat and Carbohydrate Intake as Functions of Proportion of Life Spent in a City

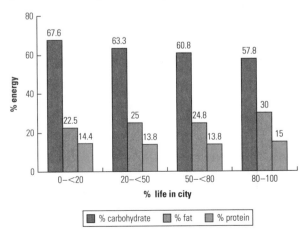

Source: Bourne, Lambert, and Steyn 2002.

traditional pattern of walking long distances, and urban employment usually entails far less physical labor than rural employment or other activities of daily living, such as chopping wood, carrying water, or tilling the fields. In the cities, high crime levels prevent people from moving about freely. In the poorest periurban settings, inhabitants watch television more frequently than their rural counterparts do. Few studies on the physical activity patterns of people in Sub-Saharan Africa have been published.

A study carried out in Cameroon comparing rural with urban people 15 years of age or older clearly illustrated lower rates of physical activity in the urban settings (Sobngwi et al. 2002). Similar differences were found for healthy, elderly people in Nigeria (Ezenwaka et al. 1997). In the urban settings, 62 percent of men and 83 percent of women age 55 years or older led a sedentary lifestyle, whereas this was the case for only 22 percent of men and 50 percent of women in the rural areas. In Nigeria it was also found that civil servants with high seniority had lower levels of physical activity than their junior counterparts, suggesting that upward social mobility was associated with less physical activity (Forrest et al. 2001).

Many studies across Sub-Saharan Africa have revealed the impact of a sedentary lifestyle on emerging NCD risk factors. The physical activity of the Nigerian civil servants studied by Forrest and colleagues (2001) was mostly attributed to occupational activities. Low levels of physical activity were correlated to weight, body mass index (BMI), waist-to-hip ratio, blood pressure, insulin levels, and total and low-density lipoprotein (LDL) cholesterol in men. Similarly, Sobngwi and colleagues (2002) in Cameroon as well as Aspray and colleagues (2000) in Tanzania concluded that physical inactivity was associated with obesity, diabetes, and hypertension in the people they studied in urban and rural settings in both Cameroon and Tanzania. A qualitative study in Cameroon also found that the reduced physical activity accompanying sedentary occupations in the cities explained the higher rate of obesity observed in people with these sedentary occupations (Treloar et al. 1999). Levitt, Steyn, Lambert, and colleagues (1999) showed an independent association between low levels of physical activity and having type 2 diabetes in a poor, periurban community near Cape Town.

In an interesting three-year prospective study in Senegal, researchers followed the unusually high physical activity level of adolescent girls between the ages of 13 and 15 years; physical activity was measured by accelerometers recording minute-by-minute movements (Benefice and Cames 1999; Benefice, Garnier, and Ndiaye 2001a, 2001b; Garnier and

Benefice 2001). The girls were spending a minimum of 3.5 hours per day doing domestic duties, including collecting water and stomping maize. The level of physical activity was higher during the rainy season. During the dry season, some of these adolescent girls were sent to the cities to work as servants. It was found that the adolescents in the city had an even higher physical expenditure than those who stayed at home. However, despite the heavier workload, those in the city had a better nutritional status. These healthy Senegalese girls all had higher physical activity levels than those reported for girls in developed countries.

A health and fitness survey of adolescent schoolchildren age 12 to 18 years in the Western Cape in South Africa conducted by Lambert and colleagues in 2000 found that a high level of fitness was inversely associated with current BMI in both boys and girls. Inactivity, defined as watching television for more than three hours a day, was associated with current BMI and a low fitness level. The use of BMI projection formulas to predict future BMI suggests that 24.5 percent of the females and 12.8 percent of the males will be overweight at the age of 18 years (Lambert et al. 2000).

Two surveys carried out seven years apart in Maputo, Mozambique, of students age 8 to 15 years in the same group of schools, showed a significant increase of mean systolic blood pressure, diastolic blood pressure, and total body fat between the 1992 and the 1999 samples for all ages and for both sexes but no changes in the mean level of cholesterol. These changes of cardiovascular risk factors were attributed to the reductions in physical activity observed concomitantly with changes in nutrition (Damasceno and Prista 2001).

One of the reasons for the small number of published studies on physical activity in Sub-Saharan Africa is the difficulty of measuring it in large epidemiological studies. For such studies researchers have to rely on physical activity questionnaires that must be accurate, valid, and reproducible. Some efforts have been made to develop questionnaires that may be useful for Sub-Saharan Africa countries or that can be shown to be reliable in all regions of the world. Sobngwi and colleagues (2001) clearly showed how necessary this validation process is for the use of physical activity questionnaires with people in Sub-Saharan Africa, as study participants' self-ranking of their physical activity did not match the tested questionnaire's quartiles of physical activity (Heini et al. 1996; Sobngwi et al. 2001).

Wareham (2001) emphasized that to develop internationally standardized questionnaires, such as the International Physical Activity Questionnaire, in all countries efforts will have to be made to ensure that validation and reliability studies take place.

OBESITY

The World Health Organization (WHO) defines obesity as a condition in which excess body fat has accumulated to such an extent that health may be adversely affected. The degree of body weight is usually expressed as BMI; this is the ratio of weight in kilograms to the square of height in meters. The BMI is used to classify a person's body weight as underweight (BMI less than 18.5), normal weight (BMI 18.5–24.9), overweight (BMI 25–29.9), or obese (BMI greater than 30) (WHO 2000).

In addition, it is customary to indicate the amount of abdominal fat mass. This can vary considerably among individuals who have the same BMI. Abdominal fat is reported by measuring the waist circumference or the waist-to-hip circumference ratio. The waist circumference is thought to provide a better correlate with abdominal fat mass than the waist-to-hip ratio. High abdominal fat mass is frequently referred to as central obesity. This form of obesity has been shown to have more morbidity than if the fat distribution is predominantly on the hips (WHO 2000).

Obesity greatly increases the risk for conditions such as type 2 diabetes, hypertension, dyslipidemia, gall bladder disease, sleep apnea, osteoarthritis, and lower back pain. It has also been shown to be associated with coronary artery disease and some cancers, and to reduce life expectancy. Central obesity has been shown to be associated with metabolic syndrome. The key features of this condition are raised blood pressure, raised insulin and triglyceride levels, reduced high-density lipoprotein (HDL)-cholesterol levels, and insulin resistance. The condition is strongly atherogenic and predisposes to an elevated risk of diabetes and cardiovascular disease (Fontaine et al. 2003; Peeters et al. 2003; Solomon and Manson 1997; WHO 2000).

In many Sub-Saharan Africa countries, an increased level of body fat is associated with beauty, prosperity, health, and prestige, despite its negative impact on health. Thinness, in contrast, is perceived to be a sign of ill health or poverty and is something to be feared and avoided, particularly in recent years, when it has been associated with AIDS (Treloar et al. 1999). In disadvantaged communities in South Africa, food is highly valued because food security has not always been ensured. Researchers found it to be socially unacceptable for an individual to refuse to eat food that was offered to them (Mvo, Dick, and Steyn 1999). Brown and Konner (1987) also reported that the majority of the less developed regions had, or still have, ideals of feminine beauty that include plumpness, which is consistent with the hypothesis that fat stores function as a cushion against food shortages during pregnancy and lactation. It is therefore unsurprising that studies have shown that black women in South Africa also do not perceive being overweight or obese as a health risk (Ndlovo and Roos 1999).

Urbanization, associated with changing dietary patterns and less physical activity and a rise in socioeconomic status, is occurring across Sub-Saharan Africa countries. All these factors lead to an increase in the prevalence of overweight and obese people in the region. This phenomena is illustrated in a study by Kruger and colleagues (2002) of the nutrition and physical activity patterns of a large sample of people from the North West Province of South Africa exposed to all levels of urbanization. The researchers found a significant association between household income and measures of obesity. They also saw a positive correlation between total energy intake, fat intake, and BMI. The physical activity index correlated negatively with BMI and waist circumference.

Cooper and colleagues (1997) also illustrated these trends when they compared the mean BMI of urban and rural West Africans with that of Jamaicans and blacks in the United States. A gradual increase in mean BMI was evident along the historical migration path of the West African diaspora that was attributed to a cross-cultural gradient of decreasing physical activity and Westernization of the diet.

Table 18.3 shows the prevalence of obesity from Sub-Saharan Africa reported in recent literature. South Africa has the highest prevalence of obesity in black men and women reported in Africa. Its prevalence among urban black women of 36 percent in South Africa already exceeds that of black women in the United States (Cooper et al. 1997; Puoane et al. 2002). The prevalence of obesity in South African and urban Tanzanian men was very similar, whereas the prevalence of obesity in South African women was almost double that of urban women in The Gambia and Tanzania.

An analysis of the mortality patterns associated with obesity in American people suggests that it has less of an impact on mortality and years of life lost in African Americans than in other Americans (Fontaine et al. 2003; Solomon and Manson 1997). Although no similar data are available on the association between obesity and mortality in Sub-Saharan Africa countries, it would be unwise to assume that obesity is benign for the people of this region. Reference has been made to the impact that obesity has on the emergence of hypertension, diabetes, and other chronic disease risk factors in Sub-Saharan Africa. Furthermore, high rates of LBW babies are common in the region, and this poses a risk to these babies in later life to develop obesity and other chronic disease risk factors.

Table 18.3 Anthropometric Indicators, by Country

Population	n	Height (cm)	Weight (kg)	BMI (kg/m^2)	Waist (cm)	Hip (cm)	Waist-hip ratio	Obese (%)	Body fat (%)
Men									
Nigeria	1,171	168.3	61.5	21.7	77.3	88.3	0.88	—	—
Cameroon[a]									
Urban	612	172.3	74.5	25.1	83.3	96.8	0.86	—	—
Rural	745	170.1	68.1	23.5	80.4	90.7	0.89	—	—
South Africa (black)	5,401	169	65.2	22.9	81.8	94.2	0.9	7.5	—
Cameroon[b]									
Urban	461	—	—	25	—	—	—	—	—
Rural	308	—	—	21	—	—	—	—	—
Zimbabwe (urban)	384	171.0	63.0	21.7	79.0	91.0	0.86	—	21.1
Gambia, The									
Urban	1,028	—	—	20.8	—	—	—	1.8	—
Rural	1,200	—	—	19.8	—	—	—	0.1	—
Tanzania (urban)	3,659	—	—	—	—	—	—	6.9	—
Women									
Nigeria	1,338	158.3	56.6	22.6	73.9	93.5	0.79	—	—
Cameroon[a]									
Urban	749	162.1	71.0	27.0	82.5	102.5	0.81	—	—
Rural	722	160.7	60.6	23.5	80.9	92.6	0.87	—	—
South Africa (black)	7,726	158	67.8	27.1	85.5	104.6	0.8	30.0	—
Cameroon[b]									
Urban	591	—	—	26.0	—	—	—	—	—
Rural	438	—	—	22.0	—	—	—	—	—
Zimbabwe (urban)	391	160	67.0	21.7	82.0	101.0	0.82	—	36.5
Gambia, The									
Urban	1,138	—	—	23.9	—	—	—	12.2	—
Rural	2,023	—	—	20.5	—	—	—	1.1	—
Tanzania (urban)	5,654	—	—	—	—	—	—	17.4	—

Source: Cooper et al. 1997; Puoane et al. 2002; Mbanya et al. 1998; Mufunda et al. 2000; van der Sande et al. 2000; Bovet et al. 2002.

Note: — = data not published; age-standardized against world population.

a. Data from Cooper et al. 1997.

b. Data from Mbanya et al. 1998.

HYPERTENSION

High blood pressure is a major risk factor for heart attacks and strokes. It also contributes to renal disease and blindness. It is estimated that between 10 million and 20 million people in Sub-Saharan Africa have hypertension. It has been estimated that adequate hypertension treatment of these people could prevent about 250,000 deaths (Cappuccio et al. 2000). However, hypertension in Sub-Saharan Africa is universally under diagnosed or inadequately treated, or both, with the result that extensive end-organ damage and premature death are often seen. Furthermore, hypertension frequently co-exists with other NCD risk factors, such as diabetes. Seedat (1999) summarized the pathophysiology of hypertension and response to treatment as follows:

Black hypertensive patients in Sub-Saharan Africa are prone to cerebral hemorrhage, malignant hypertension, kidney disease leading to uremia and congestive heart failure, whereas coronary heart disease is relatively uncommon. Responses to antihypertensive medication drugs like the beta-blockers and the angiotension-converting enzymes (ACE) inhibitors are poor unless these agents are combined with a thiazide diuretic. Black patients respond best to diuretics, vasodilators or calcium channel blockers.

Kaufman and colleagues (1996) reported that the risk of death increased by 60 percent with an increase of 20 mmHg in diastolic blood pressure in rural Nigeria. They estimated that the population-attributable risk or the reduction in mortality that would have been observed if hypertension were not present was 7 percent, showing the impact of hypertension on all-cause mortality in rural Nigeria. Malignant hypertension also occurs more frequently in black people of Sub-Saharan Africa than in other ethnic groups. Milne and colleagues (1989) showed this in black patients hospitalized for hypertension. This condition is frequently related to severe renal disease and hypertensive encephalopathy. Data from the South African Dialyses and Transplantation Registry have shown that hypertension was responsible for 35 percent of end-stage renal failure in blacks and that malignant hypertension was diagnosed in 57 percent of the black patients with essential hypertension (Veriava et al. 1990). Untreated malignant hypertension has been shown to have a five-year survival as low as 1 percent.

Earlier surveys showed that the lowest prevalence of hypertension occurred in the poorest Sub-Saharan Africa countries, and as affluence increased, the prevalence increased. The surveys also revealed that hypertension was more common in urban than in rural settings in the region (Nissinen et al. 1988). The elegant Kenyan Luo migration study of Poulter and colleagues (1990) was the first to show that migration of people living in traditional rural villages on the northern shores of Lake Victoria to the urban settings of Nairobi was associated with an increase in blood pressure. This suggests a marked change in the diet of the new arrivals in Nairobi to a higher salt and calorie intake along with a reduced potassium intake due to consuming less fruit and vegetables. Studies carried out in Nigeria that compared urban and rural people's sodium and potassium excretions observed similar findings (Kaufman et al. 1999). Higher pulse rates in the Nairobi participants suggest that mechanisms related to increased autonomic nervous system activity could contribute to the higher levels of blood pressure observed (Poulter et al. 1985, 1990). Urban Nigerians reported higher stress levels and lower social integration scores than their rural counterparts. These indicators of increased stress in the urban setting were associated with higher blood pressures (Kaufman et al. 1999).

Socioeconomic status and urbanization are good predictors of hypertension. Zimbabwean women doing traditional work-related activities on rural communal land had lower blood pressures than did those women who were working for a wage on large-scale, commercial agricultural farms. The latter group, in turn, had lower blood pressures than women who earned a living in more industrial mining areas (Hunter et al. 2000). Similarly, researchers (Steyn, Fourie et al. 1996) found in the black community of Cape Town,

South Africa, that the duration of urbanization independently predicted the presence of hypertension.

Table 18.4 shows the prevalence rate in some Sub-Saharan Africa countries from studies published since 1997. The studies reveal that although some countries still maintain large differences between urban and rural prevalence, differences are no longer apparent in many countries. The prevalence rates in the rural areas have increased to levels similar to those found only in the cities in the past. As an example, in the early 1990s Mollentze and colleagues (1995) showed that the rural community of QwaQwa in the Free State, South Africa, had rates of hypertension similar to those in the periurban community of Mangaung in the same province. The previously observed differences in hypertension prevalence between poorer and more affluent countries have also diminished.

Some dietary factors are related to hypertension, including increased salt (sodium) intake and a decrease in fruit and vegetables (potassium); a higher intake of alcohol products, particularly by men, also plays a role. The association between hypertension and obesity has been well documented in many countries in Sub-Saharan Africa. In Zimbabwe, Mufunda and colleagues (2000) found this strong association, as did Rotimi and colleagues (1995) in populations of West African descent. Despite this clear association it has been suggested that the noxious effect of obesity in black people is less than in people of other ethnic groups. Most of the supporting evidence for this viewpoint is based on studies carried out with African Americans in the United States. A small study in South Africa suggested similar findings (Walker et al. 1990). The influence of alcohol consumption, particularly heavy drinking, on increasing blood pressure levels has also been described in Nigeria (Bunker et al. 1992; Ekpo et al. 1992). The data on the association between high salt (sodium chloride) intake and hypertension in black people from Africa has been summarized by Seedat (1996) and suggests that black people have a transport mechanism of high sodium retention and a low rennin activity. Mtabaji and colleagues (1992) found salt sensitivity, measured by the blood pressure response on salt loading, in 46.2 percent of study subjects in Tanzania. A high intake of sodium is common in Sub-Saharan Africa, as it is used to preserve food or to make food tastier. For example, Cappuccio and colleagues (2000) described the diet in Ghana as consisting mostly of unprocessed food and highly salted fish and meat. Substantial amounts of salt are added to food while cooking, and monosodium glutamate–based flavoring cubes or salts are widely used to give food taste. In addition to a high salt

Table 18.4 Large Prevalence Studies on Hypertension since 1997, by Country

| Country | Age (years) | Cut-off point ≥140/90 mmHg | | | | Cut-off point ≥160/95 mmHg | | Equipment for blood pressure measurement |
| | | Males | | Females | | Males | Females | |
		(n)	(%)	(n)	(%)	(%)	(%)	
Nigeria								
Urban (adults; civil servants)	—	581[a]	—	417[a]	—	13.9	5.0	Mercury sphygmomanometer
Urban	25–55+	1,171	14.7	1,338	14.3	6.9	6.9	Mercury sphygmomanometer
Cameroon[b]								
Urban	25–55+	612	22.8	749	16.0	8.7	8.7	Mercury
Rural	25–55+	745	14.2	722	16.3	4.7	7.4	sphygmomanometer
Cameroon								
Urban	25–74	461	—	591	—	16.4	12.1	Mercury
Rural	25–74	308	—	438	—	5.4	5.9	sphygmomanometer
Tanzania								
Urban (Ihala)	15+	330	30.0	437	28.6	14.4	15.4	Mercury
Rural (Shari)	15+	401	32.2	527	31.5	17.2	15.6	sphygmomanometer
Tanzania[b]								
Urban	35–64	1,729	27.1	2,053	30.2	13.1	17.7	Visomat
Gambia, The								
Urban (Banjul)	Adults	1,028	22.0	1,138	16.9	7.5	7.3	Omron HEM-705-CP
Rural (Farafenni)	Adults	1,200	20.6	2,023	16.0	7.6	6.3	
Zimbabwe								
Urban	25+	384	28.0	391	41.0	18.0	28.0	Omron HEM-713C
South Africa[b]								
African	15–65+	4,283	23.5	6,174	25.0	12.9	15.7	Omron M1
Coloured	15–65+	772	27.3	1,008	29.6	14.9	22.7	electronic blood
White	15–65+	500	33.5	603	20.6	23.3	18.5	pressure manometer
Asian	15–65+	183	28.0	279	25.3	18.7	20.5	

Source: Olatunbosun et al. 2000; Cooper et al. 1997; Mbanya et al. 1998; Edwards et al. 2000; Bovet et al. 2002; van der Sande et al. 2000; Mufunda et al. 2000; Steyn et al. 2001.
Note: — = data not published; adjusted to the world population.
a. No rates.
b. Adjusted to the world population.

intake, people in Sub-Saharan Africa frequently eat little fruit and vegetables, resulting in low potassium intakes.

Few intervention studies have been conducted in Sub-Saharan Africa to show that a reduction in salt and an increase in potassium improve the blood pressure in its populations. A study done in Tanzania showed that a low-sodium diet leading to a low urinary excretion level of 52 millimoles per day reduced blood pressure in normotensive people significantly within four to five days (Mtabaji, Nara, and Yamori 1990). A study in Kenya reported that supplementation with potassium in newly diagnosed patients with hypertension reduced the blood pressure to a level similar to that found in patients treated with a diuretic (Obel and Koech 1991).

These data clearly suggest that many nutritional interventions are required to decrease the prevalence of hypertension. These interventions include regulation of the amount of salt used by the food industry in Sub-Saharan Africa, the promotion of increased potassium consumption in the form of fruit and vegetables, and the limitation of alcohol use.

Despite the many environmental factors related to hypertension, many studies in Sub-Saharan Africa suggest a possible genetic contribution to the origins of hypertension in black people. Van der Sande and colleagues (2001) in The Gambia and Steyn and colleagues (unpublished data) in South Africa have found that high blood pressure is associated with a strong family history of either hypertension or stroke. This could provide a cost-effective opportunity to identify people who need more detailed screening for hypertension. Rotimi and colleagues (1999) used computer models and regression analyses to estimate the degree of heritability of systolic and diastolic blood pressure in Nigerian families. The heritability estimate was 45 percent and 43 percent for systolic and diastolic blood pressure, respectively. This emphasizes interaction between environmental influences and genetic factors in the etiology of hypertension.

In populations of African ancestry, data from small case-control studies and a large case-control study conducted in South Africa with more than 700 cases phenotyped using 24-hour ambulatory blood pressure monitoring and 700 controls (G. R. Norton et al., personal communications) suggest that the angiotensin-converting enzyme (ACE) gene variant contributes little to hypertension. Nevertheless, gender-specific effects need to be excluded. In addition, angiotensinogen (AGT) gene variants that have been associated with hypertension in Caucasian groups are not implicated in subjects of African ancestry (Tiago et al. 2002). However, an alternative functional promoter region variant of the AGT gene ($-217G{\rightarrow}A$) has recently been shown to be strongly associated with hypertension in a small African American case-control study (Jain et al. 2002), data that has now been confirmed in a large case-control study conducted in black South Africans (G. R. Norton et al., personal communication). The role of the $-217G{\rightarrow}A$ AGT gene variant in contributing to the variance of blood pressure within families is now being assessed in a South African study. Furthermore, an additional functional AGT gene promoter region variant ($-20A{\rightarrow}C$; Zhao et al. 1999) has been shown to modify the impact of body size on blood pressure (Tiago et al. 2002), and the $-217G{\rightarrow}A$ variant's effect on the risk for hypertension (G. R. Norton et al., personal communications) in subjects of African ancestry, thus suggesting complex genotype-genotype and genotype-phenotype interactions of the AGT gene in people of African origins.

Other candidate gene variants implicated in blood pressure control or hypertension in those of European or African ancestry, including functional or potentially functional variants found within the guanosine triphosphate protein β3 subunit gene (Siffert et al. 1998), the sodium epithelial channel gene (Baker et al. 1998), the α-adducin gene (Cusi et al. 1997), and the β2 receptor gene (Svetkey et al. 1996), have been shown not to be associated with hypertension in all studies conducted in groups of African ancestry (Candy et al. 2000; Larson, Hutchinson, and Boerwinkle 2000; Nkeh et al. 2003), or have been shown to occur with too low a frequency to contribute substantially to population-attributable risk (Barlassina et al. 2000). Family-based linkage studies assessing blood pressure as a continuous variable and using 24-hour ambulatory blood pressure monitoring techniques are under way in South Africa to further evaluate the role for these variants as determinants of blood pressure in groups of African ancestry.

Effective management of hypertension usually requires treatments with more than one drug. In Ghana, Hesse and Nuama (1997) found that only 18 percent of a group of patients with hypertension had one drug prescribed, whereas 60 percent had two drugs and 22 percent had three or more drugs prescribed. The use of two or more drugs will inevitably result in a high cost for antihypertensive medication, especially when newer medications are used. However, there are cheaper, older, and effective medications available in resource-scarce settings in Sub-Saharan Africa. Hesse and Nuama (1997) also reported that between 1973 and 1993 a diuretic was the type of drug prescribed for initial treatment of patients with hypertension; diuretics were used in 90 percent of cases, including reserpine in 46 percent, methyldopa in 31 percent, and propranolol in 30 percent. With the exception of methyldopa all these medications are inexpensive and suited to resource-scarce settings.

The benefits of treating hypertension have been convincingly shown in many parts of the world, but relatively little data are available from Sub-Saharan Africa. One example is a study by Salako and colleagues (1999), who showed that when patients with hypertension are given effective treatment, there is a reduction in the excretion of urinary albumin, suggesting improved renal function in patients who previously had early renal impairment.

After reviewing the available data, Cooper and colleagues (1998) suggested: "Hypertension is fully treatable, but social conditions in Africa make the implementation of blood pressure control programs difficult. Lack of a clear strategy based on evidence has undermined these efforts." They also estimated that effective hypertension treatment would lead to a reduction in population-attributable risk of 2 percent in Africa compared with 0.15 percent in the United States. "Number needed to treat" analyses showed that the cost of drugs to prevent one death is US$1,800 in Africa, if the cheaper drugs are used, whereas it is US$14,000 to US$1 million in the United States, depending on which drugs are used. Cooper and colleagues (1998) concluded that the treatment of hypertension should be a health priority in Sub-Saharan Africa.

DYSLIPIDEMIA

Dyslipidemia is defined as a clinically significant alteration of the naturally occurring blood lipids and lipoproteins predisposing to cardiovascular diseases and other chronic diseases (Berger and Marais 2000). The two commonly measured blood lipids are cholesterol and triglycerides. These molecules are carried in a range of lipoprotein particles in the blood. The most important lipoprotein particles that predispose to atherosclerosis and thus cardiovascular diseases are the chylomicrons high in triglyceride and LDL particles, which carry mainly cholesterol. The LDL particle is the most atherogenic of all the lipoprotein particles. The HDL particle protects the arteries against atherosclerosis and, consequently, against cardiovascular diseases. HDL transports cholesterol away from the arteries to be excreted via the liver. The most recent international recommendations regarding lipid levels are that a total blood cholesterol level below 5.2 millimoles per liter is desirable; similarly, a level of LDL cholesterol below 2.6 millimoles per liter and a triglyceride level below 1.7 millimoles per liter are considered optimal. Persons with blood lipids below these levels do not carry a risk of developing atherosclerosis. An HDL cholesterol level below 1 millimole per liter also predisposes to atherosclerosis development, whereas a level above 1.6 millimoles per liter provides protection. The ratio of HDL cholesterol to the total cholesterol level, expressed as a percentage, is frequently reported. A level of more than 20 percent for men and 25 percent for women is considered to provide protection against developing atherosclerosis (Adult Treatment Panel III 2001).

A particularly atherosclerotic combination of lipid and other risk factors is referred to as the metabolic syndrome and leads to premature coronary heart disease. This syndrome consists of high levels of blood triglyceride, low levels of HDL cholesterol, and small dense LDL particles. It is also associated with type 2 diabetes, hypertension, abdominal obesity, insulin resistance, and physical inactivity. Van der Sande and colleagues (2000) found significant numbers of urban black people in Banju, the capital of The Gambia, with the coexistence of these conditions, suggesting that the metabolic syndrome is common in this city.

Since the level of ischemic heart disease reported in people from Africa is low, few hypertension and diabetes surveys in the region include blood lipid measurements. The available studies suggest that most people of African descent have far lower blood lipid levels than found in people of European or Indian descent in the region. These differences among the groups are present from a young age. In Johannesburg and Soweto, Steyn and colleagues (2000) found that the mean total cholesterol level in African and coloured five-year-old children was 3.9 millimoles per liter compared with 4.1 millimoles per liter for Indian and 4.4 millimoles per liter for white children. The corresponding ratios of HDL cholesterol to total cholesterol were 30.6 percent, 28.9 percent, 27 percent, and 25.8 percent, respectively. These findings in children at the age of five years correspond to the blood lipid pattern found in people of African descent in most studies carried out across Africa. These group differences in lipid profiles tend to continue into adolescence and adulthood. The lower total cholesterol and higher HDL cholesterol levels of persons of African descent indicate a protective pattern against developing atherosclerosis and, consequently, against ischemic heart disease (Steyn et al. 2000). Seftel and colleagues (1993) compared the lipid levels of male students between the ages of 15 and 20 years from different ethnic groups in South African urban and rural settings. The mean total cholesterol level was 3.2 millimoles per liter for the rural and 3.7 millimoles per liter for the urban students, differences that were statistically significant. The rural black males age 15 to 20 had the lowest total cholesterol level of all the groups studied. Only 1 percent of the rural and 2 percent of the urban black males had total cholesterol levels above 5.2 millimoles per liter.

In 1980 Knuiman, Hermus, and Hautvast (1980) reported even lower total cholesterol levels in rural and urban boys age seven to eight years in Côte d'Ivoire, Ghana, and Nigeria. The mean total cholesterol levels in these boys ranged from 2.6 millimoles per liter in rural Nigeria to 3.5 millimoles per liter in urban Ghana, and their ratio of HDL cholesterol to total cholesterol was high, varying from 30 to 36 percent. Walker and Walker (1978) also reported high levels of HDL cholesterol in African children and adults in a population free of coronary heart diseases.

Seftel, Raal, and Joffe (1995) reviewed the early studies on total cholesterol levels in South African adult populations. They found that the mean total cholesterol in middle-aged black men was about 4 millimoles per liter compared with 5 millimoles per liter in coloured men and 6 millimoles per liter in white men. Since the mean total cholesterol concentrations of newborn black and white babies were almost the same, the differences in middle-aged men were likely to be environmental in origin (Seftel, Raal, and Joffe 1995).

The findings of some recent lipid studies in Sub-Saharan African countries are shown in table 18.5. A study of 8,581 rural Tanzanians, age 15 years and older, found significantly higher mean total serum cholesterol levels in women than in men (Swai et al. 1993). Only in the economically more

Table 18.5 Mean Lipid Levels and Prevalence of Dyslipidemia in Black Subjects

Location (age in years)	n	Total cholesterol mmol/L	HDL-C mmol/L	Triglycerides mmol/L	Total cholesterol ≥5.2 mmol/L (%)	Triglycerides ≥1.7 mmol/L (%)
Tanzania						
Rural males	93	3.4	1.0	—	4.4	—
Rural females	91	4.4	1.0	—	22.5	—
Nomadic males	41	5.1	1.1	—	48.6	—
Nomadic females	61	5.3	1.3	—	53.7	—
Urban males	81	4.7	1.2	—	29.5	—
Urban females	79	5.3	1.3	—	50.0	—
Kilimanjaro (rural)						
Males (55+)	413	—	—	—	26.9	12.6
Females (55+)	478	—	—	—	35.5	11.5
Mara						
Males (55+)	198	—	—	—	6.6	8.1
Females (55+)	133	—	—	—	6.1	12.2
Morogoro						
Males (55+)	79	—	—	—	12.7	6.3
Females (55+)	74	—	—	—	9.5	12.1
Nigeria						
Males	110	—	—	—	7.3	—
Females	36	—	—	—	19.5	—
Gambia, The (normotensive)						
Urban males	1,028	4.1	—	0.68	12.5	4.0
Urban females	1,138	4.6	—	0.68	29.1	0.6
Rural males	1,200	3.6	—	0.81	2.3	4.3
Rural females	2,023	3.9	—	0.76	8.3	2.1
Gambia, The (hypertensive)						
Urban males	77	4.9	—	1.13	24.5	4.1
Urban females	85	5.0	—	0.79	39.1	4.7
Rural males	91	4.0	—	1.17	4.1	1.4
Rural females	127	4.4	—	0.83	13.7	2.9
South Africa						
Cape Town (periurban)	986	4.11	1.3	1.2	19.4	—
Free State QwaQwa (rural)	853	4.8	1.2	1.5	32.7	—
Mangaung (periurban)	758	5.3	1.4	1.2	37.4	—

Sources: Kadiri and Salako 1997; Mollentze et al. 1995; Njelekela et al. 2001; Oelofse et al. 1996; Swai et al. 1993; and Van der Sande et al. 2000.

Note: — = data not published; HDL-C = high-density lipoprotein cholesterol; mmol/L = millimole/liter.

advanced region, Kilimanjaro, did the total cholesterol levels increase with age as found in all Westernized people. The favorable lipid profile in most of Africa may be threatened by the march of time. Njelekela and colleagues (2001) surveyed people for chronic disease risk factors in three settings in Tanzania in 1987 and again in 1998. Their findings suggest that during the decade, a significant rise occurred in the mean levels and in the prevalence of many cardiovascular disease risk factors, including increases in total cholesterol levels and the prevalence of hypercholesterolemia.

Two other cross-sectional studies in Tanzania assessed the impact of nutritional factors on the lipid profiles of people living in different settings. One compared the impact of the low-salt fish and vegetable diet on the lipid profile of Tanzanians with that of the typical diets consumed by people in Brazil and Italy (Pavan et al. 1997). The Tanzanians' total blood cholesterol and their BMI were lower than that of the other two groups. Another study compared the lipid profiles of Tanzanian villagers who consumed a diet consisting predominantly of fish with those of villagers who were predominantly vegetarian (Pauletto et al. 1996). The total blood cholesterol levels were lower (3.5 millimoles per liter) in the fish-eating community than in the vegetarian community (4.1 millimoles per liter). Similarly, the blood triglyceride levels were 0.9 millimoles per liter and 1.3 millimoles per liter, and the lipoprotein little (a) levels were 201 milligrams per liter and 321 milligrams per liter in the fish-eating community and vegetarian community, respectively (Pauletto et al. 1996). This study suggests that fish-eating communities have a more protective lipid profile than vegetarian ones.

Total cholesterol levels can be favorably influenced by improved dietary changes; however, increased physical activity patterns also improved the lipid profile. Researchers in Nigeria found that patients with hypertension, exercising three times a week for 30 minutes per session over a 16-week period, decreased their total cholesterol and LDL-cholesterol levels slightly and increased their HDL-cholesterol levels (Iyawe, Ighoroje, and Iyawe 1996).

Although high total blood cholesterol levels are uncommon in Sub-Saharan Africa countries, there are some exceptions. One example is provided by the descendents of the colonists from the Netherlands who came to the southern tip of Africa in the seventeenth century and belong to the Afrikaans-speaking white community in South Africa. The phenomenon referred to by geneticists as the "founder effect" is reflected in the high concentration of familial hypercholesterolemia in this group. A small group of farmers from the Cape province trekked north into the interior regions of what later became South Africa, and tended to intermarry. The background prevalence of heterozygous familial hypercholesterolemia across the globe is 1 to 500. However, the overall prevalence of familial hypercholesterolemia in rural, white, Afrikaans-speaking people in South Africa was estimated to be 1 to 72 (Steyn, Goldberg et al. 1996).

The treatment of high total blood cholesterol levels with medication is most cost-effective in people who have the highest risk of ischemic heart disease. These are people who have had a previous heart attack or stroke or who suffer from familial hypercholesterolemia and those with a typical Westernized lifestyle and who have more than one chronic disease risk factor. Although limited data are available on the treatment status of high blood cholesterol in Sub-Saharan Africa, a survey of about 13,000 patients of general practitioners in private practice in South Africa revealed that high blood cholesterol is poorly treated in those who could benefit the most. These were 18.7 percent of men and 10.4 percent of women who had ischemic heart disease in the past and whose total blood cholesterol levels were found to be 5.9 millimoles per liter and 6.0 millimoles per liter, respectively. These patients need to lower their total blood cholesterol levels significantly for protection against a recurrence of heart disease. This is an achievable objective with the use of highly effective newer cholesterol-lowering agents (Steyn et al. 1998).

HEALTH SERVICES' REQUIREMENTS FOR THE MANAGEMENT OF NCD RISK FACTORS

Chronic disease rates are already higher than expected in Sub-Saharan Africa countries. Consequently, these patients are making significant demands on the health services. Appropriate planning to manage chronic diseases and their risk factors is of paramount importance in the region (Unwin et al. 2001). Most of the risk factors emerge during middle age as a result of an unhealthy lifestyle that has been followed for several decades. Many patients have several risk factors. In Nigeria it was found that patients may have as many as five chronic disease risk factors, as shown in table 18.6 (Ezenwaka et al. 1997). The risk factors have a synergistic effect on the total chronic disease risk. Health services planned for prevention and care must therefore take

Table 18.6 The Clustering of NCD Risk Factors in Nigerian Subjects
(percent)

Number of risk factors	Total participants n = 504	Men n = 295	Women n = 209
0	29.8	31.5	27.3
≥1	70.2	68.5	72.7
≥2	47.6	44.4	52.2
≥3	27.8	25.1	31.7
≥4	16.2	12.2	22.0
≥5	9.2	6.4	13.2

Source: Ezenwaka et al. 1997.
Note: Risk factors considered were smoking, alcohol intake, sedentary lifestyle, hypertension (≥160/95 mmHg), obesity, truncal obesity, hyperinsulinemia, insulin resistance, diabetes, hypercholesterolemia (≥5.2 mmol/L) and hypertriglyceridemia (≥2.5 mmol/L).

cognizance of the burden of multiple chronic disease risk factors in the same patient.

Data collected in large cohort studies conducted in the United States and the United Kingdom were used to assess the relationship between risk factors and cardiovascular disease (CVD) events. The studies used were the Framingham, Massachusetts, cohort data and United Kingdom cohort data (ATP III 2001; Grundy et al. 1999; Joint Task Force, 1998). Formulas were calculated that could be used to estimate a patient's chronic disease risk. These formulas usually express the patient's risk of suffering from a CVD event in the next 10 years or longer period. Health services are thus able to identify those patients who are at the highest risk of developing CVD and would benefit the most by using appropriate medication. Gaziano, Steyn, and Opie (2001) have shown that such an approach is more cost-effective than that of using single cut-off points for single CVD risk factors. Therefore, the total CVD risk-assessment approach clearly should be the one employed in settings with scarce resources, as is the case in Sub-Saharan Africa countries.

The model of health service provision prevailing across most of Sub-Saharan Africa is one that focuses on acute illnesses, the immediate needs of patients, and episodic interaction between the patient and the health services. This model does not provide adequate care for patients with chronic diseases. Consequently, millions of patients with chronic diseases in the region are undiagnosed or receiving inadequate treatment. The WHO conducted a two-year review of health care models and best practices from around the world. The findings, published in 2002, provided a comprehensive conceptual framework for the prevention and management of chronic conditions in poorly resourced settings (WHO 2002).

The WHO report focuses on the need to move away from the acute model of care to efficiently coordinated and patient-centered care. Such a move should facilitate an ongoing relationship between provider and patient and help patients to make full use of their own and their community's resources (Holman and Lorig 2000; Wagner 2000). This approach suggests that the focus should be on the patients in their own social settings and context and not only on the disease of the patient. This is of particular significance in Sub-Saharan Africa countries, where the patients' cultural beliefs and practices should be understood when prevention and management of chronic conditions are introduced. The partnership between the patient and the health care provider is not just a resource for understanding ill health, it is the basis for the prevention and management of chronic diseases and their risk factors (Swartz and Dick 2002).

POLICY INITIATIVES TO PROMOTE A HEALTHY LIFESTYLE

The need for preventive action to reduce or prevent the adoption of a less healthy lifestyle by people in Sub-Saharan Africa has never been greater. Many factors contribute to the lack of chronic disease preventive programs being adopted by governments (Yach 2002).

The global health community has taken some significant steps to support countries in Sub-Saharan Africa and elsewhere to promote a healthy lifestyle for the entire world. The WHO, a branch of the United Nations, spearheaded this initiative by negotiations to propose a framework convention on Tobacco Control between 1999 and 2003. The member states of the WHO (2003) unanimously endorsed the framework convention of Tobacco Control to the WHO's general assembly in June 2004 for endorsement. The treaty attacks tobacco use in many ways. It expects countries to provide treatment for people who smoke, to encourage cessation, and to prevent the onset of tobacco use in the young. It requires countries to protect the public from exposure to environmental tobacco smoke and expects them to ban advertising to the extent that their constitutions allow with respect to the protection of commercial free speech. Thirty percent of any tobacco product's packaging should contain health warnings of the danger of tobacco use. Misleading words such as "light" or "mild" should also be banned. It encourages countries to raise taxes to the point that will discourage smoking and to pass laws that hold tobacco companies accountable for medical and other costs incurred because of tobacco use (WHO 2003). With the exception of South Africa, very few Sub-Saharan Africa countries have adequate tobacco control legislation in place to effectively protect their populations against tobacco use. This treaty will encourage many countries in the region to initiate such a development.

In March 2003 the WHO and the Food and Agriculture Organization, another branch of the United Nations, issued a scientific report reviewing the data on diet, physical activity, and health. The WHO has embarked on an extensive process of consultations across the globe, including Sub-Saharan Africa countries, to ensure that a global strategy provides realistic guidelines for all countries. The strategy will include a broad series of nutrition-related recommendations, including dietary advice along with proposals dealing with the labeling and advertising of food. Collaboration with the food industry is seen as pivotal to improving the quality of manufactured food and processed food.

All these initiatives will provide countries with information to identify and act appropriately to promote a healthy lifestyle. However, it is necessary to prioritize chronic disease prevention in view of all the other large health demands that face the ministries of health in Sub-Saharan Africa countries. Countries with multiple burdens of disease will have to develop priority-setting programs in order to plan how to use scarce resources most effectively. The failure of countries to adopt the necessary steps to promote a healthy lifestyle, however difficult such a decision might be early in the twenty-first century, will inevitably lead to increasing levels of obesity, hypertension, hyperlipidemia, and diabetes in the populations of Sub-Saharan Africa countries. This, in turn, will be the cause of an avoidable chronic disease epidemic within a few decades.

CONCLUSION

On reviewing the extent of chronic diseases in the low-income and middle-income countries, the Institute of Medicine of the United States National Academy of Sciences recommended that, in addition to the preventive actions required to reduce the risk factors, health services should diagnose and control hypertension and diabetes and should ensure access to low-cost drugs and the development of affordable clinical care algorithms. The report also emphasized the need to build capacity to conduct research and development activities and to develop institutional frameworks that would facilitate the development of chronic disease prevention activities and the transformation of the health care services to adequately cope with the enormous, mostly unacknowledged burden of chronic diseases in Sub-Saharan Africa (Howson et al. 1998).

REFERENCES

Adult Treatment Panel III (Expert Panel on Detection, Evaluation, and Treatment of High Blood Cholesterol in Adults). 2001. "Executive Summary of the Third Report of the National Cholesterol Education Program (NCEP) Expert Panel on Detection, Evaluation, and Treatment of High Blood Cholesterol in Adults (Adult Treatment Panel III)." *Journal of the American Medical Association* 285 (19): 2486–97.

Aspray, T. J., F. Mugusi, S. Rashid, D. Whiting, R. Edwards, K. G. Alberti, and N. C. Unwin. 2000. "Rural and Urban Differences in Diabetes Prevalence in Tanzania: The Role of Obesity, Physical Inactivity and Urban Living." *Transactions of the Royal Society of Tropical Medicine and Hygiene* 94 (6): 637–44.

Baker, E. H., Y. B. Dong, G. A. Sagnella, M. Rothwell, A. K. Onipinla, N. D. Markandu, F. P. Cappuccio, et al. 1998. "Association of Hypertension with T594M Mutation in Beta Subunit of Epithelial Sodium Channels in Black People Resident in London." *Lancet* 351: 1388–92.

Barker, D. J. P. 1993. *Fetal and Infant Origins of Adult Disease*. London: British Medical Journal Publishing Group.

———. 1994. *Mothers, Babies and Diseases in Later Life*. London: British Medical Journal Publishing Group.

Barlassina, C., G. R. Norton, N. J. Samani, A. J. Woodiwiss, G. C. Candy, I. Radevski, L. Citterio, G. Bianchi, and D. Cusi. 2000. "Alpha-Adducin Polymorphism in Hypertensives of South African Ancestry." *American Journal of Hypertension* 13: 719–23.

Benefice, E., and C. Cames. 1999. "Physical Activity Patterns of Rural Senegalese Adolescent Girls during the Dry and Rainy Seasons Measured by Movement Registration and Direct Observational Methods." *European Journal of Clinical Nutrition* 53 (8) : 636–43.

Benefice, E., D. Garnier, and G. Ndiaye. 2001a. "Assessment of Physical Activity among Rural Senegalese Adolescent Girls: Influence of Age, Sexual Maturation, and Body Composition." *Journal of Adolescent Health* 28 (4): 319–27.

———. 2001b. "High Levels of Habitual Physical Activity in West African Adolescent Girls and Relationship to Maturation, Growth, and Nutritional Status: Results from a 3-Year Prospective Study." *American Journal of Human Biology* 13 (6): 808–20.

Berger, G. M. B., and A. D. Marais. 2000. "Diagnosis, Management and Prevention of the Common Dyslipidaemias in South Africa—Clinical Guideline, 2002." *South African Medical Journal* 90: 164–78.

Bourne, L. T., E. V. Lambert, and K. Steyn. 2002. "Where Does the Black Population of South Africa Stand on the Nutrition Transition?" *Public Health and Nutrition* 5 (1A): 157–62.

Bovet, P., A. G. Ross, J. P. Gervasoni, M. Mkamba, D. M. Mtasiwa, C. Lengeler, D. Whiting, and F. Paccaud. 2002. "Distribution of Blood Pressure, Body Mass Index and Smoking Habits in the Urban Population of Dar es Salaam, Tanzania, and Associations with Socioeconomic Status." *International Journal of Epidemiology* 31: 240–47.

Brown, P. J., and M. Konner. 1987. "An Anthropological Perspective on Obesity." *Annals of the New York Academy of Sciences* 499: 29–46.

Bunker, C. H., F. A. Ukoli, M. U. Nwankwo, J. A. Omene, G. W. Currier, L. Holifield-Kennedy, D. T. Freeman, E. N. Vergis, L. L. Yeh, and L. H. Kuller. 1992. "Factors Associated with Hypertension in Nigerian Civil Servants." *Preventive Medicine* 21 (6): 710–22.

Candy, G., N. Samani, G. Norton, A. Woodiwiss, I. Radevski, A. Wheatley, J. Cockcroft, and I. P. Hall. 2000. "Association Analysis of Beta2 Adrenoceptor Polymorphisms with Hypertension in a Black African Population." *Journal of Hypertension* 18: 167–72.

Cappuccio, F. P., J. Plange-Rhule, R. O. Phillips, and J. B. Eastwood. 2000. "Prevention of Hypertension and Stroke in Africa." *Lancet* 356: 677–78.

Ceesay, S. M., A. M. Prentice, T. J. Cole, F. Foord, E. M. E. Poskitt, L. T. Weaver, and R. G. Whitehead. 1997. "Effects on Birth Weight and Perinatal Mortality of Maternal Dietary Supplements in Rural Gambia: 5 Years Randomised Controlled Trial." *British Medical Journal* 315: 786–90.

Cooper, R., C. Rotimi, S. Ataman, D. McGee, B. Osotimehin, S. Kadiri, W. Muna, et al. 1997. "The Prevalence of Hypertension in Seven Populations of West African Origin." *American Journal of Public Health* 87 (2): 160–68.

Cooper, R. S., C. N. Rotimi, J. S. Kaufman, W. F. Muna, and G. A. Mensah. 1998. "Hypertension Treatment and Control in Sub-Saharan Africa: The Epidemiological Basis for Policy." *British Medical Journal* 316: 614–17.

Corrao, M. A., G. E. Guindon, N. Sharma, and D. F. Shokoohi. 2000. *Tobacco Control Country Profiles*. Atlanta: American Cancer Society.

Crowther, N. J., N. Cameron, J. Trusler, and I. P. Gray. 1998. "Association Between Poor Glucose Tolerance and Rapid Post Natal Weight Gain in Seven-Year-Old Children." *Diabetologia* 41: 1163–67.

Cusi, D., C. Barlassina, T. Azzani, G. Casari, L. Citterio, M. Devoto, N. Glorioso, et al. 1997. "Polymorphisms of Alpha-Adducin and Salt

Sensitivity in Patients with Essential Hypertension." *Lancet* 349: 1353–57.

Damasceno, A., and A. Prista. 2001. "Secular Trends in Cardiovascular Risk Factors in Children and Youth from Maputo, Mozambique." *Japanese Journal of Cardiovascular Disease Prevention* 36 (Suppl.): M024.

Edwards, R., N. C. Unwin, F. Mugusi, D. Whiting, S. Rashid, J. Kissima, T. J. Aspray, and K. G. Alberti. 2000. "Hypertension Prevalence and Care in an Urban and Rural Area of Tanzania." *Journal of Hypertension* 18: 145–52.

Ekpo, E. B., O. Usofia, N. F. Eshiet, and J. J. Andy. 1992. "Demographic, Lifestyle and Anthropometric Correlates of Blood Pressure of Nigerian Urban Civil Servants, Factory and Plantation Workers." *Journal of Human Hypertension* 6 (4): 275–80.

Ezenwaka, C. E., A. O. Akanji, B. O. Akanje, N. C. Unwin, and C. A. Adejuwon. 1997. "The Prevalence of Insulin Resistance and Other Cardiovascular Disease Risk Factors in Healthy Elderly Southwestern Nigerians." *Atherosclerosis* 128 (2): 201–11.

Fontaine, K. R., D. T. Redden, C. Wang, A. O. Westfall, and D. B. Allison. 2003. "Years of Life Lost Due to Obesity." *Journal of the American Medical Association* 289: 187–93.

Forrest, K. Y., C. H. Bunker, A. M. Kriska, F. A. Ukoli, S. L. Huston, and N. Markovic. 2001. "Physical Activity and Cardiovascular Risk Factors in a Developing Population." *Medicine and Science in Sports and Exercise* 33 (9): 1598–1604.

Garnier, D., and E. Benefice. 2001. "Habitual Physical Activity of Senegalese Adolescent Girls under Different Working Conditions, As Assessed by a Questionnaire and Movement Registration." *Annals of Human Biology* 28 (1): 79–97.

Gaziano, T. A., K. Steyn, and L. H. Opie. 2001. "Cost-Effectiveness Analysis of Hypertension Guidelines in South Africa." Abstract presented at the American Heart Association Meeting, Johannesburg, November 10–13.

Gibney, M. J., and P. G. Burstyn. 1980. "Milk, Serum Cholesterol and the Maasai. A Hypothesis." *Atherosclerosis* 35: 339–43.

Global Youth Tobacco Survey Collaborative Group. 2002. "Tobacco Use among Youth: A Cross-Country Comparison." *Tobacco Control* 11: 252–70.

Grundy, S. M., R. Pasternak, P. Greenland, S. Smith Jr., and V. Fuster. 1999. "AHA/ACC Scientific Statement: Assessment of Cardiovascular Risk by Use of Multiple-Risk-Factor Assessment Equations: A Statement for Healthcare Professionals from the American Heart Association and the American College of Cardiology." *Journal of the American College of Cardiology* 34 (4): 1348–59.

Haskell, W. L., A. S. Leon, and C. J. Caspersen. 1992. "Cardiovascular Benefits and Assessment of Physical Activity and Physical Fitness in Adults." *Medicine and Science in Sports and Exercise* 24 (Suppl.): S201–20.

Heini, A. F., G. Minghelli, E. Diaz, A. M. Prentice, and Y. Schutz. 1996. "Free-Living Energy Expenditure Assessed by Two Different Methods in Rural Gambian Men." *European Journal of Clinical Nutrition* 50 (5): 184–89.

Hesse, I. F., and I. Nuama. 1997. "Pattern of Out-Patient Drug Treatment of Hypertension in Korle-Bu Teaching Hospital, Accra." *West African Journal of Medicine* 16 (3): 133–38.

Holman, H., and K. Lorig. 2000. "Patients as Partners in Managing Chronic Disease." *British Medical Journal* 320: 526–27.

Howson C. P., K. S. Reddy, T. J. Ryan, and J. R. Bale, eds. 1998. *Control of Cardiovascular Disease in Developing Countries: Research, Development, and Institutional Strengthening.* Washington, DC: National Academy Press.

Hunter, J. M., B. T. Sparks, J. Mufunda, C. T. Musabayane, H. V. Sparks, and K. Mohamed. 2000. "Economic Development and Women's Blood Pressure: Field Evidence from Rural Mashonaland, Zimbabwe." *Social Science and Medicine* 50 (6): 773–95.

Iyawe, V. I., A. D. Ighoroje, and H. O. Iyawe. 1996. "Changes in Blood Pressure and Serum Cholesterol Following Exercise Training in Nigerian Hypertensive Subjects." *Journal of Human Hypertension* 10 (7): 483–87.

Jain, S., X. Tang, C. S. Narayanan, Y. Agarwal, S. M. Peterson, C. D. Brown, J. Ott, and A. Kumar. 2002. "Angiotensinogen Gene Polymorphism at −217 Affects Basal Promoter Activity and Is Associated with Hypertension in African-Americans." *Journal of Biological Chemistry* 277: 36889–96.

Johns, T., R. L. Mahunnah, P. Samaya, L. Chapman, and T. Ticktin. 1999. "Saponins and Phenolic Content in Plant Dietary Additives of a Traditional Subsistence Community, the Batemi of Ngorongoro District, Tanzania." *Journal of Ethnopharmacology* 66: 1–10.

Joint Task Force. 1998. "Prevention of Coronary Heart Disease in Clinical Practice." Recommendations of the Second Joint Task Force of European and Other Societies on coronary prevention. *European Heart Journal* 19 (10): 1434–1503.

Kadiri, S., and B. L. Salako. 1997. "Cardiovascular Risk Factors in Middle Aged Nigerians." *East African Medical Journal* 74 (5): 303–6.

Kaufman, J. S., E. E. Owoaje, C. N. Rotimi, and R. S. Cooper. 1999. "Blood Pressure Change in Africa: Case Study from Nigeria." *Human Biology* 71 (4): 641–57.

Kaufman, J. S., C. N. Rotimi, W. R. Brieger, M. A. Oladokum, S. Kadiri, B. O. Osotimehin, and R. S. Cooper. 1996. "The Mortality Risk Associated with Hypertension: Preliminary Results of a Prospective Study in Rural Nigeria." *Journal of Human Hypertension* 10 (7): 461–64.

Kinabo, J. L., K. Kissawke, and J. Msuya. 1997. "Factors Influencing Birth Weight in Morogoro Municipality, Tanzania." *South African Journal Food Science and Nutrition* 9: 3–8.

Knuiman, J. T., R. J. J. Hermus, and J. G. A. J. Hautvast. 1980. "Serum Total and High-Density Lipoprotein (HDL) Cholesterol Concentrations in Rural and Urban Boys from 16 Countries." *Atherosclerosis* 36: 529–37.

Kruger, H. S., C. S. Venter, H. H. Vorster, and B. M. Margetts. 2002. "Physical Inactivity Is the Major Determinant of Obesity in Black Women in the North West Province, South Africa: The THUSA Study." *Nutrition* 18: 422–27.

Lambert, E. V., W. Weitz, K. Charlton, M. I. Lambert, Z. Kukubeli, L. Keytel, N. Temple, and A. Daniels. 2000. "Health and Fitness Survey in Adolescent School Children in the Western Cape: Relationship to Body Mass Index and Obesity." Paper presented at the biannual meeting of the Nutrition Society and Association for Dietetics in Southern African, "From Lab to Land," Durban, August.

Larson, N., R. Hutchinson, and E. Boerwinkle. 2000. "Lack of Association of 3 Functional Gene Variants with Hypertension in African Americans." *Hypertension* 35: 1297–1300.

Levitt, N. S., E. V. Lambert, D. Woods, C. N. Hales, R. Andrew, and J. R. Seckl. 2000. "Impaired Glucose Tolerance and Elevated Blood Pressure in Low Birth Weight, Nonobese, Young South African Adults: Early Programming of Cortisol Axis." *Journal of Clinical Endocrinology and Metabolism* 85 (12): 4611–18.

Levitt, N. S., K. Steyn, T. De Wet, C. Morrell, P. R. Edwards, G. T. H. Ellison, and N. Cameron. 1999. "An Inverse Relation between Blood Pressure and Birth Weight among 5-Year-Old Children from Soweto, South Africa (Birth-to-Ten Study)." *Journal of Epidemiology and Community Health* 53: 264–68.

Levitt, N. S., K. Steyn, E. V. Lambert, G. Reagon, C. J. Lombard, J. M. Fourie, K. Rossouw, and M. Hoffman. 1999. "Modifiable Risk Factors for Type 2 Diabetes Mellitus in a Peri-Urban Community in South Africa." *Diabetic Medicine* 16: 946–50.

Longo-Mbenza, B., R. Ngiyulu, M. Bayekula, E. K. Vita, F. B. Nkiabungu, K. V. Seghers, E. L. Luila, F. M. Mandundu, and M. Manzanza. 1999. "Low Birth Weight and Risk of Hypertension in African School Children." *Journal of Cardiovascular Risk* 6: 311–14.

Margetts, B. M., M. G. M. Rowlands, F. A. Foord, A. M. Cruddas, T. J. Cole, and D. J. P. Barker. 1991. "The Relation of Maternal Weight to the Blood Pressure of Gambian Children." *International Journal of Epidemiology* 20: 938–43.

Marks, A. S., K. Steyn, and E. Ratheb. 2001. "Tobacco Use by Black Women in Cape Town." MRC Policy Brief 3. Parowvallei: Medical Research Council.

Mbanya, J. C .N., E. M. Minkoulou, J. N. Salah, and B. Balkau. 1998. "The Prevalence of Hypertension in Rural and Urban Cameroon." *International Journal of Epidemiology* 27: 181–85.

McBride, P., J. Einerson, P. Hanson, and K. Heindel. 1992. "Exercise and the Primary Prevention of Coronary Heart Disease." *Medicine, Exercise, Nutrition, and Health* 1: 5–15.

McCormick, J., and M. Elmore-Meegan. 1992. "Maasai Diet." *Lancet* 340: 1042–43.

Milne, F. J., Y. Veriava, S. H. James, and C. Isaacson. 1989. "Aetiology and Pathogenesis of Malignant Hypertension in Black South Africans—A Review." *South African Medical Journal* 76 (Suppl.): 22–23.

Mollentze, W. F., A. J. Moore, G. Joubert, K. Steyn, G. M. Oosthuizen, and D. J. Weich. 1995. "Coronary Heart Disease Risk Factors in a Rural and Urban Orange Free State Black Population." *South African Medical Journal* 85 (2): 90–96.

Mtabaji, J. P., Y. Moriguchi, Y. Nara, S. Mizushima, M. Mano, and Y. Yamori. 1992." Ethnic Differences in Salt Sensitivity: Genetic or Environmental Factors." *Clinical and Experimental Pharmacology and Physiology* 20 (Suppl.): 65–67.

Mtabaji, J. P., Y. Nara, and Y. Yamori. 1990. "The Cardiac Study in Tanzania: Salt Intake in the Causation and Treatment of Hypertension." *Journal of Human Hypertension* 4 (32): 80–81.

Mufunda, J., L. J. Scott, J. Chifamba, J. Matenga, B. Sparks, R. Cooper, and H. Sparks. 2000. "Correlates of Blood Pressure in an Urban Zimbabwean Population and Comparison to Other Populations of African Origin." *Journal of Human Hypertension* 14 (1) : 65–73.

Mvo, Z., J. Dick, and K. Steyn. 1999. "Perceptions of Overweight African Women about Acceptable Body Size and Children." *Curationis* 22 (2): 27–31.

Ndlovo, P. P., and S. D. Roos. 1999. "Perceptions of Black Women of Obesity as a Health Risk." *Curationis* 22 (2): 47–55.

Nissinen, A., S. Bothig, H. Granroth, and A. D. Lopez. 1988. "Hypertension in Developing Countries." *World Health Statistics Quarterly* 41 (3–4): 141–54.

Njelekela, M., H. Negishi, Y. Nara, M. Tomohiro, S. Kuga, T. Noguchi, T. Kanda, et al. 2001. "Cardiovascular Risk Factors in Tanzania: A Revisit." *Acta Tropica* 79 (3): 231–39.

Nkeh, B., N. J. Samani, D. Badenhorst, E. Libhaber, P. Sareli, G. R. Norton, and A. J. Woodiwiss. 2003. "T594M Variant of the Epithelial Sodium Channel Beta-Subunit Gene and Hypertension in Individuals of African Ancestry in South Africa." *American Journal of Hypertension* 16 (10): 847–52.

Obel, A. O., and D. K. Koech. 1991. "Potassium Supplementation versus Bendro Fluazide in Mildly to Moderately Hypertensive Kenyans." *Journal of Cardiovascular Pharmacology* 17 (3): 504–7.

Odendaal, H. J., D. L. Van Schie, and R. M. De Jeu. 2001. "Adverse Effects of Maternal Cigarette Smoking on Preterm Labour and Abruptio Placentae." *International Journal Gynecology and Obstetrics* 74: 287–88.

Oelofse, A., P. Jooste, K. Steyn, C. J. Badenhorst, L. T. Bourne, and J. Fourie. 1996. "The Lipid and Lipoprotein Profile of the Urban Black South African Community of the Cape Peninsula—the BRISK Study." *South African Medical Journal* 86: 166–69.

Olatunbosun, S. T., J. S. Kaufman, R. S. Cooper, and A. F. Bella. 2000. "Hypertension in a Black Population: Prevalence and Biosocial Determinants of High Blood Pressure in a Group of Urban Nigerians." *Journal of Human Hypertension* 14(4): 249–57.

Pauletto, P., M. Puato, M. G. Caroli, E. Casiglia, A. E. Munhambo, G. Cazzolato, G. Bittolo Bon, M. T. Angeli, C. Galli, and A. C. Pessina. 1996. "Blood Pressure and Atherogenic Lipoprotein Profiles of Fish-Diet and Vegetarian Villagers in Tanzania: The Lugalawa Study." *Lancet* 348 (9030): 784–88.

Pavan, L., E. Casiglia, P. Pauletto, S. L. Batista, G. Ginocchio, M. M. Kwankam, R. Biasin, et al. 1997. "Blood Pressure, Serum Cholesterol and Nutritional State in Tanzania and in the Amazon: Comparison with an Italian Population." *Journal of Hypertension* 15 (10): 1083–90.

Peeters, A., J. J. Barendregt, F. Willekens, J. P. Mackenbach, A. A. Mamun, L. Bonneux, for NEDCOM (Netherlands Epidemiology and Demography Compression of Morbidity Research Group). 2003. "Obesity in Adulthood and Its Consequences for Life Expectancy: A Life-Table Analysis." *Annals of Internal Medicine* 138: 24–32.

Popkin, B. M. 2001a. "Nutrition in Transition: The Changing Global Nutrition Challenge." *Asia Pacific Journal of Clinical Nutrition* 10: S13–18.

———. 2001b. "The Nutrition Transition and Obesity in the Developing World." *Journal of Nutrition* 131 (3): 871S–73S.

Poulter, N., K. T. Khaw, B. E. Hopwood, M. Mugambi, W. S. Peart, and P. S. Sever. 1985. Determinants of Blood Pressure Changes Due to Urbanization: A Longitudinal Study. *Journal of Hypertension* 3 (Suppl.): S375–77.

Poulter, N., K. T. Khaw, B. E. Hopwood, M. Mugambi, W. S. Peart, G. Rose, and P. S. Sever. 1990. "The Kenyan Luo Migration Study: Observations on the Initiation of a Rise in Blood Pressure." *British Medical Journal* 300: 967–72.

Puoane, T., K. Steyn, D. Bradshaw, R. Laubscher, J. Fourie, V. Lambert, and N. Mbananga. 2002. "Obesity in South Africa: The South African Demographic and Health Survey." *Obesity Research* 10 (10): 1038–48.

Rotimi, C. N., R. S. Cooper, S. L. Ataman, B. Osotimehin, S. Kadiri, W. Muna, S. Kingue, H. Fraser, and D. McGee. 1995. "Distribution of Anthropometric Variables and the Prevalence of Obesity in Populations of West African Origin: The International Collaborative Study on Hypertension in Blacks (ICSHIB)." *Obesity Research* 2 (Suppl.): 95S–105S.

Rotimi, C. N., R. S. Cooper, G. Cao, O. Ogunbiyi, M. Ladipo, E. Owoaje, and R. Ward. 1999. "Maximum-Likelihood Generalized Heritability Estimate for Blood Pressure in Nigerian Families." *Hypertension* 33 (3): 874–78.

Salako, B. L., S. Kadiri, F. A. Fehintola, and O. O. Akinkugbe. 1999. "The Effect of Anti-Hypertensive Therapy on Urinary Albumin Excretion in Nigerian Hypertensives." *West African Journal of Medicine* 18 (3): 170–74.

Saloojee, Y. 1995. "Price and Income Elasticity of Demand for Cigarettes in South Africa in Tobacco and Health." In *Tobacco and Health*, ed. K. Shlama. New York: Plenum Press.

———. 2000. "Regional Summary for the African Region." In *Tobacco Control Country Profiles*, ed. M. A. Corrao, G. E. Guindon, N. Sharma, and D. F. Shokoohi. Atlanta: American Cancer Society.

Seedat, Y. K. 1996. "Is the Pathogenesis of Hypertension Different in Black Patients?" *Journal of Human Hypertension* 3 (Suppl.): S35–37.

———. 1999. "Hypertension in Black South Africans." *Journal of Human Hypertension* 13 (2): 96–103.

Seftel, H., M. S. Asvat, B. I. Joffe, F. J. Raal, V. R. Panz, W. J. H. Vermaak, M. E. Loock, et al. 1993. "Selected Risk Factors for Coronary Heart Disease in Male Scholars from the Major South African Population Groups." *South African Medical Journal* 83: 891–97.

Seftel, H., F. J. Raal, and B. I. Joffe. 1995. "Dyslipidaemia in South Africa." In *Chronic Diseases of Lifestyle in South Africa*, ed. J. M. Fourie, and K. Steyn. MRC Technical Report. Parowvallei, Medical Research Council.

Siffert, W., D. Rosskopf, G. Siffert, S. Busch, A. Moritz, R. Erbel, A. M. Sharma, et al. 1998. "Association of a Human G-Protein Beta3 Subunit Variant with Hypertension." *Nature Genetics* 18: 45–48.

Sobngwi, E., J. C. N. Mbanya, N. C. Unwin, A. P. Kengne, L. Fezeu, E. M. Minkoulou, T. J. Aspray, and K. G. Alberti. 2002. "Physical Activity and Its Relationship with Obesity, Hypertension and Diabetes in Urban and Rural Cameroon." *International Journal of Obesity and Related Metabolic Disorders* 26 (7): 1009–16.

Sobngwi, E., J. C. N. Mbanya, N. C. Unwin, J. A. Terrence, and K. G. M. M. Alberti. 2001. "Development and Validation of a Questionnaire for the Assessment of Physical Activity in Epidemiological Studies in Sub-Saharan Africa." *International Journal of Epidemiology* 30: 1361–68.

Solomon, C. G., and J. E. Manson. 1997. "Obesity and Mortality: A Review of the Epidemiologic Data." *American Journal of Clinical Nutrition* 66 (Suppl.): 1044S–50S.

Steyn, K., L. T. Bourne, P. L. Jooste, J. M. Fourie, C. J. Lombard, and D. Yach. 1994. "Smoking in the African Community of the Cape Peninsula." *East African Medical Journal* 71: 784–89.

Steyn, K., D. Bradshaw, R. Norman, R. Laubscher, and Y. Saloojee. 2002. "Tobacco Use in South Africans During 1998: The First Demographic and Health Survey." *Journal of Cardiovascular Risk* 9: 161–70.

Steyn, K., T. de Wet, L. Richter, N. Cameron, N. S. Levitt, and C. Morrell. 2000. "Cardiovascular Disease Risk Factors in Five-Year-Old Urban South African Children—The Birth to Ten Study." *South African Medical Journal* 90 (7): 719–26.

Steyn, K., J. M. Fourie, C. J. Lombard, J. Katzenellenbogen, L. Bourne, and P. Jooste. 1996. "Hypertension in the Black Community of the Cape Peninsula, South Africa." *East African Medical Journal* 11: 758–63.

Steyn, K., J. M. Fourie, and J. Sheppard. 1998. "The Lipid Profile of South Africans Attending General Practitioners: The Cholesterol Monitor." *South African Medical Journal* 88: 1569–74.

Steyn, K., T. Gaziano, D. Bradshaw, R. Laubscher, and J. M. Fourie. 2001. "Hypertension in South African Adults: Results from the Demographic and Health Survey." *Journal of Hypertension* 19: 1717–25.

Steyn, K., Y. P. Goldberg, M. J. Kotze, M. Steyn, A. S. Swanepoel, J. M. Fourie, G. A. Coetzee, and D. R. van der Westhuyszen. 1996. "Estimation of the Prevalence of Familial Hypercholesterolaemia in a Rural Afrikaner Community by Direct Screening for Three Afrikaner Founder Low-Density Lipoprotein Receptor Gene Mutations." *Human Genetics* 98 (4): 479–84.

Steyn, K., D. Yach, I. Stander, and J. M. Fourie. 1997. "Smoking in Urban Pregnant Women in South Africa." *South African Medical Journal* 87: 460–63.

Steyn, N. P., M. Senekal, S. Brits, and J. H. Nel. 2000. "Urban and Rural Differences in Dietary Intake, Weight Status and Nutrition Knowledge of Black Female Students." *Asia Pacific Journal of Clinical Nutrition* 9 (1): 11–16.

St-Onge, M. P., E. R. Farnworth, and P. J. Jones. 2000. "Consumption of Fermented and Nonfermented Dairy Products: Effects on Cholesterol Concentrations and Metabolism." *American Journal of Clinical Nutrition* 71 (3): 674–81.

Svetkey, L. P., P. Z. Timmons, O. Emovon, N. B. Anderson, L. Preis, and Y. T. Chen. 1996. "Association of Hypertension with Beta2- and Alpha2c10-Adrenergic Receptor Genotype." *Hypertension* 27 (6): 1210–15.

Swai, A. B., D. G. McLarty, H. M. Kitange, P. M. Kilima, S. Tatalla, N. Keen, L. M. Chuwa, and K. G. Alberti. 1993. "Low Prevalence of Risk Factors for Coronary Heart Disease in Rural Tanzania." *International Journal of Epidemiology* 22 (4) : 651–59.

Swartz, L., and J. Dick. 2002. "Managing Chronic Conditions in Less Developed Countries." *British Medical Journal* 325: 914–15.

Teklu, T. 1996. "Food Demand Studies in Sub-Saharan Africa: A Survey of Empirical Evidence." *Food Policy* 21: 479–96.

Tiago, A. D., N. J. Samani, G. P. Candy, R. Brooksbank, E. N. Libhaber, P. Sareli, A. J. Woodiwiss, and G. R. Norton. 2002. "Angiotensinogen Gene Promoter Region Variant Modifies Body Size-Ambulatory Blood Pressure Relations in Hypertension." *Circulation* 106: 1483–87.

Treloar, C., J. Porteous, F. Hassan, N. Kasniyah, M. Lakshmanudu, M. Sama, M. Sha'bani, and F. Heller. 1999. "The Cross Cultural Context of Obesity: An INCLEN Multicentre Collaborative Study." *Health and Place* 5: 279–86.

Unwin, N., P. Setel, S. Rashid, F. Mugusi, J. C. Mbanya, H. Kitange, L. Hayes, R. Edwards, T. Aspray, and K. G. Alberti. 2001. "Noncommunicable Diseases in Sub-Saharan Africa: Where Do They Feature in the Health Research Agenda?" *Bulletin of the World Health Organization* 79 (10): 947–53.

Van der Sande, M. A. B., P. J. M. Milligan, O. A. Nyan, J. T. Rowley, W. A. S. Banya, S. M. Ceesay, W. M. Dolmans, T. Thien, K. P. W. J. McAdam, and G. E. L. Walvaren. 2000. "Blood Pressure Patterns and Cardiovascular Risk Factors in Rural and Urban Gambian Communities." *Journal of Human Hypertension* 14 : 489–96.

Van der Sande, M. A. B., G. E. L. Walvaren, P. J. M. Milligan, W. A. S. Banya, S. M. Ceesay, O. A. Nyan, and K. P. W. J. McAdam. 2001. "Family History: An Opportunity for Early Interventions and Improved Control of Hypertension, Obesity and Diabetes." *Bulletin of the World Health Organization* 79: 321–28.

Veriava, Y., E. du Toit, C. G. Lawley, F. J. Milne, and S. G. Reinach. 1990. "Hypertension as a Cause of End-Stage Renal Failure in South Africa." *Journal of Human Hypertension* 4 (4): 379–83.

Wagner, E. G. 2000. "The Role of Patient Care Teams in Chronic Care Management." *British Medical Journal* 320: 569–671.

Walker, A. R., and B. F. Walker. 1978. "High High-Density-Lipoprotein Cholesterol in African Children and Adults in a Population Free of Coronary Heart Disease." *British Medical Journal* 6148 (2): 1336–37.

Walker, A. R., B. F. Walker, B. Manetsi, N. G. Tsotetsi, and A. J. Walker. 1990. "Obesity in Black Women in Soweto, South Africa: Minimal Effects on Hypertension, Hyperlipidaemia and Hyperglycemia." *Journal of the Royal Society of Health* 110 (3): 101–3.

Wareham, J. 2001. "Commentary: Measuring Physical Activity in Sub-Saharan Africa." *International Journal of Epidemiology* 30: 1369–70.

WHO (World Health Organization). 2000. *Obesity: Preventing and Managing the Global Epidemic*. WHO Technical Report Series 894. Geneva: WHO.

———. 2002. *Innovative Care for Chronic Conditions: Building Blocks for Action*. WHO Global Report. Geneva: WHO.

———. 2003 (updated 2004/5). "WHO Framework Convention on Tobacco Control." http://www.who.int/tobacco/framework/WHO_FCTC_english.pdf (accessed January 31, 2006).

Yach, D. 2002. "Unleashing the Power of Prevention to Achieve Global Health-Gains." *Lancet* 360: 1343–44.

Zhao, Y. Y., J. Zhou, C. S. Narayanan, Y. Cui, and A. Kumar. 1999. "Role of C/A Polymorphism at −20 on the Expression of Human Angiotensinogen Gene." *Hypertension* 33: 108–15.

Chapter **19**

Jean-Claude Mbanya and Kaushik Ramiaya

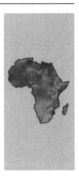

Diabetes Mellitus

The global burden of disease study of the World Health Organization (WHO) estimated that about 177 million people in the world had diabetes in the year 2000 (WHO 2003). In the second edition of the International Diabetes Federation's *Diabetes Atlas* it is estimated that 194 million people had diabetes in the year 2003, and about two-thirds of these people lived in developing countries (IDF 2003). In 1901 Albert Cook, a medical missionary in Uganda, reported that "diabetes is rather uncommon and very fatal" (Cook 1901). Over the next 50 to 60 years diabetes continued to be regarded as rare in Sub-Saharan Africa. Communicable diseases still make up the greatest disease burden, but by 2020, noncommunicable diseases, including hypertension and diabetes, will outstrip communicable diseases as a cause of death (Murray and Lopez 1997). Even allowing for the uncertainties of predicting future disease patterns posed by the unfolding of the human immunodeficiency virus (HIV) epidemic in Sub-Saharan Africa, it is clear that the relative importance of noncommunicable diseases will increase (Panz and Joffe 1999). This situation is a result of demographic change (populations with older age structures), increasing urbanization (WHO 1998), and associated changes in risk-factor levels, such as tobacco smoking, obesity, and physical inactivity (Hunter et al. 2000; Kaufman et al. 1999; Pavan et al. 1997). Countries of Sub-Saharan Africa are in various stages of the epidemiological transition with a multiple burden of diseases.

The available evidence suggests that noncommunicable diseases currently contribute substantially to the burden of mortality and morbidity in adults. Age-specific levels of diabetes and hypertension in many urban areas of Sub-Saharan Africa are as high as, or higher than, those in most Western European countries (Aspray et al. 2000; Edwards et al. 2000; Mollentze et al. 1995). In a demographic surveillance system in Tanzania they account for between one in six and one in three adult deaths (Kitange et al. 1996; Setel et al. 2000; Walker et al. 2000), with age-specific death rates from nonspecific, noncommunicable diseases being as high or higher than in developed countries (Unwin et al. 1999).

Diabetes mellitus can be classified into four principal types (WHO 1999). This includes type 1 diabetes, type 2 diabetes, other specific types of diabetes, and gestational diabetes mellitus. The most common types of diabetes seen in Sub-Saharan Africa are type 2 and type 1 diabetes mellitus.

This chapter focuses on the published data on the burden of type 1 and type 2 diabetes in Sub-Saharan Africa. Although type 1 diabetes is not caused by the adverse effects of lifestyle, as type 2 can be, the chronic complications of both type 1 and type 2 diabetes on the eyes, cardiovascular system, nerves, and kidneys are similar.

SOURCES OF DATA

The data search was limited to studies published after 1979, because data collected before 1980 may no longer reflect the current prevalence of diabetes. The Medline database and the Internet were used for the literature search, but also diabetes researchers and clinicians were asked to provide information on the burden of diabetes for their Sub-Saharan Africa country or subregion. The Medline search was undertaken for diabetes prevalence and for each complication: retinopathy, neuropathy, nephropathy, and so on. In the absence of data from any country, data were extrapolated from the socioeconomically, ethnically, and geographically most similar country. The data obtained were from prevalence studies, hospital-based studies, registry reports, hospital statistics, government estimates, and the like. Some of the specific data sources are mentioned in table 19.1. The sources of data for the 2003 estimates of diabetes mellitus and IGT are listed in table 19.2.

There is still a dearth of published studies describing the burden of diabetes in Sub-Saharan Africa. The prevalence

Table 19.1 Data Sources for the Prevalence of Type 2 Diabetes and IGT, by Year of Study

| Country, locality | Data sources | Year | Urban-rural | Age group (yrs) | N | Prevalence (%) | |
						DM	IGT
Tanzania	Ahren and Corrigan	1984	U and R	≥20	3,145	0.7	—
Kahalanga			R		996	0.5	—
Ndolage			R		1,141	2.5	—
Mwanza			U		1,008	1.9	—
Mali	Fisch et al.	1987	R	>15	7,472	0.9	—
Togo	Teuscher et al.	1987	R	>1	1,381	0.0	—
Nigeria	Ohwovoriole, Kuti, and Kabiawu	1988	U	—	1,627	1.7	—
Tanzania	McLarty et al.	1989	R	≥15	6,097	0.9	7.8
						1.1	8.4[a]
South Africa							
Cape Town	Levitt et al.	1993	U	>30	729	6.3	5.9
						8.0[a]	7.0[a]
Durban	Omar et al.	1993	U	>15	479	4.2	6.9
						5.3[a]	7.7[a]
Mangaung, OFS	Mollentze et al.	1995	U	≥25	758	6.0[a]	12.2[a]
Qwa-Qwa, OFS			R		853	4.8[a]	10.7[a]
Mauritania	Ducorps et al.	1996	U and R	>17	744	1.88	—
Cameroon	Mbanya et al.	1997	U and R	24–74	1,767	1.1	2.7
Yaoundé			U		1,048	1.3	1.8
Evodoula			R		719	0.8	3.9
Nigeria	Cooper et al.	1997	R	25–74	247	2.8	—
Tanzania	Aspray et al.	2000	U and R	≥15			
Dar es Salaam			U		770	—	—
Kilimanjaro			R		928	—	—
Ghana	Amoah, Owusu, and Adjei	2002	U	>25	4,733	6.3	10.7[a]
						6.4[a]	

Source: Authors, from data sources in table.

Note: The studies were published using the WHO 1980, 1985, or 1999 criteria. DM = diabetes mellitus (type 2 diabetes); IGT = impaired glucose tolerance; — = not available; OFS = Orange Free State.

a. Age-adjusted rates.

Table 19.2 Data Sources for Prevalence Estimates of Diabetes Mellitus and IGT, by Country, 2003

Country	Data sources	Screening method	Diagnostic criteria	Sample size	Age
Angola[a]	McLarty et al. 1989 and Aspray et al. 2000 (Tanzania)	OGTT/FBG	WHO, 1985 and 1999	7,781	15+
Benin[b]	Mbanya et al. 1997 (Cameroon) and Amoah, Owusu, and Adjei 2002 (Ghana)	OGTT	WHO, 1985 and 1999	6,500	24+
Botswana[c]	Omar et al. 1993 and Levitt et al. 1993 (South Africa)	OGTT	WHO, 1985	1,208	15+
Burkina Faso[b]	Mbanya et al. 1997 (Cameroon) and Amoah, Owusu, and Adjei 2002 (Ghana)	OGTT	WHO, 1985 and 1999	6,500	24+
Burundi[a]	McLarty et al. 1989 and Aspray et al. 2000 (Tanzania)	OGTT/FBG	WHO, 1985 and 1999	7,781	15+
Cameroon	Mbanya et al. 1997 (Cameroon)	OGTT/FBG	WHO, 1985	1,767	24–74
Cape Verde[b]	Mbanya et al. 1997 (Cameroon) and Amoah, Owusu, and Adjei 2002 (Ghana)	OGTT	WHO, 1985 and 1999	6,500	24+
Central African Republic[a]	Mbanya et al. 1997 (Cameroon) and Amoah, Owusu, and Adjei 2002 (Ghana)	OGTT	WHO, 1985 and 1999	6,500	24+
Chad	Elbagir et al. 1996 (Sudan)	2BG	WHO, 1985	1,284	25–84
Comoros	McLarty et al. 1989 and Aspray et al. 2000 (Tanzania)	OGTT/FBG	WHO, 1985 and 1999	7,781	15+
Congo, Dem. Rep. of[a]	McLarty et al. 1989 and Aspray et al. 2000 (Tanzania)	OGTT/FBG	WHO, 1985 and 1999	7,781	15+
Congo, Rep. of[a]	Mbanya et al. 1997 (Cameroon) and Amoah, Owusu, and Adjei 2002 (Ghana)	OGTT	WHO, 1985 and 1999	6,500	24+
Côte d'Ivoire	Mbanya et al. 1997 (Cameroon) and Amoah, Owusu, and Adjei 2002 (Ghana)	OGTT	WHO, 1985 and 1999	6,500	24+
Djibouti	Elbagir et al. 1996 (Sudan)	2BG	WHO, 1985	1,284	25–84
Equatorial Guinea[b]	Mbanya et al. 1997 (Cameroon) and Amoah, Owusu, and Adjei 2002 (Ghana)	OGTT	WHO, 1985 and 1999	6,500	24+
Eritrea[a]	McLarty et al. 1989 and Aspray et al. 2000 (Tanzania)	OGTT/FBG	WHO, 1985 and 1999	7,781	15+
Ethiopia	McLarty et al. 1989 and Aspray et al. 2000 (Tanzania)	OGTT/FBG	WHO, 1985 and 1999	7,781	15+
Gabon[b]	Mbanya et al. 1997 (Cameroon) and Amoah, Owusu, and Adjei 2002 (Ghana)	OGTT	WHO, 1985 and 1999	6,500	24+
Gambia, The[b]	Mbanya et al. 1997 (Cameroon) and Amoah, Owusu, and Adjei 2002 (Ghana)	OGTT	WHO, 1985 and 1999	6,500	24+
Ghana	Amoah, Owusu, and Adjei 2002 (Ghana)	OGTT	WHO, 1999	4,733	25+
Guinea[b]	Mbanya et al. 1997 (Cameroon) and Amoah, Owusu, and Adjei 2002 (Ghana)	OGTT	WHO, 1985 and 1999	6,500	24+
Guinea-Bissau[b]	Mbanya et al. 1997 (Cameroon) and Amoah, Owusu, and Adjei 2002 (Ghana)	OGTT	WHO, 1985 and 1999	6,500	24+
Kenya[a]	McLarty et al. 1989 and Aspray et al. 2000 (Tanzania)	OGTT/FBG	WHO, 1985 and 1999	7,781	15+
Lesotho[c]	Omar et al. 1993 and Levitt et al. 1993 (South Africa)	OGTT	WHO, 1985	1,208	15+
Liberia[b]	Mbanya et al. 1997 (Cameroon) and Amoah, Owusu, and Adjei 2002 (Ghana)	OGTT	WHO, 1985 and 1999	6,500	24+
Madagascar[a]	McLarty et al. 1989 and Aspray et al. 2000 (Tanzania)	OGTT/FBG	WHO, 1985 and 1999	7,781	15+
Malawi[a]	McLarty et al. 1989 and Aspray et al. 2000 (Tanzania)	OGTT/FBG	WHO, 1985 and 1999	7,781	15+
Mali[b]	Mbanya et al. 1997 (Cameroon) and Amoah, Owusu, and Adjei 2002 (Ghana)	OGTT	WHO, 1985 and 1999	6,500	24+
Mauritania	Elbagir et al. 1996 (Sudan)	2BG	WHO, 1985	1,284	25–84
Mozambique[a]	McLarty et al. 1989 and Aspray et al. 2000 (Tanzania)	OGTT/FBG	WHO, 1985 and 1999	7,781	15+
Namibia[c]	Omar et al. 1993 and Levitt et al. 1993 (South Africa)	OGTT	WHO, 1985	1,208	15+
Niger[b]	Mbanya et al. 1997 (Cameroon) and Amoah, Owusu, and Adjei 2002 (Ghana)	OGTT	WHO, 1985 and 1999	6,500	24+

(Continues on the following page.)

Table 19.2 *(Continued)*

Country	Data sources	Screening method	Diagnostic criteria	Sample size	Age
Nigeria[b]	Mbanya et al. 1997 (Cameroon) and Amoah, Owusu, and Adjei 2002 (Ghana)	OGTT	WHO, 1985 and 1999	6,500	24+
Réunion	Dowse et al. 1990 (Mauritius)	OGTT	WHO, 1985	4,929	25–74
Rwanda[a]	McLarty et al. 1989 and Aspray et al. 2000 (Tanzania)	OGTT/FBG	WHO, 1985 and 1999	7,781	15+
São Tomé and Principe[b]	Mbanya et al. 1997 (Cameroon) and Amoah, Owusu, and Adjei 2002 (Ghana)	OGTT	WHO, 1985 and 1999	6,500	24+
Senegal[b]	Mbanya et al. 1997 (Cameroon) and Amoah, Owusu, and Adjei 2002 (Ghana)	OGTT	WHO, 1985 and 1999	6,500	24+
Seychelles	Dowse et al. 1990 (Mauritius)	OGTT	WHO, 1985	4,929	25–74
Sierra Leone[b]	Mbanya et al. 1997 (Cameroon) and Amoah, Owusu, and Adjei 2002 (Ghana)	OGTT	WHO, 1985 and 1999	6,500	24+
Somalia[a]	McLarty et al. 1989 and Aspray et al. 2000 (Tanzania)	OGTT/FBG	WHO, 1985 and 1999	7,781	15+
South Africa[c]	Omar et al. 1993 and Levitt et al. 1993 (South Africa)	OGTT	WHO, 1985	1,208	15+
Swaziland[c]	Omar et al. 1993 and Levitt et al. 1993 (South Africa)	OGTT	WHO, 1985	1,208	15+
Tanzania[a]	McLarty et al. 1989 and Aspray et al. 2000 (Tanzania)	OGTT/FBG	WHO, 1985 and 1999	7,781	15+
Togo[b]	Mbanya et al. 1997 (Cameroon) and Amoah, Owusu, and Adjei 2002 (Ghana)	OGTT	WHO, 1985 and 1999	6,500	24+
Uganda[a]	McLarty et al. 1989 and Aspray et al. 2000 (Tanzania)	OGTT/FBG	WHO, 1985 and 1999	7,781	15+
Western Sahara	Elbagir et al. 1996 (Sudan)	2BG	WHO, 1985	1,284	25–84
Zambia[a]	McLarty et al. 1989 and Aspray et al. 2000 (Tanzania)	OGTT/FBG	WHO, 1985 and 1999	7,781	15+
Zimbabwe[a]	Omar et al. 1993 and Levitt et al. 1993 (South Africa)	OGTT	WHO, 1985	1,208	15+

Source: Adapted with permission from IDF 2003.

Note: See note for table 19.1; OGTT = oral glucose tolerance test; FBG = fasting blood glucose; 2BG = 2 hours blood glucose.

a. The prevalence was calculated after the combination of the data of the two studies, notwithstanding the different criteria. IGT figures were calculated from the McLarty et al. 1989 data, as the Aspray et al. 2000 study used only the FBG criteria.

b. The prevalence was calculated as the average of the two studies, as their sample sizes differed considerably.

c. The prevalence was calculated after the combination of the data of the two studies. IGT figures were based only on the study of Omar et al. 1993.

rates of diabetes and its complications (table 19.3) have been drawn from the few country data available as applied to the population distribution of that country or a similar country. Clinic-based studies have serious limitations, so their generalizability is limited. Therefore the data presented here are only general indicators of diabetes frequency and should be interpreted with caution. As new and better epidemiological data become available, it will be possible to have actual rates of diabetes in Sub-Saharan Africa.

EPIDEMIOLOGY OF DIABETES

Diabetes mellitus is a chronic metabolic disease characterized by hyperglycemia resulting from defects in insulin secretion, insulin action, or both. Uncontrolled chronic hyperglycemia results in long-term damage, particular dysfunction, and failure of the eyes, heart, blood vessels, nerves, and kidneys.

Type 1 diabetes results from autoimmune destruction of the pancreatic beta cells, causing the loss of insulin production. Children are usually affected by this type of diabetes, although it occurs at all ages and the clinical presentation can vary with age. Patients with this type of diabetes require insulin for survival.

Type 2 diabetes is characterized by insulin resistance and abnormal insulin secretion, either of which may predominate but both of which are usually present. The specific reasons for the development of these abnormalities are largely unknown. Type 2 is the most common type of diabetes. Type 2 diabetes can remain asymptomatic for many years, and the diagnosis is often made from associated complications or incidentally through an abnormal blood or urine glucose test.

Other specific types of diabetes include those due to genetic disorders, infections, diseases of the exocrine pancreas, endocrinopathies, and drugs. This last type of diabetes is relatively uncommon.

Table 19.3 Data Sources for the Prevalence of Diabetes Complications, by Disease and Year

Year	Data source	Country	Study type	Prevalence (%)
Retinopathy				
1988	Rolfe	Zambia	Clinic (secondary care)	34
1993	Lester	Ethiopia	Clinic (secondary care)	13
1995	Gill, Huddle, and Rolfe	South Africa	Clinic (secondary care)	52
1995	Moukouri et al.	Cameroon	Clinic (secondary care)	37
1996	Drabo, Kabore, and Lengani	Burkina Faso	Clinic (secondary care)	16
1997	Kalk et al.	South Africa	Clinic (secondary care)	37
1997	Levitt et al.	South Africa	Clinic (primary care)	55
1997	Rahlenbeck and Gebre-Yohannes	Ethiopia	Clinic (secondary care)	36
1999	Sobngwi et al.	Cameroon	Clinic (secondary care)	37
Nephropathy				
1996	Drabo, Kabore, and Lengani	Burkina Faso	Clinic (secondary care)	25
1997	Levitt et al.	South Africa	Clinic (primary care)	37
1997	Rahlenbeck and Gebre-Yohannes	Ethiopia	Clinic (secondary care)	33
1999	Sobngwi et al.	Cameroon	Clinic (secondary care)	46[a]
Neuropathy				
1991	Lester	Ethiopia	Clinic (secondary care)	36
1995	Gill, Huddle, and Rolfe	South Africa	Clinic (secondary care)	42
1997	Levitt et al.	South Africa	Clinic (primary care)	28
1988	Rolfe	Zambia	Clinic (secondary care)	31
Vascular disease, lower limbs				
1994	Niang et al.	Senegal	Clinic (secondary care)	28
1997	Levitt et al.	South Africa	Clinic (primary care)	—
Coronary artery disease				
1996	Drabo, Kabore, and Lengani	Burkina Faso	Clinic (secondary care)	28
1996	Nambuya et al.	Uganda	Clinic (secondary care)	5
1988	Rolfe	Zambia	Clinic (secondary care)	1

Source: Authors.
Note: — = not available.
a. Microalbuminuria.

Gestational diabetes mellitus (GDM) is defined as any degree of glucose intolerance with onset or first recognition during pregnancy. The definition applies whether insulin or only diet modification is used for treatment and whether the condition persists after pregnancy. It does not exclude the possibility that unrecognized glucose intolerance may have antedated or begun concomitantly with the pregnancy. Approximately 7 percent of all pregnancies are complicated by GDM. The prevalence may range from 1 to 14 percent of all pregnancies, depending on the population studied and the diagnostic tests employed.

Impaired glucose tolerance (IGT) is asymptomatic, and its diagnosis is confirmed by an elevated nondiabetic level of blood glucose two hours after a 75 gram oral glucose tolerance test. Impaired fasting glycemia (IFG) is an elevated nondiabetic fasting blood glucose level. Both IGT and IFG are transitional stages in the development of type 2 diabetes.

PREVALENCE AND INCIDENCE OF TYPE 1 DIABETES

There is a dearth of published studies describing the incidence and prevalence of type 1 diabetes in Sub-Saharan Africa. Type 1 diabetes is considerably rarer than type 2 disease, and large populations need to be surveyed. Also, to assess incidence, the population surveyed should be accurately known, and this is in itself difficult, as complete censuses in Africa are rare and migration in and out of study areas common. Elamin and colleagues in the Sudan in 1992 reported a survey of nearly 43,000 schoolchildren (age 7 to 11 years) and found a prevalence rate of 0.95 per 1,000 (Elamin et al. 1992). This rate is comparable to a reported prevalence rate of 0.3 per 1,000 in Nigeria (Afoke et al. 1992). The reported incidence is 10.1 per 100,000 children per year in Sudan (Elamin et al. 1992) and 1.5 per 100,000 per year in Tanzania (Swai, Lutale, and McLarty 1993). The discrepancy between the Sudanese and Tanzanian studies may be explained by ethnic differences, and perhaps problems related to the design of the studies.

The question of whether type 1 diabetes is truly rarer in Africa than elsewhere remains unsettled, and more detailed surveys are needed. Nonetheless, it emerges from careful clinic studies that the behavior of type 1 diabetes is different in Sub-Saharan Africa from that in the rest of the world. Studies indicate that the age of onset in South Africa and Ethiopia is later than elsewhere (Kalk, Huddle, and Raal 1993; Lester 1984), and the peak age of onset of type 1 diabetes in Sub-Saharan Africa is a decade later than in the West (Afoke et al. 1992; Kalk, Huddle, and Raal 1993). In addition it afflicts more females than males. In South Africa it has been reported that the peak age of onset was about 13 years in the white South Africans (similar to Europeans) but about 23 years in the black South Africans (Kalk, Huddle, and Raal 1993). The reasons for this difference are obscure, although it has been suggested that prolonged breastfeeding, which is common in Africa, may be reducing the incidence and delaying the onset of type 1 diabetes. Early introduction of cow's milk protein does seem to be a risk factor for the later development of type 1 diabetes, possibly because, in neonates, bovine albumin can raise antibodies that mimic islet cell antibodies and attack pancreatic beta cells. This is, of course, speculative, and much still remains unknown about the pathogenesis and epidemiology of type 1 diabetes in Africa.

Genetic Factors

More than 90 percent of type 1 diabetes subjects in Sub-Saharan Africa, as in the rest of the world, have one or both human leukocyte antigens (HLA) DR3 and DR4. However, there appear to be specificities in the HLA susceptibility found in certain African populations. Recent studies using allele-specific (oligonucleotide) probes from Zimbabwe, Senegal, and Cameroon show positive and negative associations with some alleles (Garcia-Pacheco et al. 1992; Chauffert et al. 1995).

Immunological Factors

The main markers of immune islet cell attack are islet cell antibodies (ICA) and glutamic acid decarboxylase antibodies (anti-GAD). These substances are found in most Caucasian type 1 diabetic patients at diagnosis, but levels gradually decline with time. Interpretation of ICA and anti-GAD levels in type 1 diabetes is dependent on duration of disease, and this may explain the variable results found in the limited African studies so far carried out. McLarty, Kinabo, and Swai (1990) found that the prevalence of ICA antibodies was only 8 to 11 percent in newly diagnosed Tanzanian patients. In South Africa, Motala, Omar, and Pirie (2000) found that 44 percent of blacks with newly diagnosed type 1 diabetes were positive for GAD antibody. It appears from these preliminary results that the genetic susceptibility and risk factors for type 1 diabetes in Sub-Saharan Africa may be different from those in the Western world. It can be speculated that non-autoimmune factors are the major determinants of type 1 diabetes in Sub-Saharan Africa.

Environmental Factors

An environmental "trigger" factor for the onset of type 1 diabetes has long been sought. Its existence is supported by the well-known seasonality of presentation in Europe, and viral infection (perhaps of the coxsackievirus group) is considered a likely candidate. A seasonality of type 1 diabetes has been reported in Tanzania (with most cases presenting between August and November) (McLarty, Yusafai, and Swai 1989). It would therefore seem likely that potential viral triggers operate also in the rest of Africa.

PREVALENCE OF TYPE 2 DIABETES

Before the 1990s, diabetes was considered a rare medical condition in Africa. Epidemiological studies carried out in that decade, however, provided evidence of a trend toward increased incidence and prevalence of type 2 diabetes in African populations (Sobngwi et al. 2001). Indeed, Africa is experiencing the most rapid demographic and epidemiological transition in world history (Mosley, Bobadilla, and Jamison 1993). It is characterized by a tremendous rise in the burden of noncommunicable diseases (NCDs), underlined by the increasing life expectancy and lifestyle changes resulting from the reduction in infectious diseases and increased fertility, as well as Westernization.

Almost all the reports published between 1959 and 1985 showed a prevalence of diabetes below 1.4 percent, except those from South Africa, where higher prevalence was reported. Differences in diagnostic methods and criteria, however, made comparison between countries difficult. Since then, uniform diagnostic criteria has become more available, allowing comparison across countries. Epidemiological studies carried out during this period show the rising prevalence of diabetes all over Africa (table 19.2).

The prevalence of diabetes in Africa was approximately 3 million in 1994; but the region is due to experience a two- to threefold increase by the year 2010 (Amos, McCarty, and Zimmet 1997). The highest prevalence is found in populations of Indian origin, followed by black populations and Caucasians. Among the population of Indian origin in South Africa and Tanzania, the prevalence is between 12 and 13 percent (Ramaiya, Swai, McLarty, and Alberti 1991). The prevalence in blacks follows a Westernization gradient, with that of rural Africa generally below 1 percent but that of urban Africa between 1 and 6 percent. In general the prevalence of type 2 diabetes is low in both rural and urban communities of West Africa except in urban Ghana, where a high rate of 6.3 percent was recently reported (Amoah, Owusu, and Adjei 2002). Moderate rates have been reported from South Africa: 4.8 percent in a semi-urban community in the Orange Free State, 6.0 percent in an urban community of the Orange Free State, 5.5 percent in Durban (mostly occupied by the Zulu tribe), and 8 percent in Cape Town (mostly occupied by the Xhosa tribe). Also, moderate rates have been reported in studies from Tanzania (table 19.1).

Estimates of the Prevalence of Type 2 Diabetes and IGT in 2003

There are marked discrepancies between the prevalence of diabetes among different communities in Sub-Saharan Africa. The studies from Tanzania (Aspray et al. 2000; McLarty et al. 1989), showing an urban-to-rural ratio of five to one, and from Cameroon (Mbanya et al. 1997), with a ratio of two to one, both confirm the urban-rural discrepancy in diabetes prevalence and suggest the consequent likely increases because of urban migration. The data used for the extrapolation of current prevalence rates (table 19.2) in distant and probably dissimilar countries and populations indicate the great need for more epidemiological

investigations in Sub-Saharan Africa. Such a need is dictated by the prevalence of undiagnosed diabetes, which accounted for 60 percent of those with diabetes in Cameroon (Mbanya et al. 1997), 70 percent in Ghana (Amoah, Owusu, and Adjei 2002), and over 80 percent in the recent study in Tanzania (Aspray et al. 2000). It would therefore appear that in Sub-Saharan Africa, for every diagnosed person with diabetes, there are one to three undiagnosed cases.

The International Diabetes Federation estimated that in 2003 the number of people age 20 to 79 years with diabetes in Sub-Saharan Africa was over 7 million for a population of more than 295 million, giving a prevalence rate of 2.4 percent. About 65 percent of those affected with diabetes lived in the urban areas, whereas 35 percent lived in the rural communities. More than 46 percent (3.3 million) of the diabetic population were 40 to 59 years old, whereas 28 percent and 26 percent, respectively, were 20 to 39 and 60 to 79 years old (table 19.4). This has serious implications for the productivity of the region, since diabetes affects the active members of the community. The top five countries with the highest number of people affected by diabetes in Sub-Saharan Africa are Nigeria (about 1.2 million people), South Africa (841,000), the Democratic Republic of Congo (552,000), Ethiopia (550,000), and Tanzania (380,000) (table 19.4).

The impact of type 2 diabetes is bound to continue if nothing is done to curb the rising prevalence of IGT, which now varies between 2.2 percent and 16.2 percent. The estimated prevalence rate of IGT in 2003 for Sub-Saharan Africa is 7.3 percent with a total population of affected individuals of over 21 million (table 19.5). Some 70 percent of these individuals are expected to develop type 2 diabetes unless something is done to reduce the risk factors associated with the development of the disease.

The projections of type 2 diabetes and IGT from 2003 to 2025 are shown in table 19.6. It is estimated that the burden of diabetes and IGT will just about double in 2025 from their 2003 levels. The rate at which new cases of diabetes are emerging poses an additional burden on countries already stretched to the limit by common life-threatening infections, such as malaria, tuberculosis, and HIV and acquired immune deficiency syndrome (AIDS).

Risk Factors for Type 2 Diabetes

There are marked differences between diabetic and nondiabetic individuals in the prevalence of some risk factors for diabetes and its complications, notably anthropometric

Table 19.4 Prevalence Estimates of Diabetes Mellitus, by Country, 2003

| Country | Population age (20–79) (thousands) | DM prevalence (%) | Number of people with DM age 20–79 (thousands) | | | | | | | |
			Rural	Urban	Male	Female	Age 20–39	Age 40–59	Age 60–79	Total
Angola	5,846	2.7	33.1	123.7	84.0	72.8	51.6	69.5	35.8	156.8
Benin	2,911	2.1	23.6	38.9	32.7	29.8	19.0	28.1	15.5	62.5
Botswana	716	3.6	3.2	22.3	8.8	16.7	4.1	13.9	7.5	25.5
Burkina Faso	4,969	2.7	90.4	44.8	67.8	67.4	40.1	55.2	40.0	135.3
Burundi	2,860	1.3	22.0	16.0	19.4	18.6	12.6	15.6	9.8	38.0
Cameroon	7,278	0.8	19.5	38.9	23.9	34.5	9.4	42.3	6.7	58.4
Cape Verde	228	2.3	1.1	4.2	2.2	3.1	2.0	1.7	1.7	5.3
Central African Republic	1,780	2.3	16.3	25.0	21.1	20.2	10.7	17.6	13.0	41.3
Chad	3,674	2.7	60.7	39.9	39.1	61.5	12.2	54.5	33.9	100.6
Comoros	355	2.5	1.9	7.0	4.8	4.1	3.2	3.9	1.8	8.9
Congo, Dem. Rep. of	22,436	2.5	136.6	415.4	294.7	257.3	182.3	237.4	132.3	552.0
Congo, Rep. of	1,403	2.6	7.6	28.3	18.4	17.6	10.5	15.2	10.3	35.9
Côte d'Ivoire	7,959	2.3	63.9	121.9	107.3	78.6	51.4	83.0	51.5	185.8
Djibouti	300	4.9	1.3	13.5	4.8	9.9	1.3	8.3	5.2	14.8
Equatorial Guinea	226	2.5	1.8	3.8	2.9	2.7	1.5	2.5	1.7	5.6
Eritrea	1,906	1.9	13.6	22.7	19.7	16.6	11.8	15.6	8.8	36.2
Ethiopia	29,562	1.9	214.6	335.8	299.4	250.9	176.6	234.9	138.8	550.4
Gabon	647	2.9	5.0	13.9	9.9	9.0	4.0	8.1	6.8	18.9
Gambia, The	703	2.2	7.4	8.0	8.3	7.0	4.1	7.2	4.0	15.4
Ghana	9,986	3.3	143.8	190.2	185.0	149.0	93.4	152.8	87.8	334.0
Guinea	3,855	2.0	37.6	41.2	42.8	36.0	23.3	35.5	20.1	78.9
Guinea-Bissau	588	2.0	7.0	4.8	6.3	5.5	3.1	5.2	3.5	11.8
Kenya	14,604	2.5	78.1	281.5	193.6	166.0	133.7	152.3	73.5	359.6
Lesotho	1,040	3.1	17.3	14.8	12.3	19.8	4.2	17.6	10.4	32.1
Liberia	1,573	2.0	10.5	21.3	17.0	14.8	11.6	11.6	8.6	31.8
Madagascar	7,782	2.5	47.3	144.6	104.3	87.5	63.2	85.5	43.2	191.9
Malawi	5,131	1.7	38.0	49.3	46.6	40.6	28.8	35.5	23.0	87.2
Mali	5,231	2.0	54.4	52.5	55.8	81.1	30.7	42.6	33.6	106.9
Mauritania	1,309	3.5	11.4	34.6	18.0	28.0	5.6	26.1	14.3	46.0
Mozambique	8,681	3.1	44.9	221.6	142.4	124.1	86.0	118.8	61.6	266.5
Namibia	831	3.1	10.1	15.4	9.5	16.0	3.9	13.6	8.0	25.5
Niger	4,728	3.1	36.4	110.3	57.7	89.0	20.8	83.9	41.9	146.7
Nigeria	54,248	2.2	439.3	779.4	655.4	563.3	354.5	528.9	335.3	1,218.7
Réunion[a]	474	13.1	10.0	51.9	29.1	32.8	11.2	29.7	21.0	61.9
Rwanda	3,645	1.1	28.3	13.1	22.7	18.7	15.2	14.7	11.4	41.4
São Tomé and Principe[b]	107	2.8	1.0	1.9	1.6	1.4	0.6	1.3	1.0	2.9
Senegal	4,607	2.3	34.9	68.9	54.7	49.0	31.3	46.8	25.6	103.7
Seychelles[a,b]	49	12.3	1.5	4.5	2.9	3.0	1.0	2.9	2.0	6.0
Sierra Leone	2,268	2.2	21.3	27.6	25.7	23.2	14.0	21.8	13.1	48.9
Somalia	4,086	2.3	24.5	67.5	49.6	42.4	32.2	40.5	19.3	92.0
South Africa	24,741	3.4	272.1	569.1	322.7	518.5	127.1	489.6	224.5	841.2
Swaziland	450	3.0	6.0	7.4	5.2	8.2	2.0	7.4	3.9	13.4
Tanzania	16,616	2.3	98.1	281.0	203.4	175.7	134.9	163.9	80.3	379.1
Togo	2,196	2.1	21.4	23.7	23.9	21.2	13.2	19.4	12.5	45.1
Uganda	10,018	1.5	71.0	83.9	84.9	70.0	56.7	60.7	37.5	154.9
Zambia	4,625	3.0	21.8	118.2	76.1	64.0	49.2	59.1	31.8	140.1
Zimbabwe	5,686	2.6	68.2	80.5	59.0	89.7	24.7	79.7	44.3	148.7
Total	295,065	2.4	2,380	4,692	3,580	3,491	1,985	3,265	1,821	7,072

Source: Adapted with permission from IDF 2003.
Note: The total may not be the exact sum of the column due to the rounding.
a. Réunion and the Seychelles were deemed to have the same ethnicity and distribution as Mauritius.
b. Population number as described in the CIA *World Factbook 2002*, with age distribution adjustment to that of the world population in 2003.

Table 19.5 Prevalence Estimates of IGT, by Country, 2003

Country	Population age (20–79) (thousands)	IGT prevalence (%)	Number of people with IGT age 20–79 (thousands)					
			Male	Female	Age 20–39	Age 40–59	Age 60–79	Total
Angola	5,846	7.5	190.2	251.0	193.9	152.4	95.0	441.2
Benin	2,911	6.9	99.3	102.7	82.9	77.5	41.5	202.0
Botswana	716	7.0	31.4	18.9	15.3	12.3	22.7	50.3
Burkina Faso	4,969	7.0	156.8	189.3	144.6	113.2	88.3	346.1
Burundi	2,860	7.5	96.2	127.0	94.4	76.5	42.4	213.2
Cameroon	7,278	2.2	104.5	56.4	23.9	86.4	50.6	161.0
Cape Verde	228	6.8	6.2	9.2	7.2	4.2	4.0	15.4
Central African Republic	1,780	7.4	63.0	69.2	47.3	49.2	35.7	132.3
Chad	3,674	2.3	29.9	53.5	21.0	38.5	23.9	83.4
Comoros	355	7.3	11.3	14.7	12.4	8.7	4.9	26.0
Congo, Dem. Rep. of	22,436	7.6	729.1	966.7	746.0	572.8	377.0	1,695.8
Congo, Rep. of	1,403	7.2	48.7	51.7	39.5	36.5	24.4	100.4
Côte d'Ivoire	7,959	7.2	308.9	262.6	219.2	219.5	132.8	571.5
Djibouti	300	2.6	2.3	5.6	1.5	3.9	2.5	7.9
Equatorial Guinea	226	7.5	8.3	8.6	6.0	6.4	4.4	16.8
Eritrea	1,906	7.6	62.6	82.0	62.7	51.5	30.3	144.6
Ethiopia	29,562	7.6	978.6	1,270.7	966.5	796.1	486.7	2,249.3
Gabon	647	8.1	25.7	26.7	15.5	20.1	16.8	52.5
Gambia, The	703	7.4	26.0	25.8	18.9	21.5	11.5	51.9
Ghana	9,986	12.0	564.8	636.3	529.4	409.1	262.6	1,201.1
Guinea	3,855	7.0	137.9	133.9	109.0	104.9	57.8	271.7
Guinea-Bissau	588	7.4	21.4	22.0	15.9	16.7	10.8	43.4
Kenya	14,604	7.2	461.0	592.7	514.6	338.9	200.2	1,053.7
Lesotho	1,040	8.5	58.7	30.1	19.7	22.5	46.5	88.8
Liberia	1,573	6.5	52.0	50.6	49.8	30.4	22.4	102.7
Madagascar	7,782	7.5	256.3	331.0	257.2	207.1	122.9	587.3
Malawi	5,131	7.5	166.1	221.0	170.5	131.6	85.0	387.2
Mali	5,231	7.2	183.2	193.8	148.2	129.0	99.9	377.1
Mauritania	1,309	2.3	10.8	18.9	7.5	14.3	7.9	29.7
Mozambique	8,681	7.6	286.0	376.5	284.6	228.3	149.6	622.5
Namibia	831	8.0	43.3	22.9	17.0	15.4	33.7	66.1
Niger	4,728	6.7	160.8	157.1	140.8	117.7	59.4	318.0
Nigeria	54,248	7.1	1,947.9	1,900.5	1,527.5	1,432.8	888.1	3,848.4
Réunion[a]	474	16.2	29.2	47.6	29.2	31.0	16.6	76.8
Rwanda	3,645	7.2	114.7	149.5	128.5	83.3	52.4	264.2
São Tomé and Principe[b]	107	8.1	4.3	4.3	2.6	3.5	2.6	8.7
Senegal	4,607	7.0	160.5	162.2	131.1	124.7	55.9	322.7
Seychelles[a,b]	49	16.1	3.2	4.7	2.9	3.2	1.7	7.9
Sierra Leone	2,268	7.2	79.8	82.8	63.2	62.5	36.9	162.6
Somalia	4,086	7.4	129.9	171.1	139.6	104.5	56.9	301.0
South Africa	24,741	7.2	1,201.8	573.4	498.6	553.8	722.8	1,775.2
Swaziland	450	7.8	23.4	11.7	9.1	8.9	17.0	35.1
Tanzania	16,616	7.3	525.5	694.8	574.2	413.1	233.1	1,220.3
Togo	2,196	7.1	77.1	78.5	62.1	57.4	36.1	155.6
Uganda	10,018	7.3	319.3	407.9	351.2	233.9	142.1	727.2
Zambia	4,625	7.4	151.4	189.5	158.8	107.2	74.9	340.9
Zimbabwe	5,686	7.2	285.0	124.2	126.9	99.6	182.6	409.2
Total	295,065	7.3	10,426	10,984	8,789	7,434	5,186	21,410

Source: Adapted with permission from IDF 2003.

Note: The totals may not be the exact sum of columns due to rounding.

a. Réunion and the Seychelles were deemed to have the same ethnicity and distribution as Mauritius.

b. Population number as described in the CIA *World Fact Book 2002*, with age distribution adjustment to that of the world population in 2003.

Table 19.6 Projections of Diabetes and IGT from 2003 to 2025 in the Age Group of 20 to 79 Years

All diabetes and IGT	2003	2025
Total population (millions)	666.6	1,107.4
Adult population (millions)	295.1	541.1
Diabetes prevalence (%)	2.4	2.8
Diabetes numbers (millions)	7.1	15.0
IGT prevalence (%)	7.3	7.3
IGT numbers (millions)	21.4	39.4

Source: Adapted with permission from IDF 2003.

variables, such as obesity. Although it is true that these data are from cross-sectional studies that have limitations in establishing causality, they at least support the hypothesis that increasing prevalence of diabetes can be attributed largely to changes in lifestyle resulting in reduced physical activity and increased calorie intake and subsequent weight gain. Such changes have important implications for the provision of health care and for health education to promote behavioral change in order to control the emergence of diabetes in Sub-Saharan Africa.

Age and Ethnicity. Age and ethnicity are the two main nonmodifiable risk factors of diabetes in Africa. Glucose intolerance in Sub-Saharan Africa, as in other regions of the world, increases with age in both men and women (figure 19.1); however, published studies lack uniformity on the age range in which the prevalence of diabetes is observed. According to King, Aubert, and Herman (1998), in most developed communities the peak of occurrence falls in the age group of 65 years or older, whereas in developing

Figure 19.1 Prevalence of Diabetes with Increasing Age in Cameroon

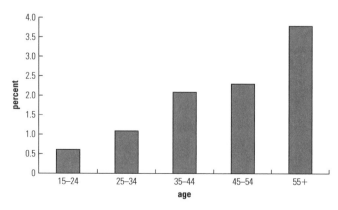

Source: Authors.

countries it is in the age group 45 to 64, and in Sub-Saharan Africa it is in the age groups 20 to 44 and 45 to 64 years. Yet data from 12 other studies from Sub-Saharan Africa indicate two peak age ranges of 45 to 64 and older than 65 years (see table 19.1 for references).

Two studies in Sub-Saharan Africa have examined ethnic differences in the prevalence of diabetes. A difference was found between Indians, blacks, and Caucasians in South Africa, where Indians had the highest predisposition and were followed by blacks and Caucasians (Levitt et al. 1999; Omar et al. 1994). In the Tanzanian study, the indigenous African population had lower diabetes prevalence than the migrant Asian group (1.1 percent as opposed to 9.1 to 7.1 percent) (McLarty et al. 1989; Ramaiya, Swai, McLarty, Bhopal, et al. 1991; Swai et al. 1990).

The prevalence of diabetes appears to be substantially higher in African-origin populations living abroad than in indigenous Africans. West Africans from Nigeria (Cooper et al. 1997) and central Africans from Cameroon (Mbanya et al. 1997) were compared with populations of West African origin in the Caribbean (Cooper et al. 1997; Mbanya et al. 1997), United Kingdom (Cooper et al. 1997; Mbanya et al. 1997), and the United States (Cooper et al. 1997). These studies suggest that environment determines diabetes prevalence in these populations of similar genetic origin.

Urban-Rural Differences. Residence seems to be a major determinant of diabetes in Sub-Saharan Africa, since urban residents have 1.5- to 4.0 times higher prevalence of diabetes than their rural counterparts. This is attributable to lifestyle changes associated with urbanization and Westernization. Urban lifestyle in Africa is characterized by changes in dietary habits involving an increase in the consumption of refined sugars and saturated fat and a reduction in fiber intake (Mennen et al. 2000). Sobngwi and colleagues (2002) have recently reported an increase in fasting plasma glucose in those whose lives have been spent in an urban environment, suggesting that both lifetime exposure to and recent migration to or current residence in an urban environment are potential risk factors for obesity and diabetes mellitus. The disease might represent the cumulative effects over years of dietary changes, decrease in physical activity, and psychological stress.

The population of Africa is predominantly rural, but the 1995–2000 urban growth rate was estimated at 4.3 percent (compared with 0.5 percent in Europe). Thus, more than 70 percent of the population of Africa will be urban residents by 2025 (UNFPA 2000). There will therefore be a tremendous increase in the prevalence of diabetes attributable to rapid urbanization. In addition, life expectancy at birth is rapidly increasing. For example, in Cameroon in 1960 it was about 35 years but in 1990 was raised to approximately 55 years. An increase in diabetes prevalence simply because of the change in the age structure of the population is therefore expected. However, the HIV pandemic may change these estimates and projections.

Family History of Diabetes. A significant proportion of the offspring of Cameroonians with type 2 diabetes have either type 2 diabetes (4 percent) or IGT (8 percent) (Mbanya et al. 2000). A positive family history seems to be an independent risk factor for diabetes, but this was not the case in the Cape Town study (Levitt et al. 1993), in which family history was not an independent risk factor.

Measure of Adiposity. Several studies from Sub-Saharan Africa have confirmed the association between the prevalence of diabetes and a surrogate of obesity, body mass index (BMI). Reports from Mali (Fisch et al. 1987), Nigeria (Cooper et al. 1997) and Tanzania (McLarty et al. 1989) have shown that the prevalence of diabetes increases with increasing BMI. BMI and obesity seem to be independent risk factors for diabetes (Levitt et al. 1993).

Physical Activity. There seems to be a significant relationship between physical inactivity and diabetes and obesity (Sobngwi et al. 2002). Physical activity is more common in rural than urban regions of Africa because rural populations rely on walking for transport and often have intense agricultural activities as their main occupation. In Sub-Saharan Africa, walking time and pace is drastically reduced (by factors of 2 to 4 for walking at a slow pace and 6 to more than 10 for walking at a brisk pace) in an urban community as compared with a rural community. The main difference in physical activity between the two types of community, however, is the use of walking in rural areas as a means of transportation.

The reduction in physical activity associated with life in a city partly explains the excess prevalence of obesity in urban areas. In a South African study, the prevalence of a sedentary lifestyle in Cape Town in subjects age 30 years and over was 39 percent for men and 44 percent for women (Omar et al. 1993). Low physical activity was normal for 22 percent of men and 52 percent of women in urban Tanzania, whereas it was usual for only 10 percent of men and 15 percent of women living in rural areas (Edwards et al. 2000). Cross-

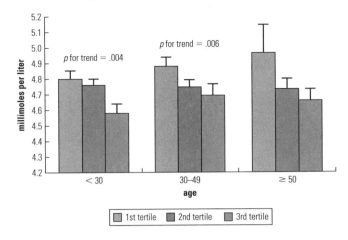

Figure 19.2 Mean Fasting Blood Glucose by Tertiles of Walking Energy Expenditure in Women: The Cameroon Study

Source: Adapted from Sobngwi, Gautier, and Mbanya 2003.

Note: Third p for trend value was not shown in the original article.

sectional data from 1,417 women age 15 to 83 years in a rural community and an urban community in Cameroon showed that in all age groups, fasting blood glucose levels were inversely associated with energy expenditure from walking (figure 19.2) (Sobngwi, Gautier, and Mbanya 2003). Rural dwellers' higher level of physical activity and related energy expenditure compared with urban subjects goes far to explain why obesity was found to be at least four times higher in urban areas than rural (Aspray et al. 2000). Thus, lack of physical activity appears to be a significant risk factor for diabetes in Sub-Saharan Africa.

COMPLICATIONS OF DIABETES

The escalating prevalence of type 1 and type 2 diabetes and their complications in Sub-Saharan Africa are a major drain on health resources in financially difficult circumstances, in addition to having a considerable physical and social impact on the individual and community.

Acute Complications of Diabetes

The three main metabolic complications of diabetes in Sub-Saharan Africa are diabetic ketoacidosis, hyperosmolar nonketotic coma, and hypoglycemia. Diabetic ketoacidosis is a common diabetic emergency in developing countries and carries with it relatively high mortality, ranging from 25 percent in Tanzania to 33 percent in Kenya. The major contributing factors to such high mortality are the chronic lack of availability of insulin, delays in seeking medical assistance by newly diagnosed type 1 patients presenting in ketoacidosis, misdiagnosis of diabetes, and poor health care in general and diabetic care in particular (Rwiza, Swai, and McLarty 1986).

Hyperosmolar nonketotic coma is usually a complication of type 2 diabetes and is less common and accounts for about 10 percent of all hyperglycemic emergencies in developing countries (Zouvanis et al. 1997). Infection is the leading precipitating factor for both diabetic ketoacidosis and hyperosmolar nonketotic coma, followed by first presentation of diabetes at a health institution and noncompliance with a medical regimen (Zouvanis et al. 1997). It carries a high mortality of up to 44 percent according to studies from South Africa, which may be because the patients are usually elderly and have other major illnesses (Rolfe et al. 1995).

Hypoglycemia is also a serious complication of treatment in patients with diabetes. Of a total of 51 episodes in 43 patients admitted at the Baragwanath Hospital, Johannesburg, South Africa, 14 cases (33 percent) were associated with sulfonylurea treatment. The major cause precipitating the event was a missed meal (36 percent), although alcohol (22 percent), gastrointestinal upset (20 percent), and inappropriate treatment (18 percent) were also important contributory factors (Gill and Huddle 1993). No mortality was associated with hypoglycemia in this study.

Chronic Complications of Diabetes

The seriousness of diabetes is largely a result of its associated complications, which can be serious, disabling, and even fatal. Prevalence studies on complications reported up to the early 1990s gave widely variable figures. These have been reviewed in two studies and include figures ranging from 9 to 16 percent for cataract, 7 to 52 percent for retinopathy, 6 to 47 percent for neuropathy, 6 to 30 percent for nephropathy, and 1 to 5 percent for macroangiopathy (Mbanya and Sobngwi 2003; Rolfe 1997). The variations are due to diagnostic criteria problems, local and geographical factors, type of diabetes, and variation in duration of diabetes. Since 1995, however, many more vigorous and well-conducted studies have taken place, giving a much clearer picture of complication prevalence; these are summarized in table 19.3. It can be seen that there is generally less wide a range between these studies and also that the figures themselves are substantial.

The prevalence of diabetic retinopathy varies from 13 to 55 percent, depending on the duration of diabetes and glycemic control, with severe retinopathy representing

15 percent of all cases (table 19.3). At diagnosis, 21 to 25 percent of type 2 patients and 9.5 percent of type 1 patients have retinopathy. Ethnic differences in the prevalence of retinopathy have been observed in multiethnic communities. In South Africa, the highest prevalence of retinopathy is observed in Africans, rather than Indians or Caucasians (whites), at diagnosis and after a similar duration of follow-up (Kalk et al. 1997). Although genetic predisposition may not be ruled out, lack of blood glucose and blood pressure control because of difficult access to health care might account for most of these differences.

The prevalence of nephropathy varies between 32 and 57 percent after a mean duration of diabetes of 5 to 10 years and between 5 and 28 percent within the first year following the diagnosis of diabetes (table 19.3). Diabetic nephropathy also occurs early in the course of diabetes, because between 32 and 57 percent of diabetic patients with a mean duration of diabetes between 5 and 10 years have microalbuminuria (Kalk et al. 1997; Rahlenbeck and Gebre-Yohannes 1997; Sobngwi et al. 1999). The diagnosis of nephropathy may, however, be faulty because of the presence of proteinuria due to renal infections and sickle-cell anemia. In Africa, diabetes mellitus accounts for a third of all patients who are admitted to dialysis units (Diallo et al. 1997), and renal replacement is both expensive and not widely available. It appears, therefore, that diabetic end-stage renal failure is the first cause of hospital mortality in diabetic patients in Africa. In South Africa, for example, 50 percent of all causes of mortality in type 1 diabetic patients may be due to renal failure (Gill, Huddle, and Rolfe 1995).

The estimates of the prevalence of neuropathy vary widely, depending on the methodology used to assess them. Macrovascular complications of diabetes are considered rare in Africa despite a high prevalence of hypertension. Lower-extremity amputation varies from 1.5 to 7 percent, and about 12 percent of all hospitalized diabetic patients have foot ulceration. A high proportion of patients have lower-limb arterial disease that contributes to the development of diabetic foot lesions. It is common to see patients with diabetic foot ulcers as the presenting complaint of diabetes. Data from Tanzania have shown that the vast majority (over 80 percent) of ulcers are neuropathic in origin and not associated with peripheral vascular disease (Abbas, Lutale, and Morback 2000). Audits of diabetes care carried out in Cape Town, South Africa; Dar es Salaam, Tanzania; and Yaoundé, Cameroon, have demonstrated poor glycemic control and inadequate foot care as risk factors for diabetic foot. Fewer than 22 percent of patients had their feet examined during a year of attendance at primary health care clinics in these three cities, even though in Cape Town, 37 percent demonstrated either peripheral neuropathy or peripheral vascular disease (Abbas, Lutale, and Morback 2000; Boulton 1990). Limited patient knowledge of proper foot care, practices relating to foot care, and cultural beliefs, including the association of diabetes, leg ulcers, and lower extremity amputation with bewitchment, are also common problems encountered in Sub-Saharan Africa countries (Abbas, Lutale, and Morback 2000; Boulton 1990).

Data on cerebrovascular disease are scarce because of the mortality associated with this complication, the low proportion of patients seen in hospitals, and the lack of death certificates or proper records of the cause of death. Recent results from the general population of Tanzania, where a morbidity and mortality surveillance system has been set up, show that stroke mortality was three to six times that of England and Wales and that 4.4 percent of type 2 diabetic patients presented with stroke at the diagnosis of diabetes (Walker et al. 2000). Coronary heart disease may affect 5 to 8 percent of type 2 diabetic patients and cardiomyopathy up to 50 percent of all patients. Whereas microvascular complications of diabetes are highly preventable and occur early during the course of the disease, macrovascular disease is rare. Late diagnosis of diabetes, poor metabolic control, and nonstandardized diagnostic procedures rather than genetic predisposition may account for this difference with other populations around the world.

MORTALITY ASSOCIATED WITH DIABETES

There have been relatively few structured mortality studies from Africa, making quantification of outcome difficult. However, a major study from Zimbabwe in 1980 (Castle and Wicks 1980) recorded follow-up of 107 newly diagnosed diabetic patients (both type 1 and type 2). In-patient mortality was 8 percent, and the survivors had a mortality rate of 41 percent within six years of follow-up. Most deaths were due to infection, hyperglycemic emergencies (ketoacidosis and nonketotic coma), or hypoglycemia. Particular risk factors for an adverse outcome were male gender, alcohol abuse, and insulin treatment.

Another outcome study was reported from Tanzania in 1990. A cohort of 1,250 newly diagnosed patients was followed from 1981 to 1987, and actuarial five-year survival rates were calculated (McLarty, Kinabo, and Swai 1990;

Swai, Lutale, and McLarty 1990). Eighty-two percent of those not on insulin survived five years, but only 60 percent of the group on insulin treatment survived that long. Once again, the causes of death were predominantly metabolic and infective. The authors concluded that in Africa "diabetes was a serious disease with a poor prognosis." One reviewer also observed that the Tanzanian study indicated that five years from diagnosis, 40 percent of those on insulin would die, whereas in Europe 40 percent of similar patients would survive more than 40 years (Deckert, Poulsen, and Larsen 1978; Gill 1997).

There is some evidence, however, that at least in some parts of Africa the prognosis of diabetes is improving. Figures reported from Ethiopia (Lester 1991, 1996), for example, are considerably better than the Zimbabwean (1980) and Tanzanian (1990) data. Interestingly, although metabolic emergencies were still the major cause of death, the mortality from renal failure was substantial, presumably from diabetic nephropathy and large vessel disease. A cohort of type 1 diabetic patients who were followed in Soweto, South Africa, has also shown relatively prolonged survival (Gill, Huddle, and Rolfe 1995). At follow-up after 10 years, with a mean diabetes duration of 14 years, only 16 percent had died. This figure was still in excess of Western rates, although almost all these deaths were due to nephropathy, a complication mostly untreatable in Africa even now.

Obviously, many factors affect mortality patterns among diabetic patients in different parts of Africa. These include provision of medical care and supply of insulin and other treatment modalities, as well as a variety of social, cultural, and ethnic factors. As seen earlier, the gradual lengthening of the duration of diabetes in itself contributes to changing patterns of mortality, to which diabetic nephropathy and macroangiopathy are rapidly playing a larger part in many areas. Large vessel disease is likely to accelerate in prevalence also because of Western influences, such as smoking, obesity, reduced exercise, and high-fat diets.

COST OF DIABETES

Studies on the economics of diabetes care in Sub-Saharan Africa are limited. A Medline search of such studies over the past 20 years yielded only the Tanzanian study (Chale et al. 1992). In Tanzania about US$4 million would have been required to take care of all patients with diabetes in 1989/90, which translates to US$138 per patient per year. This sum is equivalent to 8.1 percent of the total budgeted health expenditure for that financial year and well above the allocated per capita health expenditure in Tanzania of US$2 for the year 1989/90 (Chale et al. 1992). In Cameroon the average direct medical cost of treating a patient with diabetes in 2001 was US$489, of which 56 percent was spent on hospital admissions, 33.5 percent on antidiabetic drugs, 5.5 percent on laboratory tests, and 4.5 percent on consultation fees. The direct medical costs for treating all diabetic patients in Cameroon represented about 3.5 percent of the national budget for the year 2001/2002 (Nkegoum 2002). Estimates of diabetes care management in Malawi, based on international prices for essential drugs and Malawi hospital cost data, suggest that a type 1 diabetic patient spends about US$100 per year for the purchase of insulin, and a type 2 patient spends US$25 annually on oral hypoglycemic agents (Vaughan, Gilson, and Mills 1989).

The average age at onset of diabetes in Tanzania was 44 years and the average age at death was 46 years; population life expectancy was 53 years. The calculated number of healthy life days (HLDs) lost because of diabetes was 4,100 days per patient, of which 69 percent was because of premature mortality. This calculation was based on an average case-fatality rate after five years of 29 percent and a severe chronic disablement rate of 14 percent. The estimated HLDs lost per capita because of diabetes were 820 person-days per 1,000 people per year (Chale et al. 1992). In Ghana the average age at onset of diabetes was 40 years, with 50 percent case fatality after 15 years and an average age at death of 55 years, with 30 percent disablement before death. The total days lost were calculated as 217 per 1,000 people per year, of which 52 percent were due to premature death (Vaughan, Gilson, and Mills 1989).

Table 19.7 reports the calculated estimates of the costs of diabetes care in Sub-Saharan Africa for persons age 20 to 79 years (IDF 2003). The table uses population estimates and diabetes prevalence estimates reported in table 19.4 for those age 20 to 79 years for 2003. The total health care budget for 20- to 79-year-olds can be derived by multiplying the population figures for that age group by the per capita health expenditures. Calculations are then presented for values of R of 2 and 3. R is the ratio of the cost of care for people with diabetes compared with the cost of care of people without diabetes. The data suggest that, at least for countries with high or moderate incomes, the value of R lies between 2 and 3 (IDF 2003). The top five countries with the highest costs of diabetes care in Sub-Saharan Africa are South Africa, Kenya, Zimbabwe, Nigeria, and Ghana (table 19.7).

STRATEGIES FOR CONTROL

During the last 10 years, health care spending in the developing countries has remained low. Of the 40 heavily indebted poor countries (HIPC) defined by the World Bank, 33 of them are in Sub-Saharan Africa. The average per capita income of HIPCs, is US$310 per year. The health care spending is approximately US$8 per person per year, and pharmaceutical spending is approximately US$2 to $3 per person per year (WHO 2003).

The economic cost of diabetes and its complications is unaffordable by most Sub-Saharan Africans. Their incomes are insufficient to purchase insulin, oral hypoglycemic agents, and other supplies for management of diabetes. The limited resources of the countries in Sub-Saharan Africa are divided between fighting poverty, implementing education strategies, providing housing and appropriate sanitation, and dealing with the socioeconomic and health burden of fighting the increasing incidence and prevalence of HIV/AIDS. Diabetes poses an additional burden on the limited health care delivery system.

The problems encountered in the management of diabetes in Sub-Saharan Africa include diagnosis; medical care; insulin and other drug supplies; monitoring; infections associated with diabetes, especially the diabetic foot; dietary advice; diabetes education; and the low priority placed on noncommunicable diseases.

The training of health care providers and organizations is not focused on effective and efficient treatment of people with diabetes. With modernization, economic well-being, and a Westernized lifestyle, the burden of diabetes and its complications also increases significantly. The resource-limited countries are unable to provide even minimum care in some instances, let alone secondary and tertiary care.

Over the last 10 years several assessments of health care services for diabetes have been done, particularly in South Africa (Whiting, Hayes, and Unwin 2003). The findings from these studies have shown the following:

- Patients' attendance is poor.
- Consultation times are short, resulting in little or no time for patient education.
- Staffing levels are inadequate, and staffs' knowledge is used inappropriately.
- Staff are poorly or inadequately trained, or both, and there exist hardly any continuous education programs.
- Monitoring and evaluation of complications of diabetes are lacking.

Table 19.7 Calculated Estimates of the Costs of Diabetes Care, by Country

Country	Overall per capita health expenditure (international $[a])	Cost of diabetes care per year given values for R[b] (thousands of international $[a])	
		$R = 2$	$R = 3$
Angola	52	7,940.6	15,477.0
Benin	27	1,652.0	3,236.0
Botswana	358	8,815.1	17,044.0
Burkina Faso	37	4,873.4	9,495.1
Burundi	16	600.0	1,184.5
Cameroon	55	3,186.4	6,322.5
Cape Verde	92	476.5	932.0
Central African Republic	37	1,493.4	2,920.6
Chad	19	1,860.5	3,624.3
Comoros	35	303.9	593.3
Congo, Dem. Rep. of	21	11,313.6	22,096.7
Congo, Rep. of	25	875.1	1,737.6
Côte d'Ivoire	45	8,170.3	15,976.1
Djibouti	63	888.6	1,697.4
Equatorial Guinea	103	562.8	1,099.1
Eritrea	25	888.1	1,743.8
Ethiopia	17	9,182.5	18,035.5
Gabon	171	3,140.2	6,107.1
Gambia, The	46	693.2	1,357.4
Ghana	51	16,482.7	31,932.0
Guinea	56	4,329.8	8,489.3
Guinea-Bissau	28	323.9	653.3
Kenya	115	40,360.2	78,826.2
Lesotho	100	3,113.9	6,046.6
Liberia	3	93.5	183.4
Madagascar	33	6,180.3	12,070.1
Malawi	38	3,258.2	6,409.4
Mali	32	3,352.3	6,573.0
Mauritania	52	2,310.8	4,469.9
Mozambique	30	7,756.9	15,065.0
Namibia	366	9,055.1	17,586.6
Niger	22	3,130.3	6,077.7
Nigeria	20	23,838.5	46,651.9
Réunion	—		
Rwanda	40	1,637.4	3,238.4
São Tomé and Principe	23	64.9	126.5
Senegal	56	5,679.4	11,114.1
Seychelles	758	4,049.6	7,299.4
Sierra Leone	28	1,340.3	2,625.2
Somalia	7	629.8	1,232.5
South Africa	663	539,377.0	1,044,412.1
Swaziland	210	2,732.7	5,311.9
Tanzania	—		
Togo	36	5,491.5	10,818.3
Uganda	36	5,491.5	10,818.3
Zambia	49	6,663.1	12,945.5
Zimbabwe	171	24,779.6	48,327.5
Total		784,539	1,522,237

Source: Data on per capita health expenditure are from WHO 2003. Adapted with permission from IDF 2003.

Note: — = not available.

a. The international dollar is a common currency unit that takes into account differences in the relative purchasing power of various currencies. Figures expressed in international dollars are calculated using purchasing power parities (PPP), which are rates of currency conversion constructed to account for differences in price level between countries.

b. R = ratio of cost of care for people with diabetes and without diabetes.

- The control of blood glucose and blood pressure is poor and inadequate.
- Referral systems are almost nonexistent.
- Education of people with diabetes is lacking.
- Overall organization of the clinics is not satisfactory.
- Record keeping is poor.
- Even if treatment guidelines are available, they are hardly used and are not up to date.
- Health care systems in Sub-Saharan Africa vary widely.

A structured, organized diabetes health care system is lacking. Many people with diabetes are managed by traditional health care providers and general practitioners who are inadequately integrated into the primary care system.

Other problems with or barriers to the quality of delivery and affordable care include the following:

- inadequate infrastructure
- irregular supply of medicines
- unaffordable insulin, oral hypoglycemic agents, and antihypertensives
- disproportionate distribution of health care facilities
- lack of information and clear roles for members of diabetes health care teams
- lack of appropriate and locally adapted diabetes education programs for people with diabetes and diabetes health care professionals
- lack of government support or subsidy, resulting in unaffordable costs.

Cost of medication, especially the high cost of insulin, is a major handicap to proper diabetes care in Sub-Saharan Africa. Indeed, in a recent International Diabetes Federation survey (IDF 2003), it was observed that 80 percent of the people with diabetes were unable to obtain insulin and insulin syringes because they could not afford them. The cost of insulin preparations was higher in Sub-Saharan Africa than elsewhere (figure 19.3). Insulin and insulin syringes were accessible to only 11 percent of all people with diabetes in Africa. In addition, only 25 percent of people with diabetes monitored their blood glucose. Self-monitoring of blood glucose was rarely used, mainly because of the cost of testing supplies in 90 percent and the unavailability of testing supplies in 70 percent of the countries in Africa (IDF 2003).

It is clear that the organization of diabetes care in Sub-Saharan Africa has limitations at several levels of health delivery (box 19.1). There are solutions for each level of limitations and problems. Implementation strategies for

Figure 19.3 Cost of Different Types of Insulin in Relation to the Gross National Product

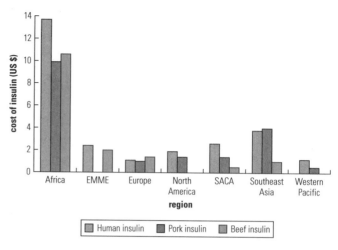

Source: Adapted from IDF 2003.

Note: EMME = Eastern Mediterranean and Middle East; SACA = South and Central America.

Box 19.1 Organization of Diabetes Care

Problem	Solution
1. Lack of resources	Diabetes associations
Financial	Twinning of diabetes
Material	associations
	Support groups
2. Prevalence	Research, studies
Magnitude of problem	
Disease complications	
3. Lack of recognition of interdependence of various levels of health care delivery	Communications
	Transport
	Trained personnel
Referrals	Drugs, equipment supply
4. Personnel	Trained manpower
	Motivation
	Continuous education
	Interpersonal communication
	Migration
5. Alternative health care provision	Confidence
	Cooperation
	Scientific research
6. Compliance	Education
	Transport
	Referrals

Source: Authors.

effecting change will vary from country to country based on several factors. Care for people with diabetes needs to begin at the primary health care level, followed by secondary and tertiary health care. In Sub-Saharan Africa, the rural-to-urban migration results in a significant increase in the geographical spread of people with diabetes. The health care for people with diabetes tends to be concentrated in large urban hospitals, too far from most of the people who need to use the services. Outreach programs in which health care workers move out into the community are feasible, affordable, and achievable and will benefit the rural population. That will probably be the long-term solution to the problems of the management of diabetes.

DIABETES HEALTH CARE

More than 50 years ago people with diabetes were mostly treated in hospitals by specialists. With limited resources and shrinking health budgets, together with a sharp rise in the prevalence of type 2 diabetes, specialist care in a hospital is not possible for everyone. An increasing number of primary and community health care professionals are responsible for managing people with diabetes. The ongoing health sector reforms in most of the countries of Sub-Saharan Africa have promoted more responsive and appropriate planning through decentralized and demand-driven health care, in which district managers decide how to divide their budgets between prevention and control of different health problems (WHO 2000).

In order to plan for proper delivery of diabetes health care, Sub-Saharan Africa countries need epidemiological and health services information. There is also a need to know the estimates of the prevalence of diabetes, its risk factors, and its complications. Finally, adequate knowledge of the overall burden of diabetes in high-risk populations and countries is a prerequisite for effective diabetes health care delivery (King et al. 1998).

Prevention

Sufficient evidence exists from countries outside Africa that weight loss, diet, and exercise can prevent or delay diabetes in people with IGT (Pan et al. 1997; Tuomilehto et al. 2001; Vijan et al. 1997) and that physical activity may exert an independent effect on the prevention and control of diabetes (Wojtaszewski et al. 2000).

The strategies for primary prevention, mostly involving support for behavior change through different forms of focused education and mass-media campaigns, are highly cost-effective (Swai et al. 1990). Prevention strategies in Sub-Saharan Africa have their own limitations. Lack of awareness by the population of and facilities for detection and monitoring contributes to the high prevalence of diabetic complications, and poorly skilled or inadequate health care staff, delay in seeking medical attention, and lack of access to affordable drugs contribute to the high rate of diabetes-related mortality. Unless these factors are taken into account when planning effective preventive strategies, the objectives will not be attainable.

The United Kingdom Prospective Diabetes Study (UKPDS 1998a) and the Diabetes Control and Complication Trial (DCCT 1993) have shown that intensive control of glucose results in a 25 to 70 percent reduction in the number and severity of microvascular complications in people with diabetes. The UKPDS also demonstrated a 12 percent reduction in mortality related to type 2 diabetes. In the UKPDS, control of high blood pressure reduced the risk of microvascular complications by 37 percent and death from type 2 diabetes–related disease by 32 percent (UKPDS 1998b), better reductions than those from tight blood glucose control (UKPDS 1998a), although the combination of blood pressure and blood glucose control was the most effective.

Health beliefs are still deeply enshrined in the healing cultures of people in Sub-Saharan Africa, thereby predisposing most patients to alternate between modern and traditional clinics. There are places in Sub-Saharan Africa where chlorpropamide and tolbutamides are still drugs of choice (and the only ones available) together with alpha methyldopa (for blood pressure control) in people affected with diabetes. The newer classes of drugs—sulfonylurea group, glinides—are unaffordable for the majority of the population.

One of the major challenges facing insulin-treated patients in Sub-Saharan Africa is the lack of a constant supply of insulin at affordable cost (Yudkin 2000). The supply of insulin in Sub-Saharan Africa is erratic, even at large hospitals, and the prospects for people with type 1 diabetes are poor (Amoah et al. 1998; Dagogo-Jack 1995). The exact burden of poor insulin access in developing countries is still unknown, because no good scientific study has been carried out in these countries. However, 16 percent of the world's population in developed countries with about 35 percent of all diabetic patients use over 40 percent of the world's total insulin each year (Jervell 1996; King 1998). Moreover, a small percentage of type 2 diabetes patients in developing countries require insulin when they become severely wasted and hyperglycemic. Therefore, insulin is underutilized in

Sub-Saharan Africa. In the second edition of *Diabetes Atlas*, the IDF's Task Force on Insulin Survey reports that no country in Africa had 100 percent accessibility to insulin. In fact two countries in Africa had the lowest accessibility in the world: the Democratic Republic of Congo, where people with type 1 diabetes had access to insulin for less than 25 percent of the time, and Zambia, where those with type 2 diabetes had access to insulin only 26 to 49 percent of the time. The high cost of insulin appears to be the most important cause of lack of access to insulin in people with type 1 diabetes in most countries of Africa (IDF 2003). There is therefore an urgent need for the initiation of international programs to alleviate the plight of insulin-treated patients in Africa. These programs may include (a) a selection of type of drug through the essential drug list; (b) improving affordability of the price charged by applying such measures as national price information, patent status, availability of generics, equity pricing schemes, review of general taxes and margins, and as a last resort, parallel import and compulsive licensing; and (c) sustainable financing of medical supplies through general tax levies, insurance schemes, copayment or full payment by the patient, loans, and donations (IDF 1998). One of the solutions to the problem being discussed is donation of insulin combined with a mechanism to support logistics, education, and monitoring. The limiting factor with this scheme is long-term sustainability.

Very few countries in Sub-Saharan Africa can afford to screen and treat the complications of diabetes (nephropathy, retinopathy, neuropathy, peripheral vascular disease) (Dagogo-Jack 1995). ACE inhibitors are a cost-effective way to reduce mortality and end-stage renal failure in people with type 1 diabetes (and type 2 diabetes) with microalbuminuria, but they are of limited use because most people cannot afford them (Hendry et al. 1997; Tooke, Thomas, and Viberti 2000). The potential for intervention and prevention of diabetic foot lesions is very high as a cost-effective strategy.

The Role of Diabetes Associations

The role of Diabetes Associations cannot be overemphasized. National Diabetes Associations should urge the government and nongovernmental organizations to ensure consistent and readily available insulin and other antidiabetes drugs and supplies at a subsidized cost. The national associations can also play a significant role in imparting education at different levels of health care and to the community at large.

The Role of the Patient

Patients must be empowered and motivated to join associations. They have to be informed about their rights. Together with the community, they would be able to remove misconceptions, mistrust, and the stigma of diabetes in Sub-Saharan Africa. The standard and quality of care being provided for people with diabetes has many limitations, which have to be overcome by a multisectoral approach.

CONCLUSION

Epidemiological data on diabetes mellitus in Sub-Saharan Africa are still limited. However, the prevalence and incidence of both type 1 and type 2 diabetes are increasing with the persistent rural-to-urban migration. Clearly, knowledge of the disease has increased since the 1990s; nevertheless, adoption of a Western lifestyle has greatly enhanced its development. The evidence shows that type 2 diabetes is a major cause of morbidity and mortality on the continent and that it is costly to manage diabetes and its complications. Given that the region still has a double and sometimes triple disease burden and that little priority is given to noncommunicable diseases like diabetes, and in the absence of a health care system adapted to this new reality and able to use costly therapeutic interventions, well-planned cost-effective methods of prevention and treatment and refined tools to assess health services and monitor progress are therefore required.

REFERENCES

Abbas, Z., J. Lutale, and S. Morback. 2000. "Outcome of Hospital Admissions for Diabetic Foot Lesions at Muhimbili Medical Centre, Dar es Salaam, Tanzania." *Diabetologia* 43 (Suppl. 1): A246.

Afoke, A. O., N. M. Ejeh, E. N. Nwonu, C. O. Okafor, N. J. Udeh, and J. Ludvigsson. 1992. "Prevalence and Clinical Picture of IDDM in Nigerian Ibo School Children." *Diabetes Care* 15: 1310–12.

Ahren, B., and C. B. Corrigan. 1984. "Prevalence of Diabetes Mellitus in North-Western Tanzania." *Diabetologia* 26: 333–36.

Amoah, A. G., S. K. Owusu, and S. Adjei. 2002. "Diabetes in Ghana: A Community Based Prevalence Study in Greater Accra." *Diabetes Research and Clinical Practice* 56: 197–205.

Amoah, A. G., S. K. Owusu, J. T. Saunders, W. L. Fang, H. A. Asare, J. G. Pastors, C. Sanborn, E. J. Barrett, M. K. Woode, and K. Osei. 1998. "Facilities and Resources for Diabetes Care at Regional Health Facilities in Southern Ghana." *Diabetes Research and Clinical Practice* 42: 123–30.

Amos, A. F., D. J. McCarty, and P. Zimmet. 1997. "The Rising Global Burden of Diabetes and Its Complications: Estimates and Projections to the Year 2010." *Diabetic Medicine* 14: S1–85.

Aspray, T. J., F. Mugusi, S. Rashid, D. Whiting, R. Edwards, K. G. Alberti, and N. C. Unwin. 2000. "Rural and Urban Differences in Diabetes Prevalence in Tanzania: The Role of Obesity, Physical Inactivity and Urban Living." *Transactions of the Royal Society of Tropical Medicine and Hygiene* 94: 637–44.

Boulton, A. 1990. *Practical Diabetes Digest* 1: 35–37.

Castle, W. N., and A. C. B. Wicks. 1980. "Follow-Up of 93 Newly Diagnosed African Diabetics for 6 Years." *Diabetologia* 18: 121–23.

Chale, S. S., A. B. M. Swai, P. G. M. Mujinja, and D. G. McLarty. 1992. "Must Diabetes Be a Fatal Disease in Africa? Study of Costs of Treatment." *British Medical Journal* 304: 1215–18.

Chauffert, M., A. Cisse, D. Cevenne, B. Parfait, S. Michel, and F. Trivin. 1995. "HLA-DR Beta 1 Typing and Non-Asp 57 Alleles in the Aborigine Population of Senegal." *Diabetes Care* 18: 677–90.

CIA (Central Intelligence Agency). 2002. *World Factbook 2002.* Washington, DC: CIA. http://www.cia.gov/publications/factbook/index.html.

Cook, A. R. 1901. "Notes on the Diseases Met with in Uganda, Central Africa." *Journal of Tropical Medicine* 4: 175–78.

Cooper, R., C. Rotimi, J. Kaufman, E. Owoaje, H. Fraser, T. Forester, R. Wilks, L. K. Riste, and J. K. Cruikshank. 1997. "Prevalence of NIDDM among Populations of the African Diaspora." *Diabetes Care* 20: 343–48.

Dagogo-Jack, S. 1995. "DCCT Results and Diabetes Care in Developing Countries." *Diabetes Care* 18: 416–17.

DCCT Research Group. 1993. "The Effect of Intensive Treatment of Diabetes on the Development and Progression of Long-Term Complications of Insulin Dependent Diabetes Mellitus." *New England Journal of Medicine* 329: 977–86.

Deckert, T., J. E. Poulsen, and M. Larsen. 1978. "Prognosis of Diabetics with Diabetes Onset before the Age of Thirty-One. I. Survival, Causes of Death, and Complications." *Diabetologia* 14: 363–70.

Diallo, A. D., D. Nochy, E. Niamkey, and B. Yao Beda. 1997. "Etiologic Aspects of Nephrotic Syndrome in Black African Adults in a Hospital Setting in Abidjan." *Bulletin Société Pathologie Exotique* 90: 342–45.

Dowse, G. K., H. Gareeboo, P. Z. Zimmet, K. G. Alberti, J. Tuomilehto, D. Fareed, L. G. Brissonnette, and C. F. Finch. 1990. "High Prevalence of NIDDM and Impaired Glucose Tolerance in Indian, Creole, and Chinese Mauritians." Mauritius Noncommunicable Disease Study Group. *Diabetes* 39: 390–96.

Drabo, P. P. Y., J. Kabore, and A. Lengani. 1996. "Complications of Diabetes Mellitus at the Hospital Center of Ouagadougou." *Bulletin Société Pathologie Exotique* 89: 191–95.

Ducorps, M., S. Baleynaud, H. Mayaudon, C. Castagne, and B. Bauduceau. 1996. "A Prevalence Survey of Diabetes in Mauritania." *Diabetes Care* 19: 761–63.

Edwards, R., N. Unwin, F. Mugusi, D. Whiting, S. Rashid, J. Kissima, T. J. Aspray, and K. G. Alberti. 2000. "Hypertension Prevalence and Care in an Urban and Rural Area of Tanzania." *Journal of Hypertension* 18 (2): 145–52.

Elamin, A., M. I. Omer, K. Zein, and T. Tuvemo. 1992. "Epidemiology of Childhood Type I Diabetes in Sudan, 1987–1990." *Diabetes Care* 15: 1556–59.

Elbagir, M. N., M. A. Eltom, E. M. Elmahadi, I. M. Kadam, and C. Berne. 1996. "A Population-Based Study of the Prevalence of Diabetes and Impaired Glucose Tolerance in Adults in Northern Sudan." *Diabetes Care* 19: 1126–1128.

Fisch, A., E. Pichard, T. Prazuck, H. Leblanc, Y. Sidibe, and G. Brucker. 1987. "Prevalence and Risk Factors of Diabetes Mellitus in the Rural Region of Mali West Africa: A Practical Approach." *Diabetologia* 30: 859–62.

Garcia-Pacheco, J. M., B. Herbut, S. Culbush, G. A. Hitman, W. Zhonglin, M. Magzoub, et al. 1992. "Distribution of HLA-DQA1 and DRBI Alleles in Black IDDM Controls from Zimbabwe." *Tissue Antigens* 40: 145–49.

Gill, G. V. 1997. "Outcome of Diabetes in Africa." In *Diabetes in Africa*, ed. G. V. Gill, J.-C. Mbanya, and K. G. M. M. Alberti, 65–71. Cambridge: FSG Communications.

Gill, G. V., and K. R. Huddle. 1993. "Hypoglycaemic Admissions among Diabetic Patients in Soweto, South Africa." *Diabetic Medicine* 10: 181–83.

Gill, G. V., K. R. Huddle, and M. Rolfe. 1995. "Mortality and Outcome of Insulin-Dependent Diabetes in Soweto, South Africa." *Diabetic Medicine* 12: 546–50.

Hendry, B. M., G. C. Viberti, S. Hummel, A. Bagust, and J. Piercy. 1997. "Modelling and Costing the Consequences of Using an ACE Inhibitor to Slow the Progression of Renal Failure in Type I Diabetic Patients." *Quarterly Journal of Medicine* 90 (4): 277–82.

Hunter, J. M., B. T. Sparks, B. Mufunda, C. T. Musabayane, H. V. Sparks, and K. Mahomed. 2000. "Economic Development and Women's Blood Pressure: Field Evidence from Rural Mashonaland, Zimbabwe." *Social Science and Medicine* 50: 773–95.

IDF (International Diabetes Federation). 1998. *Access to Insulin: A Report on the IDF Insulin Task Force on Insulin, 1994–1997.* Brussels: IDF.

———. 2003. *Diabetes Atlas.* 2nd ed. Brussels: IDF.

Jervell, J. 1996. "Variations in the Utilization and Cost of Insulin." *International Diabetes Federation Bulletin* 41: 1–2.

Kalk, W. J., K. R. L. Huddle, and F. J. Raal. 1993. "The Age of Onset of Insulin-Dependent Diabetes Mellitus in Africans in South Africa." *Postgraduate Medical Journal* 69: 552–56.

Kalk, W. J., J. Joannou, S. Ntsepo, I. Mahomed, P. Mahanlal, and P. J. Becker. 1997. "Ethnic Differences in the Clinical and Laboratory Associations with Retinopathy in Adult Onset Diabetes: Studies in Patients of African, European and Indian Origins." *Journal of Internal Medicine* 241: 31–37.

Kaufman, J. S., E. E. Owoaje, C. N. Rotimi, and R. S. Cooper. 1999. "Blood Pressure Change in Africa: Case Study from Nigeria." *Human Biology* 71 (4): 641–57.

King, H. 1998. "Insulin: Availability, Affordability, and Harmonization." *WHO Drug Information* 12(4): 230–34.

King, H., R. E. Aubert, and W. H. Herman. 1998. "Global Burden of Diabetes. Prevalence, Numerical Estimates, and Projections." *Diabetes Care* 21: 1414–31.

Kitange, H. M., H. Machibya, J. Black, D. M. Mtasiwa, G. Masuki, D. Whiting, N. Unwin et al. 1996. "The Outlook for Survivors of Childhood in Sub-Saharan Africa: Adult Mortality in Tanzania." *British Medical Journal* 312: 216–20.

Lester, F. T. 1984. "The Clinical Pattern of Diabetes in Ethiopians." *Diabetes Care* 7: 6–11.

———. 1991. Clinical Status of Ethiopian Diabetic Patients after 20 Years of Diabetes." *Diabetic Medicine* 8: 272–76.

———. 1993. "Clinical Features, Complications and Mortality in Type 2 (Non-Insulin Dependent) Diabetic Patients in Addis Abeba, Ethiopia, 1976–1990." *Ethiopian Medical Journal* 31 (2): 109–26.

———. 1996. "Mortality During Eight Years in a Cohort of Middle-Aged Ethiopian Diabetic Patients." *International Diabetes Digest* 7: 11–17.

Levitt, N. S., D. Bradshaw, M. F. Zwarenstein, A. A. Bawa, and S. Maphumolo. 1997. "Audit of Public Sector Primary Diabetes Care in Cape Town, South Africa: High Prevalence of Complications in Controlled Hyperglycaemia and Hypertension." *Diabetic Medicine* 14: 1073–77.

Levitt, N. S., J. M. Katzenellenbogen, D. Bradshaw, M. N. Hoffman, and F. Bonnici. 1993 . "The Prevalence and Identification of Risk Factors for NIDDM in Urban Africans in Cape Town, South Africa." *Diabetes Care* 16: 601–7.

Levitt, N. S., K. Steyn, E. V. Lambert, G. Reagan, C. J. Lombard, J. M. Fourie, K. Rossouw, and M. Hoffman. 1999. "Modifiable Risk Factors for Type 2 Diabetes Mellitus in a Peri-Urban Community in South Africa." *Diabetic Medicine* 16: 946–50.

Mbanya, J. C., J. Ngogang, J. N. Salah, E. Minkoulou, and B. Balkau. 1997. "Prevalence of NIDDM and Impaired Glucose Tolerance in a Rural and an Urban Population in Cameroon." *Diabetologia* 40: 824–29.

Mbanya, J. C., L. N. Pani, D. N. Mbanya, E. Sobngwi, and J. Ngogang. 2000. "Reduced Insulin Secretion in Offspring of African Type 2 Diabetic Parents." *Diabetes Care* 23: 1761–65.

Mbanya, J. C., and E. Sobngwi. 2003. "Diabetes Microvascular and Macrovascular Disease in Africa." *Journal of Cardiovascular Risk* 10: 97–102.

McLarty, D. G., L. Kinabo, and A. B. M. Swai. 1990. "Diabetes in Tropical Africa: A Prospective Study, 1981–7. II. Course and Prognosis." *British Medical Journal* 300: 1107–10.

McLarty, D. G., A. B. M. Swai, H. M. Kitange, G. Masuki, B. L. Mtinangi, P. M. Kilima, W. J. MaKene, L. M. Chuwa, and K. G. Alberti. 1989. "Prevalence of Diabetes and Impaired Glucose Tolerance in Rural Tanzania." *Lancet* (8643): 871–75.

McLarty, D. G., A. Yusafai, and A. B. M. Swai. 1989. "Seasonal Incidence of Diabetes Mellitus in Tropical Africa." *Diabetic Medicine* 6: 762–65.

Mennen, L. I., J. C. Mbanya, J. Cade, B. Balkau, S. Sharma, S. Chungong, and J. Kennedy 2000. "The Habitual Diet in Rural and Urban Cameroon." *European Journal of Clinical Nutrition* 24: 882–87.

Mollentze, W. F., A. J. Moore, A. F. Steyn, G. Joubert, K. Steyn, G. M. Oosthuizen, and D. J. V. Weich. 1995. "Coronary Heart Disease Risk Factors in a Rural and Urban Orange Free State Black Population." *South African Medical Journal* 85: 90–96.

Mosley, W. H., J. L. Bobadilla, and D. T. Jamison. 1993. "The Health Transition: Implications for Health Policy in Developing Countries." In *Disease Control Priorities in Developing Countries*, ed. D. T. Jamison, W. H. Mosley, A. R. Measham, and J. L. Bobadilla, 673–99. New York: Oxford University Press.

Motala, A. A., M. A. K. Omar, and F. J. Pirie. 2000. "Type 1 Diabetes Mellitus in Africa: Epidemiology and Pathogenesis." *Diabetes International* 10: 44–47.

Moukouri, D. T., C. McMoli, C. Nouedoui, and J. C. Mbanya. 1995. "Les aspects cliniques de la rétinopathie à Yaoundé." *Médecine d'Afrique Noire* 42 (89): 423–28.

Murray, C. J. L., and A. D. Lopez. 1997. "Mortality by Cause for Eight Regions of the World: Global Burden of Disease Study." *Lancet* 349: 1269–76.

Nambuya, A. P., M. A. Otim, H. Whitehead, D. Mulvaney, R. Kennedy, and D. R. Hadden. 1996. "The Presentation of Newly-Diagnosed Diabetic Patients in Uganda." *Quarterly Journal of Medicine* 89: 705–11.

Niang, E. H., S. N. Diop, E. A. Sidibe, M. Badiane, J. R. Lamouche, and A. M. Sow. 1994. "Echographic and Velocimetric Aspects of Arteriopathies in the Diabetic." *Dakar Medical* 39: 37–42.

Nkegoum, A. V. 2002. "Coût direct et indirect du diabéte en l'absence de complications chroniques a Yaoundé, Cameroun." MD thesis, University of Yaoundé I, Cameroon.

Ohwovoriole, A. E., J. A. Kuti, and S. I. Kabiawu. 1988. "Casual Blood Glucose Levels and Prevalence of Undiscovered Diabetes Mellitus in Lagos Metropolis Nigerians." *Diabetes Research and Clinical Practice* 4 (2): 153–58.

Omar, M. A., M. A. Seedat, R. B. Dyer, A. A. Motala, L. T. Knight, and P. J. Becker. 1994. "South African Indians Show a High Prevalence of NIDDM and Bimodality in Plasma Glucose Distribution Patterns." *Diabetes Care* 17: 70–74.

Omar, M. A. K., M. A. Seedat, A. A. Motala, R. B. Dyer, and P. Becker. 1993. "The Prevalence of Diabetes Mellitus and Impaired Glucose Tolerance in a Group of South African Blacks." *South African Medical Journal* 83: 641–43.

Pan, X. R., G. W. Li, Y. H. Hu, J. X. Wang, W. Y. Yang, Z. X. An, Z. X. Hu, et al. 1997. "Effects of Diet and Exercise in Preventing NIDDM in People with Impaired Glucose Tolerance. The Da Qing IGT and Diabetes Study." *Diabetes Care* 20: 537–44.

Panz, V. R., and B. I. Joffe. 1999. "Impact of HIV Infection and AIDS on Prevalence of Type 2 Diabetes in South Africa in 2010." *British Medical Journal* 318: 1351.

Pavan, L., E. Casiglia, P. Pauletto, S. L. Batista, G. Ginocchio, M. M. Y. Kwankam, et al. 1997. "Blood Pressure, Serum Cholesterol and Nutritional State in Tanzania and in the Amazon: Comparison with an Italian Population." *Journal of Hypertension* 15: 1083–90.

Rahlenbeck, S. I., and A. Gebre-Yohannes. 1997. "Prevalence and Epidemiology of Micro- and Macroalbuminuria in Ethiopian Diabetic Patients." *Journal of Diabetes Complications* 11: 343–49.

Ramaiya, K. L., A. B. M. Swai, D. G. McLarty, and K. G. M. M. Alberti. 1991. "Impaired Glucose Tolerance and Diabetes Mellitus in Hindu Indian Immigrants in Dar es Salaam." *Diabetic Medicine* 8: 738–44.

Ramaiya, K. L., A. B. M. Swai, D. G. McLarty, R. S. Bhopal, and K. G. M. M. Alberti. 1991. "Prevalences of Diabetes and Cardiovascular Disease Risk Factors in Hindu Indian Subcommunities in Tanzania." *British Medical Journal* 303: 271–76.

Rolfe, M. 1997. "Chronic Complications of Diabetes in Africa." In *Diabetes in Africa*, ed. G. V. Gill, J.-C. Mbanya, and K. G. M. M. Alberti, 43–50. Cambridge: FSG Communications.

———. 1988. "The Neurology of Diabetes Mellitus in Central Africa." *Diabetic Medicine* 5: 399–401.

Rolfe, M., G. G. Ephraim, D. C. Lincoln, and K. R. L. Huddle. 1995. "Hyperglycaemic Nonketotic Coma as a Cause of Emergency Hyperglycaemic Admission in Baragwanath Hospital." *South African Medical Journal* 85: 173–76.

Rwiza, H. T., A. B. M. Swai, and D. G. McLarty. 1986. "Failure to Diagnose Diabetic Ketoacidosis in Tanzania." *Diabetic Medicine* 3: 181–83.

Setel, P., N. Unwin, K. Alberti, and Y. Hemed. 2000. "Cause-Specific Adult Mortality: Evidence from Community-Based Surveillance, Selected Sites, Tanzania, 1992–1998." *Morbidity and Mortality Weekly Report* 49: 416–19.

Sobngwi, E., J. F. Gautier, and J. C. Mbanya. 2003. "Exercise and the Prevention of Cardiovascular Events in Women." *New England Journal of Medicine* 348: 77–79.

Sobngwi, E., E. Mauvais-Jarvis, P. Vexiau, J. C. Mbanya, and J. F. Gautier. 2001. "Diabetes in Africans. Part 1: Epidemiology and Clinical Specificities." *Diabetes and Metabolism* 27: 628–34.

Sobngwi, E., J-C. Mbanya, E. N. Moukouri, and K. B. Ngu. 1999. "Microalbuminuria and Retinopathy in a Diabetic Population of Cameroon." *Diabetes Research and Clinical Practice* 44: 191–96.

Sobngwi, E., J. C. Mbanya, N. C. Unwin, A. P. Kengne, L. Fezeu, E. M. Minkoulou, T. J. Aspray, and K. G. Alberti. 2002. "Physical Activity and Its Relationship with Obesity, Hypertension and Diabetes in Urban and Rural Cameroon." *International Journal of Obesity and Related Metabolic Disorders* 26: 1009–16.

Swai, A. B. M., J. Lutale, and D. G. McLarty. 1990. "Diabetes in Tropical Africa: A Prospective Study 1981–7: Characteristics of Newly Presenting Patients in Dar es Salaam, Tanzania 1981–7." *British Medical Journal* 300: 1103–7.

———. 1993. "Prospective Study of Incidence of Juvenile Diabetes Mellitus over 10 Years in Dar es Salaam, Tanzania." *British Medical Journal* 306: 1570–72.

Swai, A. B. M., D. G. McLarty, F. Sherrif, L. M. Chuwa, E. Maro, Z. Lukmanji, W. Kermali, W. MaKene, and K. G. Alberti. 1990. "Diabetes and Impaired Glucose Tolerance in an Asian Community in Tanzania." *Diabetes Research and Clinical Practice* 8: 227–34.

Teuscher, T., P. Baillod, J. B. Rosman, and A. Teuscher. 1987. "Absence of Diabetes in a Rural West African Population with a High Carbohydrate/Cassava Diet." *Lancet* (8536): 765–68.

Tooke, J. E., S. Thomas, and G. C. Viberti. 2000. "Proteinuria in Diabetes." *Journal of Royal College London* 34: 336–39.

Tuomilehto, J., J. Lindstrom, J. G. Eriksson, T. T. Valle, H. Hamalainen, P. Ilanne-Parikka, S. Keinanen-Kiukaanniemi, et al. 2001. "Prevention of Type 2 Diabetes Mellitus by Changes in Lifestyle among Subjects with Impaired Glucose Tolerance." *New England Journal of Medicine* 344: 1343–50.

UKPDS Group. 1998a. "Intensive Blood-Glucose Control with Sulphonylureas or Insulin Compared with Conventional Treatment and Risk of Complications in Patients with Type 2 Diabetes: UKPDS 33." *Lancet* 352: 837–53.

———. 1998b. "Tight Blood Pressure Control and Risk of Macrovascular and Microvascular Complications in Type 2 Diabetes: UKPDS 38." *British Medical Journal* 317: 703–12.

UNFPA (United Nations Population Fund). 2000. *State of World Population*. New York: United Nations.

Unwin, N., F. Mugusi, T. Aspray, D. Whiting, R. Edwards, J. C. Mbanya, et al. 1999. "Tackling the Emerging Pandemic of Non-Communicable Diseases in Sub-Saharan Africa: The Essential NCD Health Intervention Project." *Public Health* 113: 141–46.

Vaughan, P., L. Gilson, and A. Mills. 1989. "Diabetes in Developing Countries: Its Importance for Public Health." *Health Policy and Planning* 4: 97–109.

Vijan, S., D. Stevens, W. Hermann, M. Funnell, and C. Standiford. 1997. "Screening, Prevention, Counseling, and Treatment for the Complications of Type II Diabetes Mellitus. Putting Evidence into Practice." *Journal of General Internal Medicine* 12: 567–80.

Walker, R. W., D. G. McLarty, H. M. Kitange, D. Whiting, G. Masuki, D. M. Mtasiwa, H. Machibya, N. Unwin, and K. G. Alberti. 2000. "Stroke Mortality in Urban and Rural Tanzania." *Lancet* 355: 1684–87.

Whiting, D. R., L. Hayes, and N. C. Unwin. 2003. "Challenges to Health Care for Diabetes in Africa." *Journal of Cardiovascular Risk* 10: 103–10.

WHO (World Health Organization). 1998. *Population Ageing—A Public Health Challenge*. Geneva: WHO.

———. 1999. "Diagnosis and Classification of Diabetes Mellitus." In *Definition, Diagnosis and Classification of Diabetes Mellitus and Its Complications*. Geneva: WHO.

———. 2000. *The World Health Report 2000—Health Systems: Improving Performance*. Geneva: WHO.

———. 2003. *The World Health Report 2002—Reducing Risks, Promoting Healthy Life*. Geneva: WHO.

Wojtaszewski, J. F., B. F. Hansen, J. Gade, B. Kiens, J. F. Markuns, L. J. Goodyear, and E. A. Richter. 2000. "Insulin Signaling and Insulin Sensitivity after Exercise in Human Skeletal Muscle." *Diabetes* 49 (3): 325–31.

Yudkin, J. S. 2000. "Insulin for the World's Poorest Countries." *Lancet* 355: 919–21.

Zouvanis, M., A. C. Pieterse, H. C. Seftel, and B. I. Joffe. 1997. "Clinical Characteristics and Outcome of Hyperglycaemic Emergencies in Johannesburg Africans." *Diabetic Medicine* 14: 603–6.

Chapter **20**

Cancers

Freddy Sitas, Max Parkin, Zvavahera Chirenje, Lara Stein, Nokuzola Mqoqi, and Henry Wabinga

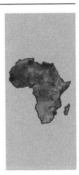

Cancer has received low priority for health care services in Sub-Saharan Africa. The reason is undoubtedly the overwhelming burden of communicable diseases, as illustrated by the proportions of deaths by major categories. Table 20.1 shows estimates, for Africa and for the whole world, made by the World Health Organization (WHO) of the percentages of deaths due to different causes in the year 2002 (WHO 2004).

From a purely objective point of view, therefore, concentration on health problems in Africa that have been largely solved in the developed world (infant and child mortality, maternal mortality, infectious diseases) appears eminently reasonable. Unfortunately, these "old" diseases coexist in Africa with the emergence of new ones, most prominently the acquired immune deficiency syndrome (AIDS), but also some of the noncommunicable diseases, such as hypertension, diabetes, accidents and violence (Motala 2002; Reza, Mercy, and Krug 2001; Seedat 2000; Walker et al. 2000), and cancer. Cancer is not a rare disease in Africa. Even ignoring the huge load of AIDS-related Kaposi's sarcoma, the probability that a woman living in present-day Kampala or Harare will develop a cancer by the

age of 65 years is only about 20 percent lower than that of her sisters in Western Europe (table 20.2). Yet the facilities for providing treatment for cancer cases in most of Africa are minimal, as illustrated by the sparse distribution of radiation therapy services in Africa (figure 20.1) (Levin, El-Gueddari, and Meghzifene 1999).

The noncommunicable diseases, such as cancers, are emerging health problems that need to be dealt with appropriately to sustain public health advances that have already been achieved. Increases in the prevalence of tobacco consumption and immunosuppression induced by the human immunodeficiency virus (HIV), coupled with such existing risk factors for cancer as alcohol; the high prevalence of cancer-associated infectious agents like human papillomaviruses (HPV), hepatitis B viruses (HBV), and human herpesvirus-8 (HHV8); and environmental exposure to toxins, such as aflatoxins, will have an important impact on future cancer patterns and incidence. Even despite declining overall life expectancy as a result of the HIV epidemic, Africans will continue to age, which will contribute to cancer's becoming an increased burden on health services, both in relative and absolute terms.

Table 20.1 Estimated Percentages of Deaths, by Cause, 2002

Cause	World	Africa
No. of deaths (all causes)	57,029,000	10,664,000
Infectious and parasitic diseases, excluding HIV/AIDS, respiratory infections	7.3	22.6
HIV/AIDS	4.9	19.6
Respiratory infections	6.9	10.5
Maternal and perinatal causes	5.2	7.4
Cancer	12.5	3.8
Cardiovascular disease	29.3	9.7
Injuries, violence	9.1	7.0
Other causes	24.8	19.4

Source: WHO 2004.

Table 20.2 Cumulative Incidence of Cancer in Women up to 64 Years of Age, 1993–97

Country	Cumulative incidence (%)
England	15.2
France[a]	14.0
Sweden	14.4
Uganda (Kampala)	11.3
Zimbabwe (Harare)	12.6

Source: Parkin et al. 2003.

Note: Kaposi's sarcoma and nonmelanoma skin cancer are excluded from table.

a. Based on data from nine cancer registries.

Figure 20.1 Distribution of Radiation Therapy Services in Africa

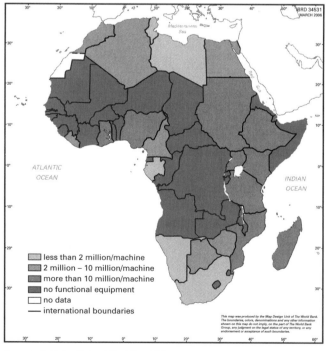

less than 2 million/machine
2 million – 10 million/machine
more than 10 million/machine
no functional equipment
no data
international boundaries

Source: Levin, El-Gueddari, and Meghzifene 1999.

Until quite recently, knowledge of cancer patterns was based primarily on clinical and pathological case series from the 1950s and 1960s, which were the subject of several reviews that drew together information on the relative frequency of different types of cancer in different areas in order to piece together an overall picture (Clifford, Linsell, and Timms 1968; Cook and Burkitt 1971; Oettlé 1964). Statistics on disease mortality are particularly sparse. Only about 0.25 percent of the population of Sub-Saharan Africa is covered by accurate death registration systems. The countries that have reasonably accurate death registration include islands like Mauritius and the Seychelles, which are unlikely to be representative of the region, and no country on the mainland of Sub-Saharan Africa has data of sufficient quality for the estimation of national mortality rates (Mathers et al. 2005). Hence, reliance has to be placed on indirect measures of mortality and on the few cancer registries that do exist across Africa, now covering roughly 8 percent (Parkin et al. 2003) of this population. An exception to this has been South Africa, which until 1990 had almost complete death notification for whites, mixed race "coloureds," and Asian Indians, comprising about 20 percent of the population. Population group identifiers on death notification forms were removed in 1991 but reintroduced in 1998. National coverage of deaths in South Africa across all populations has now increased to over 90 percent (Dorrington et al. 2001).

Since the 1990s there has been a resurgence of interest in cancer incidence in Africa, and data from cancer registries from Sub-Saharan Africa have been published from West Africa in The Gambia (Bah et al. 2001), Mali (Bayo et al. 1990), Guinea (Koulibaly et al. 1997), and Côte d'Ivoire (Echimane et al. 2000). Data from East Africa are available from cancer registries in Kampala, Uganda (Wabinga et al. 2000), and from southern Africa from the Zimbabwe Cancer Registry in Harare (Chokunonga et al. 2000), and the Malawi Cancer Registry in Blantyre (Banda et al. 2001).

Cancer registration in economically underdeveloped populations, such as all the countries of Sub-Saharan Africa, is a difficult undertaking for a variety of reasons (Parkin et al. 2003). The major challenge is to ensure that all new cases of cancer are identified. Cases can be found only when they come into contact with health services: hospitals, health centers, clinics, and laboratories. When resources are restricted, the proportion of the population with access to such institutions may be limited, and the statistics generated will thus not truly reflect the pattern of cancer. The ease with which the cases can be identified also depends on the extent of medical facilities available and the quality of statistical and record systems already in place (for example, pathology request forms, hospital discharge abstracts, treatment records, and so forth). It is impossible to know, without an extensive population survey, what proportion of those with cancer never come into contact with modern diagnostic or treatment services, instead making use only of traditional healers or receiving no care at all.

In the past, studies have suggested that some sections of the population may have been underrepresented in hospital statistics, particularly older women and young men, both of whom were more likely to return to their rural homes to seek care (Flegg Mitchell 1966). However, currently, this underrepresentation is probably rather rare in contemporary urban Africa. Most cancer patients will, eventually, seek medical assistance, although often at an advanced stage of disease. The situation in rural areas may be quite different, but almost all the present-day cancer registries are located in urban centers. From an epidemiological point of view, one must guess at how well the cancer profile from the urban areas reflects that in the country as a whole, given what is known of urban–rural differences in cancer patterns in other areas of the world.

The International Agency for Research on Cancer (IARC) has published the available data on cancer incidence and other cancer data from a variety of sources (Parkin et al. 2003). Such data have also been used to prepare a set of estimates of incidence and mortality at the national level for the year 2002 (Ferlay et al. 2005). These sources are extensively used in this chapter. We also draw upon the few available series from which it is possible to make some inferences about temporal trends in cancer incidence: the two cancer registries with data available in the 1960s—Kampala (Uganda) and Ibadan (Nigeria)—and the mortality data sets from South Africa referred to earlier.

According to the 2002 estimates of cancer incidence for the Sub-Saharan Africa region, about half a million (530,000) new cases of cancer occurred annually, 251,000 in males and 279,000 in females. Table 20.3 shows the

Table 20.3 Estimated Number of New Cases and Age-Standardized (World) Incidence Rates for the Leading Cancers in Males and Females, 2002
(per 100,000 people)

Sex/cancer	Eastern Africa		Middle Africa		Northern Africa		Southern Africa		Western Africa		Sub-Saharan Africa		Africa	
	Cases	ASR	Cases	ASR	Cases	ASR	Cases	ASR	Cases	ASR	Cases	ASR	Cases	ASR
Males														
Kaposi's sarcoma	23,094	23.0	10,097	30.0	194	0.3	3,065	13.2	3,740	4.6	39,995	16.4	40,190	12.3
Liver	14,012	21.1	7,744	27.8	2,351	4.2	1,072	7.0	10,637	15.3	33,465	18.6	35,812	14.8
Prostate	7,054	13.8	4,975	24.5	2,908	5.8	4,778	40.5	9,947	19.3	26,755	19.8	29,663	16.0
Esophagus	11,174	19.1	369	1.5	1,140	2.1	2,804	19.7	802	1.3	15,150	9.9	16,289	7.8
Non-Hodgkin's lymphoma	7,264	7.1	1,525	4.5	3,124	4.4	846	4.8	4,868	5.7	14,503	6.0	17,626	5.6
Stomach	4,687	7.4	3,283	13.4	2,550	4.4	1,183	8.2	2,131	3.4	11,287	6.9	13,836	6.2
Colon and rectum	4,019	6.1	627	2.3	3,150	5.1	1,553	11.3	3,430	5.1	9,630	5.6	12,778	5.4
All sites but skin	118,903	158.7	39,212	141.9	60,011	99.0	31,626	213.7	61,610	90.0	251,351	135.6	311,363	126.0
Females														
Cervix uteri	33,903	42.7	8,201	28	8,175	12.1	7,698	38.2	20,919	29.3	70,723	35.2	78,897	29.3
Breast	15,564	19.5	5,173	16.5	16,588	23.2	6,474	33.4	21,397	27.8	48,609	23.5	65,197	23.4
Kaposi's sarcoma	10,814	9.5	3,501	8.6	65	0.1	1,452	5.7	1,393	1.4	17,160	6.1	17,226	4.6
Liver	6,267	8.6	4,571	13.4	1,442	2.2	469	2.5	4,162	5.6	15,470	7.6	16,912	6.2
Stomach	3,883	5.5	3,780	12.6	1,671	2.5	686	3.7	2,331	3.6	10,680	5.7	12,350	4.9
Non-Hodgkin's lymphoma	4,741	4.4	2,249	6.9	1,830	2.4	614	3.0	2,995	3.5	10,598	4.4	12,428	3.9
Ovary, etc.	4,706	5.8	1,182	3.3	1,892	2.6	1,003	5.2	3,601	4.6	10,491	5.0	12,384	4.3
Colon and rectum	2,997	4.1	951	3.3	2,707	4.0	1,644	8.9	2,605	3.5	8,195	4.3	10,903	4.2
Esophagus	5,411	8.0	62	0.2	875	1.4	1,301	7.0	410	0.6	7,184	4.1	8,058	3.4
All sites but skin	129,029	156.7	38,857	121.5	59,603	85.2	32,170	163.2	78,740	104.0	278,797	133.4	338,397	121.0

Source: Ferlay et al. 2004.
Note: ASR = age-standardized rate.

Figure 20.2 Major Cancer Types in Sub-Saharan Africa, Both Sexes, All Ages

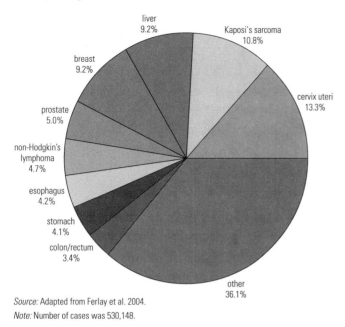

Source: Adapted from Ferlay et al. 2004.
Note: Number of cases was 530,148.

leading cancer types by region (including the northern Africa region) and by sex. Figure 20.2 shows the major cancer types in Sub-Saharan Africa; overall, world-standardized cancer rates were estimated to be 133 per 100,000 females and 136 per 100,000 males.

The top six cancers in males were the following:
- Kaposi's sarcoma (15.9 percent)
- liver (13.3 percent)
- prostate (10.7 percent)
- esophagus (6.0 percent)
- non-Hodgkin's lymphoma (5.8 percent)
- stomach (4.5 percent).

In females, the following were the leading cancers:
- cervix (25.4 percent)
- breast (17.4 percent)
- Kaposi's sarcoma (6.2 percent)
- liver (5.5 percent)
- stomach (3.8 percent)
- non-Hodgkin's lymphoma (3.8 percent).

Each of these cancers is briefly discussed in this chapter. In addition, tobacco-related cancers (especially lung cancer, which currently ranks seventh in males) and HIV-related cancers (cancers aside from Kaposi's sarcoma) are discussed, as these are likely to increase over time as both these epidemics mature.

CERVICAL CANCER

Cancer of the cervix is the leading cancer in women in Sub-Saharan Africa with an estimated 70,700 new cases occurring in 2002 (the total in the whole continent was 78,900 cases). Estimated rates for eastern and southern Africa of 30 to 60 per 100,000 are higher than those found in the rest of Sub-Saharan Africa (20 to 35 per 100,000), but the reasons for this difference are unclear. In many developed countries, such as the United Kingdom and Sweden, mortality from cancer of the cervix declined between the early 1900s and the 1960s and then declined further as a result of the introduction of national screening programs (Bergstrom, Sparen, and Adami 1999). However, in Bulawayo between 1963 and 1977 and in Kampala in the 1960s, 1970s, and 1990s, cancer of the cervix has appeared to increase in incidence over time (Skinner et al. 1993; Wabinga et al. 2000). No increases over time were observed in Nigeria and South Africa (Parkin et al. 2003).

It was noted early that cervical cancer has quite marked differences in incidence according to classical demographic variables (social class, marital status, ethnicity, religion). Later, epidemiological studies (mainly case-control studies) showed a consistent association between risk and early age at initiation of sexual activity, increasing number of sexual partners of females or of their sexual partners, and other indicators of sexual behavior. These findings were strongly suggestive of a causative role for a sexually transmitted agent. It is now recognized that certain sexually transmitted oncogenic human papillomaviruses constitute the necessary cause of cervical cancer. However, additional independent risk factors include increasing number of pregnancies, exposure to oral contraceptives, smoking, and specific dietary patterns.

At the onset of the AIDS epidemic, cancer of the cervix was classified as an AIDS-defining cancer by the U.S. Centers for Disease Control and Prevention (CDC 1993). But it is far from clear that HIV infection really increases the risk of invasive cervical cancer. No change in cervical cancer incidence has been demonstrated in some centers like Harare, where HIV/AIDS has been endemic for some time (Chokunonga et al. 1999). In Kampala the increase in cervical cancer incidence began before the advent of AIDS (Wabinga et al. 2000). With respect to cervical intraepithelial neoplasia (CIN), most studies failed to adjust for the fact that, for obvious reasons, women infected by HIV were very often also infected by HPV (with a consequently high risk of CIN). Careful adjustment for such confounding suggests that HIV has an independent effect on risk of CIN but that it is small; there is an interaction between the effects of HIV and HPV, as might be expected, if the role of HIV is indirect, through creation of immune suppression and dysfunction (Mandelblatt et al. 1999).

Case-control and descriptive studies on cancer of the cervix in Africa have shown associations of the disease similar to those observed in Western countries with respect to number of partners, level of education, high parity, and steroid contraceptives; however, genital hygiene, vaginal discharge, alcohol, and male circumcision were also found in certain studies to be important (Parkin et al. 2003). HIV was found to be associated with cervical cancer in case-control and cohort studies in South Africa and Uganda (Mbulaiteye et al., forthcoming; Newton et al. 2001; Sitas et al. 2000) with odds ratios between 1.6 and 2.4; however, such a weak association could easily be due to confounding by sexual activity, and other studies have shown no association (Newton et al. 1995; Sitas et al. 1997; ter Meulen et al. 1992). With regard to HPV, subtypes 16, 18, and 31 appear to be the leading ones, but other sexually transmitted infections causing chronic cervico-vaginal inflammation may increase the risk of cervical cancer.

Before the introduction of screening programs in the 1960s and 1970s, the incidence in most of Europe, North America, and Australia and New Zealand was much as we see it in Africa today: it was 38 per 100,000 in the Second National Cancer Survey of the United States, for example (Dorn and Cutler 1959). National screening programs have been responsible for the further decline in the incidence of cancer of the cervix. Pap test screening, with coverage of over 80 percent of the female population over 35 years of age appears to be the most effective method in reducing the incidence of cervical cancer. For example, if women were offered screening three times in their lifetime (at about ages 35, 45, and 55) the incidence of cancer of the cervix would be halved (Miller 1992).

Given the complex organization of screening programs, no organized national cervical cancer screening program exists in Africa. Reasons for this include lack of good quality cytology services, difficulty of long-term follow-up in many communities, lack of education, and lack of postal facilities and infrastructure. But many countries in Sub-Saharan Africa do not have the ability to diagnose or treat CIN. In other countries some attention has been given to the value of screening by visual inspection after acetic acid impregnation of the cervix (University of Zimbabwe/ JHPIEGO Cervical Cancer Project 1999). The high negative predictive value of this approach suggests that few significant lesions will be missed. If appropriately and safely treated by effective, affordable methods like cryotherapy

(Chirenje et al. 2001), then this method may provide a useful alternative to the conventional Pap test, not least in that treatment is provided during the same visit as the screening test, thus dispensing with the requirement to recall women for diagnosis and therapy.

Vaccines against the leading HPV serotypes have now been developed, and programs may be implemented for women before they become sexually active. However, it is unclear how long the protection will last and whether the vaccine will also be effective in reducing the incidence of cancer of the cervix among women who are infected. The ongoing trials are expected to clarify such issues. As men are also carriers of HPV, future studies ought to measure any added effectiveness of vaccination in this group.

BREAST CANCER

Breast cancer is the second most common cancer among women in Sub-Saharan Africa, accounting for 16.8 percent of all female cancers. Central, West, and East Africa appear to have lower incidence rates than southern Africa, the latter estimated at 33.4 per 100,000. An estimated total of 48,600 cases occurred in Sub-Saharan Africa in 2002.

Worldwide, risk factors for female breast cancer include menstrual and reproductive factors, high body mass index (BMI), family history of breast cancer, and certain genetic mutations, including BRCA1/2. Other suggested risk factors include, to a much lesser extent, high alcohol consumption, contraceptive use, and the use of certain postmenopausal hormone replacement therapies. Reproductive and hormonal factors appear to be the most important, with risk being increased by early menarche, late menopause, late age at first birth, and low parity (Henderson, Ross, and Bernstein 1988).

Studies in Sub-Saharan Africa have also found reproductive and hormonal factors to be important, reporting increased risk with advanced age at first pregnancy and delivery, low parity, and late age at menarche (Adebamowo and Adekunle 1999; Coogan et al. 1996; Shapiro et al. 2000; Ssali, Gakwaya, and Katangole-Mbidde 1995).

In Sub-Saharan Africa, higher incidence rates and relative frequencies of breast cancer have been reported in association with urban than with rural residence (Oettlé and Higginson 1966; Schonland and Bradshaw 1968), but data are sparse. The incidence of breast cancer is much higher among white women in Africa than among black African women; for example, in Harare between 1993 and 1995, the incidence was 127.7 per 100,000 in whites and 20.4 in blacks (Chokunonga et al. 2000). These differences may be a reflection of the distribution of lifestyle factors thought to be important in the development of breast cancer, for example, low parity and high body mass.

Breast cancer risk has been associated with socioeconomic status, with women of higher social class (as measured by education, income, housing, and so forth) having a higher risk (Kogevinas et al. 1997). Once again, such differences are most likely a reflection of different prevalences of risk factors among social classes (for example, parity, age at menstruation and menopause, height, weight, alcohol consumption).

The effect of oral contraceptive hormones on the risk of breast cancer has been the subject of much research. There appears to be a small but detectable risk in women currently using oral contraceptives, but this diminishes when contraception ceases, and after 10 years, none of the excess risk remains (Reeves 1996). A case-control study in South Africa found that combined oral contraceptives may result in a small increase in risk, confined to women below the age of 25 years, but that injectable progesterone contraceptives did not increase risk (Shapiro et al. 2000).

Dietary fat appears to be correlated with the risk of breast cancer in interpopulation studies (Prentice and Sheppard 1990), but the association has been difficult to confirm in studies of individuals (Hunter et al. 1996). However, obesity in postmenopausal women has been identified as a risk factor in Europe (Bergstrom et al. 2001) as well as in Sub-Saharan Africa (Adebamowo and Adekunle 1999; Walker et al. 1989). Although traditional diets in Africa are typically low in animal products, especially fat, and high in fiber (Labadarios et al. 1996; Manning et al. 1971), this pattern is being modified by urbanization and Westernization of lifestyles, which may lead to an increase in breast cancer incidence in African populations. A case-control study in Cape Town did not find a protective effect of breastfeeding on breast cancer (Coogan et al. 1999). However, in a meta-analysis of 47 studies from 30 countries breastfeeding appears to be protective; based on a reanalysis of about 50,302 cases and 96,973 controls, two-thirds of the difference in rates between developed and developing countries were estimated to be attributed to breastfeeding (International Collaboration on HIV and Cancer 2002).

At least part of the familial risk of breast cancer is mediated through the major susceptibility genes BRCA1 and BRCA2 (about 2 percent of breast cancer cases in Europe). Very little is known of the prevalence of these mutations in African populations, although family history of breast cancer is also a risk factor in this setting (Rosenberg et al. 2002).

About 1 percent of all breast cancer cases occur in men, with the male-to-female ratio being higher in black and African populations than among white populations (Parkin et al. 2003; Sasco, Lowels, and Pasker de Jong 1993).

A review of the literature indicates a deficit of studies on breast cancer risk in Sub-Saharan Africa, and further research could be beneficial. As certain groups become more Westernized and urbanized, with associated changes in diet, later childbirth, and reduced parity and periods of breast-feeding, breast cancer incidence may increase. Public health campaigns should encourage breastfeeding unless there are good reasons not to (for example, HIV-infected mothers where milk powder and sterile water are freely available). There is no organized mammography screening program in Sub-Saharan Africa.

KAPOSI'S SARCOMA

Prior to the HIV/AIDS era, Kaposi's sarcoma was a rare cancer in Western countries, seen mainly among immigrants from the Mediterranean littoral and African regions and in immunosuppressed transplant recipients. Meanwhile, in Africa, the incidence of Kaposi's sarcoma varied 100-fold, being most common in central and eastern Africa and rare in northern and southern Africa (IARC 1996; Oettlé 1962); in certain parts of central and eastern Africa, Kaposi's sarcoma was as common as cancer of the colon was in the West (Cook-Mozaffari et al. 1998). There appears to be some geographical association with the prevalence of human herpes virus-8, now regarded as a necessary cause for the development of Kaposi's sarcoma (Dukers and Rezza 2003). The incidence of Kaposi's sarcoma has increased over 1,000-fold in populations at high risk of HIV in some Western countries (Biggar et al. 1984; Rabkin, Biggar, and Horm 1991), but in the rest of the population the tumor still remains relatively rare (Grulich, Beral, and Swerdlow 1992; Rabkin, Biggar, and Horm 1991). In Africa, since the 1980s, areas like Malawi, Swaziland, Uganda, and Zimbabwe, where Kaposi's sarcoma was relatively common before the era of AIDS, the incidence of Kaposi's sarcoma has increased about 20-fold, such that it is now the leading cancer in men and the second leading cancer in women. In these cancer registries, overall age-standardized rates have increased by about 15 percent, mainly as a result of HIV-associated Kaposi's sarcoma (for example, Bassett et al. 1995; Wabinga et al. 1993; Wabinga et al. 2000).

According to the most recent estimates, 40,000 cases of Kaposi's sarcoma in males and 17,200 cases in females were estimated for 2002 for Sub-Saharan Africa; only 200 male and 65 female cases were estimated to occur in northern Africa. The region most affected is central Africa (age-standardized rates in males of 30 per 100,000) followed by eastern, southern, and lastly western Africa, in line with the background prevalence of HIV in each of these regions. With regard to the effect of HIV infection, three case-control studies from Africa showed increased risks of 30 to 50 in association with HIV, and these risks rise to 1,600 in HIV-positive individuals with high HHV8 antibody titers (Newton et al. 2002; Sitas et al. 1997; Sitas et al. 1999; Sitas et al. 2000). HHV8 in adults is associated with increasing age, low educational standard, and increasing numbers of sexual partners (Sitas et al. 1999). Antiretroviral therapy for treating HIV in adults has caused a decline in the incidence of Kaposi's sarcoma in Western countries (International Collaboration on HIV and Cancer 2000). HHV8 in children appears to be associated with infected mothers (Bourboulia et al. 1998). In countries with a high prevalence of HIV, Kaposi's sarcoma is now the leading cancer in children, causing almost a doubling in the childhood cancer incidence (Chokunonga et al. 1999; Wabinga et al. 1993). Antiretroviral drugs have now become more available in Botswana and recently in South Africa. If their use becomes widespread, then a decline in the incidence of Kaposi's sarcoma would be expected; however, it is unclear whether antiretrovirals (for example, zidovudine [AZT] or nevirapine) issued to mothers during delivery, which proved effective in reducing mother-child transmission of HIV, would cause a decline in Kaposi's sarcoma in children.

STOMACH CANCER

A total of 13,800 cases of stomach cancer in males and 10,700 in females was estimated in Sub-Saharan Africa in 2002. Age-standardized incidence rates in males varied, per 100,000, from 3.4 in western Africa to 7.4 in eastern, 8.2 in southern, and 13.4 in central Africa. In western Africa, where the incidence of stomach cancer is the lowest, the male-to-female ratio is 0.9 to 1; however, there is a male predominance in all other areas (table 20.3). Despite the generally low incidence rate in Africa, some populations have a particularly high incidence rate. Clusters of high incidence exist among the South African mixed race, or coloured, population of 98 per 100,000. A high incidence rate is also reported in the Great Lakes region that includes Burundi, Kivu Province of the Democratic Republic of Congo, Rwanda, northwestern Tanzania, and southwestern

Uganda. In Rwanda the age-standard incidence rate was found to be 13 per 100,000 males and 15 per 100,000 females (Newton et al. 1996). In western Uganda, stomach cancer was the second most common cancer, accounting for 12 percent of all male cancers and 6 percent of all female cancers (Wabinga et al. 2000). Bamako in Mali was another area with a high incidence rate: 18.5 per 100,000 males and 15 per 100,000 females (Bayo et al. 1990).

There is evidence of a slight but not significant increase in the incidence of stomach cancer over time in Kampala (Wabinga et al. 2000). In Kivu Province of the Democratic Republic of Congo, the incidence rates of stomach cancer among males and females were 9 and 15 per 100,000, respectively, in 1956–60, but this dropped to 6 and 4.5 per 100,000 in 1983–86 (Bourdeaux et al. 1988; Clemmensen, Maisin, and Gigase 1962). However, in rural Kenya reported incidence increased as a result of an endoscope acquired by the main hospital there (McFarlane et al. 2001). Trend data from the rest of Africa are incomplete or inconsistent; however, in South Africa, between 1948 and 1964 no real change in the relative frequency of stomach cancer was observed over time in one of the country's largest hospitals serving the predominantly black population of Soweto, Johannesburg (Robertson 1969), nor was a change observed in pathology-based cancer national registrations between 1986 and 1995 (Sitas, Madhoo, and Wessie 1998).

Helicobacter pylori infection is now recognized as an important risk factor for cancer of the stomach (IARC 1994); however, smoking and diets low in fruit and vegetables and vitamin C, and high in salts appear to play an important role. Many studies have shown the prevalence of *H. pylori* in Africa to be about 80 percent and that infection is acquired at a younger age than in Western countries (for example, Sathar et al. 1994). Chronic atrophic gastritis and intestinal metaplasia of the stomach are two key lesions in the natural history of stomach cancer. Very few studies in Sub-Saharan Africa have measured the association between gastric mucosal pathology and *H. pylori*. In summary, even in a continent where the prevalence of *H. pylori* is high, differences exist in the prevalence of *H. pylori* between those with a normal mucosa (0–33 percent) and those with gastritis of any kind. Needless to say, the prevalence of gastritis (mild or moderate) is high, but the prevalence of severe or chronic atrophic gastritis or intestinal metaplasia is low (Parkin et al. 2003). Two case-control studies from Africa show an association between *H. pylori* and stomach cancer, but the relative risks are low, probably because the mucosa of patients with gastric cancer is unfavorable to the survival of *H. pylori* (Jaskiewicz et al. 1989; Louw et al. 2001).

CagA positive strains, usually associated with more severe gastric pathology and outcomes, are the predominant strains in Africa (Ally et al. 1998), but their role in gastric carcinogenesis is unclear. Certain vacA genotypes appear to be more common in patients with gastric cancer (Kidd et al. 1999) and seem to be independent risk factors for the disease; however, no studies have been done in Sub-Saharan Africa on the relation between stomach cancer, host susceptibility (in relation to inflammatory cytokines), and the other risk factors known to be associated with stomach cancer (for example, diet, salt, smoking, and pickled foods) (see, for example, Coggon et al. 1989). There are many places in Africa where food is salted or pickled to aid preservation, but the relative importance of these risk factors in local settings is unknown.

LIVER CANCER

Early observations in Africa have always noted the high occurrence of liver cancer (for example, Oettlé 1964), and it is still one of the leading cancer types in men and women, although the relative frequency has been reduced in consequence of the large increase in the number of cases of Kaposi's sarcoma resulting from the epidemic of HIV/AIDS. Liver cancer is now the second leading cancer in men in Sub-Saharan Africa and the fourth leading cancer in women (table 20.3). There were an estimated total of 33,500 cases in males and 15,500 cases in females in 2002. Areas of high liver cancer incidence (mainly hepatocellular cancers) include countries like The Gambia, Guinea, and Senegal in West Africa, where liver cancers comprise a quarter or more of all cancer cases, with incidence rates ranging from 30 to 50 per 100,000 in men and 12 to 20 per 100,000 in women. Similarly, in central Africa, liver cancer is the leading cancer in Rwanda and in the Republic of Congo (Brazzaville); the estimated rate is 15.4 per 100,000 for men and 8.9 per 100,000 for women. Mozambique is reported to have high incidence rates, although the only data are old (Prates and Torres 1965).

Few places in Sub-Saharan Africa have information on cancer trends over time. In Ibadan, Nigeria, between 1960–69 and 1998–99, there appears to be no change in incidence, whereas in Kampala, Uganda, between the 1960s and the 1990s there appears to be a decline of liver cancer in men but not in women. However, a decline was noted in liver cancer incidence between the 1970s and the 1980s among Mozambican miners working in South Africa (Harington, Bradshaw, and McGlashan 1983).

Table 20.4 Prevalence of Hepatitis C Virus IgG Antibodies in Sub-Saharan Africa, 2000

Region	Prevalence of HCV (%)
Eastern Africa	2.7
Middle Africa	6.9
Southern Africa	0.1
Western Africa	2.4
All Africa	*3.0*

Source: Madhava, Burgess, and Drucker 2002.

Chronic carriage of HBV or hepatitis C (HCV), causing cirrhosis, or chronic hepatitis is the leading risk factor for liver cancer. The prevalence of HCV in Sub-Saharan Africa varies between 6.9 percent in central Africa to 0.1 percent in southern Africa (table 20.4). HCV transmission is probably via blood transfusion, unsterile medical and dental procedures, and traditional practices, such as scarification; sexual transmission is thought to be rare (Madhava, Burgess, and Drucker 2002).

Persistence of the HBV surface antigen (HbsAg) in blood is an indicator of chronic carriage of HBV infection. The risk of liver cancer in persons with chronic HBV infection, as indicated by the detection of HbsAg in serum, ranges from 6- to 20-fold in different studies, and it is estimated that about two-thirds of liver cancer in Africa is attributed to HBV (Pisani et al. 1997). Prevalence rates in Africa are over 10 percent in central, western, and eastern Africa and between 5 and 10 percent in southern Africa (Parkin et al. 2003).

There are relatively few African studies on the risk of HCV infection on the development of liver cancer. Those that have been conducted give relative risks ranging from 1.1 to 62 (Parkin et al. 2003). One study (Kirk et al. 2004) observed that, as has been found elsewhere, the risk of chronic infection by HCV and HBV is additive, suggesting common mechanisms of carcinogenesis.

Aflatoxin B1 (AFB1) is produced by molds of *Aspergillus* sp. that are common contaminants of poorly stored grains. AFB1 is a known liver carcinogen of animals and humans (IARC 1993, 2002). In Sub-Saharan Africa, high levels of AFB1 contamination are found in groundnuts and, to a lesser extent, corn. Contamination of groundnuts by AFB1 is quite widespread and frequently exceeds thresholds permitted in exports to most developed countries. Several geographical studies have demonstrated correlations between AFB1 levels and the incidence of hepatocellular cancer (see Parkin et al. 2003).

Iron overload, derived from food and drink preparation in iron vessels, is a common condition in rural Africa, and there have been several observations that elevated serum ferritin levels are associated with liver cancer. In one small case-control study in South Africa (Mandishona et al. 1998), liver cancer cases had higher iron overload levels than controls, corresponding to an odds ratio of 10.6 to 4.1 (depending on the control group used).

Smoking, oral contraception, and alcohol consumption (IARC 2004, 1999, and 1988, respectively) were also found to be important risk factors for liver cancer. This association, however, has not been extensively examined in Africa.

Early vaccine trials against HBV suggest that 70 to 75 percent of chronic infections could be prevented. A randomized trial to measure the effectiveness of HBV vaccination in the prevention of liver cancer is under way in The Gambia, but it will take many years before results are available. In Taiwan, however, children born after the introduction of mass vaccination had a fourfold lower incidence than those born before its introduction (Chang et al. 1997). According to the WHO Web site, by 2002, about a dozen countries in Sub-Saharan Africa had introduced hepatitis B vaccine into their infant immunization system (http://www.who.int/vaccines-surveillance/graphics/htmls/HepBvaccineUseMar02.htm).

Aflatoxin consumption could be reduced by improved education of individuals and farmers by, for example, agricultural extension officers. A trial in western Africa has shown that improved post-harvest storage of groundnuts can significantly reduce aflatoxin exposure in rural populations (Turner et al. 2005). The public could be educated to avoid contaminated peanuts sold by vendors (Wild and Hall 2000). Companies manufacturing peanut butter could be better controlled by accepting peanuts only from certified farmers and by the testing of their products by independent regulatory authorities.

PROSTATE CANCER

For the year 2002, a total of 26,800 cases of prostate cancer were estimated, comprising 10.6 percent of cancers of men in Sub-Saharan Africa (Ferlay et al. 2005). The relatively high incidence (and mortality) recorded in African populations is reflected in populations of African descent elsewhere. Thus, within the United States, the black population has the highest incidence (and mortality) rates, some 72 percent higher than whites. Southern Africa appears to have the highest rates (40.5 per 100,000). Rates of histologically diagnosed prostate cancer in South Africa are 40.1 per 100,000 in whites versus 14 per 100,000 in blacks, although for blacks, access to diagnostic facilities has been limited (Parkin et al. 2003). In Zimbabwe (defined as being part of eastern Africa), rates for whites and blacks were 70 versus 25 per 100,000 (Parkin et al. 2003). Central Africa follows with rates of 24.5 per 100,000. Surprisingly, in West Africa, where the majority of African-American men originated, the incidence rate of prostate cancer was estimated as 19.3 per 100,000 in 2002, compared with about 125 per 100,000 in the United States (Ferlay et al. 2005). High rates are observed in other places with populations that are descended from West Africa (for example, the Bahamas, Barbados, Trinidad).

Histology of the prostate in elderly men often reveals latent malignant cells, and clearly, advances in diagnostic and screening methods can cause artificial increases in reporting. This is illustrated by a fourfold increase in the incidence of histologically verified prostate cancer among whites in South Africa (most whites were covered by private health insurance) compared with no change in incidence in blacks between 1986 and 1995 (Sitas, Madhoo, and Wessie 1998). Notably, in Cape Town in the 1950s prostate cancer appeared to be more common in blacks than in whites (Muir-Grieve 1960). Increases over time have also been noted in Kampala and in Ibadan, but it is unclear how much of these increases represents a greater risk and how much can be attributed to increased awareness or a greater readiness to perform prostatectomy for urinary symptoms in elderly men (Parkin et al. 2003).

The consumption of fat and red meat has been implicated as a risk factor for prostate cancer in studies in developed countries, even though adjustment for total caloric intake was not always done. Associations with vegetable consumption have been inconclusive. Associations with anthropometric measures or a link with obesity have been inconclusive, and so have associations with numbers of sexual partners and history of sexually transmitted diseases, or STDs (Hayes et al. 2000; Key 1995; Kolonel 1996). In one case-control study from South Africa, prostate cancer was associated with high intake of fat, meat, and eggs; eating out of the house; and a low consumption of vegetables (Walker et al. 1992).

Sex hormones, modulated by polymorphisms on the long arm of chromosome X, play an important role in the development of prostate cancer (for example, Ross et al. 1998; Shibata and Whittemore 1997). Polymorphisms on the androgen receptor gene may vary by ethnic group and may provide some explanation for the geographic variation observed. However, no studies have been done on interethnic variations in androgen receptor polymorphisms in Africa.

NON-HODGKIN'S LYMPHOMA

The non-Hodgkin's lymphomas are composed of an extremely heterogeneous group of lymphoproliferative malignancies displaying distinct behavioral, prognostic, and epidemiological characteristics. Advances in molecular biology, genetics, and immunology have resulted in extensive changes in the classification of lymphoid tumors in the last few decades. The WHO classifies tumors according to cell lineage defined by immunophenotype (Jaffe et al. 2001). Three broad categories are now recognized: B-cell neoplasms, T/NK-cell neoplasms, and Hodgkin's lymphoma. Lymphocytic leukemias fall within the B-cell neoplasm group.

A total of 14,500 cases in males (5.8 percent of all cancers) and 10,600 cases in females (3.8 percent of all female cancers) were estimated for 2002 in Sub-Saharan Africa. In most African populations non-Hodgkin's lymphoma is relatively rare, but the relative frequency is above the world average in North and Sub-Saharan Africa because of the high incidence of Burkitt's lymphoma in children in the tropical zone of Africa. As in Western countries, most non-Hodgkin's lymphomas in Africa are of B-cell type. In adults, clinical series show an excess of high-grade lymphomas and a deficit of nodular lymphomas.

Human T-cell lymphotrophic viruses (for example, HTLV-I) are common in tropical Africa (IARC 1996) and are a cause of T-cell lymphomas; however, the incidence of these in Africa is low. Although Epstein-Barr virus DNA may be found in a small proportion of lymphomas, its role in causing non-Hodgkin's lymphomas is unclear (IARC 1997). HCV infection has been implicated in B-cell non-Hodgkin's lymphomas in some studies; the postulated mechanism being through the stimulation of polyclonal proliferation of B cells (reviewed by Parkin et al. 2003). HIV infection has been associated with 60-fold increased risks of developing non-Hodgkin's lymphomas in Western countries (for example, Beral et al. 1991); approximately 5 to 10 percent of HIV-infected persons will develop a lymphoma, and non-Hodgkin's lymphoma is the AIDS-defining illness in about 3 percent of HIV-infected patients (Remick 1995). In

Africa, however, the association between HIV and non-Hodgkin's lymphoma has been in the region of 2.3 to 12.3 (Mbulaiteye et al., forthcoming; Newton et al. 2001; Parkin et al. 2003; Sitas et al. 1997; Sitas et al. 2000). The reason for the discrepancy in the association between HIV and non-Hodgkin's lymphoma between developed countries and Africa is unclear. Non-Hodgkin's lymphomas were increasing in incidence in Western populations before the advent of HIV but have increased dramatically in high-risk groups affected by HIV (see, for example, Schultz, Boshoff, and Weiss 1996). In Harare, Zimbabwe (Chokunonga et al. 1999), and in Kampala, Uganda, there is now evidence of an increase in incidence between earlier cancer registration periods and periods in the 1990s (Parkin et al. 1999; Parkin et al. 2003).

Burkitt's lymphoma affects mainly children between the ages of five and nine. The jaw is affected 50 to 60 percent of the time. Burkitt's lymphoma shows a peculiar geographic distribution and has been reviewed by others (for example, Burkitt 1969; Williams et al. 1978; Wright 1973). It accounts for about a quarter to a half of childhood cancers in the eastern and central parts of Africa and in tropical West Africa, and less frequently in other places. Burkitt identified a striking distribution 15 degrees north and south of the equator, with a southern tail into Mozambique. But even within this area Burkitt's lymphoma was rarer in higher altitudes. The areas where it was most common were typified by rainfalls over 50 centimeters per year and an average of the coolest month of greater than 15.6°C, which seem associated with the distribution of malaria endemicity (Burkitt 1969; O'Conor 1970). Low socioeconomic status, family clustering, and proximity to the plant species *Euphorbia tirucalli* have been suggested as important factors in the etiology of Burkitt's lymphoma; however, the leading agent has been infection with Epstein-Barr virus (IARC 1997).

In a follow-up study of 42,000 children, those who developed Burkitt's lymphoma had higher titers of antiviral capsid antigen than in matched controls (de Thé et al. 1978; Geser et al. 1982). The link with malaria appears to be a result of the loss of cytotoxic T-cell control due to dysfunction of a subset of CD4 cells responsible for the induction of suppressor-cytotoxic CD8 cells. This may result in uncontrolled proliferation of B cells containing the Epstein-Barr virus and resultant malignant transformation (for example, Pagano et al. 1992; Whittle et al. 1990). In a five-year period of malaria suppression (when chloroquine was issued to children under 10), Burkitt's lymphoma appeared to decline in incidence. Incidence returned to the original level after the five-year program was completed (Geser, Brubaker, and Draper 1989). Burkitt's lymphoma is much rarer in adults, although Burkitt-like (or high-grade Burkitt-like) lymphomas appear to be occurring with increased frequency as a result of HIV (Sitas et al. 2000).

A prevention program for non-Hodgkin's lymphomas can be carried out only after the taxonomy and causes are further elucidated. It appears that antimalarial programs may have a significant impact on Burkitt's lymphoma in children, and as in Western countries, widespread antiretroviral therapy of HIV-positive individuals would cause a decline in the incidence of non-Hodgkin's lymphoma.

CANCER OF THE ESOPHAGUS

In 2002 a total of 15,150 cases of cancer of the esophagus were estimated to occur in males in Sub-Saharan Africa and 7,200 cases in females. Cancer of the esophagus shows a remarkable geographic distribution, being one of the leading cancers in southern and East Africa (average incidence in males about 19 per 100,000) but rare in West Africa (1 to 2 cases per 100,000). Certain areas of high risk have been reported from Kenya and the former Transkei homeland in the Eastern Cape Province of South Africa, where incidence rates as high as 76.6 per 100,000 in males and 36.5 per 100,000 in females were reported between 1991 and 1995 (Somdyala et al. 2003). Several studies between the 1950s and the 1990s in South Africa, Uganda, and Zimbabwe have demonstrated that cancer of the esophagus has increased in incidence. But the latest available data from cancer registries in these countries show a declining trend in esophageal cancer incidence, particularly in males after 1990 (Parkin et al. 2003; Somdyala et al. 2003).

Tobacco and alcohol consumption, known risk factors for the development of esophageal cancer in many countries, have also been documented as important in Africa in studies conducted from the 1980s onward; earlier studies found no such association, probably because of the low alcohol concentration of noncommercial drinks. The net effect of increasing commercial alcohol consumption, combined with increases in some places of tobacco consumption, on esophageal cancer trends is to date unclear. There is no consistent evidence of an effect of homemade brews and esophageal cancer risk in Africa.

Esophageal cancer also appears to occur in areas of extreme poverty and poor nutritional status. The high incidence of esophageal cancer in the Transkei region of the Eastern Cape Province has been associated with the monotonous consumption of corn, which contains low levels of niacin, riboflavin, vitamin C, zinc, calcium, and magnesium (Van Rensburg 1981) and is sometimes contaminated with fungal toxins produced by *Fusarium* spp. Certain studies in this region have shown a geographical association with the presence of *Fusarium moliniforme,* a common fungal contaminant of poorly stored corn. Other risk factors reported in the Transkei include infections with *Candida albicans* and the consumption of a green, leafy plant weed, *Solanum nigrum* (Sammon 1992).

OTHER HIV-ASSOCIATED CANCERS

Aside from Kaposi's sarcomas and non-Hodgkin's lymphomas, other cancers that appear to be associated with HIV immune suppression are cancer of the conjunctiva and possibly cancers of the cervix, vulva or vagina, anus, and liver (IARC 1996). However, except for conjunctival cancers, the data, at least from Sub-Saharan Africa, are not yet conclusive (IARC 1996; Parkin et al. 2003). Conjunctival cancers are increasing in incidence in Malawi (Banda et al. 2001);Uganda (Newton et al. 2001; Parkin et al. 1999), and Zimbabwe (Chokunonga et al. 2000); these countries have some of the most prolonged and highest levels of HIV prevalence in Africa, and it is anticipated that these cancers will increase in time in other places in Africa that are affected by HIV.

TOBACCO-RELATED CANCERS

Tobacco smoking is by far the most important cause of lung cancer. The evidence has been reviewed many times (IARC 1986, 2004). In 1985 it was estimated that about 76 percent of all lung cancer worldwide (84 percent of cases in men and 46 percent in women) could be attributed to tobacco smoking (Parkin et al. 1994). However, in Africa, because smoking is a relatively recent habit in most areas, the proportion of tobacco-attributed lung cancers is low.

Only where the smoking habit has been established in a significant percentage of the population for a prolonged period of time is the proportion of tobacco-attributable cancers also significant—85 percent of cases in males in certain southern African populations and 68 percent in northern Africa, for example (Parkin and Sasco 1993).

Because of the lower incidence of lung cancer in Africa (and the low prevalence of tobacco consumption in most

Figure 20.3 Number of Cigarettes Consumed per Adult

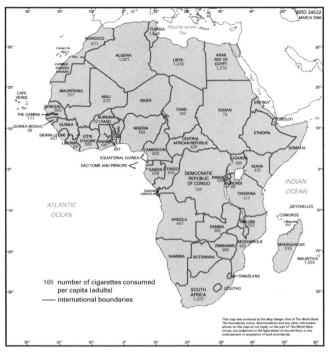

Source: http://apps.nccd.cdc.gov/nations/African_region.asp.

places in Africa) there is a widespread misconception that the hazards of tobacco are only relevant in developed countries. However, it appears that tobacco consumption, particularly of manufactured cigarettes, is increasing in Africa. Figure 20.3 shows the distribution of per capita consumption of cigarettes in Africa in countries where data exist. It is notable that aside from southern and northern Africa, consumption is low. Typical per capita consumption in the United States, for example, is 2,255 cigarettes, and in China, 1,791, per year. In a WHO survey it was found that between two decades, 1970–72 and 1990–92, 15 countries in Africa increased their consumption of cigarettes, 6 decreased, and 5 remained unchanged (WHO 1997). Data were unavailable for the rest of Africa. Adult smoking rates also vary significantly; prevalence in Africa among men varies from 10 to 50 percent, and among women from 1 to 10 percent (WHO 1997). An exception may be the mixed-race population of South Africa, where there has been a high prevalence (currently 40 to 50 percent) of smoking among women, and, indeed, lung cancer rates (and rates for other tobacco-associated cancers such as oral and esophageal cancers) are higher in southern Africa than the rest of Africa.

Evidence of the recent effect of the tobacco epidemic in Africa comes from the Northern Province (mainly rural) of South Africa (Mzileni et al. 1999) and Soweto (urban South Africa) (Pacella-Norman et al. 2002). In the Northern Province, the relative risk that males would develop lung

cancer if they smoked 15 cigarettes or more per day was 13, but in Soweto the relative risk for smoking the same number of cigarettes was 20.7. The latter relative risk is comparable to that observed in some developed countries.

In a study from South Africa, which uses the death registration system to ask the next of kin about the smoking status of the deceased, 61 percent of male and 48 percent of female deaths due to lung cancer were found to be attributed to smoking (compared with 80 to 90 percent in men and 30 to 70 percent in women in Western countries (Parkin and Sasco 1993). It was estimated that in all about 22,000 adult deaths (8 percent of total deaths compared with 15 percent of deaths in Western countries; Peto et al. 2004) were attributed to tobacco (Sitas et al. 2004). Surprisingly, more deaths from chronic obstructive pulmonary disease and tuberculosis would be expected from tobacco than deaths from lung cancer. The reason for the lower proportions of lung cancers attributed to smoking is that some of such cancers can be attributed to occupational exposures, environmental tobacco smoke, air pollution, and radon gas exposure (Parkin and Sasco 1993). Other tobacco-attributed cancers studied in Africa include those of the bladder, cervix, larynx, and esophagus and oral cancers (summarized in chapters in Parkin et al. 2003).

CONCLUSION

Over the past century, until about the 1980s (prior to the advent of HIV/AIDS), the average age of most populations in Sub-Saharan Africa has increased because of improvements in the rates of both infant and adult mortality (Timaeus 1999). Since cancer risk is strongly related to age, the aging population has experienced an increase in the numbers of cancers and in crude incidence. Cancer has therefore been an emerging public health problem. The HIV epidemic has arguably caused the biggest change in cancer patterns, with Kaposi's sarcoma now being the leading cancer type in men and the third most common cancer in women. But also, certain cancer types, such as cancer of the lung, breast, prostate, and esophagus, have increased significantly as a result of changing lifestyles and changes in exposures to common carcinogens.

Although the relative importance of many important carcinogens has been described for many cancers in most Western countries, little is known about the distribution of these and the relative importance of the major causes of cancer in Africa. Even in places with existing cancer registries, or well-resourced countries like South Africa, very few cancers or common carcinogenic exposures are being researched in a systematic fashion, and there is therefore wide uncertainty about their relative importance and their evolution over time. The relative importance of cancers and related exposures to them needs to be carefully assessed in order to formulate appropriate health promotion strategies. Given the tremendous variation in the genetics, lifestyle characteristics, and cancer patterns throughout Africa, it may be misleading to extrapolate cancer patterns from one area to the next, so better data from population-based cancer registries and from mortality statistics are needed to provide data of local relevance.

There have, however, been some positive developments. Compared with 1978–82, when no data from population-based cancer registries in Sub-Saharan Africa existed (Muir et al. 1987), the information derived from cancer registries in Sub-Saharan Africa now covers 8 percent of the population. Despite this great achievement most of these registries are staffed by a part-time director and one or two clerks, who do not know whether sufficient support will be forthcoming from their Departments of Health or other potential stakeholders. Given the short time that these registries have existed in Africa the impact of these on cancer incidence is still difficult to quantify. Yet long-term surveillance is necessary to quantify the impact of the epidemics of tobacco and AIDS and to evaluate the efficacy of cancer control measures.

Still, despite the dramatic reduction in life expectancy in many populations in Sub-Saharan Africa, age-standardized cancer incidence in these registries has remained the same, and in places where HIV prevalence is high, the overall incidence of cancer seems to have increased by up to 15 percent. This is counterintuitive to the common belief that a reduction in life expectancy due to HIV would cause a decline in chronic disease.

ACKNOWLEDGMENTS

The authors are grateful to Ruth Lawrence for preparing the manuscript.

REFERENCES

Adebamowo, C. A., and O. O. Adekunle. 1999. "Case-Controlled Study of the Epidemiological Risk Factors for Breast Cancer in Nigeria." *British Journal of Surgery* 86 (5): 665–68.

Ally, R., M. Hale, C. Hadjinicolaou, H. E. M. Sonnendecker, K. D. Bardhan, et al. 1998. "Helicobacter Pylori in Soweto South Africa. CagA Status and Histopathology in Children." Abstract. *Gastroenterology* 114: A54.

Bah, E., D. M. Parkin, A. J. Hall, A. D. Jack, and H. Whittle. 2001. "Cancer in The Gambia: 1988–1997." *British Journal of Cancer* 84: 1707–24.

Banda, L. T., D. M. Parkin, C. P. Dzamalala, and N. G. Liomba. 2001. "Cancer Incidence in Blantyre, Malawi 1994–1998." *Tropical Medicine and International Health* 6 (4): 296–304.

Bassett, M. T., E. Chokunonga, B. Mauchaza, L. Levy, J. Ferlay, and D. M. Parkin. 1995. "Cancer in the African Population of Harare, Zimbabwe in 1990–92." *International Journal of Cancer* 63: 29–36.

Bayo, S., D. M. Parkin, A. K. Koumare, A. N. Diallo, T. Ba, S. Soumare, and S. Sangare. 1990. "Cancer in Mali, 1987–1988." *International Journal of Cancer* 45 (4): 679–84.

Beral, V., T. Peterman, R. Berkelman, and E. S. Jaffe. 1991. "AIDS-Associated Non-Hodgkin Lymphoma." *Lancet* 337: 805–9.

Bergstrom, A., P. Pisani, V. Tenet, A. Wolk, and H. O. Adami. 2001. "Overweight as an Avoidable Cause of Cancer in Europe." *International Journal of Cancer* 91 (3): 421–30.

Bergstrom, R., P. Sparen, and H. O. Adami. 1999. "Trends in Cancer of the Cervix Uteri in Sweden Following Cytological Screening." *British Journal of Cancer* 81 (1): 159–66.

Biggar, R. J., J. Horm, J. F. Fraumeni, M. H. Greene, and J. J. Goedert. 1984. "Incidence of Kaposi Sarcoma and Mycosis Fungoides in the United States Including Puerto Rico, 1973-1981." *Journal of the National Cancer Institute* 73: 89–94.

Bourboulia, D., D. Whitby, C. Boshoff, R. Newton, V. Beral, H. Carrara, A. Lane, and F. Sitas. 1998. "Serologic Evidence for Mother to Child Transmission of Kaposi Sarcoma Associated Herpes Virus Infection." *Journal of the American Medical Association* 280 (1): 31–32.

Bourdeaux, L., F. Renard, P. L. Gigase, Mukolo-Ndjolo, P. Maldague, and A. De Muynck. 1988. L'incidence des cancers à l'hôpital de Katana, Kivu, Est Zaire, de 1983 à 1986. *Ann. Soc. Belg. Med Trop* 68: 141–56.

Burkitt, D. P. 1969. "Etiology of Burkitt's Lymphoma—An Alternative Hypothesis to a Vectored Virus." *Journal of the National Cancer Institute* 42: 19–28.

Centers for Disease Control and Prevention (CDC). 1993. "Revised Classification System for HIV Infection and Expanded Surveillance Case Definition for AIDS among Adolescents and Adults." *Journal of the American Medical Association* 269: 729–30.

Chang, M. H., C. J. Chen, M. S. Lai, H. M. Hsu, T. C. Wu, M. S. Kong, D. C. Liang, W. Y. Shau, and D. S. Chen. 1997. "Universal Hepatitis B Vaccination in Taiwan and the Incidence of Hepatocellular Carcinoma in Children." Taiwan Childhood Hepatoma Study Group. *New England Journal of Medicine* 336: 1855–59.

Chirenje, M., V. Rusakaniko, M. Akino, and Z. Mlingo. 2001. "A Randomised Clinical Trial of Loop Electrosurgical Excision Procedure (LEEP) versus Cryotherapy in the Treatment of Cervical Intraepithelial Neoplasia." *Journal of Obstetrics and Gynecology* 21 (6): 617–21.

Chokunonga, E., L. Levy, M. Bassett, M. Z. Borok, B. G. Mauchazo, M. Z. Chirenje, and D. M. Parkin. 1999. "AIDS and Cancer in Africa. The Evolving Epidemic in Zimbabwe." *AIDS* 13: 2583–88.

Chokunonga, E., L. M. Levy, M. T. Bassett, B. G. Mauchaza, D. B. Thomas, and D. M. Parkin. 2000. "Cancer Incidence in the African Population of Harare, Zimbabwe: Second Results from the Cancer Registry 1993–1995." *International Journal of Cancer* 85 (1): 54–59.

Clemmensen, J., J. Maisin, and P. Gigase. 1962. "Preliminary Report on Cancer in Kivu and Rwanda-Urundi." University of Louvain, Institut de Cancer, Louvain.

Clifford, P., C. A. Linsell, and G. L. Timms, eds. 1968. *Cancer in Africa*. Nairobi: East African Publishing House.

Coggon, D., D. J. Barker, R. B. Cole, and M. Nelson. 1989. "Stomach Cancer and Food Storage." *Journal of the National Cancer Institute* 81 (15): 1178–82.

Coogan, P. F., R. W. Clapp, P. A. Newcomb, R. Mittendorf, G. Bogdan, J. A. Baron, and M. P. Longnecker. 1996. "Variation in Female Breast Cancer Risk by Occupation." *American Journal of Industrial Medicine* 30 (4): 430–37.

Coogan, P. F., L. Rosenburg, S. Shapiro, and M. Hoffmann. 1999. "Lactation and Breast Carcinoma in a South African Population." *Cancer* 86: 982–89.

Cook, P. J., and D. P. Burkitt. 1971. "Cancer in Africa." *British Medical Bulletin* 27: 14–20.

Cook-Mozaffari, P., R. Newton, V. Beral, and D. P. Burkitt. 1998. "The Geographical Distribution of Kaposi Sarcoma and of Lymphomas in Africa before the AIDS Epidemic." *British Journal of Cancer* 78: 1521–28.

de Thé, G., A. Geser, N. E. Day, P. M. Tukei, E. H. Williams, D. P. Beri, P. G. Smith, et al. 1978. "Epidemiological Evidence for Causal Relationship between Epstein Barr Virus and Burkitt's Lymphoma from Ugandan Prospective Study." *Nature* 274: 756–61.

Dorn, H. F., and S. J. Cutler. 1959. *Morbidity from Cancer in the United States: Parts I and II*. Public Health Monograph 56. Washington, DC: U.S. Department of Health, Education and Welfare.

Dorrington, R., D. Bourne, D. Bradshaw, R. Laubscher, and I. M. Timaeus. 2001. *The Impact of HIV/Aids on Adult Mortality*. MRC Technical Report. Cape Town: MRC. http://www.mrc.ac.za/bod/bod.htm.

Dukers, N. H., and G. Rezza. 2003. "Human Herpesvirus 8 Epidemiology: What We Do and Do Not Know." *AIDS* 17: 1717–30.

Echimane, A. K., A. A. Ahnoux, I. Adoubi, S. Hien, K. M'Bra, A. D'Horpock, M. Diomande, D. Anongba, I. Mensah-Adoh, and D. M. Parkin. 2000. "Cancer Incidence in Abidjan, Ivory Coast: First Results from the Cancer Registry, 1995–1997." *Cancer* 89 (3): 653–63.

Ferlay, J., F. Bray, P. Pisani, and D. M. Parkin. 2004. "GLOBOCAN 2002: Cancer Incidence, Mortality and Prevalence Worldwide." Version 2.0, IARC CancerBase 5. Lyons: IARC Press.

Flegg Mitchell, H. 1966. "Sociological Aspects of Cancer Rate Surveys in Africa." *Journal of the National Cancer Institute Monographs* 25: 151–70.

Geser, A., G. Brubaker, and C. C. Draper. 1989. "Effect of a Malaria Suppression Program on the Incidence of African Burkitt's Lymphoma." *American Journal of Epidemiology* 129: 740–52.

Geser A., G. de Thé, G. Lenoir, N. E. Day, and E. H. Williams. 1982. "Final Case Reporting from the Ugandan Prospective Study of the Relationship between EBV and Burkitt's Lymphoma." *International Journal of Cancer* 29: 397–400.

Grulich, A. E., V. Beral, and A. J. Swerdlow. 1992. "Kaposi Sarcoma in England and Wales before the AIDS Epidemic." *British Journal of Cancer* 66: 1135–37.

Harington, J. S., E. M. Bradshaw, and N. D. McGlashan. 1983. "Changes in Primary Liver and Oesophageal Cancer Rates among Black Goldminers, 1964–1981. *South African Medical Journal* 64: 650.

Hayes, R. B., L. M. Pottern, H. Strickler, C. Rabkin, V. Pope, G. M. Swanson, R. S. Greenberg, et al. 2000. "Sexual Behaviour, STDs and Risks for Prostate Cancer." *British Journal of Cancer* 82 (3): 718–25.

Henderson, B. E., R. Ross, and L. Bernstein. 1988. "Estrogens as a Cause of Human Cancer: The Richard and Hinda Rosenthal Foundation Award Lecture." *Cancer Research* 48: 246–53.

Hunter, D. J., D. Spiegelman, H.-O. Adami, L. Beeson, P. A. van den Brandt, A. R. Folsom, G. E. Fraser, et al. 1996. "Cohort Studies of Fat Intake and the Risk of Breast Cancer—A Pooled Analysis." *New England Journal of Medicine* 334: 356–61.

IARC (International Agency for Research on Cancer). 1986. *Tobacco Smoking*. IARC Monographs on the Evaluation of Carcinogenic Risks to Humans, vol. 38. Lyons: IARC Press.

———. 1988. *Alcohol Drinking*. IARC Monographs on the Evaluation of Carcinogenic Risks to Humans, vol. 44. Lyons: IARC Press.

———. 1993. *Some Naturally Occurring Substances: Food Items and Constituents, Heterocyclic Aromatic Amines and Mycotoxins*. IARC Monographs on the Evaluation of Carcinogenic Risks to Humans, vol. 56. Lyons: IARC Press.

———. 1994. *Schistosomes, Liver Flukes and* Helicobacter pylori. IARC Monographs on the Evaluation of Carcinogenic Risks to Humans, vol. 61. Lyons: IARC Press.

———. 1996. *Human Immunodeficiency Viruses and Human T-Cell Lymphotrophic Viruses*. IARC Monographs on the Evaluation of Carcinogenic Risks to Humans, vol. 67. Lyons: IARC Press.

———. 1997. *Epstein-Barr Virus and Kaposi Sarcoma Herpesvirus/Human Herpesvirus 8*. IARC Monographs on the Evaluation of Carcinogenic Risks to Humans, vol. 70. Lyons: IARC Press.

———. 1999. *Hormonal Contraception and Post-menopausal Hormonal Therapy*. IARC Monographs on the Evaluation of Carcinogenic Risks to Humans, vol. 72. Lyons: IARC Press.

———. 2002. *Some Traditional Herbal Medicines, Some Mycotoxins, Naphthalene and Styrene*. IARC Monographs on the Evaluation of Carcinogenic Risks to Humans, vol. 82. Lyons: IARC Press.

———. 2004. *Tobacco Smoke and Involuntary Smoking*. IARC Monographs on the Evaluation of Carcinogenic Risks to Humans, vol. 83. Lyons: IARC Press.

International Collaboration on HIV and Cancer. 2002. "Review: Breastfeeding Is Associated with Reduced Risk of Breast Cancer." *Lancet* 20: 187–95.

Jaffe, E. S., N. L. Harris, H. Stein, and J. W. Vardiman, eds. 2001. *WHO Classification of Tumours: Pathology and Genetics of Tumours of the Haematopoietic and Lymphoid Tissues*. Lyons: IARC Press.

Jaskiewicz, K., H. D. Lowrens, C. W. Woodroof, M. J. van Wyk, and S. K. Price. 1989. "The Association of *Campylobacter pylori* with Mucosal Pathological Changes in a Population at Risk of Gastric Cancer." *South African Medical Journal* 75: 417–19.

Key, T. 1995. "Risk Factors for Prostate Cancer." In *Preventing Prostate Cancer. Screening versus Chemoprevention*, ed. R. T. D. Oliver, A. Belldegrun, and P. F. M. Wrigley. Cancer Surveys, vol. 23. Cold Spring Harbor, NY: Cold Spring Harbor Laboratory Press.

Kidd, M., A. J. Lastovica, J. C. Atherton, and J. A. Louw. 1999. "Heterogeneity in the Helicobacter Pylori VacA and CagA Genes: Association with Gastroduodenal Disease in South Africa?" *Gut* 45: 499–502.

Kirk, G. D., O. A. Lesi, M. Mendy, A. O. Akano, O. Sam, J. J. Goedert, P. Hainaut, A. Hall, H. Whittle, and R. Montesano. 2004. "The Gambia Liver Cancer Study. Infection with Hepatitis B and C: The Risk of Hepatocellular Carcinoma in West Africa." *Hepatology* 39: 211–19.

Kogevinas, M., N. Pearce, M. Susser, and P. Boffetta, eds. 1997. *Social Inequalities and Cancer*. IARC Scientific Publications 138. Lyons: IARC Press.

Kolonel, L. N. 1996. "Nutrition and Prostate Cancer." *Cancer Causes and Control* 7: 83–94.

Koulibaly, M., I. S. Kabba, A. Cisse, S. B. Diallo, M. B. Diallo, N. Keita, N. D. Camara, M. S. Diallo, B. S. Sylla, and D. M. Parkin. 1997. "Cancer Incidence in Conakry, Guinea: First Results from the Cancer Registry 1992–1995." *International Journal of Cancer* 70 (1): 39–45.

Labadarios, D., A. R. Walker, R. Blaauw, and B. F. Walker. 1996. "Traditional Diets and Meal Patterns in South Africa." *World Review of Nutrition and Diet* 79: 70–108.

Levin, C. V., B. El-Gueddari, and A. Meghzifene. 1999. "Radiation Therapy in Africa: Distribution and Equipment." *Radiotherapy Oncology* 52 (1): 79–84.

Louw, J. A., M. S. G. Kidd, A. F. Kummer, K. Taylor, U. Kotze, and D. Hanslo. 2001. "The Relationship between *Helicobacter pylori* Infection, the Virulence Genotypes of the Infecting Strain and Gastric Cancer in the African Setting." *Helicobacter* 6: 268–73.

Madhava, V., C. Burgess, and E. Drucker. 2002. "Epidemiology of Chronic Hepatitis C Virus Infection in Sub-Saharan Africa." *Lancet Infectious Disease* 2: 293–302.

Mandelblatt, J., P. Kanetsky, L. Eggert, and K. Gold. 1999. "Is HIV Infection a Cofactor for Cervical Squamous Cell Neoplasia?" *Cancer Epidemiology Biomarkers and Prevention* 8: 97–106.

Mandishona, E., A. P. MacPhail, V. R. Gordeuk, M. A. Kedda, A. C. Paterson, T. A. Rouault, M. C. Kew. 1998. "Dietary Iron Overload as a Risk Factor for Hepatocellular Carcinoma in Black Africans." *Hepatology* 27: 1563–66.

Manning, E. B., J. I. Mann, E. Sophangisa, and A. S. Truswell. 1971. "Dietary Patterns in Urbanised Blacks." *South African Medical Journal* 48: 488–98.

Mathers, C. D., D. M. Fat, M. Inoue, C. Rao, and A. D. Lopez. 2005. "Counting the Dead and What They Died From: An Assessment of the Global Status of Cause of Death Data." *Bulletin of the World Health Organization* 83: 171–77.

Mbulaiteye, S. M., E. T. Katabira, H. Wabinga, D. M. Parkin, P. Virgo, R. Ochai, M. Workneh, A. Coutinho, E. A. Engels. Forthcoming. "Spectrum of Cancers among HIV-Infected Persons in Africa: The Uganda AIDS-Cancer Registry Match Study." *International Journal of Cancer.*

McFarlane, G., D. Forman, F. Sitas, and G. Lachlan. 2001. "A Minimum Estimate for the Incidence of Gastric Cancer in Eastern Kenya." *British Journal of Cancer* 85 (9): 1322–25.

Miller, A. B. 1992. *Cervical Cancer Screening Programmes. Managerial Guidelines.* Geneva: WHO.

Motala, A. A. 2002. "Diabetes Trends in Africa." *Diabetes Metabolism Research Reviews* 18 (Suppl. 3): S14–20.

Muir, C., J. Waterhouse, T. Mack, J. Powell, S. Whelan, and F. Casset. 1987. *Cancer Incidence in Five Continents.* Vol. 5. IARC Scientific Publication 88. Lyons: IARC Press.

Muir-Grieve, J. "South Africa, Cape Province." 1960. In *Cancer Incidence in Five Continents*, vol. 2, ed. R. Doll, C. Muir, and J. Waterhouse, 98–109. Berlin: Springer Verlag.

Mzileni, O., F. Sitas, K. Steyn, H. Carrara, and P. Bekker. 1999. "Lung Cancer, Tobacco and Environmental Factors in the African Population of the Northern Province, South Africa." *Tobacco Control* 8: 398–401.

Newton, R., A. Grulich, V. Beral, B. Sindikubwabo, P.-J. Ngilimana, A. Nganyira, and D. M. Parkin. 1995. "Cancer and HIV Infection in Rwanda." *Lancet* 345 (8961): 1378–79.

Newton, R., P.-J. Ngilimana, A. Grulich, V. Beral, B. Sindikubwabo, A. Nganyira, and D. M. Parkin. 1996. "Cancer in Rwanda." *International Journal of Cancer* 66: 75–81.

Newton, R., F. Sitas, M. Dedicoat, and J. L. Ziegler. 2002. "HIV Infection and Cancer." In *AIDS in Africa*, 2nd ed., ed. M. Essex, S. Mboup, P. J. Kanki, R. G. Marlink, and S. D. Tlou. New York: Kluwer Academic.

Newton, R., J. Ziegler, V. Beral, and the Uganda Kaposi Sarcoma Study Group. 2001. "A Case-Control Study of Human Immunodeficiency Virus Infection and Cancer in Adults and Children Residing in Kampala, Uganda." *International Journal of Cancer* 92: 622–27.

O'Conor, G. T. 1970. "Persistent Immunologic Stimulation as a Factor in Oncogenesis with Special Reference to Burkitt's Tumour." *Annual Journal of Medicine* 48: 279–85.

Oettlé, A. G. 1962. "Geographical and Racial Differences in the Frequency of Kaposi Sarcoma as Evidence of Environmental or Genetic Causes." *Acta Unio Internationalis Contra Cancrum* 18: 330–63.

———. 1964. "Cancer in Africa Especially in Region South of the Sahara." *Journal of the National Cancer Institute* 33: 383–439.

Oettlé, A. G., and J. Higginson. 1966. "Age Specific Cancer Incidence Rates in the South African Bantu: Johannesburg 1953–1955." *South African Journal of Medical Science* 31: 21–41.

Pacella-Norman, R., M. I. Urban, F. Sitas, H. Carrara, R. Sur, M. Hale, P. Ruff, et al. 2002. "Risk Factors for Oesophageal, Lung, Oral and Laryngeal Cancers in Black South Africans." *British Journal of Cancer* 86 (11): 1751–56.

Pagano, J. S., G. Jimenez, N. S. Sung, N. Raab-Traub, and J. C. Lin. 1992. "Epstein-Barr Viral Latency and Cell Immortalization as Targets for Antisense Oligomers." *Annals of the New York Academy of Sciences* 660: 107–16.

Parkin, D. M., J. Ferlay, M. Hamdi-Cherif, F. Sitas, J. O. Thomas, H. Wabinga, and S. L. Whelan. 2003. *Cancer in Africa—Epidemiology and Prevention.* IARC Scientific Publications 153. Lyons: IARC Press.

Parkin, D. M., P. Pisani, A. D. Lopez, and E. Masuyer. 1994. "At Least One in Seven Cases of Cancer Is Caused by Smoking. Global Estimates for 1985." *International Journal of Cancer* 59: 494–504.

Parkin, D. M., and A. J. Sasco. 1993. "Lung Cancer: Worldwide Variation in Occurrence and Proportion Attributable to Tobacco Use." *Lung Cancer* 9: 1–16.

Parkin, D. M., H. R. Wabinga, S. Nambooze, and F. Wabwire-Mangen. 1999. "AIDS Related Cancers in Africa. Maturation of the Epidemic in Uganda." *AIDS* 13: 2563–70.

Peto, R., A. D. Lopez, J. Boreham, M. Thun, and C. Heath. 2004. *Mortality from Smoking in Developed Countries 1950–2000.* Oxford: Oxford University Press.

Pisani, P., D. M. Parkin, N. Munoz, and J. Ferlay. 1997. "Cancer and Infection: Estimates of the Attributable Fraction in 1990." *Cancer Epidemiology, Biomarkers Prevention* 6: 387–400.

Prates, M. D., and F. O. Torres. 1965. "A Cancer Survey in Lorenco Marques, Portuguese East Africa." *Journal of the National Cancer Institute* 35: 729–57.

Prentice, R. L., and L. Sheppard. 1990. "Dietary Fat and Cancer: Consistency of Epidemiologic Data and Disease Prevention that May Follow from a Practical Reduction in Fat Consumption." *Cancer Causes and Control* 1: 81–97.

Rabkin, C. S., R. J. Biggar, and J. W. Horm. 1991. "Increasing Incidence of Cancers Associated with the Human Immunodeficiency Virus Epidemic." *International Journal of Cancer* 47: 692–96.

Reeves, G. 1996. "Breast Cancer and Oral Contraceptives—The Evidence So Far." *Cancer Causes and Control* 7: 495–96.

Remick, S. C. 1995. "Acquired Immunodeficiency Syndrome-Related Non-Hodgkin Lymphoma." *Cancer Control* 2: 97–103.

Reza, A., J. A. Mercy, and E. Krug. 2001. "Epidemiology of Violent Deaths in the World." *Injury and Prevention* 7: 104–11.

Robertson, M. A. 1969. "Clinical Observations on Cancer Patterns at the Non-White Hospital Baragwanath, Johannesburg, 1948–1964." *South African Medical Journal* 26: 915–31.

Rosenberg, L., J. P. Kelly, S. Shapiro, M. Hoffman, and D. Cooper. 2002. "Risk Factors for Breast Cancer in South African Women." *South African Medical Journal* 92: 447–48.

Ross, R. K., M. C. Pike, G. A. Coetzee, J. K. Reichardt, M. C. Yu, H. Feigelson, F. Z. Stanczyk, L. N. Kolonel, and B. E. Henderson. 1998. "Androgen Metabolism and Prostate Cancer: Establishing a Model of Genetic Susceptibility." *Cancer Research* 58: 4497–4504.

Sammon, A. M. 1992. "A Case-Control Study of Diet and Social Factors in Cancer of the Oesophagus in Transkei." *Cancer* 69: 860–65.

Sasco, A., A. B. Lowels, and P. Pasker de Jong. 1993. "Epidemiology of Male Breast Cancer. A Meta-Analysis of Published Cases-Control Studies and Discussion of Selected Etiological Factors." *International Journal of Cancer* 53: 538–49.

Sathar, M. A., A. E. Simjee, D. F. Wittenberg, and A. M. Mayat. 1994. "Seroprevalence of *Helicobacter pylori* Infection in Natal/KwaZulu, South Africa." *European Journal of Gastroenterology and Hepatology* 6: 37–41.

Schonland, M., and E. Bradshaw. 1968. "Cancer in the Natal African and Indian, 1964–1966." *International Journal of Cancer* 3: 304–16.

Schultz, T. F., C. H. Boshoff, and R. A. Weiss. 1996. "HIV Infection and Neoplasia." *Lancet* 348: 587–91.

Seedat, Y. K. 2000. "Hypertension in Developing Nations in Sub-Saharan Africa." *Journal of Human Hypertension* 14: 739–47.

Shapiro, S., L. Rosenberg, M. Hoffman, H. Truter, D. Cooper, S. Rao, D. Dent, et al. 2000. "Risk of Breast Cancer in Relation to the Use of Injectable Progestogen Contraceptives and Combined Estrogen/Progestogen Contraceptives." *American Journal of Epidemiology* 151: 396–403. Erratum in *American Journal of Epidemiology* 151: 1134.

Shibata, A., and A. S. Whittemore. 1997. "Genetic Predisposition to Prostate Cancer: Possible Explanations for Ethnic Differences in Risk." *Prostate* 32: 65–72.

Sitas, F., W. R. Bezwoda, V. Levin, P. Ruff, M. C. Kew, M. J. Hale, H. Carrara, et al. 1997. "Association between Human Immunodeficiency Virus Type 1 Infection and Cancer in the Black Population of Johannesburg and Soweto, South Africa." *British Journal of Cancer* 75: 1704–7.

Sitas, F., H. Carrara, V. Beral, R. Newton, G. Reeves, D. Bull, U. Jentsch, et al. 1999. "The Seroepidemiology of HHV-8/KSHV in a Large Population of Black Cancer Patients in South Africa." *New England Journal of Medicine* 340: 1863–71.

Sitas, F., J. Madhoo, and J. Wessie. 1998. "Incidence of Histologically Diagnosed Cancer in South Africa 1993–1995." National Cancer Registry, South African Institute for Medical Research, Johannesburg.

Sitas, F., R. Pacella-Norman, H. Carrara, M. Patel, P. Ruff, R. Sur, U. Jentsch, et al. 2000. "The Spectrum of HIV-1 Related Cancers in South Africa." *International Journal of Cancer* 88: 489–92.

Sitas, F., M. Urban, D. Bradshaw, D. Kielkowski, S. Bah, and R. Peto. 2004. "Tobacco Attributable Deaths in South Africa." *Tobacco Control* 13: 396–99.

Skinner, M. E. G., D. M. Parkin, A. P. Vizcaino, and A. Ndhlovu. 1993. *Cancer in the African Population of Bulawayo, Zimbabwe, 1963–1977.* IARC Technical Report 15. Lyons: IARC Press.

Somdyala, N. I., W. F. Marasas, F. S. Venter, H. F. Vismer, W. C. Gelderblom, and S. A. Swanevelder. 2003. "Cancer Patterns in Four Districts of the Transkei Region—1991–1995." *South African Medical Journal* 93 (2): 144–48.

Ssali, J. C., A. Gakwaya, and E. Katangole-Mbidde. 1995. "Risk Factors for Breast Cancer in Ugandan Women: A Case Control Study." *Eastern and Central African Journal of Surgery* 1: 9–13.

ter Meulen, J., H. C. Eberhardt, J. Luande, H. N. Mgaya, J. Chang-Claude, H. Mtiro, M. Mhina, et al. 1992. "Human Papillomavirus (HPV) Infection, HIV Infection and Cervical Cancer in Tanzania, East Africa." *International Journal of Cancer* 51: 515–21.

Timaeus, I. M. 1999. "Mortality in Sub-Saharan Africa." In *Health and Mortality: Issues of Global Concern*, ed. J. Chamie and R. L. Cliquet, 108–31. New York: United Nations Population Division.

Turner, P. C., A. Sylla, Y. Y. Gong, M. S. Diallo, A. E. Sutcliffe, A. J. Hall, and C. P. Wild. 2005. "Reduction in Exposure to Carcinogenic Aflatoxins by Postharvest Intervention Measures in West Africa: A Community-Based Intervention Study." *Lancet* 365: 1950–56.

University of Zimbabwe/JHPIEGO Cervical Cancer Project. 1999. "Visual Inspection with Acetic Acid for Cervical Cancer Screening: Test Qualities in a Primary-Care Setting." *Lancet* 353 (9156): 869–73.

Van Rensburg, S. J. 1981. "Epidemiologic and Dietary Evidence for a Specific Nutritional Predisposition to Esophageal Cancer." *Journal of the National Cancer Institute* 67: 243–51.

Wabinga, H. R., D. M. Parkin, F. Wabwire-Mangen, and J. W. Mugerwa. 1993. "Cancer in Kampala, Uganda, in 1989–91: Changes in Incidence in the Era of AIDS." *International Journal of Cancer* 54: 26–36.

Wabinga, H. R., D. M. Parkin, F. Wabwire-Mangen, and S. Nambooze. 2000. "Trends in Cancer Incidence in Kyadondo County, Uganda, 1960–1997." *British Journal of Cancer* 82: 1585–92.

Walker, A. R. P., B. F. Walker, S. Funani, and A. J. Walker. 1989. "Characteristics of Black Women with Breast Cancer in Soweto, South Africa." *Cancer Journal* 2: 316–19.

Walker, A. R. P., B. F. Walker, N. G. Tsotetsi, C. Sebitso, D. Siwedi, and A. J. Walker. 1992. "Case-Control Study of Prostate Cancer in Black Patients in Soweto, South Africa." *British Journal of Cancer* 65: 438–41.

Walker, R. W., D. G. McLarty, H. M. Kitange, D. Whiting, G. Masuki, D. M. Mtasiwa, H. Machibya, N. Unwin, and K. G. Alberti. 2000. "Stroke Mortality in Urban and Rural Tanzania." Adult Morbidity and Mortality Project. *Lancet* 355: 1684–87.

Whittle, H. C., J. Brown, K. Marsh, M. Blackman, O. Jobe, and F. Shenton. 1990. "The Effects of *Plasmodium falciparum* Malaria on Immune Control of B Lymphocytes in Gambian Children." *Clinical and Experimental Immunology* 80: 213–18.

WHO (World Health Organization). 1997. *Tobacco or Health: A Global Status Report.* Geneva: WHO.

———. 2004. *The World Health Report 2004—Changing History.* Geneva: WHO.

Wild, C. P., and A. J. Hall. 2000. "Primary Prevention of Hepatocellular Carcinoma in Developing Countries." *Mutation Research* 462: 381–93.

Williams, E. H., P. G. Smith, N. E. Day, A. Geser, J. Ellis, and P. Tukei. 1978. "Space-Time Clustering of Burkitt's Lymphoma in West Nile District of Uganda: 1961–1975." *British Journal of Cancer* 37: 805–9.

Wright, D. H. 1973. "Lympho-Reticular Neoplasms." *Recent Results in Cancer Research* 41: 270–91.

Chapter **21**

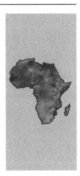

Cardiovascular Disease

Anthony Mbewu and Jean-Claude Mbanya

The burden of cardiovascular disease (CVD) in the world is enormous and growing, and the majority of those affected are in developing countries (Beaglehole and Yach 2003; Mbewu 1998). In 2002 it was estimated that 29 percent of deaths worldwide (16.7 million deaths) were due to CVD and that 43 percent of global morbidity and mortality, measured in disability-adjusted life years (DALYs), was caused by CVD (WHO 2002). Furthermore, 78 percent of global mortality and 86 percent of mortality and morbidity from CVD occurs in developing countries. By 2020 it is estimated that CVD will become the leading cause of the global health burden, accounting for 73 percent of total global mortality and 56 percent of total morbidity (Murray and Lopez 1996; Reddy and Yusuf 1998).

Africa has not been spared this global tide of CVD. In most African countries CVD is now the second most common cause of death after infectious disease, accounting for 11 percent of total deaths (WHO 1999); and CVD is a major cause of chronic illness and disability. Projections from the Global Burden of Disease Project suggest that from 1990 to 2020, the burden of CVD faced by African countries will double. A large proportion of the victims of CVD will

be middle-aged people. The poor will suffer disproportionately as a consequence of their higher disease risk and limited access to health care. The financial and social costs of this CVD epidemic are likely to have a negative impact on development and the alleviation of poverty (http://www.ichealth.org).

African countries therefore face a double burden as they struggle to cope with the burden of communicable diseases and diseases associated with lack of socioeconomic development—the "unfinished agenda." Furthermore, their predicament is only likely to worsen, because the majority of their populations are under 35 years of age, and the determinants and risk factors for CVD are already prevalent and increasing within this age group.

The relative cost of the epidemic of CVD is likely to be higher than in upper-income countries, where CVD primarily affects the elderly. In African countries more than half of CVD deaths occur among people between 30 and 69 years of age, an age 10 years or more below the equivalent group in Europe and North America (http://www.ichealth.org). In Ghana, for example, where cerebral hemorrhage is a leading cause of death, the average age at which people die from this cause is 55 years (http://www.ichealth.org). Death and disability in middle age have major social and economic consequences, depriving families of parents, workplaces of employees, and communities of leaders. Patients denied access to health care for CVD or deterred by high costs from seeking it will cause the public health systems to incur even greater health care costs in the long run as a result of the need to treat the same patients later at greater expense because the disease is more advanced.

The potential costs of this CVD epidemic for African countries are staggering. Cardiovascular disease (direct and indirect) is estimated to cost the United States about US$300 billion annually, equal to the entire gross domestic product of the African continent. Clearly, even a fraction of such cost has the potential to cause enormous damage to the economies and development trajectories of African countries. In this way, the growing CVD epidemic in Africa will increase already unacceptable levels of inequity in access to health care services.

The overall health of African nations will not improve, nor will their level of development, unless they deal with this epidemic of CVD. Furthermore, in an increasingly integrated global economy the CVD epidemic in developing countries will divert economic goods to CVD care, resulting in a reversal of developmental efforts; productivity will decline because of the loss of more productive citizens; and consumer markets will shrink as a result of loss of the purchasing power of these citizens.

THE EPIDEMIOLOGICAL TRANSITION

The process responsible for these global shifts in CVD mortality is termed the "epidemiological transition" (Omran 1971). Three main drivers fuel this transition:

- Declining infant and child mortality has led to rapid demographic changes resulting in large increases in the number of individuals surviving until middle and older age, when chronic diseases become manifest—the so-called demographic transition. By 2025 it is estimated that the number of Africans over 60 years old will increase from 39 million to 80 million.
- Falling death rates from communicable diseases have accompanied socioeconomic development and improved vaccination and other primary health care services.
- Changes have occurred in environmental and behavioral determinants of CVD, such as increasing tobacco use,

increasing fat and calorie consumption, and decreasing exercise. Longer periods of exposure to these determinants because of longer life expectancy have increased the rates of chronic disease.

Moreover, whereas European and North American populations experienced similar changes in demography, determinants, and disease rates over the course of a few centuries, African countries are passing through similar transitions in just a few decades (http://www.ichealth.org). This forced pace of globalization has resulted in the "export of risk factors" from the West such as tobacco, refined foods, and lifestyles with high CVD risk that are portrayed on television and film (Mbewu 1998).

Still, the process of epidemiological transition seems to be different in Africa than in developed and other developing countries, where it is mainly marked by the explosion of coronary heart disease (CHD). Indeed, although the epidemic of CHD was heralded in the 1980s (Ogunnowo, Odesanmi, and Andy 1986), in Africa it is still awaited, although hemorrhagic stroke is already a leading cause of mortality and morbidity (Walker et al. 2003). Furthermore, dilated cardiomyopathy is particularly prevalent in Sub-Saharan Africa, presumably owing to nutritional and viral factors. The epidemiological transition was readily apparent in the changes in causes of mortality in the Seychelles over the past 30 years (table 21.1) (Bovet 1995).

More reasons to suspect an impending epidemic of CVD in Sub-Saharan Africa include the recent finding that poor socioeconomic conditions in childhood determine CVD in middle age as strongly as do CVD risk factors in middle age in the same individuals (Lawlor, Smith, and Ebrahim 2002). Furthermore, according to the Barker Hypothesis, poor fetal growth has been shown to be associated with hypertension,

Table 21.1 The Epidemiological Transition in the Seychelles, 1976 and 1994
(percent)

Causes of death	1976	1994
Infectious and parasitic	9.9	5.5
Total CVD	26.3	39.5
Circulatory system	12.6	16.4
Hypertensive disease	—	8.4
Ischemic heart disease	—	8.0
Cerebrovascular disease	13.7	5.2
Cancer	8.2	16.2

Source: Bovet 1995.
Note: — = not available.

and CVD, in later life. However, a study carried out in Nigeria failed to demonstrate this effect (Law et al. 2001). The current impoverishment of much of Sub-Saharan Africa may paradoxically result in an epidemic of CVD in middle age for those who survive the ravages of poverty-associated communicable diseases, such as AIDS, tuberculosis, pneumonia, and malaria. Because fetal growth retardation is associated with chronic undernutrition among women, improvement in the nutrition and health of girls and young women may be important in preventing CVD in developing countries.

SOURCES OF DATA

Sources of data on CVD rates in Sub-Saharan Africa are generally lacking, and when present, are often of poor quality. Much of the available data comes from individual studies, often hospital-based, with small numbers of participants. Often the different data sources are heterogenous in methodology and cannot be compared; and systematic and regular surveillance systems are almost totally absent, making it difficult to plot changes in CVD rates over time. Nevertheless, the available data sources do give some idea of the nature and magnitude of CVD in Sub-Saharan Africa and of the changes in the nature and rates of CVD that have taken place over the past 50 years.

Measures of Cardiovascular Mortality

Globally, cause-of-death data based on the death certificate as provided to the data bank of the World Health Organization (WHO) is available in only 77 countries. There is wide regional variation in coverage by national vital registration systems, ranging from 80 percent population coverage in the European region to less than 5 percent in the Eastern Mediterranean and African regions of WHO (Sen and Bonita 2000). The most serious gap is for adult mortality, crucial if one is to gauge the true extent of CVD in the developing world and monitor trends over time.

The 10-fold variation in infant mortality between different regions of the world is largely due to communicable disease, malnutrition, and poverty, whereas the cause of death in adults age 15 to 60 is almost entirely due to noncommunicable diseases (NCDs) and injury (Murray and Lopez 1997). Men in Sub-Saharan Africa are three times more likely to die prematurely than men in Western industrial populations as a result of AIDS and violence.

Verbal autopsy has been shown to be an economical and useful way of improving the quality of cause-of-death information when health workers have minimal training. For example, in an investigation of causes of death in women of childbearing age in Guinea-Bissau, 70 percent of deaths could be attributed to a specific disease or condition (Sen and Bonita 2000).

Cardiovascular Surveillance Systems

Data on the incidence and prevalence of CVD is scanty. Surveillance should become a critical component in the strategies adopted in Sub-Saharan Africa to deal with the burgeoning epidemic of CVD. Sentinel surveillance is likely to be the preferred methodology, whereby monitoring of disease episodes is periodically conducted at sentinel sites that are broadly representative of the general population. This methodology is preferred because Sub-Saharan countries have limited resources, and their health systems cannot monitor every single disease episode. The systems set in place should include behavioral surveillance, often dubbed "second generation surveillance." Demographic health surveys are cheaper to administer but suffer from the pitfall of their cross-sectional design. Surveillance will not only monitor the prevalence of CVD but will also help gauge the impact of primary prevention strategies.

Crude Mortality versus Age-Standardized Mortality

The importance of CVD mortality in Sub-Saharan Africa countries tends to be underestimated, because crude mortality rates rather than age-standardized mortality rates are used. Thus the appalling figures for infant mortality from infectious disease and diseases of poverty tend to overshadow all other causes of death. Yet, from the perspective of citizens of Sub-Saharan countries when contemplating their own mortality, or the policy maker when considering causes of death among economically active people, age-specific mortality ratios are critical. They are also important for the planner predicting the patterns of death in years to come. Age-standardized mortality ratios make it clear that the long-heralded epidemic of CVD in Africa has, at least in some African countries, already arrived. Indeed, in some middle-income countries, such as South Africa, age-standardized mortality rates are higher than for Scotland and Finland, and they are exceeded only by rates in the former socialist economies of Europe (figure 21.1) (Bradshaw et al. 2003).

Figure 21.1 Cardiovascular Disease, Age-Standardized Rates in the World, 1994–2000

(per 100,000 people)

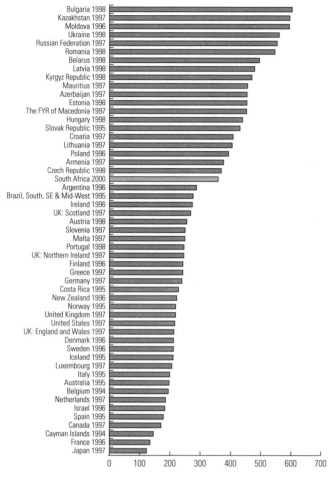

Source: Debbie Bradshaw (personal communication) and WHO Mortality Database, WHO Statistical Information System at http://www3.who.int/whosis/ (accessed June 2005).

THE CHANGING PREVALENCE, INCIDENCE, AND PATTERN OF CARDIOVASCULAR DISEASE

The relative and absolute importance of CVD in countries of Sub-Saharan Africa is thought to be increasing, but information on morbidity, mortality, and prevalence of disease and risk factors is scanty (Muna 1993b; Razum 1996). Data from 20 years ago consisted largely of hospital records, which reported that 8 to 12 percent of hospital admissions were due to heart disease in several countries in southern Africa (Vaughan 1977); hypertensive and rheumatic heart disease (RHD) accounted for 40 to 60 percent of these admissions. There were few recorded episodes of ischemic cardiac events. By 1977 such causes of death as syphilitic heart disease were rarely recorded, despite the continuing high frequency of acute syphilis. In the 1970s cardiac disease

was common among young people in Kampala, Uganda, where autopsy data demonstrated cardiac disease to be a cause of death in 15.3 percent of males older than 60 years and in 13.1 percent of males younger than 30 years (Drury 1972). In 1980 the Zambian Ministry of Health report of admissions and causes of death in all government, mining, and mission hospitals listed 2.06 percent of deaths in those under age 14 years as cardiac in origin compared with 14.50 percent in those over age 14. As regards morbidity, 0.62 percent of hospital admissions of children under 14 in that same study were cardiac in origin compared with 4.23 percent of those individuals over age 14 (Hutt 1990).

By 1990, CVD had become the third most common cause of death in a prospective autopsy study in 90 of the 167 deaths in one year at Tshepong Hospital in the North West Province of South Africa (Steenkamp, Simson, and Theron 1992). In patients over age 35, CVD was the most common cause of death.

Cerebrovascular disease accounted for 32 percent of the CVD deaths overall. Among these, intracerebral hemorrhage was found in 50 percent and cerebral infarction in 29 percent of cases. Fifty-seven percent of cardiovascular deaths were due to cardiac conditions, the most common being pulmonary hypertension (31 percent), dilated cardiomyopathy and chronic rheumatic valvular disease (17 percent each), and hypertensive heart disease (14 percent). Only 3 percent of the examined vessels had signs of severe atherosclerosis. The clinical diagnosis was the same as the final autopsy diagnosis in only 38 percent of cases, emphasizing the importance of performing autopsies to obtain reliable mortality statistics in African countries.

In a prospective study among elderly patients in Kenyatta National Hospital, Nairobi, Kenya, in 1991 to 1992, clinical evidence of CVD was present in 40 percent of the patients evaluated; 54 percent were hypertensive, 53 percent had arrhythmia, and 49 percent had congestive cardiac failure (Lodenyo, McLigeyo, and Ogola 1997). A prospective study of 708 subjects with CVD was conducted between January 1992 and December 1995 in Ghana (Amoah 2000). Participants were evaluated clinically, with ancillary laboratory tests, chest X-ray, electrocardiography, and two-dimensional echocardiography with doppler and color flow mapping. Hypertensive heart disease ($n = 133$), RHD ($n = 123$), idiopathic cardiomyopathy ($n = 103$), congenital heart disease ($n = 90$), and coronary artery disease (CAD; $n = 80$) were the major causes of cardiovascular morbidity. The mean age of the subjects was 41.6; peak incidence of CVD occurred during the decile 40–49 years of age.

A retrospective study in 1995 in Cameroon of 312 adult patients with CVD, average age 44 years, revealed high blood pressure (38.5 percent), rheumatic valvular heart diseases (25.6 percent), cardiomyopathies (22.5 percent), and other cardiovascular diseases (13.5 percent) (Kotto and Bouelet 2000). Rheumatic valvulopathies were predominant among the age group 20 to 39 years, hypertension was predominant from the age of 40 years, and cardiomyopathies were observed in the age range 20 to 60 years.

A Cameroonian study between 1992 and 1997 ranked coronary artery disease eighth among the CVDs registered with a prevalence of 1.53 percent (2.42 percent in males and 0.45 percent in females). Myocardial infarction was the most frequent clinical form of CAD observed (43 percent), followed by angina pectoris (23 percent), unstable angina (20 percent), and other forms of ischemic heart disease (13 percent). The cardiovascular risk factors were obesity (80 percent), hypertension (60 percent), dyslipidemia (43 percent), smoking (36 percent), diabetes/hyperglycemia (26 percent), and hyperuricemia (20 percent). Seventy-six percent of the patients had at least three cardiovascular risk factors (Mbanya et al. 1998).

In multiethnic South Africa, CHD is the major cause of death among white people and South Africans of Indian descent, with incidence rates of 165.3 and 101.2 per 100,000 people, respectively, but only 55.1 per 100,000 among people of mixed descent and 5.3 per 100,000 among black African people. Cerebrovascular disease is the most common cause of CVD death among those of mixed descent, followed by white people and South Africans of Indian descent, and then black African people (73.6, 62.5, and 36.5 per 100,000, respectively) (Bradshaw et al. 2003).

In South Africa 90 percent of deaths are certified; of these certifications over 70 percent are by a medical doctor, and cause-specific data are available for most deaths. A gradually shrinking proportion, currently 13 percent, are categorized as "ill-defined." It is quite possible that many deaths from CVD could masquerade as ill-defined deaths, particularly in a country where there is still a reluctance to diagnose CVD death in black people.

EPIDEMIOLOGY OF THE VARIOUS CVDS

With such inadequate data sources, it is inevitable that the epidemiology of CVD in Sub-Saharan Africa will be poorly understood.

Cerebrovascular Accidents

The prevalence and incidence of stroke in Sub-Saharan Africa have increased over the last half century, due principally to increased life expectancy and changes in environmental determinants and risk factors. The majority of cerebrovascular accidents (CVAs) occur in young and middle-aged people and are related to hypertension. Hypertension is highly prevalent in Sub-Saharan Africa and is often undetected or poorly controlled. This may be the explanation for the high proportion of hemorrhagic CVAs, whereas in developed countries most CVAs occur in older people and are thrombotic in etiology. This has been confirmed by clinical, radiological, and postmortem diagnostic methods. Overall, CVAs account for 7 percent of deaths in South Africa (Statistics South Africa 1996).

Cross-sectional, hospital-based studies of the prevalence and incidence of CHD and stroke and associated risk factors have been carried out in South Africa, central Africa, West Africa, and North Africa (Ezenwaka et al. 1997; Vorster 2002; Walker and Sareli 1997; Wiredu and Nyame 2001). In the city of Tunis in Tunisia the crude annual incidence rate of stroke has been estimated at 54 per 100,000 and the prevalence rate at 600 to 1,400 per 100,000. The incidence rate adjusted to population at risk (greater than or equal to 45 years old), is about 192 per 100,000. A door-to-door survey conducted in the town of Kelibia in Tunisia showed a prevalence rate of 720 per 100,000 when adjusted to population at risk. The crude incidence rate of stroke was estimated to be between 1 and 30 per 100,000; and the standardized rate was 68 per 100,000. Fifty percent of the stroke victims were below the age of 54 years; and one-third of them died within one week of the stroke. Overall, the age-specific rates for both sexes rose with age, with the rates for women being higher at all age strata except for the group age 45 to 54 years (Mirabet 1990). In a South African study of stroke patients in 1998, only 20 percent of the total group understood that hypertension had probably caused their stroke, although 76 percent of the older group and 56 percent of the younger group had been told at some stage that they were hypertensive (Hale, Fritz, and Eales 1998).

In a study of CVA in 21 centers in Africa, Asia, Europe, and Latin America, using computed tomography (CT) scan, magnetic resonance imaging (MRI), or cerebral angiography, the overall odds ratio of ischemic stroke was 2.99 (95 percent CI, 1.65–5.40) in Europe and 2.93 (2.15–4.00) in the non-European (developing) countries.

Table 21.2 shows data on incidence of stroke in Sub-Saharan Africa from a review of literature on hospital studies

Table 21.2 Incidence of Stroke

Author and date	Site	Incidence
Rosman 1986	Hospital based (review of literature)	101/100,000
Osuntokun et al. 1987	Population	58/100,000
Matenga 1997	Hospital based	30.7/100,000

Source: Compiled by authors.

in Africa (Rosman 1986), a population-based study in Nigeria (Osuntokun et al. 1987), and a hospital study in Zimbabwe (Matenga 1997).

In Mauritius between 1990 and 1994 (Sarti et al. 2000) the age-standardized stroke mortality for women and men age 35 to 74 years was 268 per 100,000 and 138 per 100,000, respectively.

In Tanzania, recent verbal autopsy data demonstrated that the age-adjusted stroke mortality rates were high (Walker et al. 2000). During the three-year observation period 11,975 deaths were recorded in three surveillance areas, of which 7,629 (64 percent) were of adults age 15 years or older; of these, 4,088 (54 percent) were of men and 3,541 (46 percent) were of women. CVD accounted for 421 (5.5 percent) of the deaths; of these, 225 (53 percent) were of men and 196 (47 percent) were of women. The yearly age-adjusted rates per 100,000 in the 15-to-64-year age group for the three project areas (urban, fairly prosperous rural, and poor rural) were 65 (95 percent CI, 39–90), 44 (31–56), and 35 (22–48), respectively, for men, and 88 (48–128), 33 (22–43), and 27 (16–38) for women. In a hospital-based study of 116 patients in Pretoria, one-month mortality was 33.6 percent (Rosman 1986).

Coronary Heart Disease

CHD, clinically manifested as ischemic heart disease (IHD), was formerly rare in Sub-Saharan Africa, again probably largely because the majority of Africans did not live long enough to suffer the clinical manifestations of angina, acute ischemic syndromes, myocardial infarction, and heart failure that usually develop in middle and old age. Still, even in those Africans who did live long enough for the cumulative effects of risk factors for CHD to take effect, CHD was rare up until the mid-twentieth century as evidenced by 3,500 postmortem studies in Ghana (Edington 1954) in which only three cases of CHD were found; of 635 cases of cardiac death in Uganda in 1966, 10 years later, less than 1 percent of CHD was found at autopsy (Hutt and Coles 1969). CHD

has been increasing since the 1980s (Hutt 1990), however, with reports of clinical IHD and increasing CHD prevalence (Bertrand 1992; Hutt 1990). The risk factors seem to be the same as in Europe, but the risk index is 2.1 to 2.7 compared with 3.6 in France. Myocardial infarction at 49 percent was the most common manifestation of CHD, followed by angina pectoris at 32 percent; ischemic cardiomyopathy, 7 percent; and ventricular aneurysm, 7 percent (Bertrand 1992). Myocardial infarction in black Africans under age 40 years shows characteristics similar to those seen in patients under age 40 in the West, particularly regarding the frequency of myocardial infarction as the first manifestation of the disease, low prevalence of coronary artery stenosis, and a relatively common finding of normal coronary arteriography (Nethononda et al. 2004).

The increase in CHD in Sub-Saharan Africa since the 1980s is presumably because of the increasing prevalence among African populations of the classical risk factors for CAD: smoking, a diet high in saturated fat, hypertension, obesity, diabetes mellitus, and lack of physical exercise. In addition, life expectancy in Sub-Saharan Africa has risen since the 1950s, meaning that more people are exposed to these risk factors for long enough periods to cause CAD. A study of black African patients admitted to a coronary care unit with acute myocardial infarction between 1995 and 1996 showed high rates of smoking and hypertension among the patients compared with controls matched by age and sex (Mayosi et al. 1997).

A coronary angiographic study of black African patients with acute myocardial infarction and acute ischemic syndromes admitted to Chris Hani Baragwanath Hospital in Johannesburg, South Africa, showed a clear increase in prevalence of risk factors for CHD in these patients compared with age- and sex-matched controls (Nethononda et al. 2004). In coronary angiographic studies of black Africans following myocardial infarction, mild to moderate coronary artery disease is often found rather than the moderate to severe artery disease found in their white and Indian counterparts. Indeed, CHD is the most common cause of morbidity and mortality in South Africans of Indian descent (Seedat 1998).

The risk factor profile, then, for CHD is the same in Sub-Saharan Africa countries as in Western countries, but the hemoglobin S or C trait could be a risk factor for CHD unique to Sub-Saharan Africa. The long-term outcome of infarction is severe and influenced by myocardial sequelae of imprecise origin, delayed hospitalization, absence of thrombolysis and angioplasty, and socioeconomic and literacy problems.

Mortality from CHD is much more difficult to estimate than that from stroke without a population-based study in Sub-Saharan Africa. Steinberg, Balfe, and Kustner (1988) reported a 25 percent decline in age-adjusted mortality from IHD in South Africa, from 162 per 100,000 people in 1978 to 121 per 100,000 in 1985. Bertrand (1992) reported an in-hospital mortality after myocardial infarction of 15 percent.

A recent case-control study of 98 black South Africans with CHD over 15 years culminated in 58 deaths from myocardial infarction with postmortem data available. Logistic regression analysis revealed that the classical risk factors in this cohort of patients operated in the same way as in Western populations (K. Steyn, unpublished observations). Similar results have been found in the soon-to-be published Interheart Study of risk factors for CHD among 15,152 patients around the world compared with age- and sex-matched controls. This included several hundred patients in South Africa from all ethnic groups and demonstrated that nine easily measured risk factors are associated with more than 90 percent of the risk. These results are consistent across all geographic regions and ethnic groups of the world, men and women, and young and old (Yusuf et al. 2004).

Rheumatic Heart Disease

Twenty years ago rheumatic heart disease (RHD) was the most common form of cardiac disease in Sub-Saharan Africa and still remains prevalent, with many young people in their teens and early twenties presenting with severe RHD (Ekra and Bertrand 1992). In the 1980s RHD accounted for 10 to 35 percent of hospital cardiac patients in Sub-Saharan Africa (Hutt 1990) and up to 20 percent of cardiac deaths noted at autopsy. Most of the cases occurred in young people. In Soweto, Johannesburg, South Africa, the incidence of RHD among primary schoolchildren was 6.9 per 1,000; and in Ibadan, Nigeria, the incidence was 3 per 1,000 among children (Hutt 1990).

A Ghanaian study reported the most common rheumatic valvular lesion to be mitral regurgitation (Amoah 2000). In a survey of 1,115 children in Kenya, 3 had clinical and echocardiographic evidence of RHD, giving a prevalence rate of 2.7 per 1,000 (Anabwani and Bonhoeffer 1996), whereas 6.2 percent had trivial mitral regurgitation; 0.3 percent, trivial aortic regurgitation; and 0.4 percent, isolated mild to moderate regurgitation of the pulmonary valve. Congenital heart disease was found in two children, one with secundum atrial septal defect and the other with a

ventricular septal defect and pulmonary stenosis, giving a prevalence of 1.8 per 1,000.

RHD is a disease of poverty, related to overcrowding, poor housing, and undernutrition and requires a multisectoral response for prevention and cure. It is caused by group A beta-hemolytic streptococci. The principal methods of control are primary and secondary prevention of streptococcal infection. Specifically, these preventive measures entail prompt treatment of streptococcal throat infections with penicillin in primary prevention and penicillin prophylaxis following rheumatic fever in order to prevent rheumatic heart disease in secondary prevention. The lack of these preventive measures explains the persistence of rheumatic fever and RHD in Sub-Saharan Africa, which, compared with the rest of the world, has remained poor. Countries in Sub-Saharan Africa also lack adequate health systems for managing rheumatic fever and RHD.

Heart Failure

Systemic hypertension is the most common cause of heart failure among black Africans. In a study of 52 Gambians and 55 Nigerians between ages 16 and 69 years with hypertensive heart failure, the mean duration of diagnosis of systemic hypertension among the previously known hypertensives was 4.3 years (Isezuo et al. 2000). The overall one-year survival rate was 71 percent, although it was unclear whether this was largely systolic or diastolic heart failure and whether the cases were primarily essential hypertension or included large numbers with secondary hypertension. The prognosis of hypertensive heart failure among this population is poor, with the first three months from onset of heart failure being critical for survival. Early detection and control of systemic hypertension should be more aggressively pursued.

A 1993 study of patients admitted to Kenyatta National Hospital with congestive heart failure revealed that almost 32 percent had RHD, 25 percent had cardiomyopathy, 18 percent had hypertensive heart disease, 13 percent had pericardial disease, and 2 percent had ischemic heart disease (Oyoo and Ogola 1999).

RHD remains a major cause of heart failure in Africa, especially in the young, and hypertensive heart failure is common, unlike in developed countries, where improved blood pressure control has reduced the prevalence of this condition (Mendez and Cowie 2001). However, as African countries go through the epidemiological transition and develop socioeconomically, the epidemiology of heart failure becomes increasingly similar to that of Western Europe and North America, with CHD being the most common cause of heart failure. Preventive and public health strategies need to take cognizance of the local epidemiological characteristics.

Risk factors for cardiac failure in Brazzaville, Republic of Congo, from 1975 to 1999 were found to be arterial hypertension (53 percent), hypercholesterolemia (38 percent), smoking (28 percent), obesity (24 percent), and diabetes (5 percent) (Kimbally-Kaky and Bouramoue 2000). Risk factors for ischemic cardiopathy at the Hôpital Principal in Dakar, Senegal, were hypercholesterolemia (56 percent), tobacco smoking (44 percent), arterial hypertension (41 percent), diabetes (40 percent), and overweight (27 percent) (Thiam et al. 2000). Seventy-five percent of patients presented with coronary pain, and 50 percent had symptoms of cardiac insufficiency.

Dilated Cardiomyopathy

Dilated cardiomyopathy (DCM) resulting in congestive cardiac failure is surprisingly common in Sub-Saharan Africa, accounting for up to 20 percent of cardiac cases in some regions. Occasionally the disease is familial with specific candidate genes recently identified (Sliwa, Damasceno, and Mayosi 2005). A similar picture can be seen in beriberi and alcoholic cardiac disease. There may be a whole spectrum of causes of DCM, including genetic etiology, toxins, and vitamin or micronutrient deficiency, such as selenium deficiency. Dilated cardiomyopathy is often seen as a late complication of human immunodeficiency virus (HIV) infection (Fauci and Lane 2001).

In a Ghanaian study of 708 patients in a cardiac referral center, DCM was the most common form of cardiomyopathy, followed by hypertrophic cardiomyopathy and endomyocardial fibrosis (Amoah 2000). Treatment involves nonspecific management of the congestive cardiac failure, although cardioselective beta-blockade has been increasingly used. End-stage disease often necessitates cardiac transplantation, although this is rarely feasible in most African countries because of resource constraints.

Endomyocardial Fibrosis

Endomyocardial fibrosis (EMF) was first described in detail by J. N. P. Davies in Uganda in 1948 (Davies 1948). Fibrosis of the inflow tracts of the right and left ventricles results in mitral or tricuspid incompetence and impaired ventricular function, as a result of the restrictive deficit in which the stiff fibrotic ventricles cannot contract and relax normally. Patients usually present in their twenties or thirties. The

disease is found in a broad swath across Africa, between the Sahara Desert in the north and the Zambezi River in the south. In temperate climates the disease is rare, presenting as Loeffler's endocarditis, a syndrome exhibiting marked eosinophilia. Consequently it has been suggested that EMF may be caused by an eosinophilic response to filariasis or malaria. Another hypothesis from Uganda implicates cassava protein in the etiology of EMF, but the geographical spread of the disease compared with areas where cassava is eaten does not support this as a sole etiological agent (Hutt 1990).

In a Kenyan study, patients with echocardiographically proven EMF recruited between 1993 and 1996 were found to have eosinophilia of more than 500 cells per microliter, compared with non-EMF cardiac patients, and general medical outpatients (Mayanja-Kizza et al. 2000). High eosinophilia of more than 1,000 cells per microliter was found in 38 percent of the EMF patients but only 6 percent of the non-EMF cardiac patients and in 5 percent of general medical patients. High levels of eosinophilia in the range of the hypereosinophilic syndrome (HES; over 1,500 cells per microliter) were found in 20 percent of EMF patients but in only 2 percent of the non-EMF cardiac patients and in 1 percent of the general medical patients. The prevalence of blood and stool parasites was identical in all groups and could not explain eosinophilia. More often than not the eosinophilic cells in EMF patients were abnormal.

HIV-Related Cardiomyopathy

People with AIDS have evidence of cardiac involvement at postmortem (40 percent) and by echocardiography (25 percent) (Fauci and Lane 2001). However, fewer than 10 percent ever experience symptoms. Cardiac involvement is the cause of death in only 1 to 2 percent of patients infected with HIV (Boon 2003). These figures may be higher in African populations, but good quality epidemiological data are lacking. The possibility of higher figures rests on the premises that nonischemic cardiomyopathy is more common in African populations than in Western countries and that the etiological factors that cause this high incidence of cardiomyopathy, be they nutritional deficiencies, genetic predispositions, or toxic factors, act synergistically with the effects of HIV infection on the heart.

HIV infection causes not only cardiomyopathy and heart failure but also CVA, pulmonary embolism, tuberculous pericarditis, marantic (nonbacterial) endocarditis, autonomic dysfunction, and proarrhythmic drug effects. In a recent review of 17 peer-reviewed publications covering

January 1980 to February 2003 on cardiac involvement in HIV-infected people living in Africa, Magula and Mayosi (2003) showed that cardiac abnormalities are more common in HIV-infected people than in normal controls and that about half of hospitalized patients and a significant proportion of patients followed over several years develop cardiac abnormalities. The most common HIV-related cardiac abnormalities were cardiomyopathy and pericardial disease. Tuberculosis was the major cause of large pericardial effusion in Africa. HIV-related pericardial effusions are usually exudates and tend to occur in patients with advanced disease, with an annual incidence of 10 percent among people living with HIV and AIDS. They are an independent risk factor for early death, with median survival of less than six months after occurrence of the effusion.

Myocarditis was the most common pathological abnormality in HIV-associated cardiomyopathy, and nonviral opportunistic infections, such as toxoplasmosis and *Cryptococcus,* may account for up to 50 percent of such cases in Africa. Although the mechanisms involved in cardiomyopathy in people with HIV infection are poorly defined, a role for direct retroviral action or focal infiltration of activated immune cells, or both, has been postulated. Recent studies have demonstrated cardiac myocyte protein infiltration in AIDS-related cardiomyopathies, rather than focal immune cell lesions (Magula and Mayosi 2003). In Africa, however, other factors, such as nutritional deficiencies and the cardiotoxicity of antiretroviral medications, are associated with dilated cardiomyopathy in HIV-infected patients (Magula and Mayosi 2003). Long-term cardiac side effects of antiretroviral therapy are likely to become increasingly common in Africa as antiretroviral therapy becomes more readily available through national treatment programs, such as the Plan for the Comprehensive Treatment and Care of HIV and AIDS in South Africa (http://www.doh.gov.za), the WHO "3 by 5" Initiative (WHO 2004), and the President's Emergency Plan for AIDS Relief sponsored by the United States (IOM 2005). Most African programs, however, do not include protease inhibitors, responsible for much of the long-term cardiac toxicity, in their first regimen. Antiretroviral cardiac side effects may become apparent only in several years time as protease inhibitors come off patent and become affordable to national programs in Africa.

Sickle-Cell Disease

A study of 70 children between the ages of 3 and 16 years with homozygous sickle-cell anemia in Lomé, Togo, from January 1996 to April 1997 found that 26 percent had a nor-

mal heart, 66 percent had dilated cardiac cavities and a hypocontractile left ventricle, and 9 percent had nonobstructive cardiomyopathy, dilated cardiac cavities, and a hypocontractile left ventricle (Kokou et al. 1999). A study of the left ventricular systolic function of patients with sickle-cell anemia at the University College Hospital, Ibadan, Nigeria, revealed that although the left ventricular mass index was significantly larger in the patients than in the controls, there were no significant differences in the left ventricular systolic function at rest between patients with sickle-cell anemia and age- and sex-matched normal controls (Adebiyi, Falase, and Akenova 1999). The prominent cardiovascular abnormalities seen in patients with sickle-cell anemia, therefore, are most likely to have resulted from left ventricular diastolic dysfunction. Further studies are required to evaluate the left ventricular diastolic function in patients with sickle-cell anemia as well as their cardiac function during exercise and during episodes of crisis.

Congenital Heart Disease

Ventricular and atrial septal defect, Fallot's tetralogy, and patent ductus arteriosus were the most common congenital lesions in a Ghanaian study (Amoah 2000). The major cardiovascular disorders in children were congenital heart disease and RHD. Idiopathic cardiomyopathy was rare. In a study of 13,322 schoolchildren from Sahafa Town, Khartoum, Sudan, from 1986 to 1990, the prevalence of congenital heart disease was 2.0 per 1,000, with ventricular septal defect, atrial septal defect, patent ductus arteriosus, and Fallot's tetralogy making up 85 percent of the cases (Khalil et al. 1997). Patent ductus arteriosus and atrial septal defect were twice as common in females as in males. The prevalence rate was comparable to that of similar African countries but lower than European and North American rates.

Dysrhythmias

Atrial fibrillation is the most common cardiac arrhythmia in South Africa, often related to RHD, and is responsible for significant morbidity and mortality in the general population. The incidence of atrial fibrillation in South Africa is about 8 percent of the population 70 years and older. Atrial fibrillation affects more than 5 percent of the population over 65 and 10 percent of those over 80. The incidence is higher in patients with left ventricular hypertrophy and heart failure. Intraventricular malconductions seem to exhibit a prevalence in African populations similar to that in other parts of the world (Omotoso and Kane 2000).

Pericarditis

A study carried out from 1989 to 1996 in the Republic of Congo found that 4.9 percent of patients with cardiovascular disease had nonrheumatic pericarditis with effusion (Nkoua, Tsombou, and Bouramoue 1999). Twenty-two percent were HIV positive. The principal cause of the pericarditis was tuberculosis, which accounted for about a quarter of the patients, all of whom were HIV positive; all those with benign acute pericarditis were HIV negative; and all those with lymphocytic pericarditis were HIV positive. Of those affected by cardiac tamponade, just under a third were HIV positive. The mortality rate was 11.0 percent—9.9 percent among those who were HIV negative and 15.0 percent among those who were HIV positive. This study confirms the high rate of nonrheumatic pericardial effusion, the role of HIV infection, and the leading place of tuberculosis among causes. These findings corroborate those suggesting that the outcome of pericardial effusion associated with HIV infection can be cardiac tamponade (Nkoua, Tsombou, and Bouramoue 1999).

DETERMINANTS, BEHAVIORS, AND RISK FACTORS

In the past few decades appreciation of the importance of determinants and risk factors in the etiology of CVD has grown. Determinants are the ecological factors that provide the milieu in which a disease develops and need not be directly linked to the disease causally. Most people exposed to the determinant do not inevitably develop the disease.

Genetic determinants provide the foundation on which behavioral, sociocultural, economic, and educational determinants build. As an example, the popular hypothesis that African people have a genetic predisposition for salt retention may be compounded in urban African cultures in which salt intake is high, thus causing hypertension and in part explaining the documented higher incidence of hypertension in urban than rural African societies (Steyn and Fourie 1991).

Risk factors arise from determinants and are directly linked to a disease in a causal fashion, although not everyone with the risk factor develops the disease. Risk factors include smoking, high blood pressure, malnutrition, obesity, hyperlipidemia, lack of physical exercise, and beta-hemolytic streptococcal infection. Many of the determinants of CVD are shared with cancer, diabetes, and chronic obstructive disease. Table 21.3 illustrates the relation between CVD determinants, risk factors, behaviors, and disease (Reddy 2004).

Coronary heart disease and stroke share the same risk factors, but their relative implication in the occurrence of these diseases is different. Since the middle of the twentieth century the prevalence of all risks factors for CVDs, except hyperlipidemia, has been increasing. Hyperlipidemia, although less prevalent than in developed countries, is found in patients with metabolic disorders and families with genetic susceptibility (Law 1998). Risk factors for CVD present in developed countries are the same in Sub-Saharan Africa, but their association and the possibly differing genetic susceptibilities may be responsible for the particular pattern of CVD in Africa.

Table 21.3 The Relation between CVD, Risk Factors, Behaviors, and Determinants

Disease or disorder	Risk factors	Behaviors	Determinants
Cardiovascular disease (stroke, ischemic heart disease, peripheral vascular disease)	Tobacco	Smoking tobacco Chewing tobacco	Psychosocial
			Educational
	Alcohol	Alcohol misuse	
			Environmental
	Food	Food consumption eating cooking purchasing	Economic
			Commercial
			Advertising
	Hypertension	Salt use	Marketing
		Health care–seeking behavior	Food labeling
		Medication compliance behavior	
	Obesity	Sedentary behavior	
	Lack of physical activity		

Source: Reddy 2004.

Table 21.4 Risk Factors for CHD Reported from Hospital Patients

Author and date	Age (mean or range)	Sample size	Hypertension (%)	Diabetes (%)	Obesity (%)	Smoking (%)
Bertrand 1992	45	100	25.8	12.9	29	60.0
Steyn and Fourie 1991	15–64	986	14.4 (M) 13.7 (F)	—	—	22.0 (M) 8.4 (F)
Rosman 1986	20	—	69.8	—	—	—

Source: Compiled by authors.
Note: — = not available; M = male; F = female.

A Tunisian population study estimated the prevalence of risk factors for CVD to be 19 percent for hypertension, 10 percent for diabetes, 28 percent for obesity, 36 percent for android obesity, and 21 percent for smoking (Ghanem and Fredj 1999). Total calorie intake was 2,483 kilocalories, comprised of 67 percent carbohydrates, 18 percent protein, and 15 percent fat. Among urban dwellers in Sub-Saharan Africa, intakes of food, especially fat, have risen, and intakes of high-fiber foods have fallen. The mean serum cholesterol level is significantly higher than that of rural populations living traditionally (Steyn and Fourie 1991). Obesity in females has risen enormously. The prevalence of hypertension exceeds that in developed countries. The same applies to the practice of smoking in males but not in females. The level of physical activity has fallen. Table 21.4 shows the relative prevalence of the most important risk factors for coronary heart disease in hospital patients.

Stroke and coronary heart disease occurs earlier in the lives of people in Africa, as in other low-income countries, than in the industrial world. Whereas CVDs are diseases of elderly people in developed countries, where they occur after the age of 60, they are preponderant in Africans even before the age of 40.

Hypertension

At the beginning of the twentieth century, high blood pressure was virtually nonexistent among indigenous Kenyans (Lore 1993) and Ugandans (Hutt 1990), but the reason may have been the lack of screening programs and access to care. From about 1975, high blood pressure became established in Cameroon, Côte d'Ivoire, Democratic Republic of Congo, Ghana, Kenya, Nigeria, and Uganda. As in developed countries, consumption of salt and alcohol, psychological stress, obesity, physical inactivity, and other dietary factors are thought to have played an important etiologic role in the genesis of primary hypertension in genetically predisposed

individuals. Nevertheless, communities still exist in the Democratic Republic of Congo, Kenya, Nigeria, and the Kalahari Desert in which blood pressure is low and does not seem to rise with age. Rural-to-urban migration coupled with acculturation and modernization trends have some relation to the development of high blood pressure as observed in Kenyan and Ghanaian epidemiologic studies (table 21.5).

The prevalence of hypertension is particularly high in urban settings in Sub-Saharan Africa; between 8 and 25 percent of the adult population are affected, depending on what definition of hypertension is used. The two commonly used are the Joint National Committee on Detection, Evaluation, and Treatment of High Blood Pressure VI (JNC VI) definition (JNC 1997), which is a systolic pressure above 140 and diastolic pressure above 90 millimeters of mercury (mmHg), and a more conservative cutoff of 160 systolic pressure and 100 diastolic, as used in many African control programs. Over 80 percent of hypertensive patients in clinical practice have essential hypertension (that is, primary hypertension with no known cause), with most of the remainder having a renal origin for their hypertension (Akinkugbe 1976).

Before the latter half of the twentieth century most people in most Sub-Saharan Africa countries did not live beyond 40 years, the age at which hypertension becomes increasingly more prevalent. Some earlier researchers suggested that Africans did not show the characteristic increase in blood pressure with age (Shaper 1974), but this observation may have been due to deficiencies in the design of cohort studies.

So prevalent is hypertension today in Sub-Saharan Africa that hypertensive heart disease might in fact be the most common form of CVD in Africa. Hypertension is a risk factor for both stroke and IHD (Bradshaw et al. 2003). Left ventricular hypertrophy, congestive heart failure, and stroke are common in Africans with hypertension. There is little

Table 21.5 Prevalence of Hypertension, by Country

Country	Author and date	Criteria	Population	Prevalence (%) Male	Prevalence (%) Female
Cameroon	Mbanya et al. 1998	(1)	Urban	16.4	12.1
Cameroon	Mbanya et al. 1998	(1)	Rural	5.4	5.9
Mauritius	Nan et al. 1991	(1)	Urban and rural	11.0	2.0
Nigeria	Cooper, Rotimi, Ataman et al. 1997	(2)	Urban and rural	15.0	14.0
Senegal	Astagneau et al. 1992	(1)	Urban	11.0	11.0
Senegal	Astagneau et al. 1992	(2)	Urban	24.0	22.0
South Africa	Steyn et al. 1996	(1)	Urban	13.0	2.0
South Africa	Metcalf et al. 1996	(1)	Rural	16.0	2.0
Tanzania	Berrios et al. 1997	(1)	Urban	9.0	12.0
Tanzania	Edwards et al. 2000	(2)	Urban	30.0	28.6
Tanzania	Edwards et al. 2000	(2)	Rural	32.2	31.5

Source: Compiled by authors.
Note: (1) = 160/95 mmHg or treated or self-reported; (2) = 140/90 mmHg or treated or self-reported.

published information on formal programs addressing awareness, treatment, and control. Local, regional, and national surveys are required to provide epidemiological data necessary for informed decision making and policy setting on when and whom to treat in Africa (Kapuku, Mensah, and Cooper 1998; van der Sande et al. 2001).

There seem to be marked urban-rural differences in the prevalence of the disease (table 21.5). Prevalence levels are higher in South Africa among urban Zulu people than among their rural counterparts (Mokhobo 1976; Seedat, Seedat, and Hackland 1982) and among urban Xhosa people in Cape Town than their rural relatives in the Eastern Cape (Sever et al. 1980; Steyn et al. 1993). In Cameroon, age-adjusted rates of blood pressure in urban areas were greater than or equal to 160 mmHg systolic or 95 mmHg diastolic, and treatment of hypertension rose from 5 percent in rural areas to 17 percent in urban ones (Cruickshank et al. 2001).

Few studies from Africa have reported on hypertension treatment and control. In the Black Risk Factors Study (BRISK) study in urban black townships in the Cape peninsula of Cape Town, South Africa, 61 percent of those with hypertension (greater than or equal to 160 over 95 mmHg) were aware of their hypertension, and 48 percent were treated. In an urban population in the Democratic Republic of Congo only 31 percent of those with hypertension (blood pressure greater than or equal to 160 over 95 mmHg) were aware of their diagnosis; 13 percent were treated and 3 percent of those with hypertension had their disease controlled (M'Buyamba-Kabangu et al. 1986). Nigerian studies of

hypertensive patients confirm that patients are unable to perceive changes in their blood pressure and should be taught to rely on regular blood pressure checks by their physician (Familoni and Ariba 2003).

In Western societies, such as the United States and the United Kingdom, the prevalence of hypertension and standardized mortality rates from stroke are higher for people of African origin than for whites (Cooper, Rotimi, Kaufman, et al. 1997). The same pattern is emerging in Sub-Saharan Africa. Thus in South Africa, age-adjusted hypertension prevalence and age-specific rates of death from stroke are higher among urban blacks than equivalent white populations (Opie and Steyn 1995). There is evidence that hypertension is an important cause of mortality in Sub-Saharan Africa. The Adult Morbidity and Mortality Project (AMMP 1997) showed that the probability of dying from an NCD (which is largely made up of stroke in Tanzania) between the ages of 15 and 60 years is more than six times higher in an urban area and between two and four times higher in two rural areas in Tanzania than in the United Kingdom (AMMP 1997). In the same study, NCD was the most common cause of death in the urban area and one of the rural areas for those over 60 years of age (figure 21.2).

As in other parts of the world, the prevalence of hypertension in the Sub-Saharan Africa region has increased as a manifestation of the epidemiological transition (Omran 1983). This implies that, as elsewhere in the world, environmental factors related to urbanization and increasing affluence are important determinants of the disease.

Figure 21.2 Probability of Death by Broad Cause in Men between the Ages of 15 and 60 Years in Tanzania

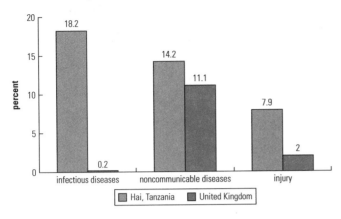

Source: AMPP 1997.

As the number of fatalities from cardiovascular diseases declines in Western industrial nations, an opposite trend is observed in East Africa (Mbaya 1998). Interregional variations in the prevalence of vascular disorders have been attributed to socioeconomic, psychosocial, and heritable physiological parameters.

Among the Luo of Kenya, increasing blood pressure within months of migrating from the rural areas to the city has been recorded, with concomitant increases in their dietary sodium and declines in their dietary potassium (Poulter 1988; Poulter et al. 1984). A prospective cross-sectional study in rural Nigeria showed the prevalence of obesity to be 2 percent, with 1.2 percent in males and 3.2 percent in females (Okesina et al. 1999). High blood pressure, observed in 15.2 percent of the subjects, occurred more among males (19.1 percent) than females (10.3 percent). Malignant hypertension is common.

Hypertensive patients whose blood pressure fails to fall at night in the normal 24-hour rhythm (nondippers) have a higher incidence of cardiovascular complication, early glomerular failure, and microalbuminuria. A Nigerian study identified 28 percent nondippers, 57.1 percent of whom had microalbuminuria (Alebiosu et al. 2004).

As regards hypertension control, the guidelines of JNC VI may be more relevant to Sub-Saharan Africa than JNC VII because of the difficulty of effecting even moderate control of hypertension in Sub-Saharan Africa.

Hyperlipidemia

Hyperlipidemia is uncommon in Africa, being present mainly in patients with metabolic disorders (hypertriglyc-

eridemia) or a family history of hypercholesterolemia. It is, however, present in 10 to 70 percent of patients with antecedent CHD or stroke. A study of black African patients admitted to a coronary care unit in Cape Town, South Africa, with acute ischemic syndromes and myocardial infarction revealed relative hyperlipidemia among the patients but not in the healthy controls (Mayosi et al. 1997).

Diabetes

Diabetes mellitus is a well-established risk factor for CVD (King, Aubert, and Herman 1998). The prevalence of type 2 diabetes in Africa is about 2.5 percent, ranging from 0.8 percent in rural Cameroon (Mbanya et al. 1997) to 13.5 percent in Mauritius (Dowse et al. 1990). Type 2 diabetes is more frequent in South Africa and North Africa than in central and West Africa, and it increases from rural to urban areas (Cooper, Rotimi, Kaufman, et al. 1997; King and Zimmet 1988). The World Bank ranks these countries as upper-middle-income countries, and they are further along the epidemiological transition than the low-income countries of Sub-Saharan Africa (table 21.6).

Tobacco Smoking and Alcohol Consumption

Tobacco consumption in South Africa has declined since 1994 due to stringent antitobacco legislation and hikes in excise duty, resulting in 25 percent reductions in both the number of people smoking and overall tobacco consumption (Reddy 1997; Steyn 1998) (see table 21.7). Alcohol consumption, however, is relatively frequent in Africa. The types of alcohol consumed include wine, beer, and locally made beverages. Alcohol has been implicated in the development of hypertension, CHD, stroke, and heart failure (table 21.8).

Lack of Physical Activity

Physical activity is more prevalent in rural than urban regions of Africa, and that partly explains the higher prevalence of obesity in urban areas. The prevalence of sedentary lifestyles in Cape Town, South Africa, among individuals 30 years of age and above was 39 percent for men and 44 percent for women (Levitt et al. 1993). Twenty-two percent of men and 52 percent of women in urban Tanzania (Edwards et al. 2000) had low levels of physical activity. Also, 10 percent of men and 15 percent of women in rural areas indicated low physical activity during the same study.

Table 21.6 Prevalence of Diabetes, by Country

Country	Author and date	Method	Site	Sample size	Prevalence (%)
Cameroon	Mbanya et al. 1997	Blood	Urban	1,048	2.8
Cameroon	Mbanya et al. 1997	Blood	Rural	719	1.1
Ethiopia	Peters 1983	Urine	Urban and rural	2,381	0.3
Lesotho	Politzer and Sachs 1967	Urine	Rural	3,000	0.2
Malawi	Davidson 1963	Urine	Urban and rural	4,725	0.1
Mali	Fisch et al. 1987	Blood	Rural	7,472	0.9
Nigeria	Ohwovoriole, Kuti, and Kabiawu 1988	Blood	Urban	1,627	1.7
Nigeria	Erasmus et al. 1989	Blood	Urban and rural	2,800	1.4
Nigeria	Owoaje et al. 1997	Blood	Urban	247	2.8
Sierra Leone	Ceesay et al. 1997	Blood	Urban	501	2.4
Sierra Leone	Ceesay et al. 1997	Blood	Rural	—	0.0
South Africa	Levitt et al. 1993	Blood	Urban	729	8.0
South Africa	Omar et al. 1993	Blood	Urban	479	5.3
South Africa	Mollentze et al. 1995	Blood	Urban	758	6.0
South Africa	Mollentze et al. 1995	Blood	Rural	853	4.8
Tanzania	Swai et al. 1993	Blood	Urban	1,255	8.8
Togo	Teuscher et al. 1987	Blood	Rural	1,381	0.0

Source: Compiled by authors.
Note: — = not available.

Table 21.7 Prevalence of Tobacco Smoking, by Country

Country	Author and date	Population	Prevalence (%) Men	Women
Ethiopia	Betre, Kebede, and Kassaye 1997	Urban	11.8	1.1
Tanzania	Bovet et al. 2002	Urban	22.0	2.6
Tanzania (Kilimanjaro)	Swai et al. 1993	Rural	42.6	2.1
Tanzania (Morogoro)	Swai et al. 1993	Rural	28.2	3.9
Tanzania (Mara)	Swai et al. 1993	Rural	8.6	2.7

Source: Compiled by authors.

Table 21.8 Prevalence of Alcohol Consumption, by Country

Country	Author and date	Population	Prevalence (%) Men	Women
Tanzania[a]	Edwards et al. 2000	Urban	6.1	2.5
Tanzania[a]	Edwards et al. 2000	Rural	3.0	0.0
Ethiopia	Betre, Kebede, and Kassaye 1997	Urban	34.0	34.0
Nigeria	Kadiri and Salako 1997	Urban	5.4	2.8
Zimbabwe[b]	Chinyadza et al. 1993	Urban	63.0	41.0

Source: Compiled by authors.
a. Heavy drinkers (more than 49 units per week for men and more than 35 units per week for women).
b. Hospital-based study.

Table 21.9 Prevalence of Obesity, by Country

Country	Author and date	Population	Prevalence (%) Male	Prevalence (%) Female
Cameroon	Sobngwi et al. 2002	Urban	17.1	3.0
Cameroon	Sobngwi et al. 2002	Rural	1.2	5.4
Gambia, The	van der Sande et al. 2001	Urban	4.0	4.0
Malawi	Msamati and Igbigbi 2000	Urban	0.0	11.4
Tanzania (Mara)	Swai et al. 1993	Rural	0.9	0.8
Tanzania (Kilimanjaro)	Swai et al. 1993	Rural	0.1	1.5
Tanzania (Morogoro)	Swai et al. 1993	Rural	0.1	1.1
Tanzania (Ilala)	Edwards et al. 2000	Urban	6.8	17.2
Tanzania (Shari)	Edwards et al. 2000	Rural	3.2	4.8
Tanzania (Dar es Salaam)	Bovet et al. 2002	Urban	6.9	17.4

Source: Compiled by authors.
Note: Obesity defined as body mass index greater than 30 kg/m^2.

Obesity

Obesity is increasing in prevalence in Sub-Saharan Africa; particularly among urban women (tables 21.9 and 21.10). However, the value of the waist-hip ratio has never been properly validated in large population-based studies in Sub-Saharan Africa in regard to their predictive value for cardiovascular outcomes. The same holds true for waist circumference of greater than 88 centimeters for females and 102 centimeters for males.

Genetic Determinants

The renin-angiotensin system and associated gene polymorphisms may be important in predicting cardiovascular

Table 21.10 Prevalence of Obesity in Women Age 15 to 49 Years, by Country

Country	Sample size	Prevalence (%) Urban	Prevalence (%) Rural
Benin	2,266	3.5	1.4
Burkina Faso	3,161	3.5	0.6
Central African Republic	2,025	2.0	0.5
Côte d'Ivoire	3,108	6.2	1.3
Ghana	1,773	8.1	1.5
Namibia	2,205	13.4	3.4
Niger	3,292	6.4	0.3
Senegal	2,895	7.2	1.9
Zimbabwe	1,968	12.5	3.4

Source: Martorell et al. 2000.
Note: Obesity defined as body mass index greater than 30 kg/m^2.

events, but the association is likely to be weak, as shown in one study of myocardial infarction in young South African Indians (Ranjith et al. 2004).

PREVENTION, REHABILITATION, AND CURE OF CARDIOVASCULAR DISEASE

Traditionally, interventions have focused on altering risk factors by, for example, eradicating streptococcal infection using antibiotics in order to prevent rheumatic fever and subsequent RHD. The health promotion approach, however, teaches that to be fully effective in curing, ameliorating, or preventing a disease, one must understand how the determinants give rise to a disease within particular settings. One can then develop determinant-based interventions. Thus, for example, rheumatic fever typically develops in situations of poverty and overcrowding, where children are malnourished, immunocompromised, and susceptible to bacterial infection. An intervention that focuses on providing penicillin for those children with streptococcal sore throat will not be fully effective in eradicating the disease. The determinants of the disease must also be dealt with by educating the caregiver to appreciate the need for prompt treatment of sore throats, educating health professionals to take a throat swab before starting antibiotic treatment, providing child support grants to caregivers so that they can buy food for the malnourished child, alleviating overcrowding so that the sick child does not sleep six to a bed with his or her siblings, thus spreading infection, and so on.

Health promotion also teaches the importance of the "settings approach" to disease prevention and control. It appreciates that the bulk of disease management does not take place in the hospital or clinic but in the home, the school, and the workplace. Understanding the etiology, natural history, and management paradigms of the disease within these settings is therefore crucial to developing prevention, rehabilitation, and cure programs.

These interventions may be tailored for the population, such as screening schoolchildren by taking throat swabs for beta-hemolytic streptococcus after an outbreak of rheumatic fever in a school or treating an infected child with penicillin for a streptococcal sore throat. Primary prevention may include the prevention and treatment of streptococcal infection by providing school feeding programs for malnourished children and providing penicillin to treat sore throats or training health personnel in the diagnosis of the condition and educating the caregiver. Secondary prevention is treating with penicillin for several years after an attack of rheumatic fever in order to prevent rheumatic heart disease; and tertiary prevention could involve treating the valvular cardiac disease of RHD symptomatically with diuretics and digoxin, curatively with balloon valvuloplasty or cardiac surgery.

A modern understanding of disease management emphasizes the importance of analyses of the cost-effectiveness of disease interventions in order to build sustainable systems for disease control. This is important for developed countries as well as for developing countries. It is particularly critical for the prevention and control of cardiovascular disease, for which secondary and tertiary interventions are often extremely expensive and require high-grade technical skills to administer. A difficult tradeoff has to be made in such CVD control programs between the different interventions, and this is best done rationally rather than emotionally. The tradeoff may be between providing antibiotics to prevent rheumatic fever versus providing surgery to babies with congenital heart disease, a difficult choice to make. The former intervention, however, may be far more cost-effective in the long run.

It is extremely difficult for policy makers and health planners to articulate and make these choices, as they often come with considerable political as well as emotional cost. Often the hard choice is masked under a "waiting list" on which children may die without an overt decision having been made to deny them lifesaving interventions. In Sub-Saharan Africa there often is no choice to make because the suffering and dying patients never even reach the clinic to demand treatment, or the facilities and surgeons to provide the surgery are nonexistent.

IMPACT ON THE HEALTH CARE SYSTEM IN AFRICA AND STRATEGIES FOR CONTROL AND PREVENTION

Options to improve monitoring of CVD morbidity and risk-factor levels include establishing community registries of stroke and repeatedly examining representative population samples. Nationwide vital registration to monitor CVD mortality would be desirable but appears not to be feasible at present, and maintaining a sample registration system would be prohibitively expensive.

In spite of the current low prevalence of hypertension in some countries, the total number of people with hypertension in the developing world is high, and a cost analysis of possible antihypertensive drug treatment indicates that developing countries cannot afford the same treatment as developed countries (Seedat 2000). Only 20 percent of the hypertension in the United States is under control, whereas in Africa only 5 to 10 percent is controlled at a blood pressure of less than 140 over 90 mmHg (Pretoria Department of Health 2002).

It is claimed that black patients respond well to thiazide diuretics, calcium channel blockers, and vasodilators such as alpha-blockers, hydralazine, and reserpine, and respond poorly to beta-blockers, angiotensin-converting enzyme inhibitors, and angiotensin II receptor antagonists unless they are combined with a diuretic. This is increasingly being brought into doubt, however. Comprehensive cardiovascular disease research programs in Africa are needed, as social, economic, and cultural factors impair control of hypertension in developing countries. Hypertension control is ideally suited to the initial component of an integrated CVD control program. Primary prevention, through a program focused on lifestyle should be synergistically linked to cost-effective methods of detection and management. The existing health care infrastructure needs to be oriented to meet the emerging challenge of CVD while empowering the community through health education.

The lipid cardiovascular risk-factor profile of African populations continues to be relatively benign, with mean total cholesterol, LDL cholesterol and HDL cholesterol, and median triglyceride levels in the "low risk" ranges, even among cohorts with established CVD. The other major risk factors, however, are significantly elevated in urban populations, particularly prevalent hypertension, increasing obesity, and type 2 diabetes mellitus, as well as growing rates of tobacco use. Furthermore, the prevalence of risk factors has risen in both urban and rural areas. A 1998 study carried out by the WHO in Tanzania found that hypercholesterolemia (total cholesterol greater than 5.2 millimeters molar per liter) was present in 21.8 percent of men and 54 percent of women; that measured weight, body mass index (BMI), and prevalence of obesity (BMI greater than or equal to 30 kilograms per square meter) had increased significantly to 22.8 percent among women in urban Dar es Salaam; and that the overall prevalence of hypertension (blood pressure higher than 160 over 95 mmHg or antihypertensive drug use) was 41.1 percent (Njelekela et al. 2001).

These classical risk factors operate in much the same way as in northern European populations with regard to being predictive of CVD (Kruger, Venter, and Vorster 2001; Yusuf et al. 2004). To date no evidence has been found that Africans have esoteric, genetically determined risk factors that differ from other populations in the world; nor do they appear to have special genetic traits that protect them from heart disease. It seems likely that the continuing socioeconomic advance in many African countries will be accompanied by the attendant increases in CVD that are seen in epidemiological transitions across the world. The challenge is to introduce primary and secondary prevention measures now, before the epidemic of CVD accelerates, particularly as such strategies may be more cost-effective than angioplasty and cardiac surgery in the cash-strapped economies of Sub-Saharan Africa.

Up to 22 percent of premature all-cause mortality and 45 percent of stroke mortality could be reduced by appropriate detection and treatment (Yusuf et al. 2004). Cheap, effective therapy is available. With mortality risk now higher from NCDs than from communicable diseases in Sub-Saharan Africa and elsewhere, systematic measurement, detection, and genuine control of hypertension once treated can go hand-in-hand with other adult health programs in primary care. In many African countries undernutrition coexists with obesity in the same communities, demonstrating a double burden of disease, such as in The Gambia, where a 1996 community-based survey demonstrated a prevalence of undernutrition (BMI less than 18 kilograms per square meter) of 8 percent, whereas prevalence of obesity (BMI greater than or equal to 30 kilograms per square meter) was 4 percent. However, obesity was higher (32.6 percent) among urban women 35 years or older (van der Sande et al. 2001). Furthermore, CVD risk factors tend to cluster, with the potential for synergistic effects, as has been described in other populations in the world (Kruger, Venter, and Vorster 2001). Differential interventions should

focus on high-risk groups, and prevention needs a multisectoral, health promotion approach.

A suitable strategy to adopt in the prevention and control of NCDs is the WHO Global Strategy for Noncommunicable Diseases, whose principal objectives are to do the following:

- Map the emerging epidemics of NCD and analyze their determinants.
- Reduce the levels of exposure of populations to common risk factors and their determinants.
- Develop norms and guidelines for effective interventions.

NCDs, including cardiovascular and cerebrovascular disease, pulmonary diseases, liver disease, cancer, diabetes, osteoporosis, and trauma, constitute the major cause of death in developed countries and are predictably emerging as significant threats to health in countries at intermediate stages of the epidemiological transition (Yusuf et al. 2004). Interventions could be designed based on the philosophy that diseases with common risk factors, such as smoking, increased fat and salt in the diet, alcohol abuse, and so on, require common preventive strategies.

Screening programs to detect hypertension in the community may be appropriate, as the disease does not become clinically manifest until it causes end organ damage, such as heart failure, heart attack, stroke, and kidney failure. Such measures would be subject to the constraints of available resources, however; and an approach that targets high-risk patients, that is, those who present with other related conditions or with multiple risk factors, may be more feasible than populationwide screening in poorer African countries (WHO 2002).

Health systems in developing countries will need to be drastically improved to deal with the burden, as they often suffer from inefficient allocation of resources and management of services. Better management must be based on both the high-risk-behaviors approach, such as detection and management of obesity, hypertension, and diabetes at the primary health care level, and the populationwide approach, such as education through the mass media and schools. Integration of the package of CVD prevention and control within the programs of ministries of health will be needed.

Increasing availability of drugs and diagnostics is a major issue in Africa, as it was for HIV/AIDS and tuberculosis. Local manufacture of off-patent CVD drugs may improve access as well as stimulate the economy, as proposed in the Initiative for Pharmaceutical Technology Transfer of

South Africa, a program of the New Partnership for Africa's Development.

Health technology for management of these CVDs will need to be appropriate, affordable, and sustainable and not simply imported from the West. The detection, prevention, and control of CVD in women is a major issue in Sub-Saharan Africa, where women may suffer inferior diagnosis of CVD and limited access to care because of adverse gender-power relations between men and women.

CVD control in Africa will probably not reach a high level of adequacy for a few decades to come, given the scant human, financial, and infrastructural resources in its countries. However, those countries cannot ignore the problem if they hold fast to the dictum of "health as a human right." They will, however, have to carefully categorize and prioritize their public health expenditure on the prevention and control of CVD. The experience of developed countries, who are further on in the course of their "epidemiological transition," suggests that primary prevention of CVD now is likely to be more cost-effective than acute care for affected patients in 20 years. In the United States, for example, the direct costs of CVD are estimated to account for 2 percent of the gross domestic product. In Canada, CVD accounts for 21 percent of total disease-classifiable costs of illness. The data for other chronic diseases in developing countries suggest that these scales of health care costs are likely to be similar. As an example, in India, the annual cost of drugs for a patient with type 2 diabetes mellitus is US$70, considerably more than the annual per capita expenditure on health care in that country. In Tanzania, diabetes care swallows up 8.1 percent of the health care budget (http://www.ichealth.org).

The costs of intersectoral, primary preventive measures to control CVD are likely to be much lower than those for acute, secondary care. As an example, the cost-effectiveness of introducing antitobacco legislation, or limiting the quantities of salt permitted in processed food, is likely to be substantially higher than building coronary care units. The evidence from developed countries since 1990 suggests that most of the decline in CVD mortality in these countries has resulted from better secondary care for CVD, but the relative cost per life saved is still high, too high for health systems in developing countries to cope with. Developed countries faced the peak in their incidence of CVD when they were already wealthy and had the resources to cope. Thus, the stratagems adopted by developing countries are likely to be different. In secondary care, African countries of the south will need to develop essential vascular packages, such as aspirin and beta-blockers for patients with angina pectoris.

The data are scanty and there is a dire need for more health economics research.

Development of a global program to provide access to CVD drugs, similar to the "3 by 5" Initiative of the WHO for antiretroviral drugs, is unlikely, because cardiovascular deaths do not have the same emotive power as AIDS deaths. Yet CVD deaths are often sudden, striking down victims in their most productive years and resulting in deep emotional and economic shock for their families. For survivors, the years lived with disability, such as heart failure or hemiplegia, are often traumatic and expensive because of health care costs and lost productivity. The prognosis for living with heart failure is like that for someone living with HIV/AIDS on antiretrovirals; the annual mortality is 5 to 15 percent. Perhaps the health systems being set up in African countries for provision of antiretroviral drugs and comprehensive AIDS care could have the beneficial side effect of providing systems and personnel for CVD surveillance and care.

In many African countries medicinal plants are used to treat cardiovascular complaints (Diallo et al. 1999). If these are truly effective, it could in part explain the low prevalence of CVD (and cancer) in rural African populations. Indigenous knowledge systems should be researched, in order to determine whether to popularize natural medicines for the prevention and cure of CVD. Cardiovascular disorders currently receive little or no attention in most African countries (Muna 1993b). Projections based on recent studies suggest that the management of these disorders will represent a major challenge for the overextended and shrinking health budgets of these poor nations in the near future. Given the prevalence of such common cardiovascular conditions as hypertension, which in some cases can be 25 percent or higher, treatment is beyond the budgetary possibilities of any of the African countries. Other conditions, including infections involving the heart and related structures, rheumatic fever and its complications, cardiomyopathies, and congenital heart disease, are also common. Recent trends suggest that ischemic heart disease may be less uncommon than was previously thought. Health planners and policy makers must be educated on the crucial role of health research in general, and cardiovascular disorders research in particular, as a basis for formulating a rational health care policy and making managerial decisions. The need for training and funding, and especially the leadership required to develop and sustain research activity, will require a multidisciplinary, multidirectional, collaborative approach at national and international levels, as well as firm local commitment. As is the case for most other important health problems, cardiovascular disorders are rapidly becoming a global issue and should be recognized as such.

Following the guidelines of JNC VI in the screening, detection, and treatment of all hypertensive patients is beyond the health budgets of most African countries (Gaziano and Opie 2001). Most countries, therefore, adopt an opportunistic approach to the identification of patients with hypertension and aim for significantly higher target blood pressures than those recommended. The result is that considerable numbers of patients continue to suffer hypertension-related strokes leading to disability or death. This inadequate detection and treatment of hypertension is the most likely explanation for the high proportion of hemorrhagic strokes in African populations.

The major challenges in the management of hypertension are therefore twofold. First is to develop cost-effective, population-based, health promotive strategies for primary prevention, and secondary amelioration of hypertension. The second challenge is to lower the costs of treatments through strategies such as the local manufacture of antihypertensive drugs that have come off patent (IPTT 2003). These are also probably the principal challenges in the management of cardiovascular disease in Africa, as hypertensive stroke is the leading cause of cardiovascular death and disability in Africa. Research is under way to develop these prevention and control strategies (http://www.ichealth.org).

Research continues into which of the two approaches to hypertensive control is most cost-effective: treating hypertension according to the absolute risk for CVD or following an arbitrary blood pressure target. The former is likely to be more cost-effective, but more research is still needed to settle the issue.

The prevention and treatment of CVDs has become a priority for some multilateral agencies. The WHO is active in promoting prevention strategies, including tobacco control and hypertension treatment. The World Bank has funded cardiovascular control initiatives in a few countries through its loans program. However, among other lenders and donors of funds for health care, such as the Asian Development Bank and most bilateral donor agencies, CVD remains a low priority (http://www.ichealth.org).

CONCLUSION

CHD and strokes share common determinants and risk factors and are more common in urban than rural areas. Any suggestion that people of black African descent are in some way immune from CVD has been dispelled by well-documented evidence from, among other countries, Cameroon, Caribbean countries, Mauritius, the Seychelles, South Africa, Tanzania, and the United States. In such countries CVD already accounts for between 15 and 40 percent of all deaths.

Data on the burden of cardiovascular disease for most African countries are, however, scanty. The estimations made in the Global Burden of Disease Study for CVD in 1990 in Africa relied on data from only 2 percent of the 700 million inhabitants of Africa (Murray and Lopez 1996). Still, studies do suggest that the prevalence of risk factors for CVD, and the behavioral, socioeconomic, and demographic determinants that underlie these risk factors, are increasing in Africa, despite the persistence of an appalling burden of communicable disease and diseases of poverty. Furthermore, the prevailing pattern of past decades, when CVD in Africa was predominantly RHD, hypertensive heart disease, stroke, and dilated cardiomyopathy, is now beginning to change, with an increasing proportion of morbidity and mortality due to ischemic heart disease.

It is probably cheaper and more effective to take population-based measures to prevent heart disease and stroke than it is to treat the people with surgery and drugs once CVD is established. RHD and heart failure also have highly effective primary and secondary interventions that can be readily applied. The time to act in prevention and control of CVD is now.

REFERENCES

Adebiyi, A. A., A. O. Falase, and Y. A. Akenova. 1999. "Left Ventricular Systolic Function of Nigerians with Sickle Cell Anaemia." *Annals of Oncology* 24 (98): 27–32.

Akinkugbe, O. O. 1976. "Epidemiology of Hypertension and Stroke in Africa." *Mongor Citation* 29: 28–42.

Alebiosu, C. O., B. Odusan, O. B. Familoni, and A. E. A. Jaiyesimi. 2004. "Pattern of Occurrence of Microalbuminuria among Dippers and Non-Dippers (Essential Hypertensives) in a Nigerian University Teaching Hospital." *Cardiovascular Journal of South Africa* 15: 9–12.

AMMP (Adult Mortality and Morbidity Project). 1997. *Policy Implications of Adult Mortality and Morbidity. End of Phase I Report.* Dar es Salaam: Department for International Development.

Amoah, A. G. B. 2000. "Spectrum of Cardiovascular Disorders in a National Referral Centre, Ghana." *East African Medical Journal* 77: 648–53.

Anabwani, G. M., and P. Bonhoeffer. 1996. "Prevalence of Heart Disease in School Children in Rural Kenya Using Colour-Flow Echocardiography." *East African Medical Journal* 73: 215–17.

Astagneau, P., T. Lang, E. Delarocque, E. Jeannee, and G. Salem. 1992. "Arterial Hypertension in Urban Africa: An Epidemiological Study on a Representative Sample of Dakar Inhabitants in Senegal." *Journal of Hypertension* 10 (9): 1095–1101.

Beaglehole, R., and D. Yach. 2003. "Globalisation and the Prevention and Control of Non-Communicable Disease: The Neglected Chronic Diseases of Adults." *Lancet* 362: 903–8.

Berrios, X., T. Koponen, T. Huiguang, N. Khaltaev, P. Puska, and A. Nissinen. 1997. "Distribution and Prevalence of Major Risk Factors of Noncommunicable Diseases in Selected Countries: The WHO Inter-Health Programme." *Bulletin of the World Health Organization* 75: 99–108.

Bertrand, E. 1992. "Coronary Disease in Black Africans: Epidemiology, Risk Factors, Clinical Symptomatology and Coronary Evolution." *Académie Nationale de Médecine Bulletin* 176 (3): 311–23; discussion 323–26.

Betre, M., D. Kebede, and M. Kassaye. 1997. "Modifiable Risk Factors for Coronary Heart Disease among Young People in Addis Ababa." *East African Medical Journal* 74: 376–81.

Boon, N. 2003. "Cardiac Disease in HIV Infection." In *Oxford Textbook of Medicine*, ed. D. A. Warrell, T. M. Cox, and J. D. Firth. Oxford: Oxford University Press.

Bovet, P. 1995. "The Epidemiologic Transition to Chronic Diseases in Developing Countries: Cardiovascular Mortality, Morbidity, and Risk Factors in Seychelles (Indian Ocean). Investigators of the Seychelles Heart Study." *Sozial- und Praventivmedizin* 40 (1): 35–43.

Bovet, P., A. G. Ross, J. P. Gervasoni, M. Mkamba, D. M. Mtasiwa, C. Lengeler, D. Whiting, and F. Paccaud. 2002. "Distribution of Blood Pressure, Body Mass Index and Smoking Habits in the Urban Population of Dar es Salaam, Tanzania, and Associations with Socioeconomic Status." *International Journal of Epidemiology* 31 (1): 240–47.

Bradshaw, D., D. Bourne, M. Schneider, and R. Sayed. 1995. "Mortality Patterns of Chronic Diseases of Lifestyle in South Africa." In *Chronic Diseases of Lifestyle in South Africa*, ed. J. Fourie, 5–31. Cape Town: South African Medical Research Council.

Bradshaw, D., P. Groenewald, R. Laubscher, N. Nannan, B. Nojilana, R. Norman, D. Pieterse, and M. Schneider. 2003. *Initial Burden of Disease Estimates for South Africa, 2000.* Cape Town: South African Medical Research Council.

Ceesay, M. M., M. W. Morgan, M. O. Kamanda, V. R. Willoughby, and D. R. Lisk. 1997. "Prevalence of Diabetes in Rural and Urban Populations in Southern Sierra Leone: A Preliminary Survey." *Tropical Medicine and International Health* 2 (3): 272–77.

Chinyadza, E., I. M. Moyo, T. M. Katsumbe, M. Chisvo, M. Mahari, D. E. Cock, and O. L. Mbengeranwa. 1993. "Alcohol Problems among Patients Attending Five Primary Health Care Clinics in Harare City." *Central African Journal of Medicine* 39: 26–32.

Cooper, R. S., C. N. Rotimi, S. Ataman, D. McGee, B. Osotimehin, S. Kadiri, W. Muna, et al. 1997. "The Prevalence of Hypertension in Seven Populations of West African Origin." *American Journal of Public Health* 87 (2): 160–68.

Cooper, R. S., C. N. Rotimi, J. S. Kaufman, E. E. Owoaje, H. Fraser, T. Forrester, R. Wilks, L. K. Riste, and J. K. Cruickshank. 1997. "Prevalence of NIDDM among Populations of the African Diaspora." *Diabetes Care* 20: 343–48.

Cruickshank, J. K., J. C. Mbanya, R. Wilks, B. Balkau, T. Forrester, S. G. Anderson, L. Mennen, A. Forhan, L. Riste, and N. McFarlane-Anderson. 2001. "Hypertension in Four African-Origin Populations: Current 'Rule of Halves,' Quality of Blood Pressure Control and Attributable Risk of Cardiovascular Disease." *Journal of Hypertension* 19: 41–46.

Davidson, J. C. 1963. "The Incidence of Diabetes in Nyasaland." *Central African Journal of Medicine* 9: 92–94.

Davies, J. N. P. 1948. "Endocardial Fibrosis in Africans." *East African Medical Journal* 25: 10.

Diallo, D., B. Hveem, M. A. Mahmoud, G. Berge, B. S. Paulsen, and A. Maiga. 1999. "An Ethnobotanical Survey of Herbal Drugs of Gourma District, Mali." *Pharmaceutical Biology* 37 (1): 80–91.

Dowse, G. K., H. Gareeboo, P. Z. Zimmet, K. G. Alberti, J. Tuomilehto, D. Fareed, L. G. Brissonnette, and C. F. Finch. 1990. "High Prevalence of NIDDM and Impaired Glucose Tolerance in Indian, Creole, and Chinese Mauritians. Mauritius Noncommunicable Disease Study Group." *Diabetes* 39: 390–96.

Drury, R. A. B. 1972. "The Mortality of Elderly Ugandans." *Tropical and Geographical Medicine* 24: 385–92.

Edington, G. M. 1954. "Cardiovascular Disease as a Cause of Death in Gold Coast Africa." *Transactions of the Royal Society of Tropical Medicine and Hygiene* 48: 419–25.

Edwards, R., N. Unwin, F. Mugusi, D. Whiting, S. Rashid, J. Kissima, T. J. Aspray, and K. G. Alberti. 2000. "Hypertension Prevalence and Care in an Urban and Rural Area of Tanzania." *Journal of Hypertension* 18 (2): 145–52.

Ekra, A., and E. Bertrand. 1992. "Rheumatic Heart Disease in Africa." *World Health Forum* 13 (4): 331–33.

Erasmus, R. T., T. Fakeye, O. Olukoga, A. B. Okesina, E. Ebomoyi, M. Adeleye, and A. Arije. 1989. "Prevalence of Diabetes Mellitus in a Nigerian Population." *Transactions of the Royal Society of Tropical Medicine and Hygiene* 83 (3): 417–18.

Ezenwaka, C. E., A. O. Akani, B. O. Akanji, N. C. Unwin, and C. A. Adejuwon. 1997. "The Prevalence of Insulin Resistance and Other Cardiovascular Disease Risk Factors in Healthy Elderly Southwestern Nigerians." *Atherosclerosis* 128 (2): 201–11.

Familoni, O. B., and A. J. Ariba. 2003. "Ability of Nigerian Hypertensive Patients to Perceive Changes in Their Blood Pressure." *Cardiovascular Journal of South Africa* 14: 195–98.

Fauci, A. S., and H. C. Lane. 2001. "Human Immunodeficiency Virus (HIV) Disease: AIDS and Related Disorders." In *Harrison's Principles of Internal Medicine*, 15th ed., 1,884. New York: McGraw-Hill.

Fisch, A., E. Pichard, T. Prazuck, H. Leblanc, Y. Sidibe, and G. Brucker. 1987. "Prevalence and Risk Factors of Diabetes Mellitus in the Rural Region of Mali (West Africa): A Practical Approach." *Diabetologia* 30: 859–62.

Gaziano, T. A., and L. Opie. 2001. "Cost-Effective Analysis of Proposed Hypertension Guidelines in South Africa; Beta-Blocker Therapy for Hypertension: Hypertension in South Africa and Efficacy of First Line Therapy." Abstract. *Cardiovascular Journal of Southern Africa* 12 (4): 223.

Ghanem, H., and A. H. Fredj. 1999. "Eating Habits and Cardiovascular Risk Factors." *Presse Medicale* 28 (19): 1005–8.

Hale, L. A., V. U. Fritz, and C. J. Eales. 1998. "Do Stroke Patients Realise That a Consequence of Hypertension Is Stroke?" *South African Medical Journal* 88 (4): 451–54.

Hutt, M. S. R. 1990. "Cancer and Cardiovascular Diseases." In *Disease and Mortality in Sub-Saharan Africa*, ed. D. T. Jamieson and R. G. Feachem. New York: Oxford University Press.

Hutt, M. S. R., and R. Coles. 1969. "Postmortem Findings in Hypertensive Subjects in Kampala, Uganda." *East African Medical Journal* 46: 342–58.

IOM (Institute of Medicine). 2005. *Scaling Up Treatment for the Global AIDS Pandemic*. Washington, DC: National Academies Press.

IPTT (Initiative on Pharmaceutical Technology Transfer). 2003. "A New Partnership for Africa's Development (NEPAD) Project for the Local Manufacture of Pharmaceuticals in Africa." http://www.iptt.net.

Isezuo, A. S., A. B. O. Omotoso, A. Gaye, T. Corrah, and M. A. Araoye. 2000. "One-Year Survival among Sub-Saharan Africans with Hypertensive Heart Failure." *Cardiologie Tropicale* 26 (103): 57–60.

JNC (Joint National Committee). 1997. "The Sixth Report of the National Committee on Prevention, Detection, Evaluation and Treatment of

High Blood Pressure (JNC VI)." *Archives of Internal Medicine* 157: 2413–46.

Kadiri, S., and B. L. Salako. 1997. "Cardiovascular Risk Factors in Middle Aged Nigerians." *East African Medical Journal* 74 (5): 303–6.

Kapuku, G. K., G. A. Mensah, and R. S. Cooper. 1998. "Hypertension in Africa." *Africa Health* 20 (2): 6–8.

Khalil, S. I., K. Gharieb, M. El-Haj, M. Khalil, and S. Hakiem. 1997. "Prevalence of Congenital Heart Disease among Schoolchildren of Sahafa Town, Sudan." *Eastern Mediterranean Health Journal* 3 (1): 24–28.

Kimbally-Kaky, G., and C. Bouramoue. 2000. "Profile and Prospects of Patients from Congo with Cardiac Insufficiency: Report of 743 Cases." *Médecine d'Afrique Noire* 47 (4): 197–203.

King, H., R. E. Aubert, and W. H. Herman. 1998. "Global Burden of Diabetes, 1995–2025: Prevalence, Numerical Estimates, and Projections." *Diabetes Care* 21: 1414–31.

King, H., and P. Zimmet. 1988. "Trends in the Prevalence and Incidence of Diabetes: Non-Insulin-Dependent Diabetes Mellitus." *World Health Statistics Quarterly* 41 (3–4): 190–96.

Kokou, O. I., A. D. Agbere, D. Y. Atakoumi, A. D. Gbadoe, E. Tsolenyanu, O. Djossou-Agbodjan, S. Baeta, K. Tatagan-Agbi, and K. Assimadi. 1999. "Cardiac Repercussions of Sickle Cell Anaemia in Children in Lomé: Report of 70 Cases." *Archives de Pediatrie* 6 (10): 1134.

Kotto, R. M., and B. A. Bouelet. 2000. "Cardiovascular Diseases in Adults in Douala (Cameroon)." *Cardiologie Tropicale* 26 (103): 61–64.

Kruger, H. S., C. S. Venter, and H. H. Vorster. 2001. "Obesity in African Women in the North West Province, South Africa Is Associated with an Increased Risk of Non-Communicable Diseases: The THUSA Study. Transition and Health during Urbanisation of South Africans." *British Journal of Nutrition* 86 (6): 733–40.

Law, C. M., P. Egger, O. Dada, H. Delgado, E. Kylberg, P. Lavin, G. H. Tang, H. Hertzen, A. W. Shiell, and D. J. Barker. 2001. "Body Size at Birth and Blood Pressure among Children in Developing Countries." *International Journal of Epidemiology* 30 (1): 52–59.

Law, M. 1998. "Lipids and Cardiovascular Disease." In *Evidence Based Cardiology*, ed. S. Yusuf, J. A. Cairns, A. J. Camm, E. L. Falen, and B. J. Gersh, 191–205. London: British Medical Journal Books.

Lawlor, D. A., G. Davey Smith, and S. Ebrahim. 2002. "Birth Weight of Offspring and Insulin Resistance in Late Adulthood: Cross Sectional Survey." *British Medical Journal* 325 (7360): 359.

Levitt, N. S., J. M. Katzenellenbogen, D. Bradshaw, M. N. Hoffman, and F. Bonnici. 1993. "The Prevalence and Identification of Risk Factors for NIDDM in Urban Africans in Cape Town, South Africa." *Diabetes Care* 16: 601–7.

Lodenyo, H. A., S. O. McLigeyo, and E. N. Ogola. 1997. "Cardiovascular Disease in Elderly In-Patients at the Kenyatta National Hospital, Nairobi, Kenya." *East African Medical Journal* 74: 647–51.

Lore, W. 1993. "Epidemiology of Cardiovascular Diseases in Africa with Special Reference to Kenya: An Overview." *East African Medical Journal* 70: 357–61.

Magula, N. P., and B. M. Mayosi. 2003. "Cardiac Involvement in HIV-Infected People Living in Africa: A Review." *Cardiovascular Journal of South Africa* 14: 231–37.

Martorell, R., L. K. Khan, M. L. Hughes, and L. M. Grummer-Strawn. 2000. "Obesity in Women from Developing Countries." *European Journal of Clinical Nutrition* 54 (3): 247–52.

Mayanja-Kizza, H., E. Gerwing, M. Rutakingirwa, R. Mugerwa, and J. Freers. 2000. "Tropical Endomyocardial Fibrosis in Uganda: The Tribal and Geographic Distribution, and the Association with Eosinophilia." *Cardiologie Tropicale* 26 (103): 45–48.

Matenga, J. 1997. "Stroke Incidence Rates among Black Residents of Harare—A Prospective Community-Based Study." *South African Medical Journal* 87 (5): 606–9.

Mayosi, B. M., A. D. Marais, A. D. Mbewu, and P. Byrnes. 1997. "Risk Factor Profile of Black Patients with Acute Coronary Syndromes." *Canadian Journal of Cardiology* 13: 242B.

Mbanya, J. C., E. Minkoulou, J. Salah, and B. Balkau. 1998. "The Prevalence of Hypertension in Rural and Urban Cameroon." *International Journal of Epidemiology* 27 (2): 181–85.

Mbanya, J. C., J. Ngogang, J. N. Salah, E. Minkoulou, and B. Balkau. 1997. "Prevalence of NIDDM and Impaired Glucose Tolerance in a Rural and an Urban Population in Cameroon." *Diabetologia* 40 (7): 824–29.

Mbaya, V. B. 1998. "Hypertension in East Africans and Others of African Descent: A Review." *East African Medical Journal* 75: 300–03.

Mbewu, A. D. 1998. "Can Developing Country Systems Cope with the Epidemics of Cardiovascular Disease?" Paper presented at the Heart Health Conference, New Delhi, India.

M'Buyamba-Kabangu, J., R. Fagard, P. Lijnen, J. Staessen, M. Ditu, K. Tshiani, and A. Amery. 1986. "Epidemiological Study of Blood Pressure and Hypertension in a Sample of Urban Bantu of Zaire." *Journal of Hypertension* 4: 485–91.

Mendez, G. F., and M. R. Cowie. 2001. "The Epidemiological Features of Heart Failure in Developing Countries: A Review of the Literature." *International Journal of Cardiology* 80 (2–3): 213–19.

Metcalf, C. A., M. N. Hoffman, K. Steyn, J. M. Katzenellenbogen, and J. M. Fourie. 1996. "Design and Baseline Characteristics of a Hypertension Intervention Program in a South African Village." *Journal of Human Hypertension* 10 (1): 21–26.

Mirabet, A. 1990. "Epidemiologic Aspects of Cerebrovascular Accidents in Tunisia. *Revue Neurologique (Paris)* 146 (4): 297–301.

Mokhobo, K. P. 1976. "Arterial Hypertension in Rural Societies." *East African Medical Journal* 52: 440–44.

Mollentze, W. F., A. J. Moore, A. F. Steyn, H. Joubert, K. Steyn, G. M. Oosthuizen, and D. J. Weich. 1995. "Coronary Heart Disease Risk Factors in a Rural and Urban Orange Free State Black Population." *South African Medical Journal* 85 (2): 90–86.

Msamati, B. C., and P. S. Igbigbi. 2000. "Anthropometric Profile of Urban Adult Black Malawians." *East African Medical Journal* 77: 364–68.

Muna, W. F. 1993a. "The Importance of Cardiovascular Research in Africa Today." *Ethnicity and Disease* 3 (Suppl.): S8–12.

———. 1993b. "Cardiovascular Disorders in Africa." *World Health Statistics Quarterly* 46 (2): 125–33.

Murray, C. J., and A. Lopez. 1996. *The Global Burden of Disease.* Washington, DC: World Bank.

———. 1997. "Mortality by Cause for Eight Regions of the World: Global Burden of Disease Study." *Lancet* 349: 1269–76.

Nan, L., J. Tuomilehto, G. Dowse, P. Zimmet, H. Gareeboo, P. Chitson, and H. J. Korhonen. 1991. "Prevalence and Medical Care of Hypertension in Four Ethnic Groups in the Newly-Industrialized Nation of Mauritius." *Journal of Hypertension* 9 (9): 859–66.

Nethononda, M. R., M. R. Essop, A. D. Mbewu, and J. S. Galpin. 2004. "Coronary Artery Disease and Risk Factors in Black South Africans—A Comparative Study." *Ethnicity and Disease* 14 (4): 515–19.

Njelekela, M., H. Negishi, Y. Nara, M. Tomohiro, S. Kuga, T. Noguchi, T. Kanda, et al. 2001. "Cardiovascular Risk Factors in Tanzania: A Revisit." *Acta Tropica* 79 (3): 231–39.

Nkoua, J. L., B. Tsombou, and C. Bouramoue. 1999. "Non Rheumatic Pericarditis with Effusion: Causes, Outcome and Relation to HIV-Infection." *Annals of Oncology* 25 (97): 3–6.

Ogunnowo, P. O., W. O. Odesanmi, and J. J. Andy. 1986. "Coronary Artery Pathology of 111 Consecutive Nigerians." *Transactions of the Royal Society of Tropical Medicine and Hygiene* 80 (6): 923–26.

Ohwovoriole, A. E., J. A. Kuti, and S. I. Kabiawu. 1988. "Casual Blood Glucose Levels and Prevalence of Undiscovered Diabetes Mellitus in

Lagos Metropolis Nigerians." *Diabetes Research and Clinical Practice* 4 (2): 153–58.

Okesina, A. B., D. P. Oparinde, K. A. Akindoyin, and R. T. Erasmus. 1999. "Prevalence of Some Risk Factors of Coronary Heart Disease in a Rural Nigerian Population." *East African Medical Journal* 76: 212–16.

Omar, M. A., M. A, Seedat, A. A. Motala, R. B. Dyer, and P. Becker. 1993. "The Prevalence of Diabetes Mellitus and Impaired Glucose Tolerance in a Group of Urban South African Blacks." *South African Medical Journal* 83 (9): 641–43.

Omotoso, A., and A. Kane. 2000. "Intraventricular Conduction Block in Adult Nigerians with Hypertensive Heart Disease; Epidemiological Study of Cardiovascular Disease and Risk Factors in Senegal: Cardiology—Out of Africa." *Cardiovascular Journal of Southern Africa* 11 (3): 173–74.

Omran, A. R. 1971. "The Epidemiological Transition: A Theory of the Epidemiology of Population Change." *Millbank Memorial Fund Quarterly* 49: 509–38.

———. 1983. "The Epidemiologic Transition Theory. A Preliminary Update." *Journal of Tropical Pediatrics* 29 (6): 305–16.

Opie, L., and K. Steyn. 1995. "Rationale for the Hypertension Guidelines for Primary Care in South Africa." *South African Medical Journal* 85 (12): 1325–28.

Osuntokun, B. O., A. O. Adeuja, B. S. Schoenberg, O. Bademosi, V. A. Nottidge, A. O. Olumide, O. Ige, F. Yaria, and C. L. Bolis. 1987. "Neurological Disorders in Nigerian Africans: A Community-Based Study." *Acta Neurologica Scandinavica* 75 (1): 13–21.

Owoaje, E. E., C. N. Rotimi, J. S. Kaufman, J. Tracy, and R. S. Cooper. 1997. "Prevalence of Adult Diabetes in Ibadan, Nigeria." *East African Medical Journal* 74: 299–302.

Oyoo, G. O., and E. N. Ogola. 1999. "Clinical and Socio Demographic Aspects of Congestive Heart Failure Patients at Kenyatta National Hospital, Nairobi." *East African Medical Journal* 76: 23–27.

Peters, V. J. 1983. "Developing In-House Audiovisual Programs For Use In Diabetes Education." *Diabetes Education* 9 (2): 11–18.

Politzer, W. M., and S. B. Sachs. 1967. "Incidence of Diabetes Mellitus in the Peri-Urban Bantu: Antenatal Surveys." *South African Medical Journal* 41 (14): 359–60.

Poulter, N. R. 1988. "Longitudinal Study of BP among Rural/Urban Immigrants in Kenya." In *Ethnic Factors in Health and Disease*, ed. D. K. Cruikshank and D. G. Beevers. Bristol: IOP Publishing.

Poulter, N. R., K. T. Khaw, B. E. C. Hopwood, M. Mugambi, W. S. Peart, G. Rose, and P. S. Sever. 1984. "Blood Pressure and Associated Factors in a Rural Kenyan Community." *Hypertension* 6: 810–13.

Pretoria Department of Health, Medical Research Council, and Measure DHS+. 2002. *South African Demographic and Health Survey 1998*. Full Report. Pretoria: Department of Health. http://www.doh.gov.za/facts/ 1998/sadhs98.

Ranjith, N., R. J. Pegoraro, L. Rom, P. A. Lanning, and D. P. Naidoo. 2004. "Renin-Angiotensin System and Associated Gene Polymorphisms in Myocardial Infarction in Young South African Indians." *Cardiovascular Journal of South Africa* 15: 22–26.

Razum, O. 1996. "Monitoring Cardiovascular Disease in Zimbabwe: A Review of Needs and Options." *Central African Journal of Medicine* 42: 120–24.

Reddy, K. S., and S. Yusuf. 1998. "Emerging Epidemic of Cardiovascular Disease in Developing Countries." *Circulation* 97: 596–601.

Reddy, P. 1997. "Selling Deception and Disease: Tobacco Control." Paper presented at the Fourth International Conference on Preventive Cardiology, Montreal, June–July 1997. Abstract. *Canadian Journal of Cardiology.*

———. 2004. "Chronic Diseases." In *South African Health Review 2003/04*, 175–90. Durban: Health Systems Trust.

Rosman, K. D. 1986. "The Epidemiology of Stroke in an Urban Black Population." *Stroke* 17 (4): 667–69.

Sarti, C., D. Rastenyte, Z. Cepaitis, and J. Tuomilehto. 2000. "International Trends in Mortality from Stroke, 1968 to 1994." *Stroke* 31 (7): 1588–601.

Seedat, Y. K. 1998. The Prevalence of Hypertension and the Status of Cardiovascular Health in South Africa. *Ethnicity and Disease* 8 (3): 394–97.

———. 2000. Hypertension in Developing Nations in Sub-Saharan Africa. *Journal of Human Hypertension* 14 (10–11): 739–47.

Seedat, Y. K., M. A. Seedat, and D. B. Hackland. 1982. "Prevalence of Hypertension in the Urban and Rural Zulu." *Journal of Epidemiology and Community Health* 36: 256–61.

Sen, K., and R. Bonita. 2000. "Global Health Status: Two Steps Forward, One Step Back." *Lancet* 356: 577–82.

Sever, P. S., D. Gordon, W. S. Peart, and P. Beighton. 1980. "Blood Pressure and Its Correlates in Urban and Tribal Africa." *Lancet* 2 (8185): 60–64.

Shaper, A. G. 1974. "Communities without Hypertension." In *Cardiovascular Disease in the Tropics*, ed. A. G. Shaper, M. S. R. Hutt, and Z. Fejfar, 77–83. London: British Medical Association.

Sliwa, K., A. Damasceno, and B. M. Mayosi. 2005. "Epidemiology and Etiology of Cardiomyopathy in Africa." *Circulation* 112: 3577–83.

Sobngwi, E., J. C. Mbanya, N. C. Unwin, A. P. Kengne, L. Fezeu, E. M. Minkoulou, T. J. Aspray, and K. G. Alberti. 2002. "Physical Activity and Its Relationship with Obesity, Hypertension and Diabetes in Urban and Rural Cameroon." *International Journal of Obesity Related Metabolic Disorders* 26 (7): 1009–16.

Statistics South Africa. 2001. *Recorded Deaths, 1996*. Report 03-09-01 (1996). Pretoria: Statistics South Africa.

Steenkamp, J. H., I. W. Simson, and W. Theron. 1992. "Cardiovascular Causes of Death at Tshepong Hospital in 1 year, 1989–1990. A Necropsy Study." *South African Medical Journal* 81 (3): 142–46.

Steinberg, W. J., D. L. Balfe, and H. G. Kustner. 1988. "Decline in the Ischaemic Heart Disease Mortality Rates of South Africans, 1968–1985." *South African Medical Journal* 74 (11): 547–50.

Steyn, K. 1998. *South Africa Demographic and Health Survey 1998*. Pretoria: National Department of Health, chaps. 11–13.

Steyn, K., and J. Fourie, eds. 1991. *BRISK Study Methodology: Coronary Heart Disease Risk Factor Study in the African Population of the Cape Peninsula*. MRC Technical Report 1. Cape Town: South African Medical Research Council.

Steyn, K., J. Fourie, C. Lombard, J. Katzenellenbogen, L. Bourne, and P. Jooste. 1996. "Hypertension in the Black Community of the Cape Peninsula, South Africa." *East African Medical Journal* 73: 758–63.

Steyn, K., J. E. Rossouw, P. L. Jooste, D. O. Chalton, E. R. Jordaan, P. C. J. Jordaan, M. Steyn, and A. S. P. Swanepoel. 1993. "The Intervention Effects of a Community-Based Hypertension Control Programme in Two Rural South African Towns: The CORIS Study." *South African Medical Journal* 83 (12): 885–91.

Swai, A. B., D. G. McLarty, H. M. Kitange, P. M. Kikima, S. Tatalla, N. Keen, L. M. Chuwa, and K. G. Alberti. 1993. "Low Prevalence of Risk Factors for Coronary Heart Disease in Rural Tanzania." *International Journal of Epidemiology* 22 (4): 651–59.

Teuscher, T., P. Baillod, J. B. Rosman, and A. Teuscher. 1987. "Absence of Diabetes in a Rural West African Population with a High Carbohydrate/Cassava Diet." *Lancet* 1 (8536): 765–68.

Thiam, M., G. Cloatre, F. Fall, X. Theobald, and J. L. Perret. 2000. "Ischaemic Cardiopathy in Africa: Experience at the Hôpital Principal in Dakar." *Médecine d'Afrique Noire* 47 (6): 281–84.

van der Sande, M. A., S. M. Ceesay, P. J. Milligan, O. A. Nyan, W. A. Banya, A. Prentice, K. P. McAdam, and G. E. Walraven. 2001. "Obesity and Undernutrition and Cardiovascular Risk Factors in Rural and Urban Gambian Communities." *American Journal of Public Health* 91 (10): 1641–44.

Vaughan, J. P. 1977. "A Brief Review of Cardiovascular Disease in Africa." *Transactions of the Royal Society of Tropical Medicine and Hygiene* 71: 226–31.

Vorster, H. H. 2002. "The Emergence of Cardiovascular Disease during Urbanisation of Africans." *Public Health and Nutrition* 5 (1A): 239–43.

Walker, A. R., and P. Sareli. 1997. "Coronary Heart Disease: Outlook for Africa." *Journal of the Royal Society of Medicine* 90 (1): 23–27.

Walker, R. W., D. G. McLarty, H. M. Kitange, D. Whiting, G. G. Masuki, D. M. Mtasiwa, H. Machibya, N. Unwin, and K. G. Alberti. 2000. "Stroke Mortality in Urban and Rural Tanzania. Adult Morbidity and Mortality Project." *Lancet* 355: 1684–87.

Walker, R. W., M. Rolfe, P. J. Kelly, M. M. George, and O. F. James. 2003. "Mortality and Recovery after Stroke in The Gambia." *Stroke* 34 (7): 1604–9.

WHO (World Health Organization). 1999. *The World Health Report 1999—Making a Difference.* Geneva: WHO.

———. 2002. *The World Health Report 2002—Reducing Risks, Promoting Healthy Life.* Geneva: WHO.

———. 2004. *The World Health Report 2004—Changing History.* Geneva: WHO.

Wiredu, E. K., and P. K. Nyame. 2001. "Stroke-Related Mortality at Korle Bu Teaching Hospital, Accra, Ghana." *East African Medical Journal* 78: 180–84.

Yusuf, S., S. Hawken, S. Ounpuu, T. Dans, A. Avezum, F. Lanas, M. McQueen, et al. 2004. "Effect of Potentially Modifiable Risk Factors Associated with Myocardial Infarction in 52 Countries (the INTER-HEART Study)." *Lancet* 364: 937–52.

Chapter **22**

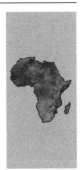

Mental Health and the Abuse of Alcohol and Controlled Substances

Florence K. Baingana, Atalay Alem, and Rachel Jenkins

Mental disorders include depression, anxiety, schizophrenia, and psychosocial and mental disorders as consequences of alcohol and substance abuse, conflicts and complex emergencies, the human immunodeficiency virus/acquired immune deficiency syndrome (HIV/AIDS), and gender-based violence; in addition, there are mental disorders of children. Standardized research instruments have been tested and widely used in Sub-Saharan Africa, and considerable attention has been paid to the transcultural performance of these instruments. However, challenges to epidemiological research still exist, including unreliable health facility records, noninclusion of mental disorders in the health management information systems (HMISs), and lack of any disease surveillance system that includes mental disorders.

This chapter discusses measurement and data sources, the burden of mental disorders and alcohol abuse in Sub-Saharan Africa, current interventions, and effective treatment strategies relevant to the context of the region. It concludes with recommendations for research as well as implications for policy formulation and development. An appendix supplies selected data on mental health disorders.

THE SCOPE OF MENTAL DISORDERS

Mental disorders are increasingly prevalent in Sub-Saharan Africa, the consequence of persistent poverty-driven conditions, such as malnutrition, malaria, and AIDS; the demographic transition; and the persistent conflicts prevalent in the region. The leading mental disorders, anxiety and depression, are often grouped together and referred to as common mental disorders (CMD).

Many of the disorders, such as depression and anxiety, are potentially preventable or treatable with currently available interventions. Increasingly, epidemiological studies carried out in Sub-Saharan Africa show that some mental disorders are more prevalent there than in other areas of the world, and some, such as depression resulting from the consequences of conflicts and HIV/AIDS, especially among orphans and other vulnerable children, are overrepresented in Sub-Saharan Africa.

Cultural and religious issues influence the value placed by society on mental health, the presentation of symptoms, illness behavior, access to services, pathways through care, the way individuals and families manage illness, the way the community responds to illness, the degree of acceptance and support experienced by the person with the illness, and the degree of stigma and discrimination experienced by that person. Therefore, cultural and other contextual issues are important considerations in developing locally appropriate mental health policy and programs.

MEASUREMENT AND DATA SOURCES

Although community surveys date from nearly 100 years ago, it is only in the last four decades that they have provided adequate diagnostic information based on standardized methods of assessment, allowing the comparison of research from different locations and from different levels.

A useful framework, originally devised for understanding the pathway by which individuals become defined as mentally ill—that is, passing through primary care and eventually reaching specialist mental health services—is the organization of epidemiological data into groupings. These groupings are defined by how far along the pathway the population under study has come, in order to ensure that like is compared with like (Goldberg and Huxley 1992). The framework comprises five levels: (a) all individuals in the community, (b) all individuals attending at the primary care level, (c) those in primary care who have been diagnosed by their doctor or nurse, (d) all those referred to specialist services, and (e) those who have been admitted to a hospital. The framework postulates a set of four filters between the five levels; the filters are influenced by the illness behavior of the patient, access to primary health care services, the ability of the primary care team to detect disorder, and the team's capacity to refer patients to higher or lower levels of care, and access to specialist services and inpatient care.

Standardized research instruments, both questionnaires and structured or semistructured interviews, have been developed, tested, and used widely around the world over the last few decades, allowing estimates of prevalence, incidence, outcome, and examination of associated risk factors (for example, Thompson Psychiatric Research Methods, Hopkins Symptom Checklist, General Health Questionnaire, Beck's Depression Inventory, Harvard Trauma Questionnaire). Whereas studies in the 1950s and 1960s showed that the reliability of psychiatric diagnoses was often low, the introduction of international diagnostic systems with guides, structured interviews, and operational definitions has transformed the situation.

Considerable attention has been given to the transcultural performance of several diagnostic tools. Goldberg and colleagues (1997) found that the widely used screening instrument the General Health Questionnaire (GHQ) performed just as well in detecting cases of depression and anxiety in low-income countries as in the Western world. Bolton (2001a), Wilk and Bolton (2002), and Bolton, Neugebauer, and Ndogoni (2002) investigated how people in an African community severely affected by HIV view the mental health effects of the epidemic, and they used the data to investigate the validity of Western concepts of depression and posttraumatic stress disorder (PTSD) in the rural Ugandan community studied. Ethnographic methods (those that take into the field certain developed viewpoints and techniques but also acknowledge that because individual cultures are unique they can be evaluated only according to their own values and standards, wary of the ethnocentric belief that one's own culture is superior in every way to all others) were used, and the participants were able to describe two, independent, depression-like syndromes resulting from the HIV epidemic. No syndromes similar to posttraumatic stress syndrome were found. The authors concluded that people recognize depression syndromes and consider them consequences of the HIV epidemic. Bolton and colleagues (2003) evaluated the feasibility of conducting controlled studies in Africa and found the controlled trial to be feasible in the local setting.

Kaaya and colleagues (2002) carried out a study to test the validity of the Hopkins Symptom Checklist-25 (HSCL-25) among HIV-positive women in Tanzania. They found the internal consistency of the HSCL-25 and the HSCL-15 to be adequate. The HSCL-25 demonstrated its usefulness as a screening tool for depression.

Epidemiological studies have been carried out in Kenya (Kiima et al. 2004) using the UK Clinical Interview Schedule (revised), and in Burundi, a survey of national welfare indicators was carried out (Baingana et al. 2004) that included the 12-item GHQ and the 5-item Alcohol Use Disorders Identification Test (AUDIT). The Kenya mental health survey also used the Core Welfare Indicators Questionnaire (CWIQ), an instrument developed by the World Bank for rapid population-level assessments of welfare indicators (World Bank 2001), and the AUDIT. In 1998, 12 psychological questions adapted from the GHQ-12 were integrated into the Burundi Household and Living Standards Survey. Analysis of the data revealed two indicators of distress, similar to those found by Goldberg and colleagues (1997) while using the GHQ-12. The two indicators were internally validated (Baingana et al. 2004).

Strauss and colleagues (1995), in assessing the predictive value of a screening questionnaire for depression and anxiety, found that general practitioners could correctly diagnose depression in 3.2 percent of patients. The screening questionnaire had a 42 percent chance of correctly identifying depression and a 97 percent chance of correctly identifying patients who did not have depression. The study confirmed the low identification rate for depression among general practitioners, highlighting how unreliable patient records are as sources for epidemiological studies.

South Africa's National Non-Natural Mortality Surveillance System, which began operation in 1998, is an excellent source for suicide mortality. "Non-natural mortality" refers to deaths from homicide, suicide, accidents, and undetermined causes. An evaluation carried out in 2001 found sensitivity to range from 65 to 95 percent for manner of death, with a positive predictive value that ranged from 74 to 80 percent for manner of death and 71 to 82 percent for mechanism of death. Maintenance costs are estimated to be R 8.00 (US$1.00) per case registered.

However, there still exist challenges to epidemiological research for mental disorders in Sub-Saharan Africa. Health facility records are not reliable, mental disorders are not included as separate items in the HMIS, and very few cross-sectional or longitudinal studies have been carried out. No disease surveillance system includes mental disorders, and no censuses, registries, or other administrative data include mental disorders.

A PubMed search was carried out with the key words "mental disorders," "depression," "suicide," and "Sub-Saharan Africa." Few epidemiological studies carried out in Sub-Saharan Africa have been published in peer-reviewed journals. The best data sources are from South Africa and Nigeria and a few from Kenya and Zambia. Additional data are potentially available in unpublished surveys, particularly in Francophone Africa.

EPIDEMIOLOGY

Major challenges to epidemiological research are limited capacity in the use of international classification systems for coding of disorders, noninclusion of mental and neurological disorders as separate categories in the HMIS, nonstandardized instruments for epidemiological research that have not been validated for use in all areas of the subcontinent, and limited capacity and resources to carry out comprehensive and scientifically sound community assessments. A large number of the studies use hospital-based data, yet many of the patients do not have access to or knowledge of the mental health services available in their vicinity.

Although prevalence studies for mental disorders in Sub-Saharan Africa are scarce, studies from the rest of the world can be extrapolated to the Sub-Saharan region. Epidemiological studies of communities (for example, Jenkins 1998; Kessler et al. 1994; Kessler et al. 2005), of people at work (Jenkins 1985), and of people in primary health care (Demyttenaere et al. 2004; Ormel et al. 1994; Sartorius et al. 1996; Ustun et al. 2004) from all regions of the world have shown that depression and anxiety are common everywhere. They contribute to sickness absence and labor turnover (Jenkins 1985) and form a significant contribution to the overall public health burden (Murray and Lopez 1996). In 1996, major unipolar depression was projected to be number two as a leading cause of disability in 2020 (Murray and Lopez 1997a); estimates of the Global Burden of Disease carried out in 2000 found depression to be the leading cause of disability, accounting for 12 percent of the global disability burden (Ustun et al. 2004).

Global Burden of Disease 2000 Study

The Global Burden of Disease was launched by the World Health Organization (WHO) in the 1990s, and the first set of data was published in 1996 (Murray and Lopez 1996). In 2000 WHO carried out the second assessment of the Global Burden of Disease, the GBD 2000 (Mathers et al. 2002). This is the most up-to-date GBD data available. The GBD 2000 study estimated the incidence and prevalence and the mortality rates of major depression, bipolar disorder, schizophrenia, panic disorder, and obsessive-compulsive disorder in the Sub-Saharan Africa WHO subregions (table 22.1). The study also estimated years lived with disability (YLDs) and disability-adjusted life years (DALYs) for these disorders (table 22.2).

Unipolar Depression. In the GBD 1996, unipolar depression, which differs from bipolar depressive disorder in that it presents with recurring depressive episodes without any manic episodes, unlike bipolar disorder, which has both manic and depressive episodes, was estimated to be the leading cause of the nonfatal disease burden in the world in 1990, accounting for 10.7 percent of total YLD. It was the fourth leading cause of total disease burden, accounting for 3.7 percent of total DALYs (Murray and Lopez 1997b). In the GBD 2000 study, unipolar depression remains the

Table 22.1 Age-Standardized Incidence, Prevalence, and Mortality Rate Estimates for WHO AFR Epidemiological Subregions, 2000
(per 100,000 people)

Disorder/Area	Incidence		Prevalence		Mortality	
	Males	Females	Males	Females	Males	Females
Schizophrenia						
AFR D	18	21	343	378	0	0
AFR E	20	24	349	418	1	0
World	19	20	422	423	0	0
PTSD						
AFR D	45	121	216	552	—	—
AFR E	44	126	212	558	—	—
World	44	121	208	559	—	—
Panic disorder						
AFR D	32	63	309	613	—	—
AFR E	32	63	309	613	—	—
World	30	61	319	631	—	—
Obsessive–compulsive disorder						
AFR D	77	83	586	790	—	—
AFR E	77	83	586	790	—	—
World	58	77	376	522	—	—
Unipolar depressive disorder						
AFR D	2,851	4,345	1,426	2,173	319	621
AFR E	2,851	4,345	1,426	2,173	319	621
World	3,199	4,930	1,607	2,552	323	630
Bipolar disorders						
AFR D	26	25	482	450	0	0
AFR E	26	25	482	450	0	0
World	26	25	467	472	0	0

Source: Mathers et al. 2002.
Note: — = not available.

leading cause of YLD, accounting for 11.9 percent of total YLD, and also remains the fourth leading cause of total disease burden, accounting for 4.4 percent of total DALYs (Mathers et al. 2002). In Butajira, Ethiopia, a demographic study site for the University of Addis Ababa and the ministry of health of Ethiopia, it was found that, using the DALY method, depression contributed 7 percent to the total disease burden (Abdulahi, Mariam, and Kebede 2001).[1]

Panic Disorder. In the GBD 1996, panic disorder was estimated to be the 27th leading cause of the nonfatal burden of disease in the world (Murray and Lopez 1996). In the GBD 2000 the estimated burden of panic disorder increased slightly, accounting for 1.2 percent of the total YLD. One of the data sources used for this estimate was a study carried out in Lesotho, which found an estimate of a one-month

prevalence of 3.7 percent for males and 15.3 percent for females in a population age 19 to 93 years. This prevalence was substantially higher than that found in other regions of the world (Mathers et al. 2002).

Bipolar Disorder. Bipolar disorder is a chronic disease with periods of depression and elevated mood and with remissions and relapses between them. In the 1990 GBD, it was estimated to be the seventh leading cause of the nonfatal burden of disease, accounting for 3 percent of the total YLD (Murray and Lopez 1996). In the GBD 2000, bipolar disorder accounts for 2.5 percent of total YLD (Mathers et al. 2002).

Schizophrenia. The seventh leading cause of YLD at the global level, schizophrenia accounts for 2.8 percent of total

Table 22.2 YLD, YLL, and DALY Estimates for WHO AFR Epidemiological Subregions, 2000

Disorder/Area	YLD per 100,000		YLL per 100,000		YLD (000s)	YLL (000s)	DALYs (000s)
	Males	Females	Males	Females			
Schizophrenia							
AFR D	250	246	2	1	828	6	834
AFR E	237	249	3	1	820	7	827
World	259	252	5	4	15,427	263	15,690
PTSD							
AFR D	27	68	—	—	160	0	160
AFR E	25	68	—	—	158	0	158
World	29	78	—	—	3,230	0	3,230
Panic disorder							
AFR D	77	152	—	—	382	0	382
AFR E	77	151	—	—	386	0	386
World	74	145	—	—	6,591	0	6,591
Obsessive–compulsive disorder							
AFR D	107	144	—	—	420	—	420
AFR E	107	146	—	—	428	—	428
World	67	90	—	—	4,761	—	4,761
Unipolar depressive disorder							
AFR D	514	786	0	0	2,172	0	2,172
AFR E	507	768	0	0	2,154	0	2,154
World	851	1,302	0	0	64,963	0	64,963
Bipolar disorders							
AFR D	261	245	—	—	845	—	845
AFR E	261	244	—	—	852	—	852
World	226	224	—	—	13,610	36	13,645

Source: Mathers et al. 2002.
Note: — = not available; YLL = years of life lost.

global YLD in the GBD 2000 study, up from 10th place (2.6 percent of YLD) in 1990 (Mathers et al. 2002; Murray and Lopez 1996). In an Ethiopian Burden of Disease study, 4 percent of the total disease burden was due to schizophrenia (Abdulahi, Mariam, and Kebede 2001). Sartorius and colleagues (1986) estimate an incidence rate for schizophrenia of 10 cases per 10,000 people. Mathers and colleagues (2002) estimate the incidence rate for Sub-Saharan Africa at 0.2 for males and 0.3 for females per 1,000 people, age-adjusted to between 0.4 and 0.53 percent. In a large semi-urban and rural population study in Ethiopia the prevalence of schizophrenia was found to be 4.7 per 1,000 people (Kebede et al. 2003).

Posttraumatic Stress Disorder. In the GBD 1990, PTSD was estimated to account for 0.4 percent of the total YLD,

about the same percentage as schizophrenia (Murray and Lopez 1996). In the GBD 2000, PTSD has increased to 0.6 percent of total YLD (Mathers et al. 2002).

Obsessive-Compulsive Disorder. Obsessive-compulsive disorder was estimated to be the 11th cause of the nonfatal burden of disease in the world, accounting for 2.2 percent of total YLD in 1990 (Murray and Lopez 1996). In the GBD 2000, obsessive-compulsive disorder now accounts for 2.5 percent of total YLD (Mathers et al. 2002).

Data Specific to Sub-Saharan Africa

Although data specific to Sub-Saharan Africa are more difficult to find, the number of epidemiological mental health studies being carried out in the last decade has increased. This is due to an increase in the number of African universities that are training psychiatrists, an increase in the number of African psychiatrists who have been trained in research methods and who are practicing in Africa, an increase in the number of African universities partnering with Western and northern universities, as well as an increasing number of African institutions participating in multi-site studies led by WHO or by U.S. research institutes. There is also a wealth of information coming out of South Africa, which had a much stronger research culture but was closed off to the rest of Africa in the apartheid years.

Depression. There have been at least three geographically localized but well-conducted epidemiological surveys of depression in Sub-Saharan Africa. Hollifield and colleagues (1990) used a two-stage approach in a rural village in Lesotho and found a prevalence of depression of 9 percent when alcohol abuse was corrected for, assuming that alcohol use preceded depressive disorder. The researchers noted that 19 percent of subjects with panic and depressive disorder had comorbid alcohol use. Rumble and colleagues (1996) note a similar high prevalence of depression in people in a rural South African village, in a study that screened for symptoms using an adapted version of the Self Report Questionnaire–25-item version (SRQ-25) and the Present State Examination (PSE) as a second-stage instrument.

The weighted prevalence for unipolar depressive disorder using the CATEGO (a computerized classification system) was 18 percent. More than half of the psychiatric morbidity detected was attributed to depressive disorders. In a homestead survey in two villages in Uganda, where the Luganda version of the PSE was used, Orley, Blitt, and Wing (1979) found that 14.3 percent of males and 22.6 percent of females among adults age 18 to 65 met criteria for depressive disorder using the CATEGO classification system. Estimated prevalence of depression in women in Harare, Zimbabwe, was reported to be 30 percent (Abas and Broadhead 1994) and the incidence rate of depression in the same population was estimated at 18 percent (Broadhead and Abas 1994). The incidence rate of major depression was found to be 15.6 percent in a rural general practice of South Africa (Strauss et al. 1995) and 15.5 percent in Rwanda five years after the genocide of April 1994 (Bolton, Neugebauer, and Ndogoni 2002).

Common Mental Disorders. *Common mental disorders* is a term used to discuss both anxiety and depression when they occur in the primary health care setting, often presenting with medically unexplained physical symptoms as well as the symptoms of depression, and anxiety (Patel et al. 1995). People with CMDs are frequent attenders at general primary health care clinics and medical and surgical inpatient beds, because they are specifically seeking help for their disorder, because they have a coexisting physical illness, or because they are somatizing their mental disorder. CMDs are significant contributors to the workload in general health clinics.

Schizophrenia. Schizophrenia is found in all countries and cultures and has a lifetime prevalence of between 7 and 9 per 1,000 people (Jablensky et al. 1992). The point prevalence varies between about 2 and 5 per 1,000. Collaborative studies by the WHO have shown that the prevalence of schizophrenia, when assessed in comparable ways, is similar in different countries (Jablensky et al. 1992). Although much rarer than depression and anxiety, it too forms a significant contribution to the overall public health burden because of the chronicity, deterioration, and extreme social disability in a significant proportion of sufferers. The outcome of schizophrenia is more favorable in developing countries than in the West, but the reasons are not yet clear (IOM 2001; Jablensky et al. 1992; Leff et al. 1992; Sartorius et al. 1986).

Jablensky recently reviewed the epidemiology of schizophrenia (IOM 2001) and concluded that there have been few systematic surveys of psychoses in Africa, although there are plenty of service-based clinical studies. An exception is a recent, well-designed community survey in an area of Ethiopia with a population of 100,000 in the age range 15 to 49 years. He concluded that the reported point prevalence of schizophrenia in most areas of the developing world where epidemiological surveys have been conducted is comparable with that in the developed world. Taking into account such factors as the higher mortality among people with serious mental disorders and incomplete ascertainment of a proportion of cases, it is likely that the reported rates are underestimates of the true prevalence of the disorder.

Posttraumatic Stress Disorder. Forty-one percent of all deaths in the WHO Sub-Saharan Africa region are from intentional injuries, the highest rates being for males age 15 to 29 years (56 percent) and 30 to 34 years (53 percent). The Sub-Saharan Africa region has the highest rates of death due to war-related injuries in the world, with a rate of 22 percent of all war-related injuries and 32 per 100,000 people (WHO 2002b). Estimates for psychosocial and mental disorders resulting from conflicts were 15.5 percent in Rwanda five years after the genocide (Bolton 2001b; Bolton, Neugebauer, and Ndogoni 2002). Studies carried out in Africa and other parts of the world indicate rates of 20 to 60 percent for depression, anxiety symptoms, and PTSD among children and women (de Jong 2002; Mollica et al. 1998; Mollica et al. 1999).

Alcohol Abuse. Adult per capita alcohol consumption is generally estimated by dividing the sum of alcohol production and imports less alcohol exports by the adult population age 15 years and older (WHO 1999b). In countries where the production is mainly home brews and spirits, thus not taxable, as in most of Sub-Saharan Africa, it becomes extremely difficult to get an accurate estimate of consumption. It is now widely accepted that the proportion of the population drinking excessively is closely related to the average consumption of that population (WHO 1999b). The increase in road traffic accidents, liver cirrhosis, and pancreatic disease as alcohol consumption increases further validates this premise.

The WHO estimates a sharp increase in per capita consumption of alcohol in Sub-Saharan Africa. Five of the 13 countries with the world's highest increase in alcohol consumption from 1970–72 to 1994–96 are in Sub-Saharan Africa. Lesotho ranked 1st, with a 1,817 percent increase; Nigeria, 5th, with a 196 percent increase; Rwanda, 10th, with a 129 percent increase; Burkina Faso, 12th, and Sudan, 13th, with 116 percent and 108 percent increases, respectively (WHO 1999b). Drinking is greater among males than females and greater among the uneducated than the formally educated. In the Seychelles, male drinkers consume eight times as much alcohol as females; among black South Africans, more than twice the men drink more regularly than women; and in Zambia, four times as many men as women drink weekly. A pattern of men drinking more frequently and to the point of intoxication is prevalent across Sub-Saharan Africa (WHO 1999b).

A worrying trend is that of consumption of alcohol by children (WHO 1999b). In Namibia, 20 percent of schoolchildren and 75 percent of young people not in school abuse alcohol on weekends. In Zimbabwe, 31 percent of those age 14 years and under report using alcohol. In Lesotho, 8.8 percent of children between the ages of 10 and 14 years and 4 percent of those between 5 and 9 years currently use alcohol.

Suicide. Suicide is an important cause of mortality in Sub-Saharan Africa. Studies have mainly been carried out in Nigeria, South Africa, and Zambia. In South Africa from 1984 to 1986 up to 0.37 percent of all admissions to hospitals (Okulate 2001) and 1.3 percent of all national mortality were suicide attempts (Flisher and Parry 1994). Parasuicide (attempted suicide) rates are much higher. In a study of 10,984 patients seen in a hospital in Durban, 17.7 percent were referred to the Department of Psychiatry because of parasuicide (Schlebusch 1985). In Nairobi, Kenya, suicide was the fourth most common cause of death due to injuries, making up 12 percent of all injury-related deaths (Muniu et al. 1994).

In a study of high school students in Addis Ababa in 1989 and 1990, Kebede and Ketsela (1993) found 14.3 percent reporting having attempted suicide. Kebede and Alem (1999) found a lifetime prevalence of 0.9 percent in Addis Ababa, and Alem et al. (1999) found a lifetime prevalence of 3.2 percent in Butajira, Ethiopia. Suicides generally occur between the ages of 13 and 50 years and peak at 20 to 29 years (WHO 1999a). Most studies reported that females generally have a higher frequency of suicide than males. Most of the suicide and parasuicide is associated with depression or alcohol abuse, or both. Dong and Simon (2001) found an increase of 320 percent in organophosphate poisoning in urban Zimbabwe for the period 1995 to 2000. Breetzke (1988) reported that in South Africa, suicide was more frequent among the white population (14 per 100,000) than among those of mixed race (3 per 100,000) and blacks (0.7 per 100,000). A study of accidental and violent death in Tanzania in women age 16 to 45 found that suicide is as common in that country as it is in the United Kingdom (CDC 2000; Setel et al. 2000). Table 22.3 summarizes some of the studies of suicide carried out in Sub-Saharan Africa.

Psychiatric Disorders among Children. Not many data are available on the burden of mental disorders among children. This is mainly because of the lack of validated testing instruments sensitive to the context of Sub-Saharan Africa; the lack of specialized personnel, such as child psychiatrists and child psychologists, able to carry out the assessments; and limited resources. Schier, Yecunnoamlack, and Tegegne (1989) found that 6.8 percent of 1,078 children treated on pediatric wards in Ethiopia had a neuropsychiatric disorder. A study carried out in Kenya found that one-third of the children referred to a psychological assessment center had emotional disorders as the cause for their learning difficulties (Dhadphale and Ibrahim 1984).

Table 22.3 Summaries of Selected Studies on Suicide and Parasuicide

Authors and year	Country and study population	Study findings
Oguleye, Nwaorgu, and Grandawa 2002	Nigeria 10-year study, 23 corrosive esophagitis patients	35% suicidal 75% of suicides in the second decade of life
Granja, Zacarias, and Bergstrom 2002	Mozambique Retrospective study 27 pregnancy-related deaths	9 deaths due to alleged suicide 59% were younger than 25 years of age
Mzezewa et al. 2000	Zimbabwe Prospective study of suicidal burns 47 patients	89% females Median age: 25 years; range: 13–50 years 64% housewives Mortality 68%
Alem et al. 1999	Ethiopia Cross-sectional survey of 10,468 adults	Lifetime suicide attempt: 3.2% of population; of these, 63% women 15–24 years most frequent age group for suicide attempt People with mental distress and problem drinking had higher lifetime prevalence for suicide attempt
Kebede and Alem 1999	Ethiopia 10,203 adults in Addis Ababa	2.7%, prevalence of current suicide ideation 0.9%, lifetime prevalence 66% under the age of 25 years Current suicidal ideation more common in men than in women Decreasing risk of suicide attempt with increasing age and educational attainment
Wilson and Wormald 1995	South Africa 27 adults who had taken battery acid	Patient had limited schooling; unemployed Male-female ratio of 2.4 to 1 9 had diagnosable psychiatric illness
Mboussou and Milebou-Aubusson 1989	Gabon 39 cases of suicide 208 attempted suicide	Higher ratio for attempted suicide among women at a female-male ratio of 3:1 More frequent among younger age groups
Odejide et al. 1986	Nigeria 39 cases of deliberate self-harm	76.9% under 30 years of age Male-female ratio of 1.4:1 51.3% students 25.6% manual workers
Cummins and Allwood 1984	South Africa 10–15-year-olds referred to a child psychiatry clinic	10% were suicide attempts Peak incidence among 13 year olds Male-female ratio of 2:1 Predisposing and antecedent causes were family stress (divorce), psychiatric illness in the patient or a family member, school problems 7% made further serious suicide attempts
Eferakeya 1984	Nigeria	Crude suicide rate of 7 per 100,000 87% of attempters under the age of 30 years Highest age group 15–19 years (39.4%) Female-male ratio of 1:1.2 64% of attempters were students, housewives, and the unemployed Major predisposing factor was mental illness (32%)

Source: Compiled by authors.

Etiology and Determinants

The major risk factors for mental disorders can be classified into genetic factors; nutritional deficiencies; infection; exposure to environmental toxins; prenatal, perinatal, and neonatal factors; poverty; and trauma.

Malnutrition. Malnutrition is prevalent in Sub-Saharan Africa; from 20 to 50 percent of all children under five years are severely malnourished. *The World Health Report 2002* estimates that 32 percent and 31 percent of children in WHO AFR D (characterized by high child and high adult mortality) and AFR E (characterized by high child and very high adult mortality), respectively, are two standard deviations below the weight for age.[2] Malnutrition is associated with mild to moderate mental retardation. Micronutrient deficiencies have also been found to be a major risk factor. These include iodine and zinc, with rates of 37 percent in AFR D and 62 percent in AFR E not consuming the recommended dietary intake. Iodine deficiency is the single most prevalent cause of mental retardation and brain damage, 25 percent of the global burden of iodine-related deficiency disorders are contributed by AFR E (WHO 2002a). Iron deficiency is prevalent in the region with hemoglobin levels of 10.6 for both AFR D and AFR E. A growing body of evidence indicates that iron deficiency anemia in early childhood is associated with reduced intelligence in mid-childhood (WHO 2002a). A study carried out in South Africa found that permanent intellectual stunting results from chronic malnutrition of infants up to four years of age (Booyens, Luitingh, and van Rensburg 1977).

Genetic Vulnerability. There is strong evidence that genetic vulnerability is an important part of the cause of schizophrenia; a person's risk of developing the disorder increases steeply with the degree of genetic relatedness (IOM 2001). Few risk factors have been specifically identified or validated in developing countries, although obstetric complications and early brain injury due to neuroinfection, toxic effects, other trauma, or maternal malnutrition during gestation are likely to be involved in a greater proportion of cases of adult schizophrenia in the developing world than in the developed world.

Incidence and prevalence studies from developing countries suggest a clustering of onset of schizophrenia in early adulthood, similar to that observed in developed countries, although it tends to occur at an earlier age in developing countries. The onset tends to be earlier in males than in females. An important difference between developing and developed countries is that in the majority of developed countries males have a higher morbidity than females, whereas in some developing countries this dominance is attenuated or inverted. Given that in many developing countries, women have higher mortality than men, this finding suggests that if adjustment for mortality could be made, the risk for schizophrenia for women in developing countries would be even higher. Causes of such a higher risk of schizophrenia among women in developing countries may involve both biological and psychosocial factors and requires further research.

Life Events. Life events that lead to the threat of loss or to actual loss, such as the death of a family member, marital separation, maternal deprivation, or loss of employment, have been shown to cluster before the onset of depressive episodes and to influence the course of depression in both developed and developing countries. Beck (1986) has described a cognitive triad that may contribute to the onset or reoccurrence of depressive episodes by increasing the risk of exposure to stressful life events: negative self view, negative interpretation of experience, and negative view of the future. Rates of depression increase in a variety of vulnerable groups, including refugees, neglected ethnic minority groups, and those exposed to war trauma (Baingana et al. 2004; Baingana, Bannon, and Thomas 2005; Barton and Mutiti 1998; de Jong 2002; Green et al. 2003; Mollica et al. 1998). Depression is also postulated to be high in Sub-Saharan Africa, resulting from the prevalent violence against women and HIV/AIDS (Baingana, Thomas, and Comblain, 2005; Bouta, Frerks, and Bannon 2004).

Poverty. A large body of evidence demonstrates the association between poverty and CMD. For example, a meta-analysis of five cross-sectional surveys carried out in Brazil, Chile, India, and Zimbabwe of people who sought treatment in primary care and the community, examining the economic risk factors for CMD, found a consistent and significant relation between low-income countries and risk for CMD. Similarly, a population-based study from Indonesia revealed that people with less education and fewer material possessions than others in their community were more likely to suffer from depression (Friedman 2004). It appears that both absolute and relative poverty are important in the genesis of depression (Friedman 2004).

Voices of the Poor, a three-volume publication of the World Bank that reports the findings from global focus group discussions with more than 60,000 poor people, notes feelings of worthlessness, hopelessness, and anxiety, as well as lack of planning for the future, as expressions of the state of being poor. These are some of the core symptoms of depression.

Gender. Both community and primary care–based studies indicate that women are often affected disproportionately by depression in both developing and developed countries (Abas and Broadhead 1997; Bean and Moller 2002; Broadhead and Abas 1994; Patel et al. 1999; Ustun et al. 2004). The multiple roles assumed by women, including the bearing and rearing of children, responsibility for the home, caring for both healthy and ill relatives, growing food, and earning income, can lead to increased exposure to life events, social adversity, and other environmental factors. Women in both developed and developing countries also encounter difficulties in relation to their social position, aspirations, social support networks, and domestic problems, which may include physical or sexual abuse.

Postpartum depression has been identified in both developed and developing countries. The greatest risk for postpartum depression is within the first 30 days of childbirth, and the condition can persist for up to two years. Certain practices in some developing countries, such as isolation of recent mothers from family and the new infant, are disruptive to the initial mother-infant relationship and eliminate the benefits of positive social supports. These practices have been identified as possible contributing factors to the onset of postpartum depression. In a study carried out in Zimbabwe, a brief screening questionnaire proved effective in identifying women in the eighth month of pregnancy who were at higher risk of postpartum depression (Nhiwatiwa, Patel, and Acuda 1998). Such a tool may be useful in devising preventive measures aimed at implementing interventions shortly after childbirth for previously identified high-risk individuals.

Violence against women, including sexual abuse of children, is linked to mental disorders of these women (Mulugeta, Kassaye, and Berhan 1998). A study carried out in Ethiopia found that in 5 percent of female high school students, completed rape had occurred and another 10 percent suffered attempted rape. Social isolation (33 percent), fear and phobia (19 percent), hopelessness (22 percent), and suicide attempts (6 percent) were the psychological sequelae. Rates of 21.1 percent have been found for domestic violence among patients presenting at a general practitioner's office (Marais et al. 1999).

Depression resulting from violence against women is postulated to be high in Sub-Saharan Africa (Marais et al. 1999). Rates of PTSD for those with a history of domestic violence were 35.3 percent versus 2.6 percent for those without such a history; rates of depression were 48.2 percent versus 11.4 percent; rates of suicide attempt were 19.0 percent versus 5.8 percent; and rates of substance abuse were 9.4 percent versus 4.7 percent. Those with major depression were also more likely to have attempted suicide and more likely to have unexplained physical symptoms and to make more visits to the general practitioner. Those with depression were also more likely to have comorbid PTSD (Marais et al. 1999).

In Butajira, Ethiopia, more than 3,000 women were systematically selected for a domestic violence study using instruments developed by the WHO (Yegomawork et al. 2003). This study showed that 59 percent of women suffered from sexual violence, and 49 percent suffered physical violence in their lifetime. Within the 12 months prior to the survey, 29 percent and 44 percent, respectively, had experienced physical and sexual violence. Very often, intimate partners are responsible for the violence. Women who suffered domestic violence reported increased lifetime mental health problems more often than those who did not suffer these adverse life events. The etiology of suicide is linked to a woman's history of sexual abuse and domestic violence; alcohol abuse; stressful life events, such as unwanted pregnancy or school-related pressures; as well as mental disorders, including depression and schizophrenia. An inverse relation has been found between suicide and education, older age, higher social class, and other indicators of well-being. Table 22.3 summarizes some of the studies carried out on suicide in Sub-Saharan Africa.

Weiss, Longhurst, and Mazure (1999), studying risk for depression in American women, found that child sexual abuse is associated with adult-onset depression in both men and women. A study of the patient profile of a clinic for child abuse and neglect in South Africa found that females made up 80 percent of the patients and that sexual abuse (90 percent) was the most common presenting complaint (de Villiers and Prentice 1996). The majority of the patients were young, 55 percent being below 10 years of age and 7 percent below 3 years. Behavior problems were recorded in 73 percent of cases, the commonest being school problems (21 percent), masturbation (19 percent), clingy behavior (12 percent), and withdrawal or depression (11.5 percent).

Similar findings were reported by Berard and Boermeester (1999). This study also found that more sexually abused patients received a diagnosis of depression than was expected, and they also scored higher on depression-rating scales. Logistic regression showed that the presence of suicidal symptoms and alcohol use were independently associated with sexual abuse. The authors concluded that "the associations of sexual abuse with suicidal symptoms, alcohol use, and troubled family circumstances, in the context of high unemployment, poverty, and gang-related violence, indicate a strong correspondence between adverse social conditions and psychological symptoms" (Berard and Boermeester 1999, 975).

HIV/AIDS. The psychiatric sequelae of HIV/AIDS are numerous and have etiologies that involve neurobiological and psychosocial factors. These include depression, anxiety disorders, manic symptoms, and atypical psychosis. Neuropsychiatric abnormalities were present in 41 percent of patients who tested positive for HIV-1 in Zaire (Perriens et al. 1992), and depression was found to be higher in symptomatic seropositive individuals than in matched seronegative individuals in the WHO Neuropsychiatric AIDS study (Maj et al. 1994). Kwalombota (2002), in a study carried out in Lusaka, Zambia, on the effect of pregnancy in HIV-infected women, found 85 percent to have major depressive episodes with suicidal thoughts. Those who knew their HIV status before becoming pregnant did not show severe depressive episodes, but those who found out while pregnant were liable to develop major depressive illness.

In Zaire, Boivin et al. (1995) studied the impact of a mother's HIV-positive status on the well-being of her children. The researchers found that "maternal HIV infection compromises the labor-intensive provision of care in the African milieu and undermines global cognitive development in even uninfected children" (p. 13).

Some research has been carried out in Sub-Saharan Africa on the links between HIV/AIDS and mental and neurological disorders. Although much of the research was done in the developed world, the data can provide information on the gaps in knowledge and the possible consequences of being HIV positive in Sub-Saharan Africa. Table 22.4 summarizes several of the studies on HIV/AIDS in Sub-Saharan Africa.

Consequences of Mental Disorders and Alcohol and Substance Abuse

Mental disorders and alcohol and substance abuse are disabling and costly. They affect productivity, impact the family and the community of the person with the disorder, and are associated with higher health care and other social services utilization, including the criminal justice system. The following is a brief discussion of some of the data available on the impact of mental disorders and alcohol and substance abuse in Sub-Saharan Africa.

Poverty. Psychiatric and neurological disorders impose a significant burden in developed and developing countries. In the West, considerable evidence links poverty and mental and neurological illness. For example, the national psychiatric morbidity surveys of 1993–94 in Great Britain showed that people with any form of mental disorder had an average income of only 46.5 percent of the average income for the general population. In countries where there are no social security payments, as is the case in many developing countries, this situation is greatly aggravated. In addition to this effect of poverty on the individual, the economy experiences a loss because of lost production from people with mental and neurological illnesses being unable to work, either in the short, medium, or long term, and reduced productivity from people being ill while at work.

There are also socioeconomic costs to families, including the cost of supporting the dependents of people with mental and neurological illnesses. Long-term consequences include unemployment, crime, and violence in young people whose childhood problems (for example, depression, conduct disorder, dyslexia, and other special educational needs) were not properly addressed in childhood.

Poor Physical Health. Poor mental and neurological health is a risk factor for many physical health problems, and emotional distress makes people more vulnerable to physical illness. Various studies carried out in the West show that depression increases the risk of heart disease fourfold (Lett et al. 2004; Nemeroff, Musselman, and Evans 1998; Zellweger et al. 2004), even though it controlled for other risk factors such as smoking (Hippisley-Cox, Fielding, and Pringle 1998). Lack of control at work is also associated with increased risk of cardiovascular disease (Marmot et al. 1997). Sustained stress or trauma increases susceptibility to viral infection and physical illness by damaging the immune system (Marmot et al. 1997; Stewart-Brown 1998). Poor mental health in mothers is a major risk factor not only for their own physical ill health but also for impaired physical, cognitive, and emotional development of children and child mortality from infectious diseases (Rutter and Quinton 1984).

Comorbidity. Comorbidity (the coexistence of two or more disorders) has been found to be common among patients suffering from depression. It typically involves a combination of general physical and mental disorders or neurological and mental disorders. In one study of patients attending primary care, of nearly 21 percent of patients with clinically significant depressive symptoms, only 1.2 percent cited depression as the reason for their visit to the physician (Broadhead and Abas 1994). Comorbidity of physical and mental illness has been found to increase with age.

Substance abuse is a frequent comorbid condition with depression. Studies in both developed and developing countries point to substance abuse as both a cause and effect of depression linked to both genetic and environmental factors. Depression has been shown to be a major factor

Table 22.4 Selected Studies on the Psychosocial and Mental Health Consequences of HIV/AIDS

Authors and year	Country, study population	Study findings
Turner et al. 2003	United States 1,827 women and 3,246 men on combination drug use Gender, depression, and ARV adherence	Women less adherent than men (13% vs. 25%) Women more likely to be diagnosed with depression (34% vs. 29%) Adherence better for those on treatment for depression
de Ronchi et al. 2000	Italy 325 subjects, 12 with DSM-IV-R criteria for organic delusional syndrome	3.7% had new-onset psychosis Generalized brain atrophy shown in CT scan of three of nine patients Remission of psychotic symptoms observed in two of the new-onset psychosis patients
Spire et al. 2002	France 445 patients on HAART	26.7% reported nonadherence at four months of follow-up Level of depression associated with nonadherence Other correlates: younger age, poor housing conditions, and lack of social support
Morrison et al. 2002	United States, Florida 93 HIV-infected women; 62 uninfected women	19.4% of infected women had depression compared with 4.8% of seronegative women Mean scores for depression higher for the HIV-infected women HIV-positive women had higher anxiety symptom scores
Evans et al. 2002	United States 63 HIV-positive women; 30 HIV-negative women Association of viral load in women with HIV	Major depression in 15.87% of HIV-positive women vs. 10.00% of HIV-negative women Higher depression scores in HIV-positive women Anxiety scores similar in the two groups Depressive and anxiety scores significantly associated with higher-activated CD8 T lymphocyte cells and higher viral loads Major depression associated with lower natural killer cell activity
Ciesla and Roberts 2001	2,596 with depression; 1,822 with dysthymic disorder Meta-analysis of 10 studies of relation between HIV infection and risk for depression	Frequency of major depression two times higher in HIV-positive individuals Depression not related to sexual orientation or disease stage of infected individuals
Drotar et al. 1999	Uganda 61 infants of HIV-infected mothers; 234 uninfected infants (seroreverters) 115 uninfected infants of uninfected mothers	Lower mental and motor development in HIV-infected infants No group differences on mean performance or growth rates on visual information processing
Carson et al. 1998	Kenya 230 subjects 34% HIV positive	No substantial differences in psychiatric morbidity or neuropsychological functioning between the HIV-positive and HIV-negative subjects
Sebit 1995	Kenya and Zaire 408 HIV-positive individuals Determining the natural history of HIV-1	Depression significantly higher in symptomatic seropositive individuals
Boivin et al. 1995	Zaire 14 asymptomatic HIV-positive children under two years of age 20 HIV-negative children born to HIV-positive mothers	Central nervous system structures affected even in seemingly asymptomatic HIV-positive children Labor-intensive provision of care in the African milieu and global cognitive development of even uninfected children compromised by maternal HIV-infection
Bleyenheuft et al. 1992	Central African Republic 292 women hospitalized for psychiatric reasons	HIV rate higher for those being hospitalized for the first time HIV appears responsible for psychiatric fragility Psychiatric symptoms apparent before the onset of symptoms of AIDS
Perriens et al. 1992	Zaire 196 patients studied 104 seropositive	Neuropsychiatric symptoms in 41% of the HIV-positive patients
Belec et al. 1989	Central African Republic 93 seropositive inpatients	Neurologic and psychiatric symptoms in 16%

Source: Compiled by authors.

Note: ARV = antiretroviral; DSM-IV-R = *Diagnostic and Statistical Manual of Mental Disorders, Revised Fourth Edition;* HAART = highly active antiretroviral therapies.

contributing to relapse in women abusing alcohol and drugs. Identifying substance abuse in patients presenting with depressive illness is an important component of management of the illness. Depression is also a common concomitant of HIV/AIDS (Ciesla and Roberts 2001; Morrison et al. 2002) and is associated with decreased compliance with medications (Turner et al. 2003), increased risk-taking behavior, putting others at risk for infection, and faster progression of the course of the illness evidenced by a rapid fall in the CD4 cell counts (Baingana, Thomas, and Comblain 2005; Evans et al. 2002).

Patients with epilepsy often present with psychological or psychotic symptoms. Sixty percent of 230 patients with epilepsy who were referred to the neurology clinic of Muhimbili Medical Center, Tanzania, had a psychological disturbance warranting intervention; 81 percent had a minor neurotic disorder, but 19 percent had schizophreniform psychosis (Matuja 1990). Other disturbances were agoraphobia and severe depression. Over 80 percent of patients with a major disturbance had epilepsy and a brain lesion; 77 percent of patients with a minor disturbance had evidence of an organic brain lesion. Organic brain lesion and psychological disturbance were overwhelmingly associated with social disadvantage.

In a study of 478 Zambian patients on a given day, all of whom were examined for goiter, 34.4 percent of all adult females and 23.2 percent of all adult males were found to have goiter (Rwegellera and Mambwe 1977). Goiter was found in 57.6 percent of females with affective illness and 77 percent of males with paranoid psychosis. Bademosi and colleagues (1976) found that 38 percent of patients with infective endocarditis had neuropsychiatric symptoms. For 75 percent of these, the neuropsychiatric symptoms were the presenting feature.

INTERVENTIONS

Possible interventions available and feasible in the context of Sub-Saharan Africa are grouped here into the traditional three: promotion, prevention, and treatment.

Promotion

The West has provided evidence about the value of interventions to strengthen individuals' mental well-being and increase emotional resilience. Such interventions are designed to promote self-esteem and improve life and coping skills, including communicating, negotiating, relating to others, and parenting. Early child interventions, as well as early recognition of any problems, have been found to be crucial to optimizing cognitive development and the future performance of children in school.

Strengthening communities—for example, increasing social inclusion and participation, improving neighborhood environments, and developing health and social services that support mental health—and reducing discrimination and inequality by promoting access to education, meaningful occupation, and adequate housing are all appropriate targets for promoting mental health. Addressing stigma in relation to mental disorders is also crucial.

Primary Prevention

Prevention is critical in reducing the impact of mental disorders and alcohol and substance abuse. On ethical grounds alone, prevention is always preferable to treatment or rehabilitation. In most instances prevention is also more cost-effective than treatment. Many potentially catastrophic disorders are now preventable. Examples include iodine supplementation to prevent mental retardation and iodine deficiency disorder, as well as immunization against tetanus, tuberculosis, measles, rubella, and polio; immunization in the perinatal and early child period prevents these infections, which can damage the central nervous system and could have epilepsy as a sequelae, and mental retardation (Down's Syndrome) is associated with rubella in the first trimester of pregnancy. Zinc, folic acid, and iron supplementation and fortification are crucial to preventing learning disabilities, mental retardation, and developmental delays. Prevention of maternal transmission of HIV is increasingly critical, thus preventing the neurological and developmental consequences associated with pediatric HIV infection. Safe motherhood initiatives, such as attendance at an antenatal clinic, tetanus vaccination during pregnancy, and delivery with a trained attendant, also greatly reduce the impact of prenatal, perinatal, and postnatal risk factors.

Preventive community-wide psychosocial programs have been shown to be effective, especially for populations affected by conflict and HIV/AIDS. These include child care centers for orphans and vulnerable children, children's clubs, school-based mental health programs, and support groups in the communities.

Recently, short-course antiretroviral prophylaxis regimens have been shown to provide a relatively low cost and effective strategy for preventing mother-to-child transmission of HIV in low-income populations by up to 30 percent

(Connor et al. 1994; Mofenson 1999). Supplemental feeding reduces the transmission through breastfeeding by a further 30 percent, thus preventing the neurological and developmental disabilities associated with HIV infection in children.

Treatment

A brief description is provided here for the treatments available for the mental disorders discussed. A concerted effort was made to provide treatment alternatives where the costs and effectiveness are known, but this is not always possible for Sub-Saharan Africa, since these studies are just being carried out. The next best alternative is to provide a discussion of what is presently being provided as treatment, even when evidence for cost-effectiveness may not be available.

Depression. Effective treatment strategies exist for depression in the form of pharmacological agents, cognitive behavioral therapy, and psychosocial treatments. Although treatment interventions may not cure all forms of depression, a large number of efficacious and low-cost treatments are available. Despite the availability of these interventions, many people in Africa remain undiagnosed and untreated. It is difficult to estimate the actual treatment gap (all those with a clinically diagnosed mental disorder who are not on treatment) because epidemiological data of diagnosed mental disorders in the community or of those who are on treatment are limited. The scant data available are often unreliable. Andrews, Henderson, and Wayne-Hall (2001), studying utilization of the Australian mental health services, found that only about 30 percent of those with a diagnosed mental disorder used the services.

Because of their efficacy and cost-effectiveness, antidepressant medications represent the mainstay of treatment for depression in developed countries. Seventy percent of patients prescribed antidepressants show significant clinical improvement. Antidepressants are also effective as prophylaxes: treatment has been shown to reduce the relapse rate for recurrent depression from 80 percent over three years to 22 percent. There has been far less research in developing countries, but the limited available evidence shows similar rates of efficacy. Tricyclic antidepressants (TCAs) and the newer selective serotonin reuptake inhibitors (SSRIs) have similar efficacy for moderate depression. The reduced side effects of SSRIs enhance patient compliance. However, the high cost of SSRIs means that they remain out of reach as a first-line treatment in Africa for all but the wealthy. Indeed, simply ensuring an adequate supply of TCAs to the

primary care level across Sub-Saharan Africa still represents a major financial challenge for these countries, even though TCAs are relatively cheaper than the SSRIs, even if the latter are now getting off patent protection. The median yearly cost for treating depression in an individual with amitriptyline in Sub-Saharan Africa was estimated at US$30.66 in 2001 and is now estimated to be US$34.38 (WHO 2001, 2005).

Bolton and colleagues (2003) tested the efficacy of group interpersonal psychotherapy in alleviating depression and dysfunction in rural Uganda and found it to be highly efficacious. Mean reduction of depression severity was 17.47 points for intervention groups and 3.55 points for controls. After the intervention, 6.5 percent of the intervention group and 54.7 percent of the control group met the criteria for major depression compared with 86 percent and 94 percent, respectively, before treatment was initiated.

Cognitive behavior therapy, problem-solving therapy, and family-focused therapy have met with success in the treatment of depression. A small number of published reports address the use of psychosocial interventions to treat depression in developing countries. Problem-solving therapy has been suggested as an effective psychosocial treatment, particularly because it seeks to provide the patient with a technique for coping with future problems, thereby potentially preventing a recurrence of depressive symptoms or enabling the patient to deal with them more effectively when they recur. Problem-solving therapy has been conducted effectively by trained community nurses in primary care settings, making the approach particularly attractive for resource-poor settings, where psychiatrists and specially trained general physicians are not available.

Schizophrenia. Evidence suggests that correct early diagnosis and initiation of treatment can have a positive impact on the subsequent course of schizophrenia. Antipsychotic medication is the mainstay of treatment and is indicated for the majority of patients over prolonged periods with no fixed limit to duration. Two classes of pharmacological agents are available. The two offer approximately equal efficacy in controlling the positive symptoms of the disorder but differ considerably in their side effects and tolerability as well as cost. The median yearly cost per person for chlorpromazine for Sub-Saharan Africa was estimated at US$40.88 in 2001 and is now estimated to be US$49.06 (WHO 2001, 2005).

Posttraumatic Stress Disorder. A combination of psychosocial and mental health interventions is recommended for PTSD. Psychosocial interventions include counseling, group support meetings, play activities, art, music, and other expressive art therapies. Mental health interventions include a short course of anxiolytics for acute distress, not to be taken for longer than two weeks. Symptoms that persist beyond the acute phase respond to smaller doses of antidepressants and antipsychotics. Drug treatment for PTSD is best combined with a psychotherapeutic intervention, such as group therapy, individual therapy, or counseling.

Mental Disorders among Children. The first step in the management of mental disorders among children is making the correct diagnosis. Management is also dependent on a collaboration between the parents or caretaker, the teachers, and the health care provider. Treatment depends on the diagnosis and the underlying causative factors. Antidepressants are effective in the management of emotional disorders of children. However, the teacher must be aware of the diagnosis and provide support within the school system. For children with learning difficulties, special needs education teachers play a crucial role in providing education tailored to the needs of the child.

For children with attention–deficit/hyperactivity disorder, Ritalin and other stimulants are not widely used in Sub-Saharan Africa, mainly because of the lack of child psychiatrists and psychologists, necessary for the close supervision required. High activity levels can be managed with behavioral methods, and a special needs education teacher can design a learning program tailored to the attention deficit. A few countries, such as Kenya, South Africa, and Uganda, have developed comprehensive special education teacher-training programs.

A FRAMEWORK FOR RESEARCH

In developing short-term, medium-term, and long-term strategies, it is clear that further research will have to be carried out in order to provide the evidence necessary to strengthen the mental health care systems of Sub-Saharan Africa. Following are some of the recommended research areas that could be pursued.

- Cross-sectional and longitudinal studies of mental disorders in Sub-Saharan Africa, including validation of the standardized testing instruments for the different populations of Africa, would establish the epidemiology and causative and risk factors, as well as links to sexual abuse, violence against women, HIV/AIDS, and conflicts. The

Butajira community laboratory (Alem et al. 1999; Kebede et al. 2003; Kebede et al. 2006), where a group of Ethiopian researchers is conducting cross-sectional and longitudinal mental health studies could be cited as a good example for such undertakings in Sub-Saharan Africa.

- Multisite studies on the mental well-being of children would establish the incidence and prevalence of mental disorders of children, links to abuse of all forms, malnutrition, conflicts, poverty and vulnerability, what interventions are available, what the burden is within the school system, and how it affects educational outcomes.

- Stigmatization confounds epidemiological studies, prevents treatment, and leads to personal and economic disaster for many affected individuals and their families. Because stigma and other cultural beliefs are locally grounded, they require local study in order to develop ways in which to deal with them constructively.

- Cost-of-illness, cost-effectiveness, cost-minimization, and cost-benefit analyses should be undertaken to provide government officials and funding agencies the necessary economic perspective in relation to mental disorders and alcohol abuse. Socioeconomic determinants of the outcome measures that could best reflect optimal care for people with mental disorders and those abusing alcohol should be identified.

- Family, twin, and adoption studies in Western countries have provided evidence of the genetic contribution to the etiology of depressive disorders. Twin studies have also demonstrated the strong role of the nonshared environment in the causation of depression. Thus, examination of gene-environment interactions is essential to future research and would benefit from a wide range of variation in the psychosocial environments, making it possible to delineate better the etiological contributions of such environmental factors as socioeconomic adversity, life events, and the breakdown of social support networks. There is a need for such studies to be carried out in Sub-Saharan Africa.

- Defective neurotransmission and neuroendocrine receptor responses are associated with depression. Three monoamines have been implicated: 5-hydroxytryptamine (serotonin), noradrenaline, and dopamine. Conclusive evidence on the impact of these defects on the course of depressive disorders remains to be found. It is still unclear whether associations with neurological function represent cause or effect in the pathogenesis of depression and whether neurological function is the major risk factor for depression in Sub-Saharan Africa.

- Additional research should be conducted in developing countries to determine the cost-effectiveness of cognitive behavioral therapy in primary health care settings. Requisite long-term follow-up studies have not been conducted in low-income countries. They would need to include attention to recovery from symptoms, dysfunction and reversal of the dysfunction following treatment, disability, the family's support of the patient, and the cost of this support to the family, as well as the social and economic burden on the family and the community. Measurements would have to be made over at least five years.

- Not enough evaluations of mental health services have been carried out in Sub-Saharan Africa, and the few that have been done are neither comprehensive nor country-wide. The process for integrating mental health into primary health care and the effectiveness of this approach needs to be documented.

POLICY ISSUES

The policy implications resulting from the epidemiology of mental health and substance abuse disorders in Sub-Saharan Africa discussed here are provided only as a menu of possible policy interventions, to be selected from, depending on the context and the needs of each country.

- As societies and economies become increasingly information oriented and dependent on highly skilled and literate workers, it is critical that children everywhere have an opportunity to reach their optimal levels of cognitive and neurological development. The persistence of excess prevalence rates of preventable mental disorders—such as depression, PTSD, and mental disorders resulting from sexual abuse of children—observed in Sub-Saharan Africa countries today is a consequence of both poverty and poor resource allocation, and it is an impediment to future social and economic development.

- To implement effective programs for community-level detection and treatment of patients with mental disorders, governments and health authorities of Sub-Saharan Africa countries must first issue clear policies articulating measures for the identification and treatment of patients with mental disorders, including children. Essential components of any strategy include the assurance of a continuous drug supply and means of distribution, prevention programs, social programs, and stigma mitigation strategies to increase employment and improve general welfare among individuals suffering from the disease. Also essential are training of health care personnel and methods for surveillance and routine data collection. Reforms in the health, social, and economic sectors need to address mental health and substance abuse clearly and in an integrated way, and programs need to be set up targeting other priority areas, such as HIV, malaria and other infectious diseases, and reproductive and child health.

Increasing the policy and service development and the clinical and research professional capacity in Sub-Saharan African countries and stemming the flow of skilled health professionals to wealthy countries (Hongoro and McPake 2004; Liese, Blanchet, and Dussault 2003; WHO, NEPAD, and ACOSHED 2005) are key to developing sustainable, locally appropriate programs.

Table 22A.1 Selected Sub-Saharan Africa Data on Mental Health Disorders

Author(s)	Disorder	Country, study population	Findings
Molteno et al. 2001	Behavioral and emotional disorders and intellectual disability	Cape Town, South Africa 355 children in special schools	31% for psychopathology, boys more affected than girls More behavioral problems among the children with severe and profound retardation Epilepsy associated with more total behavior scores
Ikeji et al. 1999	ECT and schizophrenia, mania, and severe depression	Nigeria 70 subjects Prospective open-label study	Full clinical recovery Unmodified ECT safe and effective with nonenduring subjective memory difficulty
Bolton, Neugebauer, and Ndogoni 2002	Depression	Rwanda 368 adults Community-based random sample	15.5% met criteria for DSM IV diagnosis of depression.
Kaaya et al. 2002	Depression among HIV-positive women	Tanzania 903 women Two-phase design	Internal consistency of HSCL-25 adequate HSCL-25 demonstrated utility for depression
Bean and Moller 2002	PTSD and depression	South Africa 40 battered women	63% moderately to severely depressed 59% high PTSD symptoms 38.4% anger, 54.5% guilt
Martenyi et al. 2002	PTSD	Europe, Israel, and South Africa Double-blind, randomized, placebo-controlled study Efficacy and tolerability of fluoxetine 226 patients on fluoxetine, 75 on placebo	Fluoxetine associated with greater improvement Fluoxetine effective and well tolerated in PTSD
Bolton 2001b	Mental health effects of genocide	Rwanda Free listing, key informant interviews, and pile sorts	Depression occurs in this population Supports local content validity of the depression assessment instruments
Njenga 2000	Depression	Kenya 86 professional women	22% reported depressive symptoms 30% coping less well than usual
Mkize, Nonkelela, and Mkize 1998	Depression	Transkei, South Africa 250 students randomly selected Beck's Depression Inventory	53% mild to severe depression Females more affected 3 to 1 14% moderately to severely depressed All subjects presented with somatic symptoms
Vaz, Mbajiorgu, and Acuda 1998	Stress, depression, and suicide	Zimbabwe 109 medical students Cross-sectional study	64.5% at various levels of stress or depression or both 11% very high levels of stress 12% at serious risk for suicide
Lopes and Bottino 2002	Dementia	All continents Medline and Lilacs search, 38 studies evaluated from all continents	1.17% specific prevalence rate for dementia for 65–69-year-olds 54.83% specific prevalence rate for dementia for those over 95 years Dementia more prevalent among women in 75% papers reviewed
Aina 2001	Clinical profile of patients attending psychiatric hospital	Nigeria Prospective, private hospital–based study 138 patients seen in 644 consultation sessions	Highest percentage made up of young adults 31–45 years of age 36% epilepsy 22.5% schizophrenia 18.8% affective disorders

(Table continues on the next page.)

Table 22A.1 *(Continued)*

Author(s)	Disorder	Country, study population	Findings
Molteno et al. 2001	Behavioral and emotional problems in children with intellectual disability	South Africa 355 children with intellectual disability attending special schools	31% psychopathology in children with intellectual disability More behavioral problems in boys than girls More behavioral difficulties in children with severe and profound forms of intellectual disability
Kwalombota 2002	HIV and depression	Zambia Mental health of HIV-positive women attending antenatal clinic	85% of HIV-positive women had major depressive disorder Depression more common among those diagnosed HIV positive during pregnancy
Nwosu and Odesanmi 2001	Suicide	Nigeria Study of pattern of autopsy findings in cases of completed suicides	Suicides at the rate of 0.4 per 100,000 population Higher suicide incidence in males (3.6 to 1) Majority of the victims in their 20s
Bhagwanjee et al. 1998	Minor psychiatric disorders	South Africa 354 adults Two-stage community-based epidemiological study	23.9% prevalence of generalized anxiety and depressive disorder 3.7% generalized anxiety, 4.8% major depression, 7.3% dysthymia, and 8.2% major depression with dysthymia
Okulate 2001	Suicide	Nigeria Case-control study of the characteristics of patients who attempted suicide in a military setting 51 attempted suicides	Suicide 0.37% of all admissions to the Department of Psychiatry, Military Hospital, Yaba, Nigeria 60.8% of all suicides below the age of 30 years Numbers of males and females almost equal
Dong and Simon 2001	Organophosphate poisoning	Zimbabwe Cross-sectional descriptive study of the use of organophosphate as poison Urban hospital admissions 183,569 case records studied 599 cases of organophosphate poisoning	Increase of 320% in organophosphate poisoning between 1995 and 2000 Similar male and female admission rates 82% below 31 years 74% suicide attempts
Kebede and Alem 1999	Suicide	Ethiopia Study of suicide attempts and suicide ideation 10,203 adults in Addis Ababa	Prevalence of current suicide ideation, 2.7% Lifetime prevalence, 0.9% 66% of subjects below 25 years of age Current suicide ideation more common in men than women (95% confidence interval) Hanging preferred method for men, poisoning for women
Ihueze and Okpara 1989	Psychiatric disorders of old age	Nigeria Retrospective study of 73 consecutive patients age 60 years and over admitted to a psychiatric hospital	Patients over 60 years admitted for the first time, 5% of all admissions 58% below 70 years 84% in the two lowest socioeconomic classes 49% functional psychosis 30% organic psychosis 10% neurotic disorders
Ben-Arie et al. 1983	Psychiatric disorders of old age	South Africa 139 noninstitutionalized coloured persons over 65 years old	24% some form of psychiatric disorder 16.5% depression 15% alcoholism among the men 6% on psychiatric medication
Verrier-Jones et al. 1978	Psychiatric disorders of old age	South Africa 100 patients admitted to a psychogeriatric unit	Over 50% of patients depressed, many associated with physical illness and isolation Nine patients admitted with confusion Confusion due to drugs prescribed by medical practitioners in seven of them

Source: Compiled by authors.
Note: ECT = electroconvulsive therapy.

NOTES

1. A demographic study site is a geographical area that is delineated and, after the baseline assessment of the total population is entered into a database, used for regular surveillance of health and demographic trends over time.

2. **AFR D:** Algeria, Angola, Benin, Burkina Faso, Cameroon, Cape Verde, Chad, Comoros, Equatorial Guinea, Gabon, Gambia, Ghana, Guinea, Guinea-Bissau, Liberia, Madagascar, Mali, Mauritania, Mauritius, Niger, Nigeria, São Tomé and Principe, Senegal, Seychelles, Sierra Leone, Togo. **AFR E:** Botswana, Burundi, Central African Republic, Côte d'Ivoire, Democratic Republic of Congo, Eritrea, Ethiopia, Kenya, Lesotho, Malawi, Mozambique, Namibia, Republic of Congo, Rwanda, South Africa, Swaziland, Uganda, Tanzania, Zambia, Zimbabwe.

REFERENCES

Abas, M., and J. Broadhead. 1994. "Mental Disorders in the Developing World." *British Medical Journal* 308: 1052–53.

———. 1997. "Depression and Anxiety amongst Women in an Urban Setting in Zimbabwe." *Psychology and Medicine* 27: 59–71.

Abdulahi, H., D. H. Mariam, and D. Kebede. 2001. "Burden of Disease Analysis in Rural Ethiopia." *Ethiopian Medical Journal* 39: 271–81.

Aina, F. 2001. "Socio-Demographic and Clinical Profile of Patients Attending a Private Psychiatric Hospital in Lagos, Nigeria." *West African Journal of Medicine* 20 (2): 117–22.

Alem, A., D. Kebede, L. Jacobsson, and G. Kullgren. 1999. "Suicide Attempts among Adults in Butajira, Ethiopia." *Acta Psychiatrica Scandinavica* 397 (Suppl.): 70–76.

Andrews, G., S. Henderson, and W. Wayne-Hall. 2001. "Prevalence, Comorbidity, Disability and Service Utilization: Overview of the Australian National Mental Health Survey." *British Journal of Psychiatry* 178: 145–53.

Bademosi, O., A. O. Falasae, F. Jaiyesimi, and A. Bademosi. 1976. "Neuropsychiatric Manifestations of Infective Endocarditis: A Study of 95 Patients at Ibadan, Nigeria." *Journal of Neurology, Neurosurgery and Psychiatry* 39 (4): 325–29.

Baingana, F., I. Bannon, and R. Thomas. 2005. "Mental Health and Conflicts: Conceptual Framework and Approaches." A Health, Nutrition and Population Discussion Paper, World Bank, Washington, DC.

Baingana, F., A. Dabalen, E. Menye, M. Prywes, and M. Rosholm. 2004. "Mental Health and Socio-Economic Outcomes in Burundi." A Health, Nutrition and Population Discussion Paper, World Bank, Washington, DC.

Baingana, F., R. Thomas, and C. Comblain. 2005. "HIV and Mental Health." A Health, Nutrition and Population Discussion Paper, World Bank, Washington, DC.

Barton, T., and A. Mutiti. 1998. *Northern Uganda Psycho-Social Needs Assessment (NUPSNA)*. Geneva: UNICEF.

Bean, J., and A. T. Moller. 2002. "Posttraumatic Stress and Depressive Symptomatology in a Sample of Battered Women from South Africa." Part 1. *Psychological Reports* 90 (3): 750–52.

Beck, A. T. 1986. "Hopelessness as a Predictor of Eventual Suicide." *Annals of the New York Academy of Sciences* 48: 90–96.

Belec, P. L., J. Testa, M. D. Vohito, G. Gresenguet, M. I. Martin, A. Tabo, B. Di Costanzo, and A. J. Georges. 1989. "Neurologic and Psychiatric Manifestations of AIDS in Central African Republic." *Bulletin de la Societé de Pathologie Exotique et de Ses Filiales* 82 (3): 297–307.

Ben-Arie, O., L. Swartz, A. F. Teggin, and R. Elk. 1983. "The Coloured Elderly in Cape Town—A Psychosocial, Psychiatric and Medical Community Survey." Part 2. Prevalence of Psychiatric Disorders." *South African Medical Journal* 64 (27): 1056–61.

Berard, R. M. F., and F. Boermeester. 1999. "Sexual Abuse in Adolescents: Data from a Psychiatric Treatment Center for Adolescents." *South African Medical Journal* 89 (9): 972–76.

Bhagwanjee, A., A. Parekh, Z. Paruk, I. Petersen, and H. Subedar. 1998. "Prevalence of Minor Psychiatric Disorders in an African Rural Community in South Africa." *Psychological Medicine* 28: 1137–47.

Bleyenheuft, L., P. Janne, C. Reynaert, N. Munyandamutsa, F. Verhoeven, B. Muremyangango, and L. Cassiers. 1992. "Prevalence of Human Immunodeficiency Virus Infection in a Psychiatric Population in Central Africa." *Acta Psychiatrica Belgica* 92 (2): 99–108.

Boivin, M. J., S. D. Green, A. G. Davies, B. Giordani, J. K. Mokili, and W. A. Cutting. 1995. "A Preliminary Evaluation of the Cognitive and Motor Effects of Pediatric HIV Infection in Zairian Children." *Health Psychology* 14 (1): 13–21.

Bolton, P. 2001a. "Cross-Cultural Validity and Reliability Testing of a Standard Psychiatric Assessment Instrument without a Gold Standard." *Journal of Nervous and Mental Disease* 189 (4): 238–42.

———. 2001b. "Local Perceptions of the Mental Health Effects of the Rwandan Genocide." *Journal of Nervous and Mental Disease* 189 (4): 243–48.

Bolton, P., J. Bass, R. Neugebauer, H. Verdeli, K. Clougherty, P. Wickramatne, L. Speelman, L. Ndogoni, and M. Weissman. 2003. "Group Interpersonal Psychotherapy for Depression in Rural Uganda." *Journal of the American Medical Association* 289 (23): 3117–24.

Bolton, P., R. Neugebauer, and L. Ndogoni. 2002. "Prevalence of Depression in Rural Rwanda Based on Symptom and Functional Criteria." *Journal of Nervous and Mental Disease* 190 (9): 631–37.

Booyens, J., M. L. Luitingh, and C. F. van Rensburg. 1977. "The Relationship between Scholastic Progress and Nutritional Status. Part 2. A One Year Follow-Up Study." *South African Medical Journal* 52 (16): 650–52.

Bouta, T., G. Frerks, and I. Bannon. 2004. *Gender, Conflict and Development*. Washington, DC: World Bank.

Breetzke, K. A. 1988. "Suicide in Cape Town—Is the Challenge Being Met Effectively?" *South African Medical Journal* 73 (1): 19–52.

Broadhead, J., and M. Abas. 1994. "Depressive Illness—Zimbabwe." *Tropical Doctor* 24 (1): 27–30.

Carson, A. J., R. Sandler, F. N. Owino, F. O. Matete, and E. C. Johnstone. 1998. "Psychological Morbidity and HIV in Kenya." *Acta Psychiatrica Scandinavica* 97 (4): 267–71.

CDC (Centers for Disease Control and Prevention). 2000. "Cause-Specific Adult Mortality: Evidence from Community-Based Surveillance—Selected Sites, Tanzania, 1992–1998." *Morbidity and Mortality Weekly Report* 19: 49.

Ciesla, J. A., and J. E. Roberts. 2001. "A Meta-Analysis of Risk for Major Depressive Disorder among HIV-Positive Individuals." *American Journal of Psychiatry* 15: 725–30.

Connor, E. M., R. S. Sperling, R. Gelber, P. Kiselev, G. Scott, M. J. O. O'Sullivan, et al. 1994. "Reduction of Maternal-Infant Transmission of Human Immuno-Deficiency Virus Type 1 with Zidovudine Treatment." *New England Journal of Medicine* 331 (180): 1173–80.

Cummins, R. R., and C. W. Allwood. 1984. "Suicide Attempts or Threats by Children and Adolescents in Johannesburg." *South African Medical Journal* 66 (19): 726–29.

de Jong, J. 2002. "Public Mental Health, Traumatic Stress and Human Rights Violations in Low-Income Countries." In *Trauma, War and Violence: Public Mental Health in Socio-Cultural Context*. Plenum Series in Social/Clinical Psychology. New York: Plenum.

Demyttenaere, K., R. Bruffaerts, J. Posada-Villa, I. Gasquet, V. Kovess, J. P. Lepine, M. C. Angermeyer, et al. 2004. "Prevalence, Severity, and Unmet Need for Treatment of Mental Disorders in the World Health Organization World Mental Health Surveys." *Journal of the American Medical Association* 291 (21): 2581–90.

de Ronchi, D., I. Faranca, P. Forti, G. Ravaglia, M. Borderi, R. Manfredi, and V. Volterra. 2000. "Development of Acute Psychotic Disorders and HIV-1 Infection." *International Journal of Psychiatry in Medicine* 30 (2): 173–83.

de Villiers, F. P. R., and M. A. Prentice. 1996. "Accumulating Experience in a Child Abuse Clinic." *South African Medical Journal* 86 (2): 147–50.

Dhadphale, M., and B. Ibrahim. 1984. "Learning Disabilities among Nairobi School Children." *Acta Psychiatrica Scandinavica* 69 (2): 151–55.

Dong, X., and M. A. Simon. 2001. "The Epidemiology of Organophosphate Poisoning in Urban Zimbabwe from 1995 to 2000." *International Journal of Occupational and Environmental Health* 7 (4): 333–38.

Drotar, D., K. Olness, M. Wiznitzer, C. Schatschneider, L. Marum, L. Guay, J. Fagan, et al. 1999. "Neurodevelopmental Outcomes of Ugandan Infants with HIV Infection: An Application of Growth Curve Analysis." *Health and Psychology* 18 (2): 114–21.

Eferakeya, A. E. 1984. "Drugs and Suicide Attempts in Benin City, Nigeria." *British Journal of Psychiatry* 145: 70–73.

Evans, D. L., T. R. Ten Have, S. D. Douglas, D. R. Gettes, M. Morrison, M. S. Chiappini, et al. 2002. "Association of Depression with Viral Load, CD8 T Lymphocytes, and Natural Killer Cells in Women with HIV Infection." *American Journal of Psychiatry* 159: 1752–59.

Flisher, A. J., and C. D. Parry. 1994. "Suicide in South Africa. An Analysis of Nationally Registered Mortality Data for 1984–1986." *Acta Psychiatrica Scandinavica* 90 (5): 348–53.

Friedman, E. 2004. "Mental Health Effects of the Indonesian Economic Crisis." Development Economics Group Discussion Paper, World Bank, Washington, DC.

Goldberg, D., and P. Huxley. 1992. *Common Mental Disorders.* London: Routledge.

Goldberg, D. P., R. Gater, N. Sartorius, T. B. Ustun, M. Piccinelli, O. Gureje, and C. Rutter. 1997. "The Validity of Two Versions of the GHQ in the WHO Study of Mental Illness in General Health Care." *Psychology and Medicine* 27: 191–97.

Granja, A. C., E. Zacarias, and S. Bergstrom. 2002. "Violent Deaths: The Hidden Face of Maternal Mortality." *British Journal of Obstetrics and Gynaecology* 109 (1): 5–8.

Green, B. L., M. J. Friedman, J. de Jong, S. D. Solomon, T. M. Keane, J. A. Fairbank, B. Donelan, and E. Frey-Wouters. 2003. *Trauma Interventions in War and Peace: Prevention, Practice, and Policy.* New York: Kluwer Academic/Plenum.

Hippisley-Cox, J., K. Fielding, and M. Pringle. 1998. "Depression as a Risk Factor for Ischaemic Heart Disease in Men: Population Based Case-Control Study." *British Medical Journal* 316: 1714–19.

Hollifield, M., W. Katon, D. Spain, and L. Pule. 1990. "Anxiety and Depressions in a Village in Lesotho, Africa: A Comparison with the United States." *British Journal of Psychiatry* 156: 343–50.

Hongoro, C., and B. McPake. 2004. "How to Bridge the Gap in Human Resources for Health." *Lancet* 364: 1451–56.

Ihezue, U. H., and E. Okpara. 1989. "Psychiatric Disorders of Old Age in Enugu, Nigeria. Sociodemographic and Clinical Characteristics." *Acta Psychiatrica Scandinavica* 79 (4): 332–37.

Ikeji, O. C., J. U. Ohaeri, R. O. Osahon, and R. O. Agidee. 1999. "Naturalistic Comparative Study of Outcome and Cognitive Effects of Unmodified Electro-Convulsive Therapy in Schizophrenia, Mania and Severe Depression in Nigeria." *East African Medical Journal* 76 (11): 644–50.

IOM (Institute of Medicine). 2001. *Neurological, Psychiatric, and Developmental Disorders: Meeting the Challenges in the Developing World.* Report. Washington, DC: IOM.

Jablensky, A., N. Sartorius, G. Ernberg, M. Anker, A. Korten, J. E. Cooper, R. Day, and A. Bertelsen. 1992. "Schizophrenia: Manifestations, Incidence and Course in Different Cultures. A World Health Organization Ten-Country Study." *Psychology and Medicine* 20: 1–97.

Jenkins, R. 1985. "Minor Psychiatric Morbidity in Employed Young Men and Women and Its Contribution to Sickness Absence." *British Journal of Industrial Medicine* 42 (3): 147–54.

———. 1998. "Linking Epidemiology and Disability Measurement with Mental Health Service Policy and Planning." *Epidemiologia e Psichiatria Sociale* 7 (2): 120–26.

Kaaya, S. F., M. C. Fawzi, J. K. Mbwambo, B. Lee, G. I. Msamanga, and W. Fawzi. 2002. "Validity of the Hopkins Symptom Checklist-25 amongst HIV-Positive Pregnant Women in Tanzania." *Acta Psychiatrica Scandinavica* 106 (1): 9–19.

Kebede, D., and A. Alem. 1999. "Suicide Attempts and Ideation among Adults in Addis Ababa, Ethiopia." *Acta Psychiatrica Scandinavica* 397: 35–39.

Kebede, D., A. Alem, T. Shibire, N. Deyassa, A. Negash, T. Beyero, G. Medhin, and A. Fekadu. 2006. "Symptomatic and Functional Outcome of Bipolar Disorder in Butajira, Ethiopia." *Journal of Affective Disorders* 90 (2–3): 239–49.

Kebede, D., A. Alem, T. Shibire, A. Negash, A. Fekadu, D. Fekadu, L. Jacobsson, and G. Kullgren. 2003. "Onset and Clinical Course of Schizophrenia in Butajira-Ethiopia: A Community Based Study." *Social Psychiatry and Psychiatric Epidemiology* 38: 625–31.

Kebede, D., and T. Ketsela. 1993. "Suicide Attempts in Ethiopia in Addis Abeba High School Adolescents." *Ethiopian Medical Journal* 31: 83–99.

Kessler, R. C., W. T. Chiu, O. Demler, K. R. Merikangas, and E. E. Walters. 2005. "Prevalence, Severity, and Comorbidity of 12-Month DSM-IV Disorders in the National Comorbidity Survey Replication." *Archives of General Psychiatry* 62 (6): 617–27.

Kessler, R. C., K. A. McGonagle, S. Zhao, C. B. Nelson, M. Hughes, S. Eshleman, H. U. Wittchen, and K. S. Kendler. 1994. "Lifetime and 12-Month Prevalence of DSM-III-R Psychiatric Disorders in the United States. Results from the National Comorbidity Survey." *Archives of General Psychiatry* 51 (1): 8–19.

Kiima, D. M., F. G. Njenga, M. M. Okonji, and P. A. Kigamwa. 2004. "Kenya Mental Health Country Profile." *International Review of Psychiatry* 16 (1–2): 48–53.

Kwalombota, M. 2002. "The Effect of Pregnancy in HIV-Infected Women." *AIDS Care* 14 (3): 431–33.

Leff, J., N. Sartorius, A. Jablensky, A. Korten, and G. Ernberg. 1992. "The International Pilot Study of Schizophrenia: Five-Year Follow-Up Findings." *Psychological Medicine* 22 (1): 131–45.

Lett, H. S., J. A. Blumental, M. A. Babyak, A. Sherwood, T. Strauman, C. Robins, and M. F. Newman. 2004. "Depression as a Risk Factor for Coronary Artery Disease: Evidence, Mechanisms, and Treatment." *Psychosomatic Medicine* 66 (3): 305–15.

Liese, B., N. Blanchet, and G. Dussault. 2003. "Background Paper on the Human Resource Crisis in Health Services," World Bank, Washington, DC.

Lopes, M. A., and C. M. Bottino. 2002. "Prevalence of Dementia in Several Regions of the World: Analysis of Epidemiologic Studies from 1994 to 2000." *Arquivos de Neuro-Psiquiatria* 60 (1): 61–69.

Maj, M., R. Janssen, F. Starace, M. Zaudig, P. Satz, B. Sughondhabirom, M. A. Luabeya, et al. 1994. "WHO Neuropsychiatric AIDS Study, Cross-Sectional Phase 1. Study Design and Psychiatric Findings." *Archives of General Psychiatry* 51 (1): 39–49.

Marais, A., P. J. T. De Villiers, A. T. Moller, and D. Stein. 1999. "Domestic Violence in Patients Visiting General Practitioners, Prevalence, Phenomenology and Association with Psychopathology." *South African Medical Journal* 89 (6): 635–40.

Marmot, M., H. Bosma, H. Hemingway, E. J. Brunner, and S. A. Stansfield. 1997. "Contribution of Job Control and Other Risk Factors to Social Variations in Coronary Heart Disease Incidence." *Lancet* 350: 235–39.

Martenyi, F., E. B. Brown, H. Zhang, S. C. Koke, and A. Prakash. 2002. "Fluoxetine v. Placebo in Prevention of Relapse in Post-Traumatic Stress Disorder." *British Journal of Psychiatry* 181: 315–20.

Mathers, C. D., C. Stein, D. Ma Fat, C. Rao, M. Inoue, N. Tomijima, C. Bernard, A. D. Lopez, and C. J. L. Murray. 2002. "Global Burden of Disease 2000: Version 2, Methods and Results." Global Program on Evidence for Health Policy Discussion Paper 50, WHO, Geneva.

Matuja, W. B. 1990. "Psychological Disturbance in African Tanzanian Epileptics." *Tropical and Geographical Medicine* 42 (4): 359–64.

Mboussou, M., and L. Milebou-Aubusson. 1989. "Suicides and Attempted Suicides at the Jeanne Ebori Foundation, Libreville (Gabon)." *Medicina Tropical* 49 (3): 259–64.

Mkize, L. P., N. F. Nonkelela, and D. L. Mkize. 1998. "Prevalence of Depression in a University Population." *Curationis* 21 (3): 32–37.

Mofenson, L. M. 1999. "Short Course Zidovudine for Prevention of Perinatal Infection." *Lancet* 353: 766–67.

Mollica, R., K. McInnes, C. Poole, and S. Tor. 1998. "Dose-Effect Relationships of Trauma to Symptoms of Depression and Post-Traumatic Stress Disorder among Cambodian Survivors of Mass Violence." *British Journal of Psychiatry* 173: 482–88.

Mollica, R., K. McInnes, N. Sarajlic, J. Lavelle, I. Sarajlic, and M. P. Massagli. 1999. "Disability Associated with Psychiatric Co-Morbidity and Health Status in Bosnian Refugees Living in Croatia." *Journal of the American Medical Association* 282 (5): 433–39.

Molteno, G., C. D. Molteno, G. Finchilescu, and A. R. Dawes. 2001. "Behavioural and Emotional Problems in Children with Intellectual Disability Attending Special Schools in Cape Town, South Africa." Part 6. *Journal of Intellectual Disabilities Research* 45: 515–20.

Morrison, M. F., J. M. Petitto, T. Ten Have, D. R. Gettes, M. S. Chiappini, A. L. Weber, P. Brinker-Spence, R. M. Bauer, S. D. Douglas, and D. L. Evans. 2002. "Depressive and Anxiety Disorders in Women with HIV Infection." *American Journal of Psychiatry* 159: 789–96.

Mulugeta, E., M. Kassaye, and Y. Berhan. 1998. "Prevalence and Outcomes of Sexual Violence among High School Students." *Ethiopian Medical Journal* 36 (3): 167–74.

Muniu, E., M. N. Katsivo, L. W. Mwaura, and M. Amuyunzu. 1994. "Fatal Non-Transport Injuries in Nairobi, Kenya." *East African Medical Journal* 71 (6): 346–49.

Murray, C. J. L., and A. D. Lopez. 1996. *Global Health Statistics: A Compendium of Incidence, Prevalence, and Mortality Estimates for over 200 Conditions.* Cambridge, MA: Harvard School of Public Health.

———. 1997a. "Alternative Projections of Mortality and Disability by Cause, 1990–2020: Global Burden of Disease Study." *Lancet* 349: 1498–1504.

———. 1997b. "Global Mortality, Disability, and the Contribution of Risk Factors: Global Burden of Disease Study." *Lancet* 349: 1436–42.

Mzezewa, S., K. Jonsson, M. Aberg, and L. Salemark. 2000. "A Prospective Study of Suicidal Burns Admitted to the Harare Burns Unit." *Burns* 26 (5): 460–64.

Narayan, D. 2000. *Voices of the Poor: Can Anyone Hear Us?* London: Oxford University Press.

Narayan, D., R. Chambers, M. K. Shah, and P. Petesch. 2000. *Voices of the Poor: Crying Out for Change.* London: Oxford University Press.

Nemeroff, C. B., D. L. Musselman, and D. L. Evans. 1998. "Depression and Cardiac Disease." *Depression and Anxiety* 8 (Suppl. 1): 71–79.

Nhiwatiwa, S., V. Patel, and W. Acuda. 1998. "Predicting Post-Natal Mental Disorder with a Screening Questionnaire: A Prospective Cohort Study from Zimbabwe." *Journal of Epidemiology and Community Health* 52 (4): 262–66.

Njenga, F. 2000. "Depression in Kenyan Professional Women." *International Clinical Psychopharmacology* 15 (Suppl. 3): S35–36.

Nwosu, S. O., and W. O. Odesanmi. 2001. "Pattern of Suicides in Ile-Ife, Nigeria." *West African Journal of Medicine* 20 (3): 259–62.

Odejide, A. O., A. O. Williams, J. U. Ohaeri, and B. A. Ikuesan. 1986. "The Epidemiology of Deliberate Self-Harm: The Ibadan Experience." *British Journal of Psychiatry* 149: 734–37.

Oguleye, A. O., G. B. Nwaorgu, and H. Grandawa. 2002. "Corrosive Oesophagitis in Nigeria: Clinical Spectrums and Implications." *Tropical Doctor* 32 (2): 78–80.

Okulate, G. T. 2001. "Suicide Attempts in a Nigerian Military Setting." *East African Medical Journal* 78 (9): 493–96.

Orley, I., D. M. Blitt, and I. K. Wing. 1979. "Psychiatric Disorders in Two African Villages." *Archives of General Psychiatry* 36: 513–21.

Ormel, J., M. Von Korff, T. B. Ustun, S. Pini, A. Korten, and T. Oldehinkel. 1994. "Common Mental Disorders and Disability across Cultures. Results from the WHO Collaborative Study on Psychological Problems in General Health Care." *Journal of the American Medical Association* 272 (22): 1741–48.

Patel, V., R. Araya, M. de Lima, A. Ludermir, and C. Todd. 1999. "Women, Poverty and Common Mental Disorders in Four Restructuring Societies." *Social Science and Medicine* 49 (11): 1461–71.

Patel, V., F. Gwanzura, E. Simunyu, K. Lloyd, and A. Mann. 1995. "The Phenomenology and Explanatory Models of Common Mental Disorders: A Study in Primary Care in Harare, Zimbabwe." *Psychology and Medicine* 25 (6): 1191–99.

Perriens, J. H., M. Mussa, M. K. Luabeya, K. Kayembe, B. Kapita, C. Brown, P. Piot, and R. Janssen. 1992. "Neurological Complications of HIV-1-Seropositive Internal Medicine Inpatients in Kinshasa, Zaire." *Journal of the Acquired Immune Deficiency Syndrome* 5 (4): 333–40.

Rumble, S., L. Swartz, C. Parry, and M. Zwarenstein. 1996. "Prevalence of Psychiatric Morbidity in the Adult Population of a Rural South African VIllage." *Psychological Medicine* 26: 997–1007.

Rutter, M., and D. Quinton. 1984. "Parental Psychiatric Disorder: Effects on Children." *Psychological Medicine* 14 (4): 853–80.

Rwegellera, G. G., and C. C. Mambwe. 1977. "Psychiatric Status and the Disorders of Thyroid Function. 1. Prevalence of Goiter in a Group of Psychiatric Patients." *Medical Journal of Zambia* 11 (3): 78–83.

Sartorius N., A. Jablensky, A. Korten, G. Ernberg, M. Anker, J. E. Cooper, and R. Day. 1986. "Early Manifestations and First-Contact Incidence of Schizophrenia in Different Cultures. A Preliminary Report on the Initial Evaluation Phase of the WHO Collaborative Study on Determinants of Outcome of Severe Mental Disorders." *Psychological Medicine* 16 (4): 909–28.

Sartorius, N., T. B. Ustun, Y. Lecrubier, and H. U. Wittchen. 1996. "Depression Comorbid with Anxiety: Results from the WHO Study on Psychological Disorders in Primary Health Care." *British Journal of Psychiatry* 168 (Suppl. 30): 38–43.

Schier, E., T. Yecunnoamlack, and T. Tegegne. 1989. "Neuropsychiatric Syndromes in Childhood and Adolescence among Patients at a Neuropsychiatric Ambulatory Care and Pediatric Unit of a Teaching Hospital in Ethiopia" (in German). *Arztliche Jugendkunde* 80 (3): 140–46.

Schlebusch, L. 1985. "Self-Destructive Behaviour in Adolescents." *South African Medical Journal* 68 (11): 792–95.

Sebit, M. B. 1995. "Neuropsychiatric HIV-1 Infection Study: In Kenya and Zaire Cross-Sectional Phase I and II." *Central African Journal of Medicine* 41 (10): 315–22.

Setel, P. W., N. Unwin, K. G. M. M. Alberti, and Y. Hemed. 2000. "Cause-Specific Adult Mortality: Evidence from Community-Based Surveillance—Selected Sites, Tanzania, 1992–1998." *Morbidity and Mortality Weekly Report* 49: 416–19.

Spire, B., S. Duran, M. Souville, C. Leport, F. Raffi, J. P. Moatti, and APRO-CO Cohort Study Group. 2002. "Adherence to Highly Active

Antiretroviral Therapies (HAART) in HIV-Infected Patients: From a Predictive to a Dynamic Approach." *Social Science and Medicine* 54: 1481–96.

Stewart-Brown, S. 1998. "Emotional Well-Being and Its Relation to Health. Physical Disease May Well Result from Emotional Distress." *British Medical Journal* 317: 1608–9.

Strauss, P. R., C. A. Gagiano, P. H. J. J. van Rensburg, K. J. de Wet, and H. J. Strauss. 1995. "Identification of Depression in a Rural General Practice." *South African Medical Journal* 85 (8): 755–59.

Turner, B. J., C. Laine, L. Cosler, and W. W. Hauck. 2003. "Relationship of Gender, Depression, and Health Care Delivery with Antiretroviral Adherence in HIV-Infected Drug Users." *Journal of General Internal Medicine* 18: 248–57.

Ustun, T. B., J. L. Ayuso-Mateos, S. Chatterji, C. Mathers, and C. J. L. Murray. 2004. "Global Burden of Depressive Disorders in the Year 2000." *British Journal of Psychiatry* 184: 386–92.

Vaz, R. F., E. F. Mbajiorgu, and S. W. Acuda. 1998. "A Preliminary Study of Stress Levels among First Year Medical Students at the University of Zimbabwe." *Central African Journal of Medicine* 44 (9): 214–19.

Verrier-Jones, P., F. D. Pascoe, L. S. Gillis, and J. B. King. 1978. "The First 100 Patients in the Valkenberg Psychogeriatric Assessment Unit." *South African Medical Journal* 54 (3): 113–15.

Weiss, E. L., J. G. Longhurst, and C. M. Mazure. 1999. "Childhood Sexual Abuse as a Risk Factor for Depression in Women: Psychosocial and Neurobiological Correlates." *American Journal of Psychiatry* 156: 816–28.

WHO (World Health Organization). 1999a. *Facts and Figures about Suicide.* Geneva: WHO.

———. 1999b. *Global Status Report on Alcohol.* Geneva: WHO.

———. 2001. *Atlas: Country Profiles on Mental Health Resources.* Geneva: WHO.

———. 2002a. *World Health Report 2002—Reducing Risks, Promoting Healthy Life.* Geneva: WHO.

———. 2002b. *World Report on Violence.* Geneva: WHO.

———. 2005. *Mental Health Atlas: Revised Edition.* Geneva: WHO.

WHO, NEPAD (New Partnership for Africa's Development), and ACOSHED (African Council for Sustainable Health Development). 2005. *Taking the Human Resources for Health Agenda Forward at the Country Level in Africa.* Report on the Consultative Meeting, Brazzaville, Republic of Congo, July.

Wilk, C. M., and P. Bolton. 2002. "Local Perceptions of the Mental Health Effects of the Uganda Acquired Immunodeficiency Syndrome Epidemic." *Journal of Nervous and Mental Disease* 190 (6): 394–97.

Wilson, D. A., and P. J. Wormald. 1995. "Battery Acid—An Agent of Attempted Suicide in Black South Africans." *South African Medical Journal* 85 (6): 529–31.

World Bank. 2001. *Core Welfare Indicators Survey: Handbook and CD-ROM.* Africa Operational Quality and Knowledge Services. Washington, DC: World Bank.

Yegomawork, G., N. Deyessa, Y. Berhane, M. Ellsberg, M. Emmelin, M. Ashenafi, A. Alem, et al. 2003. "Women's Health and Life Events Study in Rural Ethiopia." Special issue, *Ethiopian Journal of Health Development* 17.

Zellweger, M. J., R. H. Osterwalder, W. Langewitz, and M. E. Pfisterer. 2004. "Coronary Artery Disease and Depression." *European Heart Journal* 25 (1): 3–9.

Chapter **23**

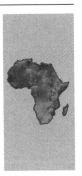

Neurological Disorders

Donald Silberberg and Elly Katabira

Neurological disorders are increasingly prevalent in Sub-Saharan Africa. The factors that are producing this increased burden include malnutrition, adverse perinatal conditions, malaria, the human immunodeficiency virus and the acquired immune deficiency syndrome (HIV/AIDS) and other causes of encephalitis and meningitis, demographic transitions, increased vehicular traffic, and persistent regional conflicts. Leading neurological disorders include cerebral palsy, mental retardation and other developmental disorders, epilepsy, peripheral neuropathy, stroke, and, increasingly, the nervous system complications of HIV/AIDS, trauma, and alcohol abuse. The disabling rather than fatal nature of many neurological disorders, the stigma associated with brain disorders, and the enormous difficulty in gathering epidemiologic data have resulted in their being underreported and neglected in Sub-Saharan Africa. This neglect represents an unfortunate paradox, since neurological (and psychiatric) disorders make up at least 25 percent of the global burden of disease and are responsible for an even greater proportion of persons living with disability.

Among the hundreds of specific disorders, some common and some uncommon, many are potentially preventable or treatable. For example, most developmental disorders and many strokes are preventable. Epilepsy, a common problem, is potentially treatable with currently available low-cost medications. Disorders such as HIV/AIDS and the dementia that often accompanies HIV infection are currently untreatable, but their prevalence can be drastically reduced with antiretroviral therapy intervention (Sacktor 2002). Although few epidemiological studies have been carried out in Sub-Saharan Africa, it is clear that some disorders of the nervous system are more prevalent in this World Bank region than elsewhere in the world. Examples of such overrepresentation include epilepsy, stroke in younger individuals, and neurological complications related to HIV infection.

Cultural and religious issues and beliefs are important in Sub-Saharan Africa. They influence the value placed by society on neurological health, the presentation of symptoms, illness behavior, access to services, pathways through care, the way individuals and families manage illness, the way the community responds to illness, the degree of acceptance and support—and stigma and discrimination—experienced by the person with neurological illness. Because of this, cultural and other contextual factors are important considerations in developing locally appropriate health care policies, programs, and services.

MEASUREMENT AND DATA SOURCES

One of the most challenging public health problems in Africa is data collection. Although community surveys date from nearly 100 years ago, it is only in the last four decades that these and other epidemiological methods have provided adequate diagnostic information based on standardized methods of assessment that permit the comparison of research from different locations and from different levels.

Major challenges to epidemiological research are the limited capacity of international classification systems for coding disorders and the noninclusion of neurological disorders as separate categories in health management information systems. Additionally, systems and instruments for epidemiological research of neurological disorders have not been standardized and validated for use in all areas of Sub-Saharan Africa. The existing capacity and resources to carry out comprehensive and scientifically sound community assessments are limited. Many studies have used hospital-based data, even though many of the patients do not have access to or knowledge of the availability of these services.

Further challenges to epidemiological research of neurological disorders in Sub-Saharan Africa are the often unreliable health facility records, the noninclusion of neurological disorders as separate items in the health management information system, and the paucity of cross-sectional studies. No disease surveillance system and no censuses, registries, or other administrative data include neurological disorders.

Few of the epidemiological studies of developmental disorders, Parkinson's disease, stroke, peripheral neuropathies, dementia, or other disorders carried out in Sub-Saharan Africa have been published in peer-reviewed journals. Similarly, few studies have been carried out that specifically quantify the neurological complications of HIV/AIDS in Sub-Saharan Africa in spite of the overwhelming burden of the disease in the region.

In 1998 South Africa began pilot operation of its National Non-Natural Mortality Surveillance System, a useful method of accumulating data. "Nonnatural mortality" refers to deaths from homicide, suicide, accidents, and undetermined causes. Evaluation carried out in 2001 found sensitivity to range from 65 to 95 percent for manner of death, with a positive predictive value that ranged from 74 to 80 percent for manner of death, and 71 to 82 percent for mechanism of death. The maintenance cost of this system is estimated to be R 8.00 (US$1.00) per case registered (Gill et al. 2001).

Another useful tool for accumulating data is period prevalence studies, such as those that can be registered at a single health facility. These are relatively inexpensive studies to conduct, and they are informative regarding outpatient or hospital use at a particular point of service (Birbeck 2001).

Newer epidemiological methods, such as capture-recapture methodology and log linear modeling, do not seem to have been introduced into investigations of neurologic disease in Sub-Saharan Africa at this time. The basic problems of data acquisition must first be solved, including designing valid screening instruments that will allow population-based screening. However, the International Clinical Epidemiology Network has fostered the development of clinical epidemiology research units in Cameroon, Ethiopia, and Uganda, each of which seeks to apply appropriate methods to their country's challenges.

A PubMed search carried out with the key words "neurological disorders," and "Sub-Saharan Africa" also confirmed that few epidemiological studies have been carried out and published in peer-reviewed journals. The best data sources are from South Africa and Nigeria and a few from Kenya and Zambia, whereas others, such as those from Uganda, are very old. Additional data are potentially available in unpublished surveys, particularly in Francophone Africa.

EPIDEMIOLOGY

In a unique study, Jelsma and colleagues (2002) conducted house-to-house screening visits of 10,839 residents in a "high density suburb" of Harare, Zimbabwe. Visits were followed up by medical examination and interview of those identified as having a functional limitation. The rate of disability and morbidity was 5.6 percent for the whole sample. Headaches, including migraine, were the most common problem. These were followed by back pain, hypertension, and osteoarthritis. HIV/AIDS was the fifth most common condition. Depression, based on responses to a screening tool, was evident in one-third of the subjects. Common activity limitations included difficulty with the performance of housework and with walking. HIV/AIDS resulted in the most severe activity limitation, in that cognitive functions were also affected.

Developmental Disorders

Few data exist on developmental disorders, other than such reports as that on the pediatric neurology clinic in The Gambia, which indicated that developmental delay, speech disorders, and learning difficulties were present among 128 children during a six-month period (Burton and Allen 2003). A three-year study of a child neurology clinic in Ibadan, Nigeria, found that cerebral palsy accounted for 16.2 percent of new referrals. Sixty-three percent of these cases were judged to have had potentially preventable causes, not including intracranial infections (Nottidge and Okogbo 1991). Anecdotal evidence suggests that the prevalence and incidence of mental retardation, cerebral palsy, and other serious developmental disturbances are much higher in Sub-Saharan Africa than in wealthy countries. Studies carried out in other low-income regions, which show rates up to 24 times higher than in similar studies carried out in Europe or North America, support this probability (Durkin 2002).

Epilepsy

Published figures for prevalence of epilepsy in Sub-Saharan Africa range from 2.2 to 58.0 per 1,000 people. Rates are higher in rural areas, reflecting the higher prevalence of predisposing factors, such as higher rates of birth trauma and repeated malaria or other parasitic infections. Hospital-based studies underestimate the prevalence of epilepsy at the community level by at least 30 percent. For comparison, the available community-based prevalence data on epilepsy for industrial countries range from 3.3 per 1,000 people in England to 6.6 per 1,000 in the United States (IOM 2001, p. 184).

Community-based surveys are the best way to evaluate the magnitude and distribution of epilepsy (IOM 2001 p. 186). As one of the few published examples, Osuntokun et al. (1978) used an instrument developed for the World Health Organization (WHO) by Bruce Schoenberg. At the University of Limoges, a questionnaire in French has been developed for the assessment of epilepsy prevalence in tropical countries (Preux 2000). However, the results of such surveys are influenced by local cultural factors. Where epilepsy is regarded as a social stigma, which is common, family members hide patients suffering from the condition from researchers. Because of the difficulties and the expense of implementing door-to-door surveys, increased attention is being focused on the use of key community informants to identify patients suffering from epilepsy. This strategy was applied successfully in an urban marginal and rural region in Kenya (Feksi et al. 1991). The WHO publication *Epilepsy in the African Region* provides a more complete account of epidemiological studies (WHO 2004).

Furthermore, epilepsy is a much more frequent cause of death in Sub-Saharan Africa than in wealthy countries. A community-based study done in Ethiopia revealed that 6.3 percent of people with epilepsy had died over a two-year period, and one-third in 20 years (Tekle-Haimanot, Forsgren, and Ekstedt 1997). In Africa, epilepsy mortality is primarily due to status epilepticus, falls, drowning, and burns in addition to the sudden death that is known throughout the world.

Infections

Few studies from Sub-Saharan Africa document the impact of the many infections on neurological morbidity and mortality. Bacterial meningitis, particularly that due to pneumococcal and meningococcal organisms, is still common. The neurological outcomes of these readily treatable infections depend on the availability of and access to health services, which differ tremendously across the region. The situation is made worse where populations are displaced by conflicts. Epidemics of meningococcal disease are particularly frequent in the "meningococcal belt," which extends from Guinea to the Sudan and northern Uganda and where, every 5 to 10 years, up to 100,000 cases occur. Viral encephalitis is on the increase, particularly where the prevalence of HIV infection is high as well.

The HIV virus enters the nervous system within hours of an individual's becoming infected. Acute inflammatory demyelinating polyneuropathy (Guillain-Barré syndrome), which can cause paralysis leading to death from respiratory failure, often accompanies this initial HIV infection and occurs with greater frequency in those infected with HIV/AIDS than in uninfected populations. As HIV/AIDS progresses, all the neurological complications appear to occur with the frequencies similar to those that were reported in wealthier countries prior to the advent of treatment with antiretroviral agents. Opportunistic infections of the nervous system occur in about 30 to 40 percent of those with AIDS (McArthur, Brew, and Nath 2005). An example is the common cryptococcal meningitis that often develops as immune suppression occurs. Other complications include toxoplasmosis; herpes zoster; central nervous system (CNS) lymphoma; several varieties of peripheral neuropathies; myelopathy, causing paraplegia; strokes; retinal infection, leading to blindness; and the dementia that develops in approximately 40 percent of those with AIDS. The fact that most infants and children who acquire HIV from their mothers develop cognitive delay, seizures, and opportunistic nervous system infections is barely recognized in most reviews.

As a result of the HIV pandemic in Sub-Saharan Africa, the neurological complications of HIV infection have become major, often overwhelming components of the overall health burden. These complications are among the most common, and often *the* most common neurologic disorders in a population. This is particularly true in East, central, and southern Africa. Opportunistic infections overwhelm many facilities, some of which have developed policies that permit only one hospital admission in a patient's lifetime. CNS lymphoma, a relatively uncommon tumor ordinarily, is now the most commonly found brain tumor in many regions. It is important to note that where highly active antiretroviral therapy has become available, the incidence of these complications among those with HIV has decreased significantly (Sacktor 2002).

Due to the widespread prevalence of (often unrecognized and untreated) sexually transmitted diseases, the neurological complications of syphilis remain common. These include meningovascular syphilis, causing strokes; tabes dorsalis, causing pain and paraparesis; and luetic encephalitis ("general paresis of the insane"), which is rapidly fatal if not treated. All these manifestations of infection with *Treponema pallidum* are preventable by treatment with antibiotics.

Malaria rivals AIDS for its impact on the nervous system. In addition to the hundreds of thousands of children who die each year from cerebral malaria, many more survive (often repeated attacks) and develop sequelae that have yet to be quantified. These include cognitive disorders and epilepsy. Similarly, tuberculous meningitis, and spinal tuberculosis (TB), leading to spinal cord compression and paraplegia (Pott's disease), are leading causes of death and disability. Additionally, in many regions leprosy continues to cause deforming peripheral neuropathy, and it may be becoming more common as the result of the redirection of resources in response to the HIV/AIDS epidemic.

Stroke

Stroke is a leading cause of death and disability in Sub-Saharan Africa. To date, most data on mortality have been hospital-based, although the majority of stroke deaths in the region are thought to occur at home (Kahn and Tollman 1999). More accurate measures of stroke mortality have

been attempted in urban and rural Tanzania (Walker et al. 2000). Among adults, 5.5 percent of deaths were attributed to cerebrovascular disease. The yearly age-adjusted rates per 100,000 people in the 15 to 64 age group averaged 49 per 100,000, four times the rates in England and Wales. In South Africa, stroke accounts for 8 to 10 percent of all reported deaths and 7.5 percent of deaths among people of prime working age, between 25 and 64 years old (Kahn and Tollman 1999). A prospective community survey in rural South Africa reported that stroke accounted for 25 percent of all noncommunicable disease, including in many younger individuals. Stroke was responsible for 5.5 percent of all deaths and 10.3 percent in those age 35 to 64 years. Stroke ranked second as the cause of death in those age 35 to 64 years, first in those age 55 to 74 years (11 percent of all deaths), and second among those age 75 and older (6 percent of all deaths) (Kahn and Tollman 1999). In a rural hospital in Zambia, stroke accounted for 9 percent of admissions, but used 14 percent of the intensive care unit's bed days (Birbeck 2001). The mortality following stroke was 50 percent, far higher than in wealthy countries, reflecting the lack of resources for early recognition and access to treatment.

Dementia

Available data indicate that the age-specific prevalence of Alzheimer's disease in Nigeria is similar to that among African Americans (Hendrie et al. 2001). However, age-related dementia becomes less common as HIV/AIDS lowers life expectancy. Those who live long enough to develop dementia are often regarded culturally as not sick and thus do not seek medical care. However, HIV/AIDS has made dementia a major issue because the associated dementia is common and often occurs in young people.

Movement Disorders

Parkinson's disease is known to occur in the region, but there is little documentation as to its prevalence and impact on morbidity and mortality. At the neurology clinic in Mulago Hospital, the teaching hospital for the Faculty of Medicine, Makerere University, Uganda, about two to three new cases are seen every month. However, most of the afflicted never seek medical care, particularly in the rural areas. Sydenham's chorea, now uncommon in wealthy countries, remains a common problem in Sub-Saharan Africa, due to the high rates of streptococcal infection and poor access to antibiotics. Additionally, the full spectrum of common movement disorders (such as essential tremor) and uncommon movement disorders (such as chorea gravidarum and focal dystonias) occur.

Headache

From the limited available studies in the region, headache is one of the most common neurological complaints encountered by health workers. Matuja (1991), at Muhimbili Medical Center, Dar es Salaam, Tanzania, found that recurrent headaches accounted for 20.6 percent of all new referrals to the adult neurology clinic over a period of two years. Thirty-four percent of the individuals had migraine, 27 percent had psychogenic (mostly anxiety and depression) disorders, and 13 percent had posttraumatic headache (Matuja 1991). Similarly, migraine accounted for 5.7 percent of all new patients seen in the child neurology clinic at Estate Specialist Hospital, in Kano, Nigeria (Okogbo 1991). Similarly, data from Zimbabwe indicated that headaches were the most common problem encountered in a large door-to-door survey (Jelsma et al. 2002). These prevalence rates for headache do not differ significantly from those in the United States and Europe.

Trauma

In some countries in Sub-Saharan Africa, trauma rivals infections and vascular disorders as the most important cause of neurological disease. Moreover, increasing motorized transportation, violence, and persistent armed conflicts in the region are rapidly changing the pattern of this trauma. Head trauma, if not immediately fatal, often leads to cognitive impairment or epilepsy or both. Spinal cord trauma often produces quadriparesis, paraparesis, or paralysis. In the absence of skilled rehabilitation services, the average life span following significant spinal cord injury is no more than several years.

ETIOLOGY AND DETERMINANTS

The major risk factors for neurological disorders can be classed as genetic factors; nutritional deficiencies; infection; exposure to environmental toxins; prenatal, perinatal, and neonatal factors; poverty; and trauma.

In Sub-Saharan Africa, by far the leading causes of neurological disorders are preventable. These include infections during pregnancy, such as syphilis and rubella; perinatal conditions, such as difficult, unassisted deliveries; and neonatal infections, including tetanus, meningitis, and septicemia. Preventable infections resulting in the extremely high under-five mortality in the region are often the cause of neurological sequelae for those that survive. The frequency and adequacy of care for epilepsy and cerebral palsy can be used as indicators of the available quality of the health care systems.

In children, febrile convulsions are reported in every African health structure as a major cause of seizures. Prevalent causes of fever are similar across the region and include malaria, pneumonia, and measles. Other infections, such as meningitis, encephalitis, and bacterial septicemia, may directly affect the brain and cause epilepsy. Other etiologies of epilepsy include such obvious causes as head injury, parasitic infestations of the nervous system (such as cysticercosis), congenital CNS abnormalities, tumors, and vascular and metabolic disorders.

A review of the neurological disorders seen at the pediatric neurology clinic of the University of Nigeria Teaching Hospital in Enugu revealed that perinatal problems, such as birth asphyxia, severe neonatal jaundice, and infections, were the most common etiological factors identified (Izuora and Iloeje 1989).

Studies from Côte d'Ivoire, Nigeria, and Zimbabwe found hypertension to be the main risk factor for both ischemic and hemorrhagic stroke (Matenga 1997; Walker 1994). Hypertension is an increasingly important public health problem in African countries, where it may affect up to 10 percent of the population and contributes to coronary heart disease, as well as to hemorrhagic and thrombotic stroke. The condition frequently goes unrecognized, however, in part because many African health care providers lack reliable equipment for measuring blood pressure (Birbeck 2000). In addition, the limited and erratic supply of and access to appropriate drugs for the management of hypertension contributes to the related high morbidity and mortality. Sickle-cell disease is a major cause of stroke among children and young adults in West, East, and central Africa, affecting at least 1 percent of those with sickle-cell disease per year. An analysis of 320 adult stroke patients in Durban, South Africa, revealed that HIV/AIDS, tuberculosis, cysticercosis, and syphilis were the most common causes of stroke in the young adult age groups. Additionally, emboli from streptococcal infection–induced cardiac disease (rheumatic heart disease) are a common cause of stroke in young adults.

CONSEQUENCES OF NEUROLOGICAL DISORDERS

Neurological disorders in Sub-Saharan Africa impose a significant burden on the family and community, as well as on the affected individual. Some disorders, such as epilepsy, are well recognized but are not socially and culturally acceptable. The enormous stigma attached to epilepsy often leads to the patient's being denied access to proper care. Lack of care then leads to severe complications, social isolation, and early death. Other disorders, such as dementia, paraplegia, and stroke, put undue stress on the caring family because institutional or community care support is limited or nonexistent. This stress leads to further neglect of the afflicted person and eventually his or her premature death. Protein-calorie and micronutrient malnutrition contribute to impaired cognitive development, which compromises the future productivity of a nation's workforce. Although the more complete epidemiology and cost analyses have yet to be done, there seems little doubt that neurological disorders impede economic development in many Sub-Saharan Africa countries.

RESOURCE ISSUES

Virtually all of the excess morbidity and mortality that occur as a consequence of neurological disorders in Sub-Saharan Africa result from scarcities of resources. Two major subsets of resource scarcities that are particularly important to neurological health and disease are the numbers of specifically trained health care workers, and the diagnostic (and therapeutic) resources available to them.

Human Resources

Countries in Sub-Saharan Africa do not have sufficient qualified staff in the clinical neurosciences (neurologists, neurosurgeons, psychiatrists). Except for South Africa, the mean ratios for countries that have these medical specialists are 1 neurologist for 1 million to 2.8 million people (versus 4 per 100,000 in Europe); 1 psychiatrist for 900,000 people (versus 9 per 100,000 in Europe); and 1 neurosurgeon for 2 million to 6 million people (versus 1 per 100,000 in Europe). Most of the clinical neuroscience services are located in the capital cities, often the largest urban areas, where the professionals also often lecture at the medical schools. Neurology patients often must travel long distances to consult with a doctor in the city.

Osuntokun (1975) noted that because of the gross shortage of "Western-trained" health personnel, Nigerians frequently turn to traditional native medicine and native herbalists (as do many in other countries in Sub-Saharan Africa). Although the training of these native doctors is arduous and lasts an average of 8 to 10 years, their shortcomings often interfere with administration of effective treatments in community clinics. These doctors are excellent psychotherapists and maintain good relationships with their patients. Yoruba native doctors recognize several classical neurological diseases, including epilepsy, cerebrovascular disease, fever and headache, migraine, and ataxic neuropathies. However, the scientific basis of their pharmacotherapeutics is for the moment mostly unknown. Their practice is thus partially based on the very large body of knowledge of herbal medicines in Africa that has yet to be explored scientifically.

The role of the traditional healer is sometimes problematic. People who would without hesitation go to their local health care center with a severe cough, fever, or burn may seek care for epilepsy through their local healer for years, never revealing their problem to the health care workers treating their other problems, and thus not receiving appropriate treatment.

In a personal communication, Gretchen Birbeck, an associate professor of neurology and epidemiology at Michigan State University, had this to say, based on her extensive experience in Zambia:

> It is important also to recognize that traditional healers may fail to recognize or refer urgent treatable conditions and that their therapies can have adverse effects. Children whose parents attribute their malaria-associated seizures to supernatural causes suffer from higher parasite counts and require longer lengths of hospital stays than their peers, likely associated with initially seeking care from local healers. Until traditional healers can become more connected to the biomedical healthcare system and/or the public becomes a great deal more educated, traditional healers will continue to care exclusively for patients who would benefit greatly from medications and treatments that are routinely available in most Sub-Saharan Africa hospitals.

Physicians are too scarce to provide routine outpatient care in most settings. The nurses and community health workers who are the frontline providers receive little or no training in how to diagnose and treat the common neurologic conditions that present to their clinic every day

(Birbeck and Munsat 2002). Their inability to respond to neurologic complaints reinforces the patients' inclination to seek care from traditional healers. In addition, as neurology has evolved into a subspecialty separate from general medicine, fewer generalists receive neurologic training. The adequate supply of physicians in wealthier countries has resulted in greater use of neurologic consultations. However, where neurologists are lacking, as in Sub-Saharan Africa, this segregation of neurology from general medicine leaves a vacuum. Because it may take many years to increase the number of neurologists, better training for primary care providers is essential.

Diagnostic Facilities: Instrumentation

The most important diagnostic measures are through interviews and by the usual clinical examination, looking for signs and symptoms of disturbed neurologic functions. This can be accomplished in any health structure. However, accurate diagnosis and management often requires diagnostic means that are usually found in secondary and tertiary health care facilities. In Sub-Saharan Africa, with the exception of South Africa, the specialized diagnostic tools for brain disorders, necessary for such purposes, consist of 79 EEG machines, 65 CT scanners, and 9 MRIs. In contrast, South Africa has 60 EEG machines, 214 CT scanners, and 46 MRIs (WHO 2004).

To compound the problem, this equipment is often badly maintained or out of order. Further, most of the patients referred to capital city hospitals cannot afford the price and therefore cannot benefit from the technological progress.

The few neurological surgeons practicing in Sub-Saharan Africa not only face these shortages in diagnostic equipment but must cope with a scarcity of needed surgical instruments as well as with a general paucity of the institutional resources needed to carry out major procedures successfully.

INTERVENTIONS: WHAT HAS WORKED?

Despite the problems enumerated above, many avenues are open to reduce the impact of neurological disorders in Sub-Saharan Africa. The potential advances start with prevention, and proceed to treatment and rehabilitation.

Primary Prevention

Prevention is critical in reducing the incidence of brain disorders. Impairment caused by these disorders is often irreversible. On ethical grounds alone, prevention is always preferable to treatment or rehabilitation. In most instances prevention is also more cost-effective than treatment. Many potentially catastrophic disorders are now preventable. Preventive measures include immunization against tetanus, tuberculosis, measles, rubella, and polio, all of which produce neurological dysfunction as their primary route of attack, or as a very common complication; early and effective management of childhood fevers to prevent febrile convulsions; and the use of zinc, folic acid, and iron supplementation and fortification to facilitate normal brain development. Prevention of HIV transmission through effective health education strategies and programs to prevent mother to child transmission are critical. Short-course antiretroviral prophylaxis regimens are becoming widely used in such programs in Sub-Saharan Africa and, in conjunction with supplemental feeding, are likely to significantly reduce HIV transmission. The situation will improve still further when antiretroviral therapy becomes universal in the region. Safe motherhood initiatives also greatly reduce the impact of prenatal and perinatal risk factors.

The potential for prevention of stroke is illustrated by the fact that in wealthy countries the incidence of stroke has been reduced by 25 to 40 percent, largely because of early recognition and treatment of hypertension and the reduction in tobacco use (Rothwell et al. 2004; Whisnant 1984). Other preventive strategies include increased exercise, adopting healthy eating habits, and regular monitoring of cholesterol. Prevention programs, although highly cost-effective, have not been undertaken in Sub-Saharan Africa.

Treatment

The WHO recommends phenobarbital as the first-line drug for the treatment of partial and generalized tonicoclonic epilepsy in developing countries. The use of this old and simple drug is encouraged because its efficacy for a wide range of seizure types and its low cost make it suitable for use in primary health care in developing countries. The majority of affected individuals can be treated successfully with phenobarbital at a cost of about US$5 per year, thereby avoiding disability and the risk of premature death. Phenytoin, which may be more effective for some individuals, has few side effects and cost US$20.59 in Sub-Saharan Africa in 2000 (WHO 2001). The publication *Epilepsy in the African Region* (WHO 2004) provides a more complete account of the availability and cost of treatment, by country.

The current global effort to make antiretroviral drugs readily available and affordable to a much larger infected population in the region will reduce morbidity and mortality related to neurological complications due to HIV/AIDS.

A FRAMEWORK FOR RESEARCH

Although disability-adjusted life years (DALYs) have been computed for some of the specific causes of developmental disability, such as meningitis and iodine deficiency,[1] these figures do not convey the full proportion of cases within a given category of disorder that result in early and lifelong disability or death (see IOM 2001). DALY estimates are not currently available for developmental disability as a whole. What is needed before useful DALY or other measures of impact can be calculated for developmental disability is accurate and up-to-date information from Sub-Saharan Africa countries on the prevalence and impacts of long-term functional limitations originating early in life, as a result of both known and unknown causes.

Stigmatization of those with epilepsy, and often their families, is widespread. Some cultural beliefs, such as the fear that epilepsy is contagious and that the individual is possessed of demons, confound epidemiological studies, prevent treatment, and lead to personal and economic disaster for many affected individuals and their families. Because stigma and other cultural beliefs are locally grounded, they require local study in order to develop ways in which to deal with them constructively.

The full picture of the epidemiology of epilepsy remains sketchy. In addition to descriptive studies, analytical research is needed to ascertain specific risk factors for the development of the disease with an emphasis on its relation to infectious disorders, such as pneumonia, meningitis, and tetanus; its links to the common causes of under-five and neonatal mortality; and its links to birth trauma. Environmental and genetic causes should be explored in various geographic locations and among different ethnic groups. Information gathered through such efforts would be critical to the formulation of effective preventive strategies.

Most econometric studies of epilepsy in developing countries await implementation. Cost-of-illness, cost-effectiveness, cost-minimization, and cost-benefit analyses should be undertaken to provide government officials and funding agencies with the necessary economic perspective. Furthermore, quality of life should be measured for epileptic patients receiving treatment in an economically constrained environment. Socioeconomic determinants of the outcome measures that could best reflect optimal care for epilepsy patients should be identified.

Most of the same observations can be made about stroke prevention and treatment, largely unrecognized major problems in Sub-Saharan Africa, and the many other disorders that affect the nervous system. For example, the direct and indirect costs of stroke are enormous, including loss of wage-earning capacity and the need for the family's provision of care for survivors.

Evaluations of cost-effectiveness of neurological interventions have not been extensively carried out in the region. They depend on the actual costs of specific drugs and other treatments, which vary among countries and will decrease as newer drugs come off patent.

POLICY ISSUES

Among brain disorders, epilepsy stands out, not only because of its high prevalence and incidence rates and the potential for successful treatment, but because of the myths and beliefs attached to it in various cultures and the resulting impact on the individual, family, and the community. Epilepsy commonly attacks children and young adults in the most productive years of their lives and frequently leads to unemployment, which confounds not only the problems of the afflicted but often the family that relies on their financial support.

To implement effective programs for the community-level detection and treatment of patients with epilepsy, governments and health authorities of developing countries must first issue clear policies articulating measures for the identification and treatment of patients with epilepsy. Essential components of any strategy are a continuous drug supply and means of distribution, prevention programs, social programs and stigma mitigation strategies to increase employment and improve the general welfare of individuals suffering from the disease, training of health care personnel, and methods for surveillance and routine data collection.

Increasing the clinical and research professional capacity in developing countries is key to developing sustainable, locally appropriate programs. Approaches to addressing these deficits include the following:

- Capacity building through training via on-site education, exchange programs, and distance learning using modern information technology

- Development of local networks that link centers with expertise to their surrounding communities
- Development of regional networks of centers with expertise
- Development of educational programs to enable primary care health workers to recognize, and when appropriate, treat brain disorders
- Introduction of locally relevant basic, clinical, and health care policy research that will lead countries to choose to increase capacity.

Clinical neuroscientists should be part of the teams that address the issues of the health care systems in Sub-Saharan Africa, so as to be certain that the prevention, recognition, treatment, and rehabilitation of brain disorders are adequately addressed.

NOTE

1. The most recent DALY figures in low- and middle-income countries for risk factors for neurological disorders discussed in this chapter include HIV/AIDS, 5.5 percent; polio, 0 percent; measles, 2.4 percent; tetanus, 1.0 percent; meningitis, 0.4 percent; malaria, 3.1 percent; Japanese encephalitis, 0 percent; trachoma, 0.1 percent; protein-energy malnutrition, 1.2 percent; iodine deficiency, 0.1 percent; Vitamin A deficiency, 0.2 percent; anemias, 1.9 percent; road traffic accidents, 2.7 percent; homicide and violence, 1.6 percent; war, 1.7 percent.

REFERENCES

Birbeck, G. 2000. "Barriers to Care for Patients with Neurologic Disease in Rural Zambia." *Archives of Neurology* 57 (3): 414–17.

———. 2001. "Neurologic Disease in a Rural Zambian Hospital." *Tropical Doctor* 31: 82–86.

Birbeck, G., and T. Munsat. 2002. "Neurologic Services in Sub-Saharan Africa: A Case Study among Zambian Primary Healthcare Workers." *Journal of the Neurological Sciences* 200: 75–78.

Burton, K. J., and S. Allen. 2003. "A Review of Neurological Disorders Presenting at a Paediatric Neurology Clinic and Response to Anticonvulsant Therapy in Gambian Children." *Annals of Tropical Paediatrics: International Child Health* 23 (2): 139–43.

Durkin, M. 2002. "The Epidemiology of Developmental Disabilities in Low-Income Countries." *Mental Retardation and Developmental Disabilities Research Reviews* 8: 206–11.

Feksi, A., J. Kaamugisha, J. Sander, S. Gatiti, and S. Shorvon. 1991. "Comprehensive Primary Health Care Antiepileptic Drug Treatment Programme in Rural and Semi-Urban Kenya." *Lancet* 337: 406–9.

Gill, G., B. Scott, N. Beeching, D. Wilkinson, and A. Ismail. 2001. "Enumeration of Non-Communicable Disease in Rural South Africa by Electronic Data Linkage and Capture-Recapture Techniques." *Tropical Medicine and International Health* 6: 435–41.

Hendrie, H. C., A. Ogunnii, K. S. Hall, O. Baiyewu, F. W. Unverzagt, O. Gureje, S. Gao, et al. 2001. "The Incidence of Dementia and AD in Two Communities: Yoruba Residing in Ibadan, Nigeria, and African Americans Residing in Indianapolis, USA." *Journal of the American Medical Association* 285: 739–47.

IOM (Institute of Medicine). 2001. *Neurological, Psychiatric, and Developmental Disorders: Meeting the Challenges in the Developing World*. Report. Washington, DC: Academy Press.

Izuora, G. I., and S. O. Iloeje. 1989. "A Review of the Neurological Disorders Seen at the Paediatric Neurology Clinic of the University of Nigeria Teaching Hospital, Enugu." *Annals of Tropical Paediatrics* 9 (4): 185–90.

Jelsma, J., J. Mielke, G. Powell, W. De Weerdt, and P. De Cock. 2002. "Disability in an Urban Black Community in Zimbabwe." *Disability and Rehabilitation* 24 (16): 851–59.

Kahn, K., and S. Tollman. 1999. "Stroke in Rural South Africa—Contributing to the Little Known about a Big Problem." *South African Medical Journal* 89 (1): 63–65.

Matenga, J. 1997. "Stroke Incidence Rates among Black Residents of Harare—A Prospective Community-Based Study." *South African Medical Journal* 87: 606–9.

Matuja, W. B. 1991. "Headache: Patterns and Features as Experienced in a Neurology Clinic in Tanzania." *East African Medical Journal* 68 (12): 935–43.

McArthur, J., B. Brew, and A. Nath. 2005. "Neurological Complications of HIV Infection." *Lancet Neurology* 4: 543–55.

Nottidge, V. A., and M. E. Okogbo. 1991. "Cerebral Palsy in Ibadan, Nigeria." *Developmental Medicine Child Neurology* 33: 241–45.

Okogbo, M. E. 1991. "Migraine in Nigerian Children—A Study of 51 Patients." *Headache* 31 (10): 673–76.

Osuntokun, B. 1975. "The Traditional Basis of Neuropsychiatric Practice among the Yorubas of Nigeria," *Tropical Geographic Medicine* 27: 422–30.

Osuntokun, B. O. 1978. "Epilepsy in Africa. Epidemiology of Epilepsy in Developing Countries in Africa." *Tropical Geographic Medicine* 30: 23–32.

Preux, P. M. 2000. "Questionnaire des investigations de l'épilepsie dans les pays tropicaux." *Bulletin Société Pathologique Exotique* 93: 276–78.

Rothwell, P., A. Coull, M. Giles, S. Howard, L. Silver, L. Bull, S. Gutnikov, et al. 2004. "Change in Stroke Incidence, Mortality, Case-Fatality, Severity, and Risk Factors in Oxfordshire, UK from 1981 to 2004 (Oxford Vascular Study)." *Lancet* 363: 1925–33.

Tekle-Haimanot, R., L. Forsgren, and J. Ekstedt. 1997. "Incidence of Epilepsy in Rural Central Ethiopia." *Epilepsia* 38: 541–46.

Sacktor, N. 2002. "The Epidemiology of Human Immunodeficiency Virus-Associated Neurological Disease in the Era of Highly Active Antiretroviral Therapy." *Journal of Neurovirology* 8 (Suppl. 2):115–21.

Walker, R. 1994. "Hypertension and Stroke in Sub-Saharan Africa." *Transactions of the Royal Society of Tropical Medicine and Hygiene* 88: 609–11.

Walker, R. W., D. G. McLarty, H. M. Kitange, D. Whiting, G. Masuki, D. M. Mtasiwa, H. Machibya, N. Unwin, and K. G. Alberti. 2000. "Stroke Mortality in Urban and Rural Tanzania-Adult Morbidity and Mortality Project." *Lancet* 355: 1684–87.

Whisnant, J. P. 1984. "The Decline of Stroke." *Stroke* 15: 160–68.

WHO (World Health Organization). 2001. *Atlas Country Profiles on Mental Health Resources*. Geneva: WHO. http://www.who.int/mental_health/management/epilepsy_in_African-region.pdf.

———. 2004. *Epilepsy in the African Region*. Geneva: WHO.

Chapter **24**

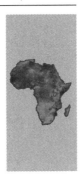

Violence and Injuries

Brett Bowman, Mohamed Seedat, Norman Duncan, and Olive Kobusingye

Historically, injuries have been understood as inescapable realities of everyday life. Increasingly, the timely and accurate collection and analysis of data in various parts of the world has encouraged a revision of these assumptions. Careful scrutiny of such data has revealed that both intentional and unintentional injuries are preventable and in many respects subject to elements of control.

An injury may be defined as "the physical damage that results when a human body is suddenly or briefly subjected to intolerable levels of energy" (Holder et al. 2001, 5). Injuries are traditionally grouped according to two broad categories: intentional and unintentional. Conventionally, intentional injuries are comprised of interpersonal violence (spousal abuse, child abuse, other assaults), self-inflicted injuries (attempted and completed suicides), as well as collective violence and war-related injuries. Motor vehicle injuries, burns, falls, drownings, and other injury classifications in which intentionality is understood to be absent constitute the broad unintentional injuries category. Thus, whereas intentional injuries are associated with violence, as defined by the World Health Organization (WHO), unintentional injuries are not. Such a distinction may be valuable for conceptual

and analytical clarity, but recent evidence points to a cluster of shared risks across intentional and unintentional injuries. Furthermore, intentionality cannot always be ascertained in particular circumstances, and violence may indirectly contribute to the prevalence of unintentional injuries (Berger and Mohan 1996). The "intentionality divide" is thus established as a useful concept for injury prevention programs, but risk factors appear porous across it.

Whatever the conceptual ambiguities may be, the WHO estimates that injuries constitute 16 percent of the global burden of disease (WHO 2002a). This translates into 5.8 million injury-related deaths at a rate of 97.9 per 100,000 worldwide. Injuries further account for between 10 and 30 percent of all hospital admissions and render at least 78 million people disabled each year (Berger and Mohan 1996). In 1998, unintentional injuries accounted for just under 3.5 million deaths worldwide (WHO 2000b). The burden resulting from unintentional injuries tends to be higher in low- to middle-income countries (LMICs) and communities. For instance, 87.9 percent of all road traffic deaths, and 88.3 percent of lost disability-adjusted life years (DALYs) were from LMICs (Mathers et al. 2001).

Despite the heavy burden from the human immunodeficiency virus and the acquired immune deficiency syndrome (HIV/AIDS), malaria, and other infectious diseases, injuries were still responsible for 19.93 percent of all deaths of those between the ages of 15 and 59 years, and for nearly one in every four deaths of those between 15 and 29 years. Most of these deaths resulted from road traffic injuries, wars, and interpersonal violence. According to the WHO (2002a), road traffic injuries, war, and homicide, respectively, were the 10th, 11th, and 14th leading causes of mortality in Africa during 2000.

In the year 2000, an estimated 1.6 million people died from various forms of violence (WHO 2002a). Although violence manifests as a worldwide public health concern, the epidemiology of violence indicates that the majority of violent deaths occur in LMICs. Less than 10 percent of all violence-related deaths occurred in high-income countries (HICs) in 2000 (WHO 2002a). The WHO (2002a, 5) defines violence as "the intentional use of physical force or power, threatened or actual, against oneself, another person, or against a group or community, that either results in or has a high likelihood of resulting in injury, death, psychological harm, maldevelopment or deprivation."

This chapter covers the incidence, prevalence, and magnitude of intentional (violent) and unintentional mortality resulting from injuries at the global and continental (African) levels. The injury profiles of South Africa and Uganda are examined to demonstrate the merits of establishing a country-level injury surveillance system. The chapter also includes an overview of the risk factors and determinants that are associated with intentional and unintentional injuries resulting in mortality in Africa. In conclusion, generic recommendations are listed for the control, prevention, and elimination of injuries and violence in Africa, with a view to encouraging injury control and safety promotion practice and policy.

DATA SOURCES

The global, regional, and national burden of nonfatal injury is exceedingly difficult to measure. Perhaps the most reliable indicators of the magnitude of violence and injury are national mortality data sets. The mandatory recording and certification of deaths in most countries renders mortality information an adequate source from which to calculate the frequency and prevalence of violence and injuries within national and global contexts. Despite the various obstacles

(Smith and Barss 1991) to the effective execution of this mandatory recording and the poor or absent record keeping among most vulnerable populations and communities, such as refugees, displaced persons, and communities afflicted by civil and armed conflict, national mortality data sets make for sound starting points from which to describe the prevalence and magnitude of injury in Africa. These figures, however, represent the tip of the injury iceberg, because although nonfatal injuries are estimated to exceed the global fatal injury profile by as much as 20 times (WHO 2002a), surveillance systems for capturing and reporting nonfatal injury are far less developed than those recording fatal injury (WHO 2002a). Most of the data on injury are acquired from surveys and specialized studies within relatively limited population groups. These studies provide a patchwork picture of the injury profile of Africa. The African injury profile provided here is thus made up of a full supplement of smaller studies extracted from the literature that complement the Africa-specific data subsets gleaned from information provided by the WHO.

INTENTIONAL INJURIES

Intentional injuries (violence) resulted in the deaths of some 311,000 people in Africa in the year 2000. This translates into a rate of 60.9 deaths per 100,000 people in Africa as a direct result of intentional injury alone. This figure dwarfs the unintentional injury mortality rates of both the WHO European and American regions with rates of 32.0 (WHO 2002a) and 27.7 unintentional injury deaths per 100,000 people, respectively. As indicated earlier, morbidity and disability due to intentional injury have a prevalence that exceeds mortality by at least 20 times. Intentional injuries therefore resulted in the disability or incapacitation of at least 6.2 million people on the African continent in the year 2000. Data collected and analyzed in some selected African states indicate the dire burden that injury exerts on these countries. In Zimbabwe, injuries were reported to account for 15 percent of all deaths for the year 1988 (Zwi et al. 1993). Survey data suggest that the injury contribution to mortality is as significant in both Ghana and Kenya (Forjuoh, Zwi, and Romer 1996).

Homicide

According to the WHO (2002a) over half a million (520,000) people died as a direct result of homicide at a rate of 8.8 per 100,000 in the year 2000. More than three-quarters

(77 percent) of these victims were male (WHO 2002a). Globally, the highest levels of homicide occurred among males 15 to 29 years old, closely followed by those 30 to 44 years old. The gender disparity in the worldwide distribution of homicide is most apparent through a rate comparison. For every female victim of homicide, 3.4 males are killed per 100,000 people globally. Conversely, more women than men are the victims of intimate partner violence, and women are more likely than men to die from such violence (NCIPC 2003). Homicide rates vary according to region and income levels (WHO 2002a). Recent results from the South African National Injury Mortality Surveillance System (NIMSS) indicate that homicide contributed 36 percent to all nonnatural injury deaths in that country in 2000 (Burrows et al. 2001) and that homicide continues to be the leading cause of premature death among South African males (Bowley, Parmar, and Boffard 2004).

Suicide

Suicide was the cause of death for an estimated 815,000 people worldwide in 2000 (WHO 2002a). The age-adjusted rate of 14.5 per 100,000 attests to the global magnitude of self-directed violence. Suicide among males is more frequent than among females, with over 60 percent of all suicides being male (WHO 2002a). An analysis of African and global suicide reveals that there is a proportionate increase in suicide with age, suicide reaching its peak among individuals 60 years of age or older. In this age cohort, male suicide rates are twice those of females. Suicide is most pronounced in the European, Southeast Asian, and Western Pacific regions of the WHO database coverage, where suicide rates are 19.1 per 100,000, 12.0 per 100,000, and 20.8 per 100,000, respectively. The suicide rate for African males in 2000 was 6.7 per 100,000, whereas the rate for females was 3.1 per 100,000. Africa appears to be the least frequently represented region in studies of suicide, but a number of national, regional, and citywide comparative studies do serve to provide a (limited) profile of the African suicide injury burden (Burrows et al. 2003; Meel 2003; Schlebusch and Bosch 2000).

War-Related Injury

The number of armed conflicts worldwide has grown exponentially over the past century. In the 1950s there were no more than 20 armed conflicts in progress across the globe. This number rose to 50 in the late 1980s and doubled to 100 armed conflicts worldwide during the 1990s (Stohl 2002).

Recent studies estimate that 310,000 people died as a direct result of injury incurred during warfare in 2000 (WHO 2002a). Injuries resulting from collective violence have been concentrated in Sub-Saharan Africa, Latin America, and the Caribbean (Jansson and Svanstrom 1999). The highest rates of these wartime injuries occurred in Africa, where war-related deaths numbered 32 per 100,000 people. Africa thus contributed 167,000, or 53.8 percent, of war-related injury mortality to the WHO injury data in 2000. Colonial and postcolonial Africa has been an epicenter for collective violence over the last 100 years. Indeed, civil strife and political instability have characterized the continent throughout its modern history. Moreover, the wars in Africa have tended to have increasingly long durations. The increased sophistication of weaponry has changed the nature of global conflicts. Examples of wars on the African continent are numerous. The WHO has estimated that the war between Ethiopia and Eritrea toward the concluding years of the twentieth century resulted in the deaths of tens of thousands of people. Besides the obviously direct mortality consequences for African states, wars undermine health and political infrastructures, indirectly resulting in many more deaths from outbreaks of communicable disease (WHO 2002a).

Many injury studies in the literature focus on the injury consequences of African war on children (Cliff and Noormohamed 1993; Stohl 2002). Others concentrate on the direct and indirect health outcomes of war for the continent in general (Elliot 2000; Elliot and Harris 2001; Marysse 2003). Although the bulk of lives lost to war injuries in Africa have resulted from armed conflicts in the Democratic Republic of Congo (Marysse 2003), Liberia, and Rwanda, the legacy of war continues to contribute to African mortality through, for example, the detonation of redundant landmines in Mozambique (Elliot 2000; Elliot and Harris 2001). The indirect war-mortality figures are equally as devastating as the casualties resulting from direct combat. Estimates of the indirect war-mortality figures vary; some studies estimate 2.5 million Congolese deaths as an indirect consequence of the civil strife that characterized the Democratic Republic of Congo from 1998 to 2003 (Marysse 2003).

UNINTENTIONAL INJURIES

The magnitude, prevalence, and severity of unintentional injury mortality (bar deaths resulting from natural disasters) are often underpublicized. Such mortality imposes, however, a significant burden on global and African health systems.

Traffic-Related Fatal Injuries

According to the WHO (Peden, McGee, and Sharma 2002), the overwhelming majority (90 percent) of all fatal road traffic injuries (RTIs) occurred in LMICs in 2000. In that year 1.26 million people across the globe died as a direct result of these injuries. This figure translates into a rate of 20.8 people dying from RTIs per 100,000 worldwide. Again, males are at higher risk of dying in this manner than their female counterparts. For every female traffic-related death, there are at least three male victims (Peden, McGee, and Sharma 2002). Globally, males in Africa have the second highest RTI fatality rate of 35.8 per 100,000, superseded only by the male RTI fatality rate of 42.4 per 100,000 in Southeast Asia. Worldwide, over 50 percent of all fatal RTIs occur among young adults between the ages of 15 and 44 years. This trend is replicated in Africa (Peden, McGee, and Sharma 2002).

A study focused on describing the prevalence and magnitude of RTI fatalities in Kenya (Odero, Khayesi, and Heda 2003) reported that the country has one of the highest road fatality rates in relation to vehicle ownership in the world, and a number of South African studies (De Wet 1993; Peltzer 2003; Venter 1998) have confirmed the significant contribution of RTIs to the country's nonnatural mortality burden. A recent injury epidemiological study conducted in Tanzania again revealed RTIs to be the leading cause of injury mortality in the areas of Dar es Salaam, Hai, and Morogoro (Moshiro et al. 2000). A study comparing transport-related injuries in urban and rural settings in Ghana found that the "nature of transport injury in both urban and rural areas is fundamentally different from that in developed countries" (Mock, Forjuoh, and Rivara 1999, 367). This difference is most pronounced in the contribution of minibus taxis and other public transport vehicle crashes and motor vehicle crashes involving pedestrians (Mock, Forjuoh, and Rivara 1999) to transport-related injuries in Ghana.

Burns, Falls, and Drowning

Fire-related burn injuries resulted in the death of some 238,000 people in 2000 (Peden, McGee, and Sharma 2002). Ninety-five percent of these occurred in LMICs. Africa had the second highest rate of fatal burn injuries in that year. Most notably, fire-related burns are the only cause of injury

in which global female rates of death outnumber those of men. This is, however, not the case in Africa, where males are more frequently the victims of burn fatalities. Young children and the elderly are the most vulnerable to burn injuries. This seems to be the case in all forms of burn mortality in particular African countries. A study conducted in Tanzania (Mbembati, Maseru, and Leshabari 2002) found that children younger than 15 years constitute a particularly vulnerable group for domestic burn injuries. Children in the same age cohort have been identified as especially vulnerable to burn injuries in South Africa (Lerel 1994). Forjuoh (1996) confirmed that children were a vulnerable unintentional (and in 5.4 percent of cases, intentional) burns cohort in the Ashanti region of Ghana. The most frequently represented external causes of the initial epidemiological investigation (Forjuoh 1995) included scalds (44 percent), contact with hot objects (30 percent), and flames (20 percent).

Falls accounted for more than 280,000 deaths globally in the year 2000 (Peden, McGee, and Sharma 2002). Almost a quarter of all falls occurred in high-income WHO regions. Globally, females over 70 years of age constitute the most vulnerable group to fall fatalities. This is particularly pronounced in Africa, where female fall fatalities in the age group 80 years and older are approximately twice that of males.

Deaths due to drowning are almost exclusively an injury problem of LMICs. Ninety-seven percent of all drownings worldwide occur in LMICs, and thus Africa, where the drowning mortality rate is 113.1 per 100,000 people (Peden and McGee 2003), has been identified as a region at risk for drownings. Males in Africa have the highest drowning mortality rates in the world with a drowning rate of 19.2 per 100,000 population. Children are unquestionably most at risk for death from drowning; more than 50 percent of all global drowning mortalities occur in children up to 14 years old. This trend is emphasized in Africa, where the highest rate of drowning fatalities (18.9 per 100,000) occurs among children between zero and four years (Peden, McGee, and Sharma 2002).

THE EXPERIENCES OF SOUTH AFRICA AND UGANDA

Both South Africa and Uganda are countries that can provide examples of the benefits of developing sound injury measurement systems. Such systems are aimed at establishing or implementing African context-specific "best-practices" for the prevention of injury and can be of use in the various African states. According to collated international data, South Africa contributes significantly to the burden of injury in Africa. A sound South African injury mortality surveillance system could, however, bias the injury-mortality contribution of the country to the continent. Nonetheless, a socioeconomic profile that describes significant disparities between rich and poor measured by a Gini coefficient of 0.58 (Nattrass and Seekings 2001) and a complex political history make South Africa a good country to analyze as an injury control and prevention case example. The South African NIMSS, which captures approximately 34 percent of all nonnatural deaths nationally, reported 18,876 people to have died as a direct result of injuries in 2000 (Matzopoulos 2002). Homicide was the leading manner of death (44.5 percent), followed by transport-related fatalities (34.5 percent) and suicide (9.4 percent). Figures extracted from the 2001 NIMSS annual report reveal no significant decrease in the magnitude and prevalence of mortality due to injury in South Africa (Matzopoulos 2002). Again these figures represent the tip of the injury iceberg, as they do not describe the preponderant morbidity prevalence of the country.

The NIMSS statistics to a large extent reflect the gender trends in international injury statistics, indicating that in South Africa males are more likely than females to be the victims of nonnatural deaths. Indeed, it would appear that the gender divide in terms of injury prevalence is even more pronounced in South Africa than internationally. Specifically, the NIMSS statistics indicate that, in the cities participating in the NIMSS, 80 percent of all victims of non-natural deaths are males (Donson and Van Niekerk 2002). These statistics also indicate that during 2001, males accounted for 82.4 percent of all suicide cases.

In the South African cities of Pretoria, Durban, Cape Town, and East London, where injury-mortality surveillance systems provide full coverage, injury rates indicate the dire magnitude of injury as a disease burden. Pretoria, the capital city of South Africa and home to a population of 2,043,500 (Sukhai and Matzopoulos 2002) had an all-injury death crude rate of 136 per 100,000 in 2001. Although this figure pales in comparison to injury death estimates in Kampala (the capital city of Uganda), the rate attests to the prevalence of injury resulting in death in one of South Africa's cities with the most resources. Such figures continue to call attention to the burden of injury in other South African cities, where crude injury mortality rates are equally disturbing. In the west coast city of Cape Town, the tourist hotspot of South Africa, the all-injury mortality rate of 170 per 100,000 is a serious source of concern. The injury death rate of 160 per 100,000 in Durban further emphasizes the burden of injury on another one of South Africa's coastal cities. In the southwest city of East London, the rate of injury death was 203 per 100,000 for the year 2000.

Transport-related deaths and homicide collectively account for the majority of deaths in the urban centers of South Africa (Sukhai and Matzopoulos 2002); East London showed a homicide rate of 100 per 100,000 in 2001 and Cape Town revealed a transport-related fatality crude rate of 42 per 100,000 in 2001 (Sukhai and Matzopoulos 2002). Although nontransport unintentional injury deaths are overshadowed by violent and transport-related causes of death in South Africa, their contribution to the injury burden of the country is significant; in 2001 alone, East London had an unintentional, nontransport-related injury mortality rate as high as 27 per 100,000.

Focusing on cities that yield data like those presented above have proved of use in injury prevention and safety promotion in South Africa for many reasons. Census data that yield accurate population denominators for calculating rates of injury in most cities in South Africa provide decision and policy makers with quality information for mobilizing resources toward the prioritization of injury prevention and safety promotion at both national and local levels of government. The experience of South Africa has indicated that although national data collection is imperative for the development of national injury profiling, a city focus appears to expedite data collection, analyses, and delivery to decision makers aiming at preventive action. Injury prevention practitioners have therefore reversed earlier attempts to secure full coverage at the national level and refigured their targets to data-driven prevention in cities. Ultimately, injury prevention researchers and practitioners believe that illustrating the utility of injury surveillance at the city level will inform the prioritization of a national injury prevention agenda.

In Uganda, as in South Africa, violence and unintentional injury are a major cause of disease burden and constitute the fifth leading cause of premature death nationally (Uganda, Ministry of Health 2000). The magnitude of these burdens was measured in a survey conducted in Kampala by the Ministry of Health. In one section of Kampala 119 fatal injuries were reported for a population of 10,982 for the five-year period 1992 to 1996, resulting in a mortality rate of 220 per 100,000 people per year. In the preceding six months, 138 injuries leading to disabilities were reported, giving an incidence of injuries leading to disabilities of

23 per 1,000 people per year. The incidence of nonfatal injuries was 114 per 1,000 per year. Furthermore, 312 disabilities as a direct result of injury were recorded by the survey. This translates into an injury-caused disability rate of 2.8 per 1,000 per year. The overall incidence of all the injuries was 116 per 1,000 per year. Road traffic crashes constituted the primary cause of injury deaths and disabilities. Interpersonal violence involving the use of firearms was the second leading cause of injury mortality in this urban community. Burns were the leading cause of severe (fatal or disabling) injuries in children age 10 years or younger. Burns also constituted 51 percent of all injuries from which this age group fully recovered, pointing to the importance of burns in the population (see tables 24.1 to 24.5).

In the rural district of Mukono, in the southern part of the country, 34 fatal injuries were reported to have occurred in a population of 7,427 people during the five-year period preceding the ministry's survey. These figures translated into an average annual injury mortality rate of 92 per 100,000 persons (see table 24.1). The prevalence rate of disabilities due to injury was 0.7 percent. Drowning was the leading cause of injury mortality in this rural district, followed by

Table 24.1 Cause of Injury by Outcome: Mukono District, Uganda

| | Outcome of injury | | | | | |
| | Fatal injuries, 1994–98 (n = 34) | | Prevailing disabilities due to injury (n = 55) | | Fully recovered injuries past 6 months (n = 575) | |
Cause	(no.)	(%)	(no.)	(%)	(no.)	(%)
Traffic	6	18.0	19	35.0	72	13.0
Burns	2	6.0	6	11.0	71	12.0
Stabs/cuts	4	6.0	9	16.0	197	34.0
Blunt force	5	15.0	6	11.0	109	19.0
Poison	1	3.0	0	0.0	2	0.3
Drowning	9	27.0	0	0.0	3	0.5
Animal bites	2	6.0	0	0.0	29	5.0
Falls	1	3.0	13	24.0	73	13.0
Gunshots	2	6.0	0	0.0	0	0.0
Other	2	6.0	2	4.0	19	3.0

Source: Kobusingye, Guwatudde, and Lett 2001.

Table 24.2 Cause of Injury by Outcome: Kawempe Division, Kampala District, Uganda

| | Outcome of injury | | | | | |
| | Fatal injuries, 1992–96 (n = 119) | | Prevailing disabilities due to injury (n = 312) | | Fully recovered injuries past 6 months (n = 478) | |
Cause	(no.)	(%)	(no.)	(%)	(no.)	(%)
Traffic	55	46.0	122	39.0	139	29.0
Burns	11	9.0	36	12.0	113	24.0
Stabs/cuts	1	0.8	21	7.0	73	15.0
Blunt force	4	3.0	15	5.0	30	6.0
Poison	9	8.0	7	2.0	4	0.8
Animal bites	6	5.0	18	6.0	14	3.0
Falls	4	3.0	39	13.0	85	18.0
Gunshots	24	20.0	35	11.0	7	1.0
Other	5	4.0	19	6.0	13	3.0

Source: Kobusingye, Guwatudde, and Lett 2001.

Table 24.3 Cause of Injury by Outcome: Gulu District, Uganda

Cause of injury	Death rate per 10,000 (no.)	Death rate per 10,000 (rate)	Disability rate per 10,000 (no.)	Disability rate per 10,000 (rate)	Injury rate per 10,000 (no.)	Injury rate per 10,000 (rate)
Gunshots	168	32.8	87	17.0	288	56.2
Stabs/cuts	71	13.9	59	11.5	183	35.7
Blunt force	41	8.0	112	21.9	201	39.2
Land mines	26	5.1	36	7.0	70	13.7
Poisoning	22	4.3	24	4.7	58	11.3
Dog, snake, etc., bites	9	1.8	16	3.1	63	12.3
Traffic	8	1.6	55	10.7	88	17.2
Burns	7	1.4	19	3.7	63	12.3
Drowning	5	1.0	0	0.0	5	1.0
Falls	1	0.2	76	14.8	117	22.8
Other	39	7.6	95	18.5	171	33.4
All causes	397	77.5	579	113.0	1,307	255.1

Source: Kobusingye, Guwatudde, and Lett 2001.

Table 24.4 Top Three Causes of Injury, by Age, Rural District (Mukono), Uganda

Age group	Severe injuries n	Severe injuries Causes	Severe injuries No.	Severe injuries %	Recovered injuries n	Recovered injuries Causes	Recovered injuries No.	Recovered injuries %
<10	15	Falls	5	33	182	Burns	45	25
		Traffic	4	27		Cuts/stabs	42	23
		Burns	2	13		Falls	36	20
10–19	17	Burns	5	29	126	Cuts/stabs	36	29
		Traffic	3	18		Blunt force	24	19
		Drowning	3	18		Traffic	17	13
20–29	17	Traffic	5	29	103	Cuts/stabs	49	48
		Cuts/stabs	3	18		Blunt force	21	20
		Drowning	3	18		Traffic	16	16
30–39	11	Traffic	5	45	84	Cuts/stabs	34	40
		Falls	2	18		Traffic	19	23
		Drowning	2	18		Blunt force	17	20
40–49	7	Traffic	3	43	40	Cuts/stabs	18	45
		Cuts/stabs	2	29		Blunt force	6	15
		Burns	1	14		Traffic	5	13
≥50	15	Traffic	5	33	37	Cuts/stabs	17	46
		Blunt force	4	27		Falls	6	16
		Cuts/stabs	3	20		Traffic	5	14
Not stated	n.a.	n.a.	n.a.	n.a.	3	Falls	1	33
						Cuts/stabs	1	33
						Blunt force	1	33
Total	82	Traffic	25	30	575	Cuts/stabs	196	34
		Falls	13	16		Blunt force	108	19
		Cuts/stabs	11	13		Falls	72	13

Source: Kobusingye, Guwatudde, and Lett 2001.
Note: n.a. = not applicable.

Table 24.5 Top Three Causes of Injury, by Age, Urban Division (Kawempe), Uganda

Age group	Severe injuries				Recovered injuries			
	n	Causes	No.	%	*n*	Causes	No.	%
<10	58	Burns	24	41	168	Burns	85	51
		Traffic	14	24		Falls	31	19
		Falls	7	12		Cuts/stabs	24	14
10–19	71	Traffic	25	35	90	Traffic	28	31
		Falls	1	15		Falls	22	24
		Burns	8	11		Cuts/stabs	20	22
20–29	126	Traffic	56	44	105	Traffic	48	46
		Gunshots	27	21		Cuts/stabs	14	13
		Animal bites	10	8		Blunt force	13	12
30–39	96	Traffic	50	52	61	Traffic	27	44
		Gunshots	20	21		Falls	12	20
		Falls	5	5		Cuts/stabs	6	10
40–49	40	Traffic	19	48	25	Traffic	11	44
		Gunshots	6	15		Falls	4	16
		Falls	4	10		Burns	3	12
≥50	33	Traffic	11	33	13	Traffic	4	39
		Falls	9	27		Falls	4	39
		Cuts/stabs	3	9		Cuts/stabs	3	23
Not stated	7	Traffic	2	29	16	Cuts/stabs	4	25
		Burns	1	14		Traffic	3	19
		Blunt force	1	14		Falls	2	13
Total	431	Traffic	117	27	478	Traffic	139	29
		Gunshots	59	14		Burns	113	24
		Burns	47	11		Cuts/stabs	73	15

Source: Kobusingye, Guwatudde, and Lett 2001.

road traffic accidents. Falls were the most common cause of severe injuries in children below 10 years of age (33 percent), followed by traffic (27 percent) and burns (13 percent).

In Gulu, a rural district in northern Uganda that is experiencing a protracted armed rebellion, 1,475 households with 8,595 people were surveyed. Seventy-three percent of the population lived in temporary housing, 46 percent were internally displaced persons living in camps, and 81.3 percent of the total population was under 35 years. These conditions are being experienced in several countries in Africa, and the pattern of injuries has not been well described. Fourteen percent of the population were injured annually, gunshots being the leading cause of injury mortality. The annual injury mortality rate was 7.7 per 1,000 (95 percent confidence interval [CI], 7.01–8.49), and the annual injury disability rate was 11.3 per 1,000 (95 percent CI, 10.4–12.2). Only 4.5 percent of the injured were reported to be combatants. Fifty percent of the injured received first aid, whereas only 13 percent of those who died reached the hospital. The injury fatality rate is three and a half times higher than that in urban Uganda, and more than eight times the global average (Lett, Kobusingye, and Ekwaru 2006).

These figures serve well as a picture of the alarmingly high prevalence and magnitude of death due to injury in Uganda and South Africa. Furthermore, these statistics describe and underscore the importance of data as the basis for prioritizing interventions aimed at the prevention of violence and injury in Africa. The establishment of similar injury surveillance systems in other parts of the continent would thus contribute to a more complete profile of continental injury patterns. This more comprehensive picture would allow for inclusively prioritizing prevention programs for those countries not yet identified as primary injury prevention targets in Africa.

RISK FACTORS

Throughout this review of the magnitude of injury mortality, the data have implied various risk factors. In response to the range of injury risk factors identified within myriad studies, the WHO has developed a factor matrix that captures its typology of injury risk. These risk factors, which the WHO, in its ecological typology for grouping risk factors, refers to as "individual" factors, do not remain discreet through the complex causal paths that result in violence. So, for example, being a male is associated with being a risk factor for being both the perpetrator and the victim of a violent (and in the case of the victim) fatal act. These risk factors are enmeshed within the complex relational exchanges in the production of fatal injury. They interact both within and between the broader matrices of the risk factors of fatal injury. Following the ecological typology proposed by the WHO (2002a), relationships, community, and society form another set of risk factors.

Relationship Risk Factors

Relationship factors can be defined as those factors related to close personal relationships, such as family, peer, and intimate partner relationships, that increase the likelihood of violence and injury.

Family Relationships. Family relationships appear to be central to the development and occurrence of a broad range of injuries and acts of violence. For example, violent behavior during adolescence has been linked to conflictual parental relationships (WHO 2002a). Furthermore, research has found that the physical abuse and neglect of children were strong predictors of the latter's later arrest for violence. Similarly, other studies have found that the harsh physical punishment of children by their parents at the age of eight years appeared to increase the former's chances of arrest for violence up to the age of 30 years (WHO 2002a). Moreover, it also appeared to increase the likelihood that these children would become physically abusive parents themselves.

Peer Relationships. Peer relationships, particularly during adolescence, appear to be strongly related to violent behavior and intentional injuries. For example, researchers have found a strong relationship between violence and having delinquent friends (WHO 2002a). However, the causal direction of this relationship, that is, whether having delinquent friends leads to violence or whether violence results in the establishment of friendships with delinquent friends is not clear.

Community Factors

This repertoire of risk factors includes those related to various community contexts that may increase the likelihood of violence and injury, such as the neighborhood, the workplace, places of worship, and schools. These factors include community integration or cohesion, the availability of firearms, the presence of gangs, neighborhood density, policing, and drug trafficking.

Social Cohesion. The degree of community cohesion and functionality is strongly related to the rates of various forms of violence and injury. Studies have found a cyclical relation between the levels of violence and community dysfunction and lack of cohesion in Jamaica (WHO 2002a). Along similar lines, other studies have found that communities with the lowest levels of intimate partner violence were those characterized by levels of cohesion and functionality that allowed for sanctions against intimate partner violence and effective victim support (WHO 2002a). In South Africa, Keikelame and Ferreira (2000) also found a strong relationship between community dysfunction and elder abuse.

Drug Trafficking. Internationally, violence has been found to be closely associated with drug trafficking. For example, in Brazil, research has shown that drug trafficking is responsible for a significant proportion of homicides and injuries (WHO 2002a). In other parts of South and Central America, studies have also found that adolescents involved in drug dealing exhibit higher levels of violence than their peers who are not (WHO 2002a).

Societal Factors

This set of risk factors are those broad social factors "that create an acceptable climate for violence, those that reduce inhibitions against violence, and those that create and sustain gaps [and tensions] between different groups or countries" (WHO 2002a, 13). These include health, educational, economic, and political factors and social policies and practices that result in high levels of social, political, and economic inequality. Prevailing cultural values and practices also form part of this set of societal risk factors.

Economic Inequalities. The WHO (2002a) argues that there is a manifest relationship between poverty and levels of violence and injury. This position is borne out by a range of studies. For example, various studies conducted in Africa report a link between poverty and the risk of childhood burns (Mbembati, Maseru, and Leshabari 2002). Additionally, as reported earlier, 87.9 percent of all road traffic deaths occur in LMICs (WHO 2002a). Then too, the WHO (2002a) indicates that although the composite rate of homicide, suicide, and war-related deaths for high-income countries is 14.4 per 100,000, the rate for LMICs is 32.1 per 100,000, more than twice as high as that for HICs. In this regard, studies have found that the gross domestic product across countries is negatively related to violence (WHO 2002a). In South Africa, Budlender (2000) has also reported a link between poverty and death and injury due to crime. However, in many cases, this relationship is substantially moderated by income inequalities. In effect, significant income inequalities are associated with high rates of violence, even in high-income contexts. To a certain extent, this finding could perhaps account for the high levels of violence in South Africa, given its substantial income disparities (May, Woolard, and Klasen 2000).

Culture. To a large extent, people's responses to their environment are influenced by culture, which is reflected in the values and norms of a society. For this reason, culture is also considered to play an important role in the levels of violence in a particular society. Research shows that cultures that support values that endorse violence and that do not provide nonviolent alternatives to resolve conflicts appear to have higher rates of violence. More specifically, a number of studies have found that the risk of violence against women is increased in cultures that endorse male dominance and aggression (WHO 2002a). Additionally, the WHO (2002a) argues that contemporary cultural norms that valorize youthfulness is a significant contributory factor in the elevated levels of elder abuse.

STRATEGIES FOR CONTROL: WHAT PRACTICES EXIST?

The preceding analysis and the work of international agencies, including the WHO, point to the importance of establishing injury surveillance systems that can provide timely, accurate, and quality data for informing prevention policies and practices and serve as the backbone of national prevention programs. Without surveillance as a method and a process, health care planners are unable to prioritize the allocation of resources. Thus, a national program may focus on strengthening capacities for data collection and prevention methodologies, encouraging research on the determinants and costs of injuries and their prevention, encouraging intersectoral and cross-disciplinary collaboration, and enhancing responses for the prevention, control, and management of injuries.

Prevention of Road Traffic Injuries

In the prevention of RTIs the focus could be on proven measures, such as encouraging pedestrians to walk facing traffic, introducing bright and visible clothing, enacting speed limits, persuading drivers to use headlights during the daytime, and promoting the use of approved disc brakes. Environment-based measures for the prevention of RTIs include vigilant and consistent policy and enforcement measures; the introduction of red light cameras; the use of traffic circles; the bright illumination of crossings; and the provision of adequate sidewalks for pedestrians, who are among the most vulnerable road users. Other prevention measures include segregating public vehicles from private transport vehicles; providing adequate separate lanes for heavy vehicles, cyclists, and pedestrians; and introducing a flexible time arrangement for car-free zones for pedestrians (Mohan 2003).

Control measures aimed at reducing the severity of RTIs may include requiring the use of protective clothing and helmets for cyclists, the use of seatbelts, and the development of safer dashboards in motor vehicles. Key measures for the effective management of traffic-related injuries include rapid responses to crashes in the form of first aid for the injured, elimination of fuel leakage, and clearance of accident scenes, in addition to effective policing systems and accessible hospital and rehabilitation centers for the injured (Forjuoh 1996).

Violence Prevention

Violence prevention measures may be universal, selected, or indicated in nature. Whereas universal interventions are aimed at the total population without consideration of individual risks (for example, community-wide media campaigns), selected interventions target those at risk for violence (for example, training single parents in parenting skills and anger management). Other interventions should be directed at those who have already engaged in violent behavior (for example, rehabilitation programs for perpetrators of domestic violence).

Selected interventions that are keenly attuned to risk factors that include biological factors, psychological and behavioral characteristics, family influences, peer influences, income, gender, age, geographical location, and various other context-specific variables have been shown to be effective in preventing violence (Berger and Mohan 1996). Following the ecological approach of the WHO (2002a), violence prevention targeting the vulnerable 12-to-19-year age cohort may, for instance, include social development programs, academic enrichment programs, mentoring initiatives, extracurricular activities, and attempts to reduce poverty and income inequality (WHO 2002a). The causal pathways of violence are complex, and the prevention of interpersonal violence should be multisectoral and multidimensional and therefore include all the identified risk factors that are specific to the context in which such violence occurs (Zwi et al. 1996). A survey study conducted by Butchart, Kruger, and Lekoba (2000), in which community perceptions of violence yielded qualitative information, provides an alternative means of gaining rich information on the causes and possible prevention of violence. This information lends itself to analysis that may uncover the nuances and context specificities often overlooked by more broadly based epidemiological studies.

Burns, Falls, and Drowning Prevention

The WHO (2002b) has provided the most comprehensive set of recommendations and guidelines for the prevention of burns, falls, and drowning to date. Although most of these prevention suggestions are formulated in relation to the Southeast Asia region, their generic applicability to other LMICs cannot be underestimated. Country-specific factors must, however, be included in prevention strategies that take local risk factors and available resources into account. Country-specific studies should tailor these guidelines to their local contexts; for example, studies in South Africa suggest that the unsafe use of paraffin is significantly associated with burn injuries (Steenkamp, van der Merwe, and de Lange 2002). Paraffin management strategies must therefore inform burn prevention strategies for the country.

Recommendations for the prevention of burn injuries include the provision of stable lamps and stoves in LMIC contexts, effective training of personnel in evacuation processes following fires in the workplace, the installation of fire and smoke alarms in public buildings, the regulation or elimination of dangerous fireworks, the greater use of flame-resistant fabrics, and the promotion of the use of cold water in the treatment of burns at the tertiary prevention level (WHO 2002b).

Falls could be best prevented through the use of accommodating and soft materials, such as mud and sand, in the design of playgrounds; the provision and implementation of safety regulations for places in which children most frequently play; legislating for safer designs for fall-vulnerable structures, such as railings and grab bars on balconies; and

the stimulation and encouragement of safer working techniques in the workplace (WHO 2002b).

Measures for the prevention of drowning as recommended by the WHO (2002b) include the development of strategies to ensure safe water transport and commutation, the sensitization of policy makers to the benefits of life jackets and other flotation devices to the protection of children and other vulnerable users near water, and the provision of adequate life protection services (in the form of adult supervision or qualified life guards) for recreational swimming times and places (WHO 2002b).

CONCLUSION

Violence and injury are salient and definitive threats to the health of African nations, and the globe. Consequently, the inclusion of violence and injury prevention curricula across the full spectrum of primary, secondary, and tertiary education platforms, as well as the training of African injury prevention specialists, should be seen as vitally important. Fortunately, it appears as though these areas are receiving growing attention in some African countries. For instance, in a positive development, the WHO Injuries and Violence Prevention Department collaborates with Mozambican counterparts to enhance the safety and security of Mozambique's 20 million people. The Mozambique Project, as a national action plan, includes the development of national violence prevention policies, the detailed countrywide analysis of injuries, the development of a network of prevention practitioners through training and awareness campaigns, and an initiative aimed at controlling the supply and distribution of small arms. Perhaps the most powerful illustration of the recent prioritization of injury prevention and safety promotion for combating the devastating social and economic effects of injuries and violence on the African continent is embodied by a resolution passed by the heads of states of the African Union (signed in Maputo in 2003). The resolution declared 2005 the African Year of Violence Prevention and endorsed the nine recommendations of the *World Report on Violence and Health* (WHO 2002a), which urged states to implement multisectoral national plans of action to limit injury and violence and to enhance data collection systems.

In South Africa, the presidential Lead Programme on Crime, Violence and Injury is focused on the development of injury surveillance methods; good practices for the prevention, control, and management of injuries; the implementation of injury prevention strategies through training; the strengthening of current bottom-up and top-down initiatives; and the stimulation of prevention policies. A major focus of the program is to chart the contextual, social, process, and content factors that influence data uptake and the stimulation of prevention policies and practices (Seedat 2002).

Injury prevention may thrive while a national program focuses on developing systems to record the magnitude and risks of injuries, evaluating and documenting promising and effective practices, stimulating the wide-scale implementation of these practices, and encouraging the development of evidence-led policies and associated funding decisions. To ensure the long-term development of the injury and violence prevention sector in Africa, however, intersectoral and multidisciplinary collaboration, technical cooperation, and partnerships between government and civil society are vital.

REFERENCES

Berger, L., and D. Mohan. 1996. *Injury Control: A Global View*. New York: Oxford University Press.

Bowley, D. M. G., N. K. Parmar, and K. D. Boffard. 2004. Burdens of Disease in Southern Africa. *Lancet* 363: 1508–9.

Budlender, D. 2000. "Human Development." In *Poverty and Inequality in South Africa: Meeting the Challenge*. Cape Town: David Philip.

Burrows, S., B. Bowman, R. Matzopoulos, and A. van Niekerk, eds. 2001. *A Profile of Fatal Injuries in South Africa 2000: Second Annual Report of the National Injury Mortality Surveillance System*. Cape Town: MRC Press.

Burrows, S., M. Vaez, A. Butchart, and L. Laflamme. 2003. "The Share of Suicide in Injury Deaths in the South African Context: Sociodemographic Distribution." *Public Health* 117 (1): 3–10.

Butchart, A., J. Kruger, and R. Lekoba. 2000. "Perceptions of Injury Causes and Solutions in a Johannesburg Township: Implications for Prevention." *Social Science and Medicine* 50: 331–44.

Cliff, J., and A. R. Noormohamed. 1993. "The Impact of War on Children's Health in Mozambique." *Social Science and Medicine* 36 (7): 843–48.

De Wet, B. 1993. "Reflect to Be Seen." *Trauma Review* 1 (3): 2.

Donson, H., and A. Van Niekerk. 2002. "Suicide." In *A Profile of Fatal Injuries in South Africa: Third Annual Report of the National Injury Mortality Surveillance System*, ed. R. Matzopoulos, 31–34. Cape Town: MRC Press.

Elliot, G. 2000. "Mozambique: Development through De-Mining." *South African Journal of International Affairs* 7 (1): 97–105.

Elliot, G., and G. Harris. 2001. "A Cost-Benefit Analysis of Landmine Clearance in Mozambique." *Development Southern Africa* 18 (5): 625–33.

Forjuoh, S. N. 1995. "Pattern of Intentional Burns to Children in Ghana." *Child Abuse and Neglect* 9 (7): 837–41.

———. 1996. "Burn Repetitions in Ghanaian Children: Prevalence, Epidemiological Characteristics and Socioenvironmental Factors." *Burns* 22 (7): 539–42.

Forjuoh, S. N., A. B. Zwi, and C. J. Romer. 1996. *Injury Control in Africa: Proceedings of Round Table Session and Associated Meetings Held at the Third International Conference on Injury Prevention and Control, Melbourne, Australia, February 18–22, 1996*. Pittsburgh: University of Pittsburgh.

Holder, Y., M. Peden, E. Krug, J. Lund, J. Gururaj, and O. Kobusingye, eds. 2001. *Injury Surveillance Guidelines*. Geneva: WHO.

Jansson, B., and L. Svanstrom. 1999. "Injury as a Public Health Problem: Looking Behind the Figures." In *Safety Promotion Research*, ed. L. Laflamme, L. Svanstrom, and L. Schelp, 43–62. Kristianstads: Kristianstads Boktryckeri AB.

Keikelame, J., and M. Ferreira. 2000. "Mpathekombi, ya Bantu abadala: Elder Abuse in Black Townships on the Cape Flats." Human Sciences Research Council and University of Cape Town Centre for Gerontology, Cape Town.

Kobusingye, O., D. Guwatudde, and R. Lett. 2001. "Injury Patterns in Rural and Urban Uganda." *Injury Prevention* 7: 46–50.

Lerel, L. 1994. "The Epidemiology of Fatal Childhood Burns." *South African Medical Journal* 84 (3): 169–70.

Lett, R. R., O. C. Kobusingye, and P. Ekwaru. 2006. "Burden of Injury during the Complex Political Emergency in Northern Uganda." *Canadian Journal of Surgery* 49 (1): 51–57.

Marysse, S. 2003. "Regress and War: The Case of the DR Congo." *European Journal of Development Research* 15 (1): 73–98.

Mathers, C. D., R. Sadana, J. A. Salomon, C. J. L. Murray, and A. D. Lopez. 2001. "Healthy Life Expectancy in 191 Countries, 1999." *Lancet* 357: 1685–91.

Matzopoulos, R., ed. 2002. *A Profile of Fatal Injuries in South Africa: Third Annual Report of the National Injury Mortality Surveillance System*. Cape Town: MRC Press.

May, J., I. Woolard, and S. Klasen. 2000. "The Nature and Measurement of Poverty and Inequality." In *Poverty and Inequality in South Africa: Meeting the Challenge*, ed. J. May. Cape Town: David Phillip.

Mbembati, N. A., L. M. Maseru, and M. T. Leshabari. 2002. "Childhood Burn Injuries in Dar es Salaam: Patterns and Perceptions of Prevention." *African Safety Promotion* 1 (1): 42–45.

Meel, B. 2003. "Determinants of Suicide in the Transkei Sub-Region of South Africa." *Journal of Clinical Forensic Medicine* 10: 71–76.

Mock, C. N., S. N. Forjuoh, and F. P. Rivara. 1999. "Epidemiology of Transport-Related Injuries in Ghana." *Accident Analysis and Prevention* 31: 359–70.

Mohan, D. 2003. "Typical Crash Analysis." Paper presented at the Fifth Injury Control and Traffic Safety Training Course, Johannesburg, July 21–25.

Moshiro, C., R. Mswia, K. Alberti, D. Whiting, N. Unwin, and P. Setel. 2000. "The Importance of Injury as a Cause of Death in Sub-Saharan Africa: Results of a Community-Based Study in Tanzania." *Public Health* 115: 96–102.

National Center for Injury Prevention and Control (NCIPC). 2003. "Intimate Partner Violence Fact Sheet." Atlanta: NCIPC. http://www.cdc.gov/ncipc/factsheets/ipvfacts.htm, accessed September 12, 2003.

Nattrass, N., and J. Seekings. 2001. "Two Nations? Race and Economic Inequality in South Africa Today." *Daedalus* 130: 45–70.

Odero, W., M. Khayesi, and P. M. Heda. 2003. "Road Traffic Injuries in Kenya: Magnitude, Causes and Status of Intervention." *Injury Control and Safety Promotion* 10 (1–2): 53–61.

Peden, M., and K. McGee. 2003. "The Epidemiology of Drowning Worldwide." *Injury Control and Safety Promotion* 10 (4): 195–99.

Peden, M., K. McGee, and G. Sharma. 2002. *The Injury Chart Book: A Graphical Overview of the Global Burden of Injuries*. Geneva: WHO.

Peltzer, K., and W. Renner. 2003. "Superstition, Risk-Taking, and Risk Perception of Accidents among South African Taxi Drivers." *Accident Analysis and Prevention* 35: 619–23.

Schlebusch, L., and B. A. Bosch, eds. 2000. "Suicidal Behaviour." 4. *Proceedings of the Fourth South African Conference on Suicidology.* Durban: University of Natal.

Seedat, M. 2002. "Extending the Boundaries of Injury Prevention Theory, Research and Practice in Africa." *African Safety Promotion* 1 (1): 5–15.

Smith, G. S., and P. Barss. 1991. "Unintentional Injuries in Developing Countries: The Epidemiology of a Neglected Problem." *Epidemiology Reviews* 13: 228–66.

Steenkamp, W. C., A. E. van Der Merwe, and R. de Lange. 2002. "Burn Injuries Caused by Paraffin Stoves." *South African Medical Journal* 92 (6): 445–46.

Stohl, R. J. 2002. "Under the Gun: Children and Small Arms." *African Security Review* 11 (3): 17–25.

Sukhai, A., and R. Matzopoulos. 2002. "Appendix 1: Inter-city and Regional Comparisons." In *A Profile of Fatal Injuries in South Africa: Third Annual Report of the National Injury Mortality Surveillance System,* ed. R. Matzopoulos, 31–34. Cape Town: MRC Press.

Uganda, Ministry of Health. 2000. *Health Management Information System Report.* Kampala: Ministry of Health.

Venter, P. 1998. "The Young Pedestrian in Traffic." *Trauma Review* 6 (3): 8–9.

WHO (World Health Organization). 2002a. *World Report on Violence and Health.* Geneva: WHO.

———. 2002b. *Injuries in South-East Asia Region: Priorities for Policy and Action.* Geneva: WHO.

Zwi, A., S. Murugusampillay, B. Msika, et al. 1993. "Injury Surveillance in Zimbabwe: A Situation Analysis." Ministry of Health and Child Welfare, Zimbabwe, and London School of Hygiene and Tropical Medicine, London.

Zwi, A., S. Forjuoh, S. Murugusampillay, W. Odero, and C. Watts. 1996. "Injuries in Developing Countries: Policy Response Needed Now." *Transactions of the Royal Society of Tropical Medicine and Hygiene* 90: 593–95.

Index

Boxes, figures, and tables are indicated by b, f, and t, respectively.

breastfeeding
cancer and, 294
diabetes and, 272
transmission of HIV and, 242
undernutrition of children and, 92, 93, 100, 101*f*
burden of disease. *See specific diseases and conditions*
Burden of Malaria in Africa (BOMA) project, 200, 208
Burkina Faso
adult mortality rates in, 38
alcohol consumption in, 335
HIV/AIDS in, 71
malaria in, 206
onchocerciasis control program in, 217
Burkitt's lymphoma, 298
burn-related injuries, 364, 371
Burundi
Household and Living Standards Survey, 330
malaria in, 202
stomach cancer in, 295
undernutrition of children in, 101

Cameroon
adult mortality rates in, 37
cardiovascular disease in, 309
diabetes in, 272, 276, 277, 278, 280
HIV/AIDS in, 240
hypertension in, 315
life expectancy in, 277
noncommunicable disease burden in, 252
physical activity in, 277
urban lifestyle and lack of physical activity in, 252
cancer, 289–301
See also specific types
burden of, 2
data sources on, 290–291, 300–301
epidemiological estimates of deaths caused by, 52
HIV/AIDS and, 4, 299
incidence of, 289, 290*t*, 291–292, 292*f*
male vs. female, 291–292, 291*t*
screening, 293
tobacco-related cancers, 299–300
women and, 292–294
cardiovascular disease (CVD), 305–323
age of onset, 315
alcohol consumption and, 317
burden of, 2–3, 305
as cause of death, 56, 305
measurement of, 307
cerebrovascular accidents, 309–310
clustering of multiple risks, effect of, 261

coronary heart disease, 310–311, 314, 315, 315*t*
costs of interventions, 322, 323
crude mortality vs. age-standardized mortality, 307, 308*f*
data sources on, 307
diabetes and, 317
diet contributing to, 253
See also obesity
dilated cardiomyopathy, 312
drug treatment of, 321–322
dyslipidemia and, 258–260, 259*t*
dysrhythmias, 313
endomyocardial fibrosis, 312
epidemiological transition in, 306–307, 306*t*, 316
epidemiology of, 309–314
genetic determinants of, 314, 319
HIV-related, 4, 312–313
hyperlipidemia, 317
hypertension, 254–257, 256*t*, 315–317
cost-effectiveness of interventions for, 257, 323
interventions for, 256, 257, 320, 322, 323
prevalence of, 315–316, 316*t*, 355
stroke and, 355
urbanization and, 255, 315–316, 316*t*
interventions, 319–320
pericarditis, 314
physical activity and, 317
prevalence and incidence of, 308–309
prevention, 319–320
rheumatic heart disease (RHD), 311
risk factors for, 314–315*t*, 314–319
low birthweight and, 248
screening for, 320, 321
sickle-cell disease, 313
smoking and, 317
causes of death, 43–58, 290*t*
cause-specific estimating, 52–53, 53*f*
data sources on, 43–53, 76
epidemiological estimates of, 49–52, 317*f*
cancer, 52
CVD, 305, 307, 308
diarrheal diseases, 50, 50*t*
epilepsy, 353
HIV/AIDS, 51–52
lower respiratory infections, 51
malaria, 50, 50*t*
maternal mortality, 51
suicide, 363
vaccine preventable diseases, 50–51
war and violence, 52, 362–363
epidemiological literature, review of, 44–45, 44*t*

GBD process for estimating, 44, 47–48, 48*f*, 52
leading causes of death
by age, 54–55, 55–56*t*
regional comparisons, 54, 54*t*
by sex, 53–54, 53*t*, 55–56, 56*t*
life tables, construction of, 48–49, 49*f*, 61
verbal autopsies and. *See* verbal autopsies
vital records showing, 45–47, 46–47*t*
census data. *See* U.S. Census Bureau
Center for International Earth Science Information Network (CIESIN) on distribution of child undernutrition, 93–94, 94*f*
cerebral malaria, 136, 200, 203, 354
cerebral palsy, 140–141, 353
See also neurological disorders
cerebrovascular disease, 279, 309–310, 354
See also stroke
cervical cancer, 292–293
Chad
adult mortality rates in, 38
malaria in, 206
refugee populations of, 9
child abuse, 338, 369
childbirth
See also maternal conditions
access to skilled attendance, 231, 231*f*, 233
emergency obstetric care, 233–234
low birthweight. *See* low birthweight
maternal death. *See* maternal mortality
neonatal death. *See* child mortality rates
preterm birth and malaria, 204–205
projected rates of, after AIDS, 63
childhood health
See also specific diseases and conditions
burns, 364
cancer and, 298
developmental disabilities, 126–128
See also developmental disabilities
diabetes, 270, 272
diarrheal diseases. *See* diarrheal diseases
drownings, 364
epilepsy. *See* epilepsy
malnutrition. *See* stunting; undernutrition of children
mental disorders, 335
treatment of, 343
neurological disorders, 355, 358
perinatal conditions. *See* perinatal conditions
respiratory disease. *See* respiratory diseases of children
stunting. *See* stunting
TB and, 182

child mortality rates, 15–30
under age 5 mortality, 11
annual rate of change in, 19–20, 20*f*
causes of, 44, 44*t*, 46, 46*t*
diarrheal disease and, 107, 108*f*,
109*f*, 117
estimated levels, 18–19, 18*f*, 25–29,
26*f*, 27–29*t*
HIV/AIDS and, 159, 239
interventions to reduce, 22
lower respiratory tract infections and,
149, 152, 159
malaria and, 202
malnutrition and, 95–96, 96*f*
MDGs for, 15, 117
measurement of, 78–80, 80*f*, 80*t*
trends in, 19–20, 19*f*, 22, 107,
126–127
causes of death, 44, 44*t*, 56–57
leading causes of death, 54–55, 55*t*
vital records on, 46–47, 46–47*t*
data available on, 15–16, 16*f*
measurement of, 78–80, 80*f*, 80*t*
sources and methods for, 16–18
study data used, 17
infant and neonatal mortality, 11
comparison of Sub-Saharan Africa
with other regions, 12, 13*f*, 13*t*
malaria and, 204
MDGs on, 234
measurement of, 78–80, 80*f*, 80*t*
tetanus and, 168
trends in, 126–127
malaria and, 202, 206
methodology for estimation of trends,
17–18, 22–25
application of, 25
linear splines and "knots," 23–24, 23*f*
weighted least squares with linear
splines, 23
weights, 24
chloroquine, 208
cholera, 115, 116*t*
cholesterol levels, 258–260, 259*t*
CVD and, 260, 315, 320
lifestyle and, 251
chronic diseases
See also specific diseases
burden of, 247
interventions recommended, 261–262
risk factors for, 246–262
See also risk factors for
noncommunicable diseases
cigarette smoking. *See* tobacco use
clean drinking water. *See* safe water,
access to

climate determinants of malaria, 153,
197, 198*f*
cognitive function
fetal alcohol syndrome and, 139
malnutrition's effect on, 139
communicable diseases. *See* infectious and
communicable diseases
community-based rehabilitation and
developmental disabilities, 142–143
community-directed treatment with
ivermectin (CDTI), 219–220,
220*t*, 221
community violence, 369
comparison of Sub-Saharan Africa with
other regions and countries
developmental disabilities prevalence,
129, 130*t*
HIV/AIDS prevalence, 238–239, 239*t*
mortality rates, 12, 12*t*, 13, 13*t*, 14*f*
TB prevalence, 183, 184*f*
Comprehensive Africa Agriculture
Development Programme, 104
condoms. *See* HIV/AIDS
conflicts. *See* wars and conflicts
congenital disorders, 132–134, 133*t*
heart disease, 313
congenital rubella, 135
congestive heart failure. *See* cardiovascular
disease (CVD)
Congo, Democratic Republic of
cancer in, 295, 296
cardiovascular disease in, 312, 314
low birthweight and, 248
child mortality rates in, 15, 15*f*
conflict in, 8
diabetes in, 273
hypertension in, 315, 316
immunization rates in, 9
infant mortality rates in, 13
malaria in, 203, 206
TB recurrence in HIV-infected
individuals in, 188
undernutrition of children in, 101
war in, 363
consanguineous marriages and congenital
abnormalities, 132, 134
Core Welfare Indicators Questionnaire
(CWIQ), 330
coronary heart disease, 310–311, 314,
315, 315*t*
See also cardiovascular disease (CVD)
cost-effective interventions. *See specific
diseases and conditions*
Côte d'Ivoire
adult mortality rates in, 38
cancer in, 290

hypertension in, 315
TB in, 190
cotrimoxazole treatment, 190
cultural beliefs. *See* religious and
cultural customs
CVD. *See* cardiovascular disease

DALYs. *See* disability-adjusted life years
data collection, 7–8
See also vital events registration
adult mortality rates, 32–33
on cancer, 290–291, 300–301
on causes of death, 43–53, 76
child mortality rates, 16–18
on CVD, 307
on developmental disabilities, 128–129,
129–130*t*
on diabetes, 268–270, 269–271*t*
on diarrheal diseases, 108–110, 117–119
on injuries, 362
maternal mortality rates, 32, 223–226
on mental disorders, 330–331
model life tables, use of, 76
on mortality rates, 32–33
on neurological disorders, 352
population projections after AIDS, 59–61
recommendations for improving, 41
on undernutrition of children, 92
deafness. *See* hearing loss
death. *See* child mortality; mortality rates;
specific diseases
dehydration. *See* diarrheal diseases
dementia, 354
Democratic Republic of Congo. *See* Congo,
Democratic Republic of
Demographic and Health Surveys (DHS),
12, 76
diarrheal diseases, 108, 115
maternal mortality, 228, 229
undernutrition of children, 92
demographic context, 5–6, 6*f*
See also population trends
demographic surveillance systems (DSS)
malaria monitoring, 200, 206, 208
mortality measurement, 75, 76, 85
depression. *See* mental disorders
developmental disabilities, 2, 125–147
accidents as cause of, 140
bacterial meningitis as cause of, 136–137
burden of disease in childhood, 126–128
measurement of, 127–128
causes of, 135–137
cognitive disabilities, 130
community-based rehabilitation and, 142
cost-effectiveness of, 143
congenital disorders, 132–134

polio
    burden of, 164–165
    global elimination, goal of, 165, 173
    vaccine for, 163, 165
    See also vaccine-preventable diseases
population trends, 5–6, 6*f*
    projections after AIDS, 59–74
        birth rate projections, 63–64, 64*f*
        data sources, 59–61
        effects on, decomposed, 61–65, 62*f*, 63*t*
        fertility projections, 62–63
        HIV prevalence and, 68–71, 70*f*, 71*t*, 74
        life expectancy projections, 65–70*f*, 65–74
        sex and age ratios for life expectancy, 67–68, 68*f*
postpartum depression, 338
posttraumatic stress disorder (PTSD), 333
    specific data on Sub-Saharan Africa, 334–335
    treatment of, 342–343
poverty
    CVD and, 305
    developmental disabilities and, 126, 138–139
    diarrheal diseases and, 114
    injuries and, 369–370
    lower respiratory tract infections and, 151
    malaria and, 206–207
    maternal mortality and, 230
    mental disorders and, 337, 339
    reduction, 4–5
    undernutrition and, 87–88
    violence and, 369–370
Poverty Reduction Strategy approach, 230
pregnancy
    See also childbirth; maternal mortality; prenatal care programs
    developmental disabilities and, 134
    malaria and, 196, 204–205
    nutrition during, 247
    risk factors for chronic diseases from, 247–248
    smoking during, 247–248
    vaccines during, 169, 169*f*
premature births. *See* childbirth; low birthweight
prenatal care programs
    See also maternal conditions
    access to, 98, 99*f*
    nutritional care, 91–92, 102–103
prescriptions. *See* drugs
prevention. *See specific diseases and conditions*
prostate cancer, 297–298, 300
protease inhibitors, 243

psychiatric disorders. *See* mental disorders
PTSD. *See* posttraumatic stress disorder
public health
    malaria, effect of, 196, 196*f*
    prenatal and infant care, effect of, 91–92, 102–103
    surveillance. *See* surveillance

radiation therapy for cancer, 290*f*
RAMOS (Reproductive Age Mortality Studies), 225
rape, 9, 338
Rapid Epidemiological Mapping of Onchocerciasis, 216
refugee populations, 8–9
    diarrheal diseases and, 115
    malaria and, 199
regional comparisons
    adult mortality, 35–39, 38–39*f*
    child mortality under age of five, 18–21, 18–21*f*
    leading causes of death, 54, 54*t*
registration of births, deaths, marriages, etc. *See* vital events registration
religious and cultural customs
    maternal mortality and, 230
    neurological health and, 351, 358
    violence and, 370
Reproductive Age Mortality Studies (RAMOS), 225
research and development
    mental disorders, 343–344
    vaccines, 173
respiratory diseases of children
    as causes of death, 51
    cost of interventions, 158
    Hib conjugate vaccine and, 156–157, 159
    lower respiratory tract infections, 3, 149–162
        See also lower respiratory tract infections (LRTI)
    pneumonia, 151–152, 153
    S. pneumoniae conjugate vaccine and, 157–158
retroviruses. *See* HIV/AIDS
rheumatic heart disease (RHD), 311
    See also cardiovascular disease (CVD)
risk factors for noncommunicable diseases, 2, 247–262
    See also specific risks (e.g., cholesterol levels, obesity)
    antenatal influences on, 247–248
    clustering of multiple risks, effect of, 260–261, 260*t*
    CVD and, 314–315*t*, 314–319
    diabetes and, 273–277

    dyslipidemia and, 258–260, 259*t*
    health services' requirements for management of, 260–261, 260*t*
    injuries and, 368–370
    obesity and, 253, 254*t*
    physical activity, lack of, 251–252
    promotion of healthy lifestyle to counter, 261–262
    smoking and, 248–250, 249–250*t*
river blindness. *See* onchocerciasis
road traffic injuries. *See* traffic-related injuries
Roll Back Malaria movement, 208
Romania and abortion, 231–232, 232*f*
rotavirus, 113–114, 113–114*t*
    See also diarrheal diseases
    immunization for, 172
rubella
    See also vaccine-preventable diseases
    congenital rubella, 135
    vaccination, 135
Rwanda
    adult mortality rates in, 37
    alcohol consumption in, 335
    cancer in, 295, 296
    conflict in, 8, 9
    depression in, 334
    diarrheal diseases in refugees from, 115
    infant mortality rates in, 13
    malaria in, 206
    PTSD in, 335
    war in, 363

Safe Motherhood Initiative (1987), 228
safe water, access to, 98, 98*f*, 114
sanitation improvements
    diarrheal diseases and, 114–115, 115*f*, 115*t*
    undernutrition of children and, 98, 98*f*
schizophrenia. *See* mental disorders
Senegal
    diabetes in, 272
    liver cancer in, 296
    malaria in, 202
    pertussis in, 167, 168
    physical activity of adolescent girls in, 252
severe malaria anemia (SMA), 200, 203
sexually transmitted infections
    HIV/AIDS. *See* HIV/AIDS
    neurological impact of, 354
sexual violence and abuse, 338
    See also rape
shigella. *See* diarrheal diseases
sibling survival as source of mortality data, 32
sickle cell anemia and related disorders, 134, 313, 355